# Complications of Cancer Management

'The next greatest misfortune to losing
a battle is to win such a victory as this'.

Duke of Wellington
(after Waterloo)

# Complications of Cancer Management


**P.N. Plowman** MA, MD, FRCP, FRCR
Consultant in Radiotherapy and Oncology, St. Bartholomew's Hospital and The
Hospital for Sick Children, Great Ormond Street, London

**T.J. McElwain** MB, BS, FRCP
Professor of Medical Oncology, University of London; Head, Section of
Medicine, Institute of Cancer Research and Royal Marsden Hospital, Sutton,
Surrey

**Anna T. Meadows** MD
Professor of Pediatrics, University of Pennsylvania School of Medicine; Senior
Oncologist, Children's Hospital of Philadelphia, Philadelphia, Pennsylvania,
USA


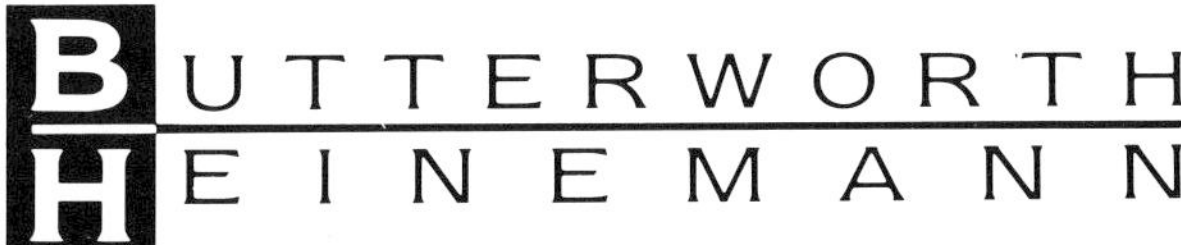

**Butterworth–Heinemann Ltd**
**Halley Court, Jordan Hill, Oxford OX2 8EJ**

 PART OF REED INTERNATIONAL P.L.C.

Oxford  London  Guildford  Boston  Munich  New Delhi  Singapore  Sydney
Tokyo  Toronto  Wellington





First published 1991

© Butterworth–Heinemann Ltd, 1991



**British Library Cataloguing in Publication Data**

Complications of cancer management
  1.  Man.  Cancer.  Therapy,  Complications
  I.  Plowman, P. N.  II.  McElwain, T.J. (Timothy John)
616.9946

  ISBN 0–7506–13416



**Library of Congress Cataloging-in-Publication Data**

Complications of cancer management / edited by P.N. Plowman, T.
  McElwain, Anna Meadows.
    p.   cm.
  Includes bibliographical references.
  Includes index
  ISBN 0 7506 13416
  1.  Cancer--Treatment--Complications and sequelae.
  I.  Plowman, P.N.  II.  McElwain, T. J.
  III.  Meadows, Anna T.
  [DNLM:  1. Drug Therapy--adverse effects.  2. Morbidity.
3. Neoplasms--complications.  4. Neoplasms--therapy.
5. Radiotherapy--adverse effects.    QZ266 C737]
RC270.8.C63    1990
616.99'406--dc20
DNLM/DLC                         90-12479
for Library of Congress              CIP



Phototypeset by Scribe Design, Gillingham, Kent
Printed in Great Britain at the University Press, Cambridge

# Preface

In the opening few pages of this book, the reader will find a quotation from the Duke of Wellington, made as he surveyed the carnage of Waterloo and contemplated the cost of victory. I believe this quotation to be an entirely apt introduction for this book. For too long, cancer specialists have shrugged off the late sequelae of their therapy as 'the morbidity of survival'. However, in the last decade, led by 'Late Effects Groups' set up by paediatric oncologists, and looking backwards from the late clinical problems and through recent radiobiological and chemobiological observations and advances in surgery, many new treatment strategies have evolved, aimed at reducing morbidity without jeopardizing cancer control. This book has provided a wonderful opportunity to review the scientific observations alongside the clinical problems, such that state-of-the-art policies for reduced morbidity in cancer treatment may be available to practising oncologists of all disciplines. Whilst the consequences of ignoring these observations may be most severe in the paediatric cancer population, the conclusions have very great relevance for adult patients too – particularly as numerically the complications of cancer management are much commoner in adults.

P.N. Plowman

# Professor T J McElwain, FRCP

As this book was going to press, we were deeply saddened to learn of the death of Tim McElwain.

He will be missed by friends, colleagues and patients, past and present, for his dedication and his contribution to the progress of cancer medicine.

As his co-editors, we hope this book will be one fitting memorial to this famous cancer physician. We dedicate the volume to him.

Nick Plowman
Anna Meadows
January 1991

# List of contributors

**Ulrik Abildgaard** MD
Senior Registrar, Department of Cardiology, Rijshospitaliet, Copenhagen, Denmark
**E.M. Alstead** MD, MRCP
Senior Registrar, Department of Gastroenterology, St. Bartholomew's Hospital, London, UK
**Julianne Byrne** PhD
Senior Staff Fellow, Clinical Epidemiology Branch, National Cancer Institute, Bethesda, Maryland, USA
**Bruce A. Chabner** MD
Director, Division of Cancer Treatment, National Cancer Institute, Bethesda, Maryland, USA
**Bruce H. Cohen** MD
The Cleveland Clinic Foundation, Cleveland, Ohio, USA
**C. Norman Coleman** MD
Professor and Chairman, Harvard Medical School, Joint Center for Radiation Therapy, Boston, Massachusetts, USA
**Christopher H. Collis** MD(Cantab), MRCP, FRCR
Consultant in Radiotherapy and Oncology, Royal Free Hospital, London, UK
**Louis S. Constine** MD
Associate Professor of Radiation Oncology and Pediatrics, University of Rochester Cancer Center, Rochester, New York, USA
**Giulio D'Angio** MD
Childrens Cancer Research Center, Children's Hospital of Philadelphia, Philadelphia, Pennsylvania, USA
**Gedske Daugaard** MD
Senior Registrar, Department of Oncology, Rijshospitaliet, Copenhagen, Denmark

**Cynthia DeLaat** MD
Assistant Professor of Clinical Pediatrics, Division of Hematology/Oncology, Children's Hospital Medical Center, Cincinnati, Ohio, USA
**H. Brendan Devlin** MA, MD, MCh, FRCS, FRCSI, FRCSEd, FACS
Consultant Surgeon, North Tees General Hospital; Lecturer in Clinical Surgery, University of Newcastle-upon-Tyne, Newcastle-upon-Tyne, UK
**G.S.E. Dowd** MB, ChB, MChOrth, FRCS
Consultant Orthopaedic Surgeon, St Bartholomew's Hospital, London, UK
**Richard G. Evans** PhD, MD
Professor and Chairman, Department of Radiation Oncology, University of Kansas Medical Center, Kansas City, Kansas, USA
**M.J.G. Farthing** BSc, MD, FRCP
Reader in Gastroenterology and Honorary Consultant Physician, St Bartholomew's Hospital, London, UK
**J.A. Fixsen** MChir, FRCS
Consultant Orthopaedic Surgeon, St. Bartholomew's Hospital, London, UK
**Alan S. Gamis** MD
Fellow of Paediatrics, University of Minnesota, Minneapolis, Minnesota, USA
**Steven Greer** MD, FRCPsych, FRANZCP
Director, CRC Psychological Medicine Group, Royal Marsden Hospital, Sutton, Surrey, UK
**Ashley Grossman** BA, BSc, MD, MRCP
Senior Lecturer in Endocrinology and Honorary Consultant Physician, St Bartholomew's Hospital, London, UK
**A.N. Harnett** MB, BS, MRCP, FRCR
Beatson Oncology Centre, Western Infirmary, Glasgow, Scotland
**Eric Heiligenstein** MD
Clinical Assistant Professor, Department of Psychiatry, University of Wisconsin Medical School, Madison, Wisconsin, USA
**Jimmie C. Holland** MD
Chief, Psychiatry Service; Professor, Department of Psychiatry, Cornell University Medical Center, New York, New York, USA
**J.W. Hopewell** PhD
CRC Normal Tissue Radiobiology Research Group, Research Institute (University of Oxford), The Churchill Hospital, Oxford, UK
**J.L. Hungerford**
Moorfields Eye Hospital, London, UK
**Alison Jones** MRCP
Division of Medicine, Institute of Cancer Research and Royal Marsden Hospital, Sutton, Surrey, UK
**Mark W. Kissin** MChir, FRCS
Senior Surgical Registrar, Bristol Royal Infirmary, Bristol, UK
**Hans-Jochem Kolb** Prof Dr Med
Klinikum Grosshadern, Universität München, Munich, W. Germany

**E.D. Kramer** MD
Cooper Hospital, Camden, New Jersey, USA
**Beatrice C. Lampkin** MD
Professor of Pediatrics; Director, Division of Hematology/Oncology, Children's
Hospital Medical Center, Cincinnati, Ohio, USA
**Mark P. Langer** MD
Instructor, Harvard Medical School, Joint Center for Radiation Therapy, Boston,
Massachusetts, USA
**David A. Larson** MD, PhD
Assistant Professor and Vice Chairman, Department of Radiation Oncology,
University of California, San Francisco, California, USA
**Ilene B. Lefkowitz** MD
Assistant Professor of Clinical Pediatrics, Children's Hospital Medical Center,
Cincinnati, Ohio, USA
**T. A. Lister** MB, BChir, MRCP, MRCS, LRCP
Department of Medical Oncology, St. Bartholomew's Hospital, London, UK
**T.J. McElwain** MB, BS, FRCP
Professor of Medical Oncology, University of London; Head, Section of
Medicine, Institute of Cancer Research and Royal Marsden Hospital, Sutton,
Surrey, UK
**Margaret Masterson** MD
Third Year Fellow, Division of Hematology/Oncology, Children's Hospital
Medical Center, Cincinnati, Ohio, USA
**Anna T. Meadows** MD
Professor of Pediatrics, University of Pennsylvania School of Medicine; Senior
Oncologist, Children's Hospital of Philadelphia, Philadelphia, Pennsylvania,
USA
**John L. Millar** PhD, MRCPath
Team Leader, Section of Medicine Research Laboratories, Institute of Cancer
Research and Royal Marsden Hospital, Sutton, Surrey, UK
**J. Mulvihill** MD
National Cancer Institute, Bethesda, Maryland, USA
**J.P. Neglia** MD, MPh
Assistant Professor of Pediatrics, University of Minnesota, Minneapolis,
Minnesota, USA
**R.J. Packer** MD
Children's Hospital of Philadelphia, Philadelphia, Pennsylvania, USA
**P.N. Plowman** MA, MD, FRCP, FRCR
Consultant in Radiotherapy and Oncology, St Bartholomew's Hospital and The
Hospitals for Sick Children, Great Ormond Street, London, UK
**C.G.A. Price** MB, BS, MRCP
Department of Medical Oncology, St Bartholomew's Hospital, London, UK
**Simon A. Raimes** FRCS
Senior Registrar in General Surgery, North Tees General Hospital, Stockton on
Tees, UK

**Leslie L. Robison** PhD
Associate Professor, Departments of Pediatrics and Epidemiology, University of Minnesota, Minneapolis, Minnesota, USA

**M.E.C. Robbins** PhD
CRC Normal Tissue Radiobiology Research Group, Research Institute (University of Oxford), The Churchill Hospital, Oxford, UK

**Mace Rothenberg** MD
Special Assistant for Clinical Science, Division of Cancer Treatment, National Cancer Institute, Bethesda, Maryland, USA

**P. Rubin** MD
Chairman, Department of Radiation Oncology; Professor of Radiation Oncology, University of Rochester Cancer Center, Rochester, New York, USA

**J.E. Sanders** MD
The Fred Hutchinson Cancer Research Center, Seattle, Washington, USA

**Stephen R. Smalley** MD
Assistant Professor, Department of Radiation Oncology, University of Kansas Medical Center, Kansas City, Kansas, USA

**Elisabeth J. Shakin** MD
Associate Director Division Consultation-Liaison, Jefferson Medical College, Philadelphia, Pennsylvania, USA

**Elizabeth L. Travis** PhD
Professor, M.D. Anderson Cancer Center, Department of Experimental Radiotherapy, Houston, Texas, USA

**Klaus-Rüdiger Trott**
Department of Radiobiology, Medical College of St Bartholomew's Hospital, London, UK

**William M. Wara** MD
Professor and Vice Chairman, Department of Radiation Oncology, University of California, San Francisco, California, USA

**David O. Waterhouse** MD
Assistant Professor, Pediatrics, North Western University, Chicago; Hematologist/Oncologist, Children's Memorial Hospital, Chicago, Illinois, USA

**G. Westbury** MB, FRCP, FRCS
Formerly Professor of Surgery, Institute of Cancer Research and Royal Marsden Hospital, Sutton, Surrey, UK

**Wyndham Wilson** MD
Special Assistant for Preclinical Science, Division of Cancer Treatment, National Cancer Institute, Bethesda, Maryland, USA

**S. Venitt** BSc, PhD
Section of Molecular Carcinogenesis, Institute of Cancer Research, Sutton, Surrey, UK

# Contents

# Section 1

# 1

# Complications of drug therapy for cancer: general review

**M. Rothenberg, W. Wilson and B.A. Chabner**

The goal of any modality of cancer treatment may be simply stated: the complete and permanent elimination of all neoplastic cells from the patient. For tumors localized to one anatomical site or region, local treatment modalities such as surgery or radiotherapy may succeed in eradicating all malignant cells. However, many patients with clinically localized disease are not cured by local treatment modalities because of the presence of microscopic metastases, frequently resulting in recurrence if systemic treatment is not administered. For example, recurrence rates in patients with early-stage breast cancer and Dukes' B or C colon and rectal cancers can be significantly reduced by the administration of adjuvant chemotherapy [1–5].

Since the first clinical use of systemic therapy by Gilman and Philips in 1946 [6] and Farber *et al.* in 1947 [7], chemotherapy continues to be the most effective systemic therapy available. Over the past decade, however, recognition of the antitumor activity of biological response modifiers and immunotherapeutic agents has expanded the armamentarium of systemic therapy for cancer. But even with an expanded arsenal of cytotoxic agents, interferons, lymphokines and cytokines, the success of systemic therapy is still limited by normal tissue toxicity. This chapter will provide a brief review of the principles of cancer chemotherapy and will consider how the toxicity associated with systemic therapy influences treatment decisions.

## Principles of cancer chemotherapy

Many of the principles applied to the design of chemotherapeutic regimens have been empirically derived. For example, the use of multi-agent therapy (i.e. combination chemotherapy) to treat malignancies grew out of the observation that, with the exception of Burkitt's lymphoma and gestational choriocarcinoma, single-agent therapy rarely produced complete remissions or cures. Although attempts in the 1950s to combine agents on a rational biochemical or pharmacological basis were hampered by the few available drugs and limitations on controlling drug-induced toxicity, by the early 1960s combination chemotherapy had achieved its first successes in Hodgkin's disease (MOPP) and childhood acute lymphoblastic leukemia (VP) [8]. Further experimental work clearly established the importance of using multiple agents with different mechanisms of action to obtain optimal effects and, more recently, the use of agents that modulate antitumor activity of other drugs through biochemical or pharmacological interactions has provided an additional rationale for combination therapy. The theoretical work of Goldie and Coldman [9] has stressed an additional factor in the design of combination therapy regimens – the use of agents that do not share common mechanisms of drug resistance. The experience gained with these and subsequent combination regimens has provided the foundation upon which the following practical and theoretical guidelines for modern combination chemotherapy have been derived [10]:

1. Only drugs that have significant single-agent activity or that have an enhancing effect on other active agents should be included in a combination regimen. Consideration should be given to drugs that have different mechanisms of action that do not share a common mechanism of drug resistance and that have synergistic activity. In general, the use of drugs that have questionable

activity will only add toxicity and will usually reduce the ability to administer adequate doses of effective drugs.

2. Drugs with minimal overlapping toxicity should be used whenever possible in order to avoid dose reductions of other drugs that share similar toxicities.

3. Schedules of drug administration should be designed to allow maximal exposure to each agent as early in the treatment regimen as possible to prevent outgrowth of drug-resistant populations. Dose intensity (the dose administered per unit time) should be maximized for all cytotoxic agents.

## Toxicities of chemotherapy

The adherence to these tenets of chemotherapy is tempered by normal tissue tolerance to the toxic effects of chemotherapy. This factor influences virtually every aspect of chemotherapy administration, including drug selection, drug dosing, combinations of agents, schedule of administration, and combinations of drugs with other modalities.

In a clinical context, it is impossible to speak of the antitumor activity of a drug without consideration of its therapeutic index, i.e. the ratio of the dose producing unacceptable toxicity to the dose required for antitumor activity [11]. Clearly, in order for a drug to be clinically useful, this ratio must be sufficiently high to allow administration of effective drug doses without unacceptable side effects. It is important to recognize that the therapeutic index for a drug given alone may be significantly altered by the co-administration of other drugs or by co-morbid conditions present in the patient at the time of treatment. For example, the therapeutic index of methotrexate may be markedly reduced by the presence of significant third-space fluid (ascites, pleural effusion, etc.) which delays drug excretion [12]. The volume of distribution of methotrexate may be sufficiently altered due to sequestration of the drug into the third-space fluid that a prolongation of the terminal half-life of the drug occurs, resulting in a significantly increased risk of myelosuppression and mucositis. In this case, toxicities may be reduced by adequate drainage of third-space fluid prior to treatment or modifying drug dose and administration schedules. Age, in and of itself, should not be considered an absolute contraindication to high-dose chemotherapy. Although older patients often have co-morbid conditions that increase toxicity to therapy, in their absence such patients generally tolerate therapy quite well. In fact, the inferior response rates and survival frequently reported for older individuals who receive cancer chemotherapy are more often due to inadequate treatment than to a fatal complication of chemotherapy.

Finally, there are some rare genetic predispositions to increased toxicity to some chemotherapeutic agents, including increased neurotoxicity from vinca alkaloids in Charcot-Marie-Tooth disease and myelosuppression and stomatitis from fluorouracil in patients lacking dihydropyrimidine dehydrogenase [13,14]. Such predispositions, however, are very rare. Thus, a knowledge of the therapeutic index of a drug and how it is influenced by other factors is essential to help the clinician avoid these kinds of toxicities.

## Dose intensity

The dose rate or dose intensity refers to the amount of drug administered over a given period of time. Both time and schedule are important determinants of response to and toxicity of therapy. In animal models of high growth-rate tumors, a linear–log relationship between drug dose and cell kill has been observed. In some models, doubling drug doses may increase cell kill by as much as ten-fold, while reductions of 20% may decrease the cure rate by 50% [10]. Since the fraction of cells killed by a cycle of chemotherapy is rarely, if ever, 100% it is not surprising that the dose per unit time is of critical importance to the ultimate response from chemotherapy. The importance of dose rate has recently been clinically demonstrated for a number of tumors. Meta-analyses performed by Hryniuk *et al.* [15,16] in clinical trials in breast and ovarian cancers have demonstrated a remarkably linear correlation between dose rate and response, duration of disease-free survival and, in the case of ovarian cancer, survival. Similar analyses in intermediate-grade lymphomas have shown a positive correlation as well [17]. However, when applying this concept to protocol design, it is important to keep in mind that a steep dose-response curve exists for both the therapeutic and toxic effects of many anticancer drugs. Clearly, excessive doses of a drug may result in unacceptably severe or permanent damage to normal tissues, and too frequent administration of chemotherapy may not allow normal tissue recovery, resulting in increased toxicity with each subsequent cycle of chemotherapy. Thus, dose rate must be balanced against toxicity when determining the dose and rate at which chemotherapy is to be delivered.

## Normal tissue protection

The toxicity that occurs from chemotherapy may be altered or reduced by specific techniques such as changes in the method of treatment (e.g. aggressive hydration and chloride loading for cisplatin) [18], schedule of administration (e.g. constant infusion versus bolus), and use of drugs that ameliorate specific toxicities (e.g. colony-stimulating factors [19], WR-2721 to reduce bone marrow suppression [20]) and bone marrow transplant.

When specific drug toxicities are dose-limiting, measures that provide regional protection – such as the use of mesna to prevent hemorrhagic cystitis due to metabolites of cyclophosphamide or ifosfamide [21], or the use of systemic thiosulfate with intraperitoneal cisplatin [22] – allow increases in dose. A second example of regional protection comes from the clinical experience with cisplatin. In the early 1970s great enthusiasm was generated by the excellent antitumor activity of cisplatin against several solid malignancies but, because of the severe nausea, vomiting and nephrotoxicity encountered, doses rarely exceeded $100\,mg/m^2$. However, with the development of more effective antiemetics such as metoclopramide, and kidney-protective manoeuvers such as aggressive hydration and forced chloruresis, significantly higher doses of cisplatin could be safely administered. An important clinical finding was that the higher doses of cisplatin were generally more effective against tumors such as ovarian and testicular cancers [15]. This was a clinical confirmation of *in vitro* experiments that demonstrated that alkylators, including platinum compounds, exhibit steep tumoricidal dose-response curves.

Another approach to increasing the dose rate is through the protection of normal, but not malignant, tissues from the toxic effects of chemotherapy. The earliest experimental data come from experiments in mice, where it was demonstrated that a usually lethal dose of cyclophosphamide could be administered if the mice were pretreated 2–4 days earlier with a lower priming dose of the same or different cytotoxic drug [23,24]. In this setting the priming dose exerted a protective effect on normal tissues such as bone marrow, uroepithelium and intestinal epithelium, but less so on malignant tissues, although this differential effect is dependent on the tumor type. Even though the mechanism(s) for this protection are unclear, it was shown that the priming dose induced a transient resting state $(G_0)$ in highly proliferating tissue, thereby reducing its sensitivity to the subsequent high dose of chemotherapy and, in addition, could increase the important detoxification enzymes, intracellular glutathione and glutathione transferase.

These approaches have laid the ground for other approaches. For example, biologics such as interleukin 1 (IL-1) and γ-interferon are potent bone marrow protectors against radiation and possibly chemotherapy in murine systems [25,26]. These agents will soon be entering clinical trials and, if effective, may significantly reduce the toxicity of chemotherapy. The rate at which the bone marrow recovers is also an important determinant of toxicity and, consequently, the interval between chemotherapy cycles. Unfortunately, delays in drug administration due to hematopoietic recovery may allow regrowth of that fraction of tumor cells not killed by the previous dose of chemotherapy, even though the cells are not necessarily drug resistant. Clearly, this will have the greatest impact on tumors with high growth fractions, such as lymphomas, so that the intervals between cycles are usually kept to a minimum. There are now some potentially exciting new approaches to improving hematopoietic recovery and minimizing cycle length through the use of the recombinant colony-stimulating factors GM-CSF, G-CSF and IL-3, which are necessary for the normal proliferation and differentiation of hematopoietic cells [27–29]. Preliminary studies have demonstrated that these factors shorten the period of neutropenia by stimulating bone marrow recovery, and they are undergoing clinical investigation in the setting of multiple cycles of chemotherapy. Ultimately, a combination of bone marrow protector with a colony-stimulating factor might have the greatest impact on reducing bone marrow toxicity.

Finally, techniques such as autologous or allogeneic bone marrow transplantation have allowed major increases in dose by overcoming the dose-limiting effect of myelosuppression. Over the past decade, high-dose chemotherapy with bone marrow support has been used to treat an expanding number of malignancies, and results demonstrate its effectiveness in a number of relapsed malignancies, including leukemias, lymphomas and testicular and breast malignancies [30,31]. For this reason, bone marrow transplant is being studied as consolidation therapy in the initial treatment of the advanced stages of these malignancies, and early results are very encouraging. However, one must keep in mind that these gains are not achieved without significant toxicities. Because myelosuppression is no longer dose-limiting in bone marrow transplant, chemotherapy and radiotherapy are escalated to the maximum tolerance of other major organ systems, resulting in toxicity. Thus, when developing a new ablative regimen, it is imperative to select drugs that are effective and that have minimal overlapping toxicities, and to dose escalate to the maximum tolerated dose in a phase I setting.

Unfortunately, even with the aforementioned approaches to decreasing toxicity of chemotherapy, significant toxicity inevitably occurs as doses of chemotherapy are maximized. In clinical practice there is an unfortunate tendency among some oncologists to reduce drug doses and delay cycles of chemotherapy, even when treating potentially curable diseases, in order to minimize toxicity, without taking into account the adverse impact this may have on a successful clinical outcome. Clearly, a balance between toxicity and maximization of dose rate must be achieved and, in the case of potentially curable tumors such as lymphomas and testicular carcinomas, significant treatment toxicity will often be incurred in order to achieve an adequate dose rate. Ultimately, the achievement of this balance must depend upon the clinical experience and judgment of the oncologist.

## Drug–drug and drug–radiation interactions

One must recognize both the favorable and unfavorable drug interactions resulting from the concurrent use of multiple anticancer drugs that may involve pharmacokinetic, cytokinetic or biochemical interactions. For example, a drug that impairs renal function, such as cisplatin, may result in delayed excretion of drugs cleared by the kidney, such as methotrexate or bleomycin, resulting in increased toxicity. Hence, regimens that include nephrotoxic drugs require concurrent monitoring of renal function and dose adjustment for changes in creatinine clearance. In the case of methotrexate, serial serum drug level monitoring and leucovorin rescue in patients with delayed drug excretion provide added margins of safety.

The sequential or concurrent use of two or more drugs may enhance the cytotoxic effect of the drugs through specific biochemical interactions. The best example of this is the combination of 5-fluorouracil and leucovorin where the addition of leucovorin acts to stabilize the ternary compound formed by fluoro-deoxyuridine monophosphate (FdUMP), thymidylate synthase and the cofactor 5,10-methylene-tetrahydrofolate [32]. Failure to form and maintain a stable ternary complex results in incomplete inhibition of thymidylate synthetase, DNA synthesis, and relative resistance to 5-fluorouracil. The addition of leucovorin to 5-fluorouracil increases the gastrointestinal mucosal toxicity of the antimetabolite, necessitating a 25% reduction in 5-fluorouracil dose, but the combination has resulted in significantly improved response rates in patients with metastatic colon cancer as compared with those seen with 5-fluorouracil alone. Other drug–drug interactions that alter clinical toxicity are listed in Table 1.1.

Certain chemotherapeutic agents may interact with other modalities of cancer therapy in both advantageous and disadvantageous ways. A well recognized interaction is the enhancement of local effects of ionizing radiation by systemically administered cytotoxic drugs. Clinical protocols designed to exploit this interaction have utilized such drugs as 5-fluorouracil, actinomycin D, hydroxyurea or doxorubicin. Drug–radiation combinations have

**Table 1.1 Drug interactions in combination chemotherapy**

Transport:
1. Calcium channel blockers block efflux of antitumor antibiotics

Enhancement of activity:
1. Methotrexate increases 5-fluorouracil activation
2. Methotrexate increases cytosine arabinoside activation
3. Leucovorin increases 5-fluorouracil inhibition of thymidylate synthase
4. Inhibitors of *de novo* pyrimidine synthesis enhance 5-fluorouracil incorporation into RNA and formation of active nucleotides
5. Nitroimidazoles enhance alkylating agent activity

Antagonism of antitumor effect:
1. 5-Fluorouracil pretreatment prevents antifolate action of methotrexate
2. L-Asparaginase pretreatment blocks antitumor effect of methotrexate

Reversal of toxicity (rescue):
1. Leucovorin prevents methotrexate toxicity
2. Deoxycytidine prevents toxicity of cytosine arabinoside
3. Allopurinol blocks 5-fluorouracil activation by normal tissues

yielded promising clinical results in patients with head and neck cancer and small cell lung cancer [33–35]. Of course, some normal tissues are susceptible to enhanced toxicity with the combined approach, including bone marrow, lung, gastrointestinal tract, skin, heart and brain.

Drug toxicity may be enhanced by prior radiotherapy. For example, a patient who received radiotherapy many years earlier may later require chemotherapy due to recurrent or progressive disease. Although peripheral blood counts may be normal, the proliferative response of the bone marrow stem cells is chronically impaired by the radiotherapy, and chemotherapy may induce more severe and prolonged myelosuppression than would be seen in the absence of prior pelvic radiation [36].

Another interaction between radiation and chemotherapy is that of radiation recall. Some chemotherapeutic agents, particularly methotrexate and doxorubicin, produce local inflammatory reactions in sites of previous radiation. These reactions may range from localized skin erythema to severe cardiomyopathy or pulmonary fibrosis.

## Guidelines to chemotherapy toxicity

At present there are no therapeutic agents that have toxicity limited to neoplastic cells, primarily because no drug target, whether a metabolic pathway, surface protein or mechanism of growth and division, is found exclusively in cancer cells. Therefore, current therapy must generally exploit qualitative differences between normal and malignant cells, such as substrate requirements or growth fraction, in order to attempt eradication of the malignancy without causing unacceptable normal tissue toxicity. One must be familiar not only with the spectrum of clinical activity of a given drug, but also with its toxicity. Before any chemotherapy is administered, one should be aware of the full ramifications of this action. The following questions should be addressed and answered before embarking on a course of treatment:

1. What is the spectrum of organ toxicity associated with each drug? Which organs are most sensitive to the effects of this drug; which are most resistant and how is this related to dose?
2. When is the toxicity most likely to appear and how long will it last? How will this affect the frequency with which this therapy can be administered?
3. How will drug route and duration of administration affect toxicity? Will the different pharmacokinetic profiles affect the nature of the toxicity (e.g. bolus *versus* infusional therapies, interperitoneal *versus* intravenous routes)?
4. What are the clinical implications of this toxicity? Will it require specific monitoring or supportive measures? Is it reversible?
5. Is the toxicity preventable? What measures may be taken to minimize or avoid the toxicity, and will they interfere with the antitumor activity of the drug?
6. What drug or radiation interactions may occur? What are the mechanisms of these interactions (e.g. alterations in drug metabolism, or alterations in end-organ function), and will previous therapy lead to different or more severe toxicity than otherwise expected?
7. Is the patient at increased risk for toxicity from this drug? Does the patient have any specific characteristics that puts him/her at increased risk, such as age, genetic traits, type of malignancy, or concurrent medical conditions of more severe or uncommon drug toxicity?
8. Has the patient been fully informed of the risks associated with the therapy and are there specific psychological and social conditions that may impact on his/her ability to tolerate the toxicity?

These questions are not merely presented for rhetorical purposes. Careful consideration of each of these points will result in the design and administration of therapy most likely to optimize benefit and minimize risk to the patient.

## References


1. Fisher, B., Redmond, C., Dimitrov, N.V. *et al.* A randomized clinical trial evaluating sequential methotrexate and fluorouracil in the treatment of patients with node-negative breast cancer who have estrogen-receptor-negative tumors. *New England Journal of Medicine*, **320**, 473–478 (1989)
2. Fisher, B., Costantino, J., Redmond, C. *et al.* A randomized clinical trial evaluating tamoxifen in the treatment of patients with node-negative breast cancer who have estrogen-receptor-positive tumors. *New England Journal of Medicine*, **320**, 479–484 (1989)
3. Mansour, E.G., Gray, R., Shatila, A.H. *et al.* Efficacy of adjuvant chemotherapy in high-risk node-negative patients. *New England Journal of Medicine*, **320**, 485–490 (1989)
4. Fisher, B., Wolmark, N., Rockette, H. *et al.* Postoperative adjuvant chemotherapy for rectal cancer: results from NSABP protocol R-01. *Journal of the National Cancer Institute*, **80**, 21–29 (1988)
5. Wolmark, N., Fisher, B., Rockette, H. *et al.* Postoperative adjuvant chemotherapy or BCG for colon cancer: results from NSABP protocol C-01. *Journal of the National Cancer Institute*, **80**, 30–36 (1988)
6. Gilman, A. and Philips, F.S. The biological actions and therapeutic applications of the b-chloroethyl amines and sulfides. *Science*, **103**, 409–415 (1946)
7. Farber, S., Cutler, E., Hawkins, J.W. *et al.* The action of pteroyl-glutamic conjugates in man. *Science*, **106**, 619–621 (1947)
8. Nathanson, L., Hall, T.C., Schilling, A. and Miller, S. Concurrent combination chemotherapy of human solid tumors: experience with a three-drug regimen and review of the literature. *Cancer Research*, **29**, 419–425 (1969)
9. Goldie, J.H. and Coldman, A.J. A mathematical model for relating the drug sensitivity of tumors to their spontaneous mutation rate. *Cancer Treatment Reports*, **63**, 1727–1733 (1979)
10. DeVita, V.T. Principles of chemotherapy. In *Cancer: Principles and Practice of Oncology*, 2nd edn (eds V.T. DeVita, S. Hellman and S.A. Rosenberg), J.B. Lippincott, Philadelphia, pp. 257–285 (1985)
11. Chabner, B.A. and Myers, C.E. Clinical pharmacology of cancer chemotherapy. In *Cancer: Principles and Practice of Oncology*, 2nd edn (eds V.T. DeVita, S. Hellman and S.A. Rosenberg), J.B. Lippincott, Philadelphia, pp. 287–328 (1985)
12. Chabner, B.A. Methotrexate. In *Pharmacologic Principles of Cancer Treatment* (ed. B.A. Chabner), W.B. Saunders, Philadelphia, pp. 229–255 (1982)
13. Griffiths, J.D., Stark, R.J., Ding, J.C. and Cooper, I.A. Vincristine neurotoxicity in Charcot-Marie-Tooth syndrome. *Medical Journal of Australia*, **143**, 305–306 (1985)
14. Diasio, R.B., Beavers, T.L. and Carpenter, J.T. Familial deficiency of dihydropyrimidine dehydrogenase. Biochemical basis for familial pyrimidinemia and

severe 5-fluorouracil-induced toxicity. *Journal of Clinical Investigation*, **81**, 47–51 (1988)

15. Levin, L. and Hryniuk, W.M. Dose intensity of chemotherapy regimens in ovarian cancer. *Journal of Clinical Oncology*, **5**, 756–767 (1987)

16. Hryniuk, W. and Bush, H. The importance of dose-intensity in chemotherapy of metastatic breast cancer. *Journal of Clinical Oncology*, **2**, 1281–1288 (1984)

17. DeVita, V.T., Hubbard, S.M., Young, R.C. and Longo, D.L. The role of chemotherapy in diffuse aggressive lymphomas. *Seminars in Hematology*, **25**, 2–10 (1988)

18. Ozols, R.F., Corden, B.J., Jacob, J. *et al.* High-dose cisplatin in hypertonic saline. *Annals of Internal Medicine*, **100**, 19–24 (1984)

19. Weisbart, R.H., Gasson, J.C. and Golde, D.W. Colony-stimulating factors and host defense. *Annals of Internal Medicine*, **110**, 297–303 (1989)

20. Glover, D., Glick, J.H., Weiler, C. *et al.* WR-2721 protects against the hematological toxicity of cyclophosphamide: a controlled phase II study. *Journal of Clinical Oncology*, **4**, 584–588 (1986)

21. Bryant, G.M., Ford, H.T., Jarman, M. *et al.* Prevention of isophosphamide-induced urothelial toxicity with 2-mercaptoethane sulphonate sodium (mesnum) in patients with advanced carcinoma. *Lancet*, **ii**, 657–659 (1983)

22. Markman, M., Cleary, S. and Howell, S.B. Nephrotoxicity of high-dose intracavitary cisplatin with intravenous thiosulfate protection. *European Journal of Cancer and Clinical Oncology*, **21**, 1015–1018 (1985)

23. Millar, J.L., Hudspith, B.N. and Blackett, N.M. Reduced lethality in mice receiving a combined dose of cyclophosphamide and busulphan. *British Journal of Cancer*, **32**, 193–198 (1975)

24. Carmichael, J., Adams, D.J., Ansell, J. and Wolf, C.R. Glutathione and glutathione transferase levels in mouse granulocytes following cyclophosphamide administration. *Cancer Research*, **46**, 735–739 (1986)

25. Neta, R., Douches, S. and Oppenheim, J.J. Interleukin 1 is a radioprotector. *Journal of Immunology*, **136**, 2483–2590 (1986)

26. Neta, R. and Oppenheim, J.J. Cytokines in therapy of radiation injury. *Blood*, **72**, 1093–1095 (1988)

27. Koike, K., Stanley, E.R., Ihle, J.N. and Ogawa, M. Macrophage colony formation supported by purified CSF-1 and/or interleukin 3 in serum-free culture: evidence for hierarchical difference in macrophage colony-forming cells. *Blood*, **67**, 859–864 (1986)

28. Santoli, D., Yang, Y.C., Clark, S.C. *et al.*, Synergistic and antagonistic effects of recombinant human interleukin (IL) 3, IL-1α, granulocyte and macrophage colony-stimulating factors (G-CSF and M-CSF) on the growth of GM-CSF-dependent leukemic cell lines. *Journal of Immunology*, **139**, 3348–3354 (1987)

29. Antman, K.S., Griffin, J.D., Elias, A. *et al.* Effect of recombinant human granulocyte-macrophage colony-stimulating factor on chemotherapy-induced myelosuppression. *New England Journal of Medicine*, **319**, 593–598 (1988)

30. Frei, E. III, Antman, K., Teicher, B. *et al.* Bone marrow autotransplantation for solid tumors – prospects. *Journal of Clinical Oncology*, **7**, 515–526 (1989)

31. Cheson, B.D., Lacerna, L., Leyland-Jones, B. *et al.* Autologous bone marrow transplantation. Current status and future directions. *Annals of Internal Medicine*, **110**, 51–65 (1989)

32. Grem, J.L. 5-Fluorouracil plus leucovorin in cancer therapy. In *Principles and Practice of Oncology – Updates*, Vol. 2 (eds V.T. DeVita, S. Hellman and S.A. Rosenberg), J.B. Lippincott, Philadelphia, pp. 1–12 (1988)

33. Taylor, S.G. IV. Integration of chemotherapy into the combined modality therapy of head and neck squamous cancer. *International Journal of Radiation Oncology, Biology, Physics*, **13**, 779–783 (1987)

34. Turrisi, A.T. III, Glover, D.J. and Mason, B.A. A preliminary report: concurrent twice-daily radiotherapy plus platinum-etoposide chemotherapy for limited stage and small cell lung cancer. *International Journal of Radiation Oncology, Biology, Physics*, **15**, 183–187 (1988)

35. Johnson, B.E., Grayson, J., Woods, E. *et al.* Limited stage small cell lung cancer treated with concurrent etoposide/cisplatin plus b.i.d. chest radiotherapy. *Proceedings of the American Society of Clinical Oncology*, **8**, 228 (abstract 888) (1989)

36. Kjellgren, O. and Jonsson, L. Bone marrow depression in the pelvis after megavoltage irradiation for ovarian carcinoma. *Obstetrics and Gynecology*, **105**, 849–855 (1969)

# 2

# Complications of radiotherapy: general concepts and historical review

G. D'Angio

Wilhelm Roentgen made his epochal discovery in November 1895 [1]. It is both sobering and amazing to recognize how rapidly the biological effects of X-radiation became recognized. Holmes and Schulz summarized well the biological observations that were made in late 1895 and early 1896 [2]. Radiation dermatitis and epilation secondary to X-radiation were reported within weeks of the date of Roentgen's paper; indeed, X-radiation had been used therapeutically for the first time in Chicago by Grubbé for cancer of the breast on 29 January 1896 [2]. Radiobiological experiments started early, too; disturbance in bone growth had already been reported by Perthes in 1903 in experiments conducted in chicks [3]. Meanwhile parallel observations were being made concerning gamma radiation, discovered by Becquerel in 1896, and soon leading to the discovery of radium [4].

Early therapists tried to exploit the damaging effects before the turn of the century, applying them to orthopedic problems (scoliosis) and to various dermatological conditions from hypertrichosis to cancer of the skin [5,6]. The perspicacity as well as the ingenuity of the pioneering workers is remarkable; the fact that many of the early attempts had disastrous consequences (e.g. carcinogenesis) was recognized and already published by Codman in 1900 [2]. Thus, research in radiobiology was being conducted both in the clinic and the laboratory, where astute observers recorded both the beneficial and untoward consequences of X-radiation.

This heritage has been carried forward by radiation therapists to this day. Always aware that their therapeutic modality has its dark side, radiotherapists have been among the most assiduous reporters of both the benefits and the risks associated with ionizing radiations. They have also been very well aware of the fact that, unlike other forms of treatment, many years sometimes are needed before the full extent of radiation-induced tissue damage becomes apparent. Abundant literature has resulted, and 'tolerance doses' for the various tissues and structures of the body are known within reasonably precise limits [7]. This body of knowledge has had to be revised drastically in recent years because of the advent of combined modality care. Some of the chemotherapeutic agents used for cancer management have direct toxic effects on specific organs, e.g. the heart or lungs [8]. Other drugs are radiation enhancers and reactivators [9,10], i.e. when used together with radiation they produce reactions in various tissues at much lower doses than those required when X radiation is used alone. Moreover, administration of these agents after completion of radiation therapy can 'recall' latent radiation damage within irradiated tissues. Discussion of radiation damage *per se* is therefore becoming increasingly complex because of these interplays, especially in pediatrics where combined chemoradiation therapy has become the 'norm' [11].

Radiation injuries can be divided into two major categories: functional impairments and oncogenesis. Each of these topics with its various sub-headings is treated extensively elsewhere in this volume. Here, general radiobiological and anatomical principles will be discussed.

## Mechanisms and interplays

Many radiation workers over the years have studied effects of varying doses on specific tissues. These pioneering investigators made land-mark discoveries, resulting in certain general principles. The 'law' of Bergonié and Tribondeau was based on studies by them and other French investigators using the rodent testicle as a target organ [12]. The 'law' states that the more rapidly dividing and the more immature the cell, the more 'radiosensitive' it is. This general precept is largely correct as far as relatively quick responses to irradiation are concerned, but not necessarily for the prediction of long-term effects [13,14].

First, it is important to recognize that radiation does not directly destroy the irradiated cell [13,14]; rather, it severely affects the ability of the cell to reproduce normally and to give rise to a continuing line of progeny. (The normal lymphocyte and the dysgerminoma cell are exceptions to this general rule and appear to undergo rapid destruction when irradiated.) It can be inferred that in other cells the target molecule is the DNA, and this view is supported by numerous very precise experiments based on cells in tissue culture [13,14]. It also is clear that effects at the molecular level are not mediated directly through 'direct hits' of the ionizing radiation on the target molecule. Rather, they are mediated through changes in the ambient environment. It is interesting to note that these effects were anticipated in the very early days. Some of the earliest radiobiological studies were performed within a few days of the discovery of X-rays on the potential bactericidal effects of X-radiation. By 1898 it had been shown that X-radiation did not affect bacteria in culture, but did suppress their proliferation in living tissues. Thus, it became obvious that X-radiation effects required mediating influences. Free radicals, highly reactive molecules and atoms, are probably responsible. At the molecular level it is established that radicals are activated in the adjacent milieu by ionizing radiations and that they damage portions of the DNA molecule. At the cellular level it can be inferred that radicals are implicated in the immune response, perhaps through chemotaxis.

Further discusssion of these intricate physico-chemical-biological effects is beyond the scope of this chapter. At the tissue level, however, radiation effects on target tissues also are often indirect. Ellis, in a land-mark formulation, proposed that radiation responses in normal structures are largely based on damage to the stroma in which functional cells lie, i.e. the blood vessels and connective tissue that form the essential framework for more specialized cells and tissues [15]. He reasoned that, since the stroma is not tissue- or organ-specific, a formula could be written that would predict normal tissue damage anywhere in the body, excepting brain and possibly bone. The elements of the Ellis formula incorporated total dose, fraction size and overall time of therapy. The details of the formula, and the concept itself, have been much debated and modified for different tissues and for early and late reactions, but the importance of relating tissue damage to time,

dose and fraction size is nonetheless recognized as being correct [13,14].

These interplays can be extended to encompass organ–organ interactions. Damage produced in one organ can have serious consequences in another, whether closely adjacent or remote. An example is the scoliosis produced by asymmetric radiation of the soft tissues of the juvenile trunk. This leads to subsequent fibrosis of the soft tissues, asymmetric growth through a 'bow string effect' and eventual spinal curvature [16]. Another example in pediatrics is the radiation suppression of pituitary function with predictable consequences on normal growth [17]. Severe radiation fibrosis of a lung can cause cardiac failure because perfusion of the non-functioning lung gives rise to what amounts to an arteriovenous fistula with resultant cardiac strain. Radiation nephropathy leading to hypertension and cardiac failure is another example of radiation damage in one organ causing life-threatening, if not lethal, expressions in another organ system [18].

## Phases of radiation injury

Radiation complications can be seen early, at an intermediate time, or late [7]. By 'early' is meant during treatment itself or within a few days or weeks after completion; 'intermediate' is taken to mean several weeks or months after the completion of treatment, and 'late effects' are encountered after the passage of years.

### Early

These reactions can be very brisk but seemingly heal completely, e.g. severe oropharyngeal radiation mucositis. However, significant residual damage is often present, despite what seems to be total recovery. This can be manifest in many ways. In the example cited, residual damage to the salivary glands is expressed as a change in the character of the saliva, if not xerostomia. Other changes possible include osteitis, disruption of normal dentition in children, and eventual radiogenic neoplasms of the skin and the salivary and thyroid glands, which are the most susceptible tissues of the region [19].

### Intermediate

Reactions may occur with or without antecedent early responses. Examples are the somnolence syndrome after cranial irradiation, which appears 4–6 weeks after completion of radiation therapy [17]. Another example is radiation pneumonopathy, manifest as pulmonary edema. Again, these changes may disappear with or without medical intervention with what seems to be a return to a normal state.

Here too, however, the appearance may be illusory. Careful pulmonary function studies in irradiated patients show functional impairments even though there may be no overt clinical evidence.

## Late effects

The spectre of malignant change in any of the irradiated structures is ever-present. After cranial irradiation, for example, not only the skin and the underlying bone are at risk but also the brain itself, where gliomata and other tumors of the brain and its coverings may appear in later years [19].

Functional impairments may take many months to years before they become apparent. Cranial irradiation in children and in adults is associated with short-term memory problems and often difficulties with arithmetic and mathematics that appear 2 or more years after therapy [17,20]. Long delays between treatment and the expression of radiation damage are exemplified in the case reported by O'Malley *et al.* [18]. A girl, treated when 3 months old for stage IV-S neuroblastoma, was given radiation to the enlarged liver. The fields included both kidneys which received an estimated dose in the 1400 cGy range. Twenty years later she developed fulminant hypertension and cardiac failure, died, and at autopsy was found to have changes consistent with radiation nephropathy. This patient provides another example of how damage in one organ can have adverse effects on another. She also had developed a cancer in the irradiated skin at age 18, demonstrating in her short life both the dysfunctional and carcinogenic sequelae of irradiation.

Other irradiated children have subsequently developed coarctation of the treated portion of the abdominal aorta, leading to secondary effects in the kidneys with resultant hypertension [16]. Any arterial trunk can be affected similarly with resultant peripheral ischemic changes.

## Comment

The above discussion has emphasized that there is an interdependence at all levels – from atoms to complex tissues – between the delivery of ionizing radiations and subsequent biological events. It also has given examples of radiation effects that may be expressed in sequence from acute to intermediate to late changes, omitting clinical evidence at one or two of these three stages. However, there always are residua, even though they may be subclinical. It remains only to be stressed that combination chemoradiation therapy very often accelerates, intensifies and reactivates radiation reactions, and that 'tolerance doses' of radiation therapy are not valid under those circumstances.


## References

1. Roentgen, W.C. Ueber eine neue Art von Strahlen Sitzungsberichte der physikal-medicin. *Gesselschaft, Wuerzburg*, **137**, 132–141 (1895)
2. Holmes, G.W. and Schulz, M.D. *Therapeutic Radiology*, Lea and Febiger, Philadelphia (1950)
3. Perthes, G. Ueber den Einfluss der Roentgen-strahlen auf epithelial Gewebe insbensondere auf das Carcinom. *Archiv fuer Klinische Chirurgie*, **71**, 955–1000 (1903)
4. Curie, P., Curie, P. and Bemont, G. Sur une nouvelle substance fortement radioactive continue dans la pecheblende. *Comptes Rendus de l'Academie des Sciences*, **127**, 1215–1217 (1898)
5. Daniel, J. Depilatory action of X-rays. *Medical Record*, **49**, 595–596 (1896)
6. Freund, L. Ein mit Roentgen-Strahlen behandelter Fall von Nevus pigmentosus piliferus. *Wiener Medizinische Wochenschrift*, **47**, 427–429 (1897)
7. Rubin, P. and Casarett, G.W. *Clinical Radiation Pathology*, Vols 1 and 2, W.B. Saunders, Philadelphia (1968)
8. Perry, M.C. and Yarbro, J.W. (eds). *Toxicity of Chemotherapy*, Grune and Stratton, Orlando (1984)
9. D'Angio, G.J. Clinical and biologic studies of actinomycin-D and roentgen irradiation. *American Journal of Roentgenology*, **87**, 106–109 (1962)
10. Donaldson, S.S., Glick, J.M. and Wilbur, J.R. Adriamycin activating a recall phenomenon after radiation therapy (letter to the editor). *Annals of Internal Medicine*, **81**, 407–408 (1974)
11. Pizzo, P.A. and Poplack, D.G. (eds). *Pediatric Oncology*, J.B. Lippincott, Philadelphia (1989)
12. Bergonié, J. and Tribondeau, L. Interpretation de quelques résultats de la radiotherapie. *Comptes Rendus de l'Academie des Sciences*, **143**, 983–988 (1906)
13. Suit, H.D. Radiation biology: the conceptual and practical impact on radiation therapy. *Radiation Research*, **94**, 10–40 (1983)
14. Withers, H.R. Biologic basics of radiation therapy. In *Principles and Practice of Radiation Oncology* (eds C.A. Perez and L.W. Brady), J.B. Lippincott, Philadelphia (1987)
15. Ellis, F. Dose, time and fractionation: a clinical hypothesis. *Clinical Radiology*, **20**, 1–7 (1969)
16. Littman, P.S. and D'Angio, G.J. Growth considerations in the radiation therapy of children with cancer. In *Annual Review of Medicine: Selected Topics in the Clinical Sciences* (eds W.B. Creger, C.H. Coggins and E.W. Hancock), Annual Reviews, Inc., Palo Alto, CA, **30**, 405–415 (1979)
17. Packer, R.J., Meadows, A.T., Rorke, L.B. *et al.* Long-term sequelae of cancer treatment of the central nervous system in childhood. *Medical and Pediatric Oncology*, **15**, 241–253 (1987)
18. O'Malley, B., D'Angio, G.J. and Vawter, G.F. Late effects of roentgen therapy given in infancy. *American Journal of Roentgenology*, **89**, 1067–1074 (1963)

19. Modan, B., Baidatz, D., Mart, H. *et al.* Radiation-induced head and neck tumours. *Lancet*, **i**, 277–279 (1974)

20. Ron, E., Modan, B., Floro, S. *et al.*, Mental function following scalp irradiation during childhood. *American Journal of Epidemiology*, **116**, 149–160 (1982)

# 3

# Morbidity of combined chemotherapy and radiotherapy

L.S. Constine and P. Rubin

The primary goal of the oncologist is to eradicate local and systemic cancer without severely compromising the patient's potential for a normal quality of life. The optimal combination of chemotherapy and radiotherapy is thus based on its tumoricidal effectiveness weighed against its normal tissue morbidities. Ideally chemotherapy will sterilize micrometastases outside the radiotherapy field and increase the likelihood of radiotherapy achieving local control of the primary tumor. Radiation will, in addition, sterilize areas not effectively controlled by drugs. The aggressiveness of therapy can only be determined by knowledge of the acute tolerance of the normal tissues and debilitating late effects which might ensue. In this era of combined therapy adverse effects occur in patients who have received seemingly 'safe' doses of each mode, below the generally accepted threshold levels for toxicity when used alone [1]. Untoward reactions can occur at unexpected time intervals and in an unpredictable fashion.

The variety of possible interactions between these two therapies accounts for the breadth of the spectrum of potential morbidities [2]. These include the following:

1. The damaging effects of radiation on a target tissue can be increased by chemotherapy (e.g. radiation pneumonitis intensified by dactinomycin [3], or esophagitis exacerbated by doxorubicin (Adriamycin) [4]).
2. The damaging effects of chemotherapy on the target cell can be increased by irradiation (e.g. bone marrow suppression or second malignancies in the treatment of Hodgkin's disease [5,6], lung fibrosis in patients treated with high-dose cyclophosphamide followed by thoracic irradiation [7]).
3. The independent injuries which each causes in the same organ can combine to increase the degree of resulting dysfunction (e.g. cardiomyopathy after radiation and doxorubicin (Adriamycin) [8], cystitis after radiation and cyclophosphamide [9]).
4. An injury can be produced which is not commonly seen with either modality alone (e.g. leukoencephalopathy after low doses of irradiation and methotrexate in patients with leukemia [10], hepatopathy in children with Wilms' tumor treated with irradiation and doxorubicin [11]).

The difficulty inherent in understanding these consequences is furthermore complicated by the number of chemotherapeutic agents generally combined in treatment protocols, and newer unconventional radiotherapy techniques (e.g. hyperfractionated and intraoperative therapy). Although laboratory approaches toward examining the normal tissue effects of each chemotherapeutic agent and radiation are in progress, reliable dose-response data are generally lacking. The bulk of useful information available to the clinician is derived from clinical observations. This chapter will attempt to provide a framework for understanding the morbid effects of combined therapy by examining the basis for injury after each modality alone and then as they interact.

## Definitions of acute and chronic morbidity

While the concepts of acute and chronic adverse effects are generally well appreciated, specific definitions are lacking. An operational definition proves to be useful. Acute or early appearing complications are those appearing during or within days following a course of therapy. Those which appear during treatment can sometimes be managed by modifying therapy. Late or chronic complications are those sequelae which have their onset months or years following the cessation of treatment. This definition implies that therapeutic decisions intended to obviate late effects can only be based on the probability but not the certainty that such events will occur [12]. In general, the chemotherapist has been predominantly concerned with acute and subacute effects because it is this toxicity that determines the tolerance of and the ability to administer chemotherapeutic regimens. Conversely, the radiation therapist has traditionally been more concerned with late toxic effects since the overall duration of the treatment course is less but the late sequelae can be dramatic.

The relationship between acute injury and late effects is unpredictable. Although it might be expected that therapy which is sufficiently intense to cause acute morbidity would lead to chronic effects, the characteristics of certain tissues are such that this sequence may not occur. Moreover, the absence of any acute difficulties does not preclude the occurrence of late effects [13,14]. The relationship between acute and late effects, and the role that combined modality therapy plays in their occurrence, is best appreciated by recognizing the difference between subclinical and clinical reactions. It is obvious that reactions must occur above a subclinical threshold in order to be readily observed. As a corollary, clinical reactions must have a subclinical basis. As illustrated in Figure 3.1 [15], the administration of either drugs or radiation causes cellular injury (mechanisms will be more completely addressed in the next section), the repair of which is unlikely to be complete. Depending on the severity of the initial injury (a function of radiation dose, drug type and dose) to the vital organ or tissue, residua of damage is present. This subclinical injury may not be recognized until the subsequent use of a seemingly safe dose of the other therapeutic mode. Thus, classically, when radiation therapy is administered first and causes subclinical injury (Figure 3.1a), treatment with drugs leads to its clinical expression. One of the best examples of this phenomenon was, in fact, one of the earliest appreciations of the interaction between radiation and chemotherapy. Children with Wilms' tumor treated with irradiation and then dactinomycin developed a so-called 'recall' skin reaction (Figure 3.2) and pneumonitis if the lungs had been treated [16]. The skin reaction appeared months after irradiation and only in the treatment field, was often worse than at the time of irradiation, and reappeared at the time of subsequent dactinomycin courses. It is unlikely that this clinical finding is actually a recall of radiation damage; it is more

likely added cell kill in the basal skin layer beyond that caused by irradiation [17]. Another example is the occurrence of liver failure in children with Wilms' tumor treated with hepatic irradiation in the setting of concomitant and subsequent dactinomycin and vincristine [18].

The manifestation of clinical following subclinical injury also occurs when radiation follows chemotherapy (Figure 3.1b). Moreover, recognized late effects can shift to a severe or life-threatening, if not fatal, level as in the case of radiation/dactinomycin pneumonitis [3], or severe proctitis or enteritis, and fatal small bowel obstruction in children treated for rhabdomyosarcoma with vincristine, dactinomycin, cyclophosphamide and doxorubicin followed by abdominal irradiation [19]. It is the current inability to detect morphological changes in a variety of tissues following administration of one therapeutic modality that has falsely given the impression that immediate cellular and ultrastructural changes are temporary and reversible. It is only when these treated tissues are challenged with additional therapy that the persistent residual defects are clinically demonstrated [20].

Efforts to both define and quantify the toxic effects of radiation and chemotherapy on normal tissues are long-standing. Organs and tissues in radiation oncology have been characterized in terms of their tolerance doses (TD 5/5 and TD 50/5 = the 5% and 50% likelihood of a complication 5 years after treatment). Doses below the TD 5/5 are considered to be 'safe doses' but are affected by the relative volume of the organ irradiated [15]. Thus, the concept of dose-volume histograms is helpful in weighing 'volume' in the prediction of a safe dose. This, however, assumes that no other competing modalities such as chemotherapy are used. Attempts at quantifying chemotherapeutic doses engendering injury are more recent and exist in terms of cumulative doses administered within a certain time period. Doxorubicin and carmustine are examples of drugs for which maximal accumulated dose levels are identified in terms of tolerance [21]. Quantifying the relative combined effects of irradiation and chemotherapy on normal tissue reactions has been performed in the laboratory according to a dose-effect factor (DEF) proposed by Phillips and Fu [1]. The enhancement as measured by this DEF is described by the formula:

$$DEF = \frac{\text{radiation dose for biological effect without drug}}{\text{radiation dose for biological effect with drug}}$$

As an example, mice undergoing unilateral nephrectomy, irradiation to the remaining kidney, and doxorubicin exhibit renal and body growth inhibition as well as renal functional disturbances. The dose of irradiation in the absence of doxorubicin

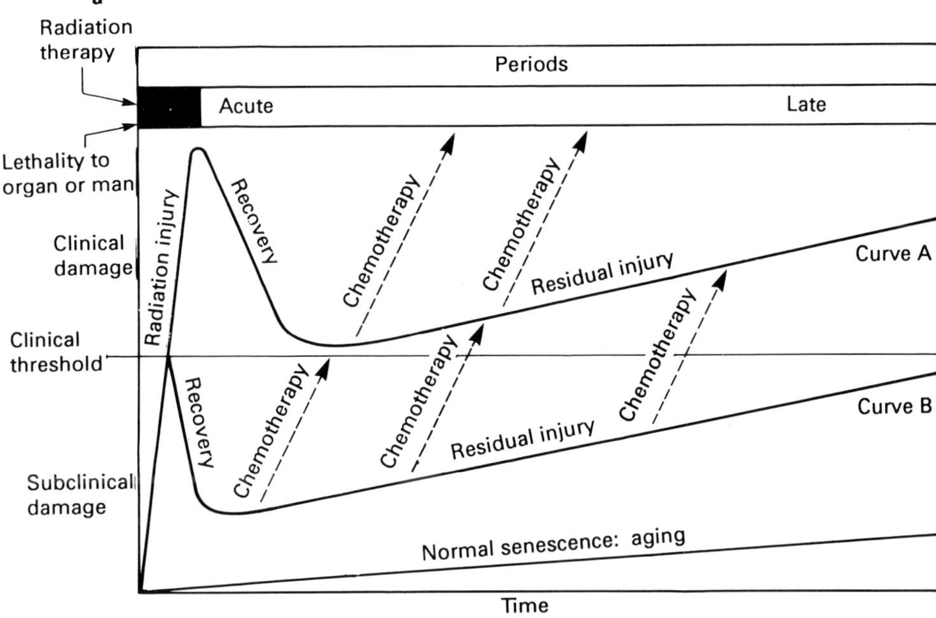


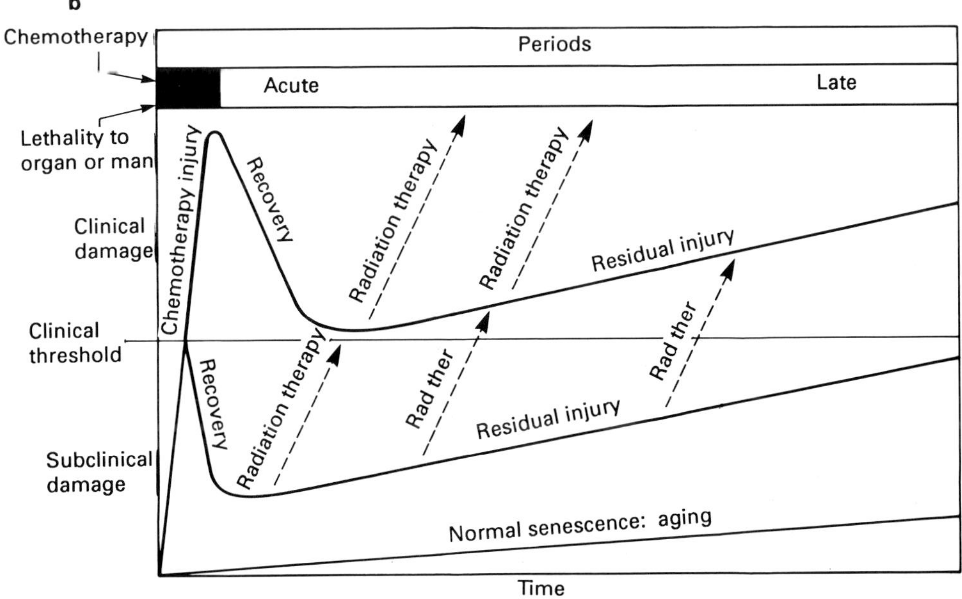


**Figure 3.1** Clinical pathological course of events **a** when radiation therapy precedes chemotherapy and **b** when chemotherapy precedes radiation therapy; –––––, complications (infection, trauma, stress) leading to clinical symptoms and signs. Reprinted with permission from ref. [15]

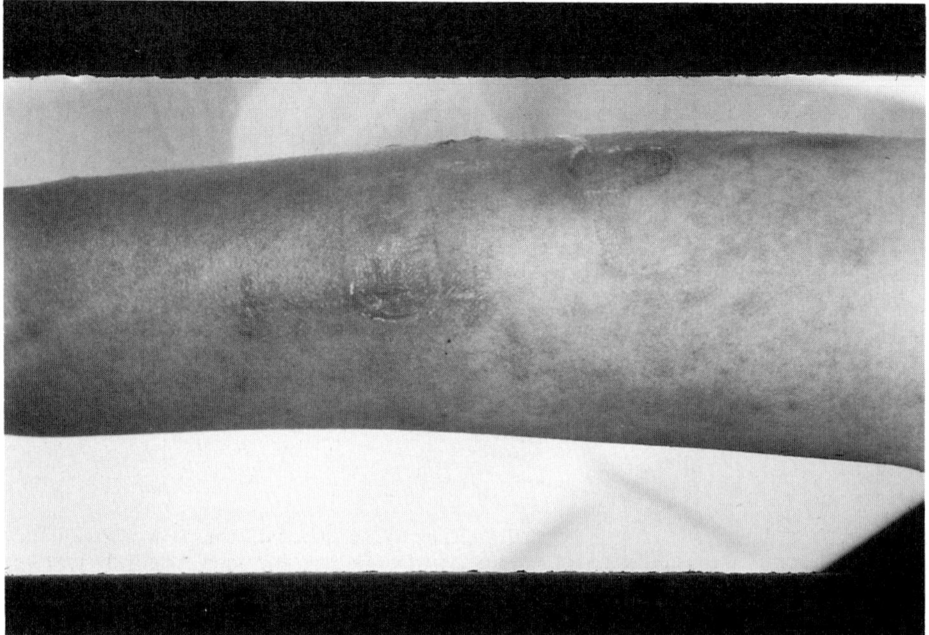

**Figure 3.2** Dactinomycin-induced 'recall' reaction in a 10-year-old boy treated with 45 Gy and combination chemotherapy (vincristine, cyclophosphamide and dactinomycin). One month following completion of irradiation, at a time when the associated skin erythema had resolved, dactinomycin was administered. Three days later a brisk erythema and small area of skin breakdown occurred, upon which dressings were placed. The edge of the radiation field can be seen on the proximal portion of the forearm (right of the photograph). Less intense reactions continued to occur following dactinomycin in subsequent months

causing the same effect was 33% greater, giving a DEF of 1.33 [22]. Such a formula can also be applied to clinical responsiveness, both for tumors and normal tissues. The renal disturbances described above have been encountered in children treated for Wilms' tumor [22a], although sufficient data to determine a DEF are not yet available. For tumors, a DEF >1 is desired; i.e., tumor cell kill will ideally be accomplished at a lower radiation dose in the presence of chemotherapy than in its absence. Conversely, for normal tissues, the lowest possible DEF is desired, certainly one that is lower than the DEF for tumors. It is this relative difference between the two DEFs which provides for a therapeutic gain – the combination of irradiation and drugs has a greater relative effect on the tumor compared with important normal tissues than when either modality is used alone. Although the DEF formula was specifically devised to address the effects of drugs on the radiation dose causing a particular event, a similar formula could be devised to address the alteration in drug dose occasioned by the use of irradiation. In considering the potential for a therapeutic gain from the addition of one mode to the other, it is important to remember that an increase in tumor cell kill is only of value if normal tissue dose limits are not simultaneously exceeded.

# Definitions relevant to chemotherapy/radiation interactions

Variables relevant to normal tissue reactions in general are listed in Table 3.1 and include patient, therapy and tumor factors (to be further discussed in a later section). An additional therapeutic variable specifically relevant to drug/radiation interactions is the relative timing of the administration of each mode. Several temporal strategies with different rationales are used [2]:

1. Simultaneous: radiation and chemotherapy are given concomitantly.
2. Adjuvant: chemotherapy follows definitive local irradiation.
3. Neoadjuvant: chemotherapy precedes definitive local irradiation.

**Table 3.1 Parameters which determine the effects of combined modality therapy**

Patient factors:
1. Underlying genetic predispositions, illnesses, structural abnormalities
2. Developmental status (age)
3. Inherent normal tissue sensitivites, repair capacities

Therapy factors:
1. Chemotherapeutic agent(s), dose, schedule, route
2. Radiation dose (total, fractional and rate), overall treatment time, treatment volume, dose distribution, machine energy
3. Sequencing of and time interval between chemotherapy and radiotherapy
4. Other biological response modifiers (e.g. sensitizers, protectors, immunotherapy)

Tumor factors:
1. Inherent tumor sensitivity, repair capacity
2. Direct effects on tissue (such as extent of invasion)
3. Indirect effects on tissues (such as chemical secretion, mechanical obstruction of a kidney, etc.)

4. Alternating: chemotherapy and radiation cycles are alternated ('ping-ponged', sandwiched, etc.).

A variety of possible interactions between the two modes can now be considered, the intent of which is to improve the therapeutic ratio [1,17,23,24].

1. Independent activity (spatial cooperation): each mode acts in isolation in different parts of the body – radiation locally eradicates the primary tumor while chemotherapy addresses occult disease beyond the local tumor volume. This spatial cooperation occurs without any intended interaction between the two modes. It is the most frequent rationale behind 'adjuvant' chemotherapy.
2. Increased activity: tumor cell kill is in excess of that which would be achieved by either mode alone, while normal tissue morbidities are not. Mechanisms for tumor cell kill can be the same or different, but for normal tissue toxicities should ideally be different for each mode so that no dose reduction of either is required. Included in this category are the following:
   (a) subadditive effects: tumor cell kill is greater than that seen with either mode alone but less than that expected from the combination;
   (b) additive effects: tumor cell kill is that expected from the strict addition of that which would result from each mode alone;
   (c) enhanced effects: true synergism (supra-additivity) has occurred with cell kill beyond that which would result from addition of the effects of each mode alone.

In practice it is often difficult to identify which of the above actions has transpired since specific dose-response curves for each treatment are not clearly known, i.e. both modes cause cell death and individual dose-effect curves are not linear [23]. It is, in fact, likely that true supra-additivity, for example, is a rare phenomenon.
3. Diminished activity: interference of the effects of one mode by the other has occurred such that tumor cell kill is less than that expected from either of the two modes alone. Included in this category are:

   (a) inhibition: the net effectiveness of the combination is somewhere between that of the lesser and more effective of the two modes;
   (b) antagonism: the net effectiveness of the combination is below that of the least active of the modes.

In the above scheme, true 'sensitization' and 'protection' are not included since these terms denote the effect of an otherwise inactive agent – that is, not a cytotoxic chemotherapeutic agent – on the biological effect of either of the therapeutic modes. Thus hypoxic cell sensitizers (nitroimidazoles) or oxic cell sensitizers (halogenated pyrimidines) which do not have independent cell kill capabilities are not considered. Similarly, chemicals that selectively protect normal tissues from injury (e.g. sulfhydryl compounds such as WR2721) are not included.

## Cellular basis for early and late tissue damage

Cell cycle kinetics, mitotic behavior, and differentiation underlie the chemo- and radiosensitivity of normal tissues. Thus the basis for determining the risks for normal tissue morbidity, both acute and chronic, is the action and interaction of chemotherapy and radiotherapy on the cells of these tissues. Tissue and organ dysfunction are the ultimate expression of this underlying cellular injury. The vitality of the organ and the severity of the damage determine the resulting clinical morbidity. The cellular characteristics which dispose a cell to injury by radiation are generally different from those relevant for drugs.

### *Chemotherapy*

Cell cycle kinetics and the relatively greater growth fraction of the population of cells in neoplasms as compared with most normal renewing tissues are considered in explaining the effects of chemotherapeutic agents. The killing effect of different drugs varies depending on whether they act during a specific phase of the cell cycle (cell cycle specific) or affect cells in the resting phase as well (cell cycle non-specific) [25]. The most vulnerable cells are actively cycling stem cells as compared with those in $G_0$ or prolonged $G_1$, which may escape the effects of S phase specific drugs. The tumor cell population with its relatively greater growth fraction and reduced repair capacity is more vulnerable than those normal tissues which have more quiescent cells with greater repair capabilities. Nevertheless, normal tissues, such as the bone marrow and gastrointestinal tract may be rapidly proliferating, and in this situation cell kill is expressed clinically as an acute injury. The slow renewal tissues with more post-mitotic, fully differentiated cells were previously thought to be relatively resistant to the effects of cytotoxic drugs and late adverse effects were thought not to occur in this setting. It is now known that drug action is so diverse that such assessments are inaccurate. For example, consider the effect of doxorubicin on mature myocytes in which ADP-stimulated respiration is reduced and oxidative phosphorylation is inhibited, thereby decreasing mitochondrial ATPase activity of cardiac mitochondria [26]. It is clear that cell injury may occur, depending on the chemotherapeutic agent, at different levels of cell cycle activity or cell differentiation. The expression of this injury may not be frank cell death but instead a depletion of stem cell reserve, i.e. the loss of their normal mitotic potential. This concept is illustrated by studies on the reduction in the regenerative capacity of bone marrow hematopoietic progenitor cells following

cytotoxic therapy [27]. A set of events can thus be pictured which describes the competition between cellular repopulation and depletion following chemotherapy (Figure 3.3). In most multidrug regimens, the number of normal tissue cells is progressively reduced as the induction, consolidation and maintenance phases of regimens are completed. As an increasing number of stem cells are killed, first reversible and then irreversible injury occurs.

## Radiotherapy

The sequential changes in normal tissues following irradiation are also based upon the mitotic behaviour of the cell and its state of differentiation [15]. The dividing cell is more vulnerable to irradiation than the quiescent cell, particularly if functionally mature. Except for the small lymphocyte, radiation cell death is mitotically linked, occurring only when the cell divides. The development of radiation injury in any given tissue is thus based on its cell renewal characteristics (Figure 3.4). The parenchymal cell compartments of various tissues are predominantly either rapidly or slowly renewing. Rapid renewal tissues tend to have stem cells that rapidly proliferate and differentiate. Conversely, the functional cell has completed this process and is rarely capable of further mitotic activity. Slow renewal tissues are characterized by a parenchymal cell compartment that turns over slowly but often has the capacity, when challenged by injury, to dedifferentiate and proliferate [28], i.e. a mature appearing parenchymal cell may revert to

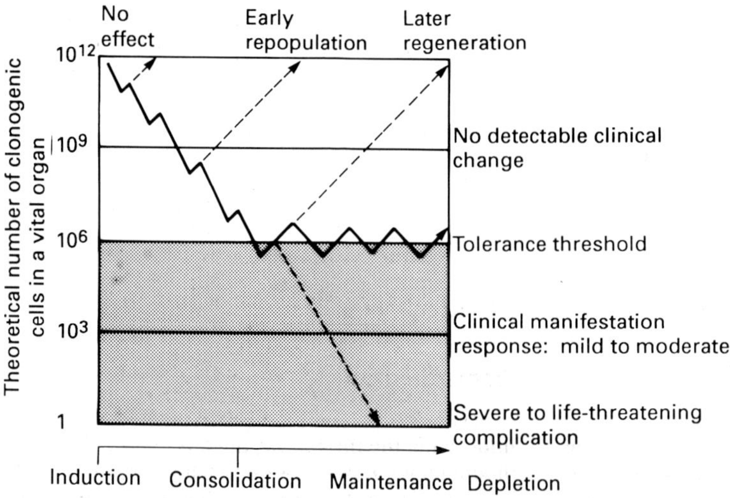


**Figure 3.3** Diagrammatic presentation of the reduction of normal tissue cells. Reprinted with permission from ref. [32]

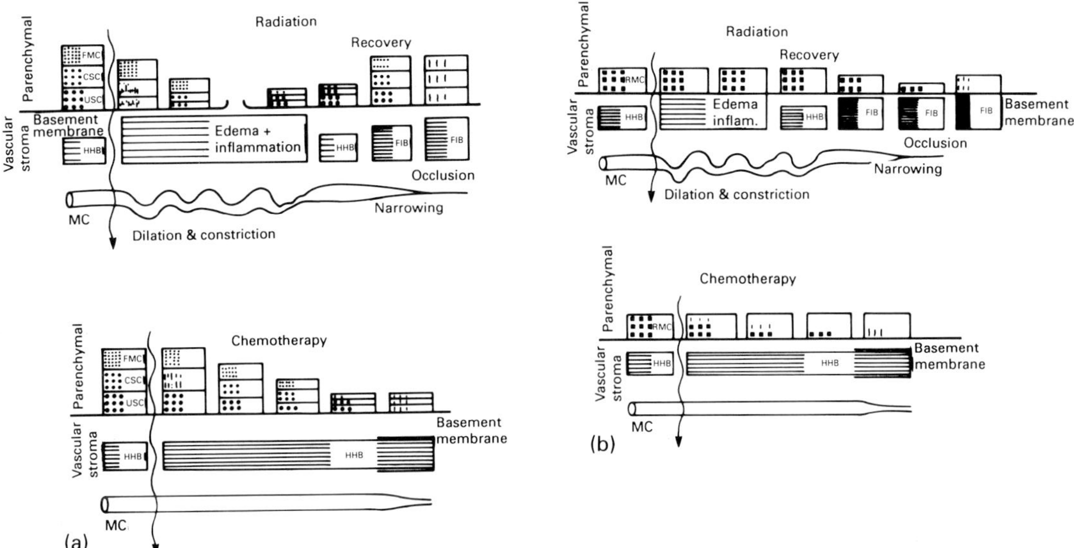



**Figure 3.4** Kinetics or sequence of cell changes following exposure to radiation or drugs in **a** a rapid renewal system and **b** a slow renewal system. FMC, fixed mitotic cells; CSC, committed stem cells; USC, uncommitted stem cells; HHB, histochematic barrier; FIB, increased fibrosis; MC, micro-circulation; RMC, reverting mature cells. Reprinted with permission from ref. [15].

a stem cell and repopulate the lost parenchymal cells. However, many organs have little capacity in this regard.

The acute and late effects of radiotherapy on normal tissues are explained in terms of these concepts. Acute local effects result from parenchymal cell hypoplasia, usually in the epithelial linings such as mucous membranes. It is not inactivation of functional cells but rather an impairment in regeneration of clonogenic stem cells in sufficient numbers which accounts for the acute reactions to radiotherapy [29]. Typical early-reacting tissues include the gastrointestinal tract, skin and bone marrow. When the radiation dose which exceeds the threshold for damage has been delivered, the time to expression of this damage is dependent on the rate of cell turnover and not additional dose. The chronic damage which occurs is based on both inactivity of functional (committed) parenchymal cells and the impairment of their replacement over time. Moreover, beyond the ability of any tissue to recover due to parenchymal cell replacement is the progressive damage which results from injury of the underlying vasculature [30–32]. This arterio-capillary fibrosis predominates in the late irreparable injury and accentuates the cellular depletion of the parenchyma. In late-reacting tissues (e.g. brain,

heart, kidney) the latent period to the expression of injury is dose-dependent, progressively decreasing with higher doses.

It is the vascular changes that follow irradiation, but not chemotherapy, which partially account for the differences in the late effects of the two modes of treatment. The distribution of late radiation damage reflects vascular injury primarily and cannot be explained simply as an indirect effect of parenchymal cell loss resulting in underlying vascular injury. It is this vascular injury which accounts for the devastating late effects of radiation in either rapidly or slowly proliferating normal tissues when there has been no clinically recognizable acute phase.

## Combined chemotherapy and radiotherapy

Again, the obvious goals of combining the modes is to enhance the tumor response for the same level of normal tissue toxicity, or to reduce toxicity without compromising tumor response. The mechanisms underlying the interaction are less clear than for the independent action of each. As suggested by Phillips [17] and Fu [33], several possible mechanisms which result in an enhanced effect can be identified (Table 3.2). Although they are primarily directed towards

**Table 3.2 Mechanisms by which chemotherapy and radiotherapy might interact. Modified from Phillips [17]**

Physiological:
1. Improved drug delivery after irradiation
2. Altered pharmacokinetics after irradiation
3. Reoxygenation of cells following chemotherapy
4. Decreased cell–cell interaction enhancing cell sensitivity

Cell kinetics:
1. Recruitment of quiescent cells into a proliferative phase
2. Redistribution of cells into a sensitive phase

Cell survival/repair
1. Modification of the slope of the dose-response curve
2. Inhibition of repair or decreased accumulation of sublethal damage
3. Inhibition of recovery from potentially lethal damage

explaining effects on tumor cells, they can be extended to normal tissues in several instances.

Physiological mechanisms primarily relate to increasing tissue drug concentration and exposure time, and to the physical environment of cells. It is likely that radiation increases blood flow to both the tumor (particularly after shrinkage) and normal tissues in some instances, thereby improving drug distribution and concentration [34]. The hypoxic cell fraction may also decrease with improved blood flow, partially as a result of reoxygenation of previously hypoxic cells [35]. As tumor bulk decreases after treatment with one modality, responsiveness to the other may increase [36]. Explanations include those mentioned above as well as a possible increase in cell sensitivity resulting from alterations in cell–cell interactions as cell numbers decrease [17]. Changes in drug pharmacokinetics with an increase in delivery or uptake may also occur, such as the penetration of systemically administered methotrexate into the central nervous system after irradiation [37]. Alterations in drug metabolism resulting from enzyme induction, for example, are speculative.

A change in cell kinetics effected by one mode can influence the sensitivity to the other. Following irradiation, cells are recruited from a quiescent to a proliferative phase and the cycling time may also be decreased [38]. An increased sensitivity to cell cycle specific drugs would be expected. Radiotherapy and chemotherapy can each synchronize cells from tumors and normal tissues into a common cycling sequence, thereby increasing the sensitivity to a modality which preferentially kills cells in a particular cell cycle phase. For example, hydroxyurea causes a transitory block at the $G_1/S$ phase. If radiation is then delivered at a proper interval as cells emerge from this block, increased cell death

would be expected [39]. This strategy has been used clinically [40].

Although cell survival and repair characteristics following irradiation have been extensively described, little is known about them following individual chemotherapeutic agents [2]. Information is available on the effects of drugs on radiation dose-response curves (comprehensive reviews by Fu [33], Steel [41] and Kelland and Steel [42]). For example, DNA intercalators such as dactinomycin and cisplatin can increase the steepness of such curves [43–45], and this presumably is an explanation for the enhanced effect of these drug–radiation combinations in tumors and normal tissues [46,47]. Another mechanism by which drugs can enhance a radiation effect is through an alteration in the repair capabilities of cells. In fact, this is exceedingly difficult to determine [48]. Drug inhibition of the repair of radiation damage is most easily conceived as (or determined by demonstrating) a progressive increase in the DEF as the number of radiation fractions increases. Dactinomycin and cisplatin have this capacity [49,50], while doxorubicin appears to decrease the amount of damage a cell can sustain before dying [51,52], thereby enhancing the radiation effect in normal tissues [53]. Recent data also suggest that both bleomycin and ifosfamide may produce greater than additive effects, at least on tumor cells [54–56].

The complexity of the interactions is nicely illustrated by studies on the alteration in hematopoietic reserve which is seen following combined drugs and irradiation. Kovacs has assessed the effects of different chemotherapeutic agents on the acute, delayed and residual effects on hematopoietic stem cells (HSC). Doxorubicin was shown to affect the more primitive HSC subpopulations, resulting in enhanced radiosensitivity of the marrow both immediately and progressively over prolonged (and perhaps permanent) intervals. 5-Fluorouracil and cyclophosphamide were more selectively harmful to the mature HSC and resulted in a more acute enhancement of marrow radiosensitivity. Cyclophosphamide, in addition, produced a prolonged stromal effect resulting in a second, though transient, interval of enhanced radiosensitivity. Taken together, the data showed that drugs have selective specificity for different hematopoietic cell subpopulations, and that these sensitivities determine the temporal consequences of drug treatment on subsequent radiation tolerance of the marrow. The drugs that influence long-term radiation tolerance do so in a dose-dependent manner and initially affect the more primitive stem cells. Thus the initial drug-induced lesion in the stem cell compartment, resulting in long-term sensitization to radiation damage involves a major restriction (either in cell number or intrinsic proliferative potential) of the capacity for recovery from subsequent radiation insult [57].

Ideally dose-response curves for both chemotherapeutic agents and irradiation could be constructed, providing a means for quantitating the effect of one mode on the other, both in terms of cell survival and repair capabilities. As previously stated, formulations of this nature for drugs are lacking. However, they do exist in the radiation biology literature. When multiple radiation doses are administered, producing a certain injury, a dose-response curve is constructed based on the assumption that each radiation fraction produces a similar biological effect. The resulting curves derived from a number of normal tissues closely fit a linear quadratic equation of the form [2,48,58]:

$$\text{effect} = \alpha D + \beta D^2$$

The two types of injury described by this equation include one that is proportional to dose ($D$) and thus irreparable, and one that is proportional to the square of the dose and has some capacity for repair. This model is of value in predicting the effects of fractionated irradiation on normal tissues. The $\alpha/\beta$ ratio is substantially higher for late reacting tissues than early reacting tissues. Perhaps the best method currently to determine drug-induced changes in survival curve shape which also reflect underlying changes in repair capacity, is to determine how drugs change this $\alpha/\beta$ ratio. As shown in Figures 3.5a and b, the effect of drugs on the value of this ratio for late reacting tissues provides information on the modification of important radiation effects by chemotherapeutic agents.

# Parameters determining the effects of combined modality therapy on normal tissues and tumors

The likelihood of an acute or chronic effect will depend on an interplay of patient, therapy and tumor factors (Table 3.1) [59]. Patient factors primarily relate to the underlying 'health' of the normal tissues, i.e. the absence of inherent abnormalities, and to the cellular activity and maturation of the target tissue exposed to the therapeutic modes. In children, different tissues develop at different rates and in different temporal sequences, making it more difficult to discern sensitivities to cytotoxic therapy [60]. For example, the brain is most sensitive during its rapid growth phase in the first 3 years of life, while the skeleton is most sensitive both in these early postnatal years and to a lesser degree during puberty, and the gonads just before and during puberty. Thus the vulnerability of

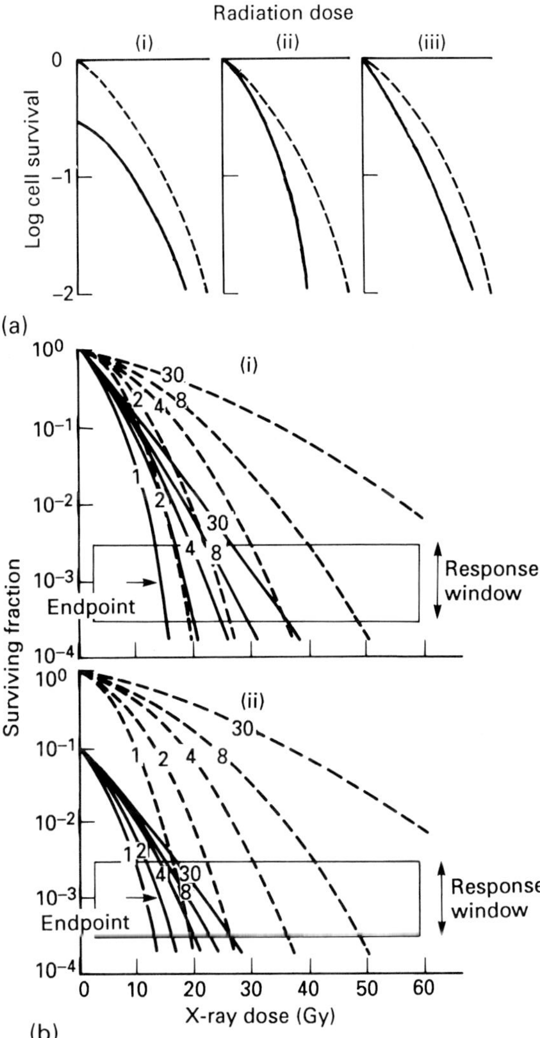

Figure 3.5 a Possible modification of linear quadratic dose-response curve by various forms of interaction between radiotherapy and chemotherapy acting on normal tissue: (i) independent cell killing, no change in dose-response curve; (ii) radiosensitization, predominantly increase in final slope; (iii) inhibition of repair of sublethal damage, mainly reduction of shoulder. Reprinted with permission from ref. [2]. b Survival curves for radiation alone (- - - - -) and radiation + drug (—) calculated using an $\alpha/\beta$ value of 2 Gy and 10 Gy respectively: (i) no drug killing; (ii) killing by drug alone by factor of 10. Reprinted with permission from ref. [48]

these tissues to therapy is increased during the periods of rapid proliferation, whereas in adults these same tissues may be more resistant since they are in a mature steady state with slow cell renewal kinetics.

As discussed in Chapters 1 and 2, tolerance doses for normal tissues to chemotherapy alone or radiotherapy alone are reasonably well established. Tissues vulnerable to the effects of either are also those most susceptible to the effects of the combined modes. Depending on the tissue, and the target cells for injury in that tissue, adverse effects from the combination may be seen at therapeutic doses which might otherwise be 'safe'. The mechanisms for injury in this setting are not always known, despite the previous discussion in this chapter as to the possibilities. In fact, more than one mechanism may be relevant. For example, cyclophosphamide and bladder irradiation can cause cystitis at doses which would independently be clinically tolerable; in this case, the effects are presumed to be additive and the target cells for damage the same [61]. Doxorubicin and irradiation injure different target cells in the heart. When clinically tolerable doses of each are administered, the overall damage caused by the combination may surpass the compensatory ability of the heart [62]. Dactinomycin and pulmonary irradiation cause pneumonitis at otherwise tolerable radiation doses; since dactinomycin alone is unassociated with pneumonitis, it is likely that the threshold for radiation damage to the important target cell(s) (the type II pneumocyte and the endothelial cell) has been lowered by dactinomycin [63].

Therapy factors are essentially the drug and radiation characteristics which influence the likelihood of an adverse event. Although laboratory and clinical data supporting this exist for each mode alone, the influence of a particular therapeutic parameter of one mode on the other has been systematically studied only in the laboratory, as will be illustrated. Nevertheless, clinical experience supports the importance of these therapeutic factors on the consequences of the modes as they interact. Some drugs (dactinomycin and doxorubicin) appear to place all tissues at risk for enhanced toxicity from irradiation [64], while others appear to be more selective (e.g. the nitrosoureas for skin and gut [65,66]). Drugs which are cell cycle or phase dependent (e.g. methotrexate, 5-fluorouracil) primarily place rapidly proliferating tissues at risk. For most drugs, the tissue at greatest risk is the tissue for which each mode has independent toxicity, e.g. bleomycin and lung, cyclophosphamide and bladder.

Not only is increasing drug dose associated with increasing toxicity, but the duration and route of administration is relevant. Some drugs are most effective when given intravenously while others may be effectively administered orally. A long continuous exposure through a continuous intravenous infusion is optimal for some drugs in some settings, while a single intense exposure or a pulsatile exposure is most appropriate for the same drug in other settings or for other drugs. The toxicities vary accordingly, which in turn affect those seen after combined therapy. Fu has documented this effect in the laboratory for cisplatin and continuous low-dose rate irradiation. A continuous cisplatin infusion was associated with a supra-additive effect in contrast to an additive effect with bolus injection [67]. An example of the relevance of the route and duration of drug exposure in the clinic is shown by doxorubicin, where a prolonged intravenous infusion rather than bolus injection appears to reduce cardiac toxicity while maintaining antitumor activity [68].

Radiation dose and fraction size are related to the likelihood of an adverse effect, as discussed previously. Dose rate is yet another important factor. As the dose rate is lowered and the exposure time extended, the biological effect of a given dose is generally reduced [69]. This effect is a consequence of the increase in repair of sublethal damage that occurs during the longer exposure. Yet the effects of drugs on the repair of radiation damage is relatively greater at these low dose rates as compared with high dose rates, presumably because drugs which inhibit the repair of radiation damage have a greater opportunity to express this effect at the lower dose rates (or more prolonged period of dose administration). Sherman has demonstrated this effect in mice treated with doxorubicin and thoracic irradiation, using pulmonary and oroesophageal toxicity as the end points. In this setting the DEF was greater at a low dose rate (5 cGy/min) than at a higher rate (70 cGy/min). Despite this relative effect, the total radiation dose causing a particular level of injury was lower at the higher dose rate because of the importance of radiation dose rate, independent of the drug, in causing normal tissue injury [70]. Among patients treated with varying preparatory regimens for bone marrow transplantation, the dose rate clearly influenced the frequency and severity of pulmonary toxicity [71].

The importance of the volume of tissue irradiated in the occurrence of radiation injury has recently been reviewed by Rubin [72]. The destruction of a certain volume may or may not be tolerated, depending on the ability of the affected organ to compensate through regeneration or hypertrophy and thereby remain functional, though impaired. For example, high doses to small portions of the liver may be tolerated, whereas fatal hepatitis and cirrhosis are seen at the same dose level to larger volumes [73]. Recognition of this relationship has led to an increasing use of dose-volume histograms. The technique of irradiation determines the distribution of dose within the target tissue which in turn determines the likelihood of a complication. In the early years of treating Hodgkin's disease, weighted mantle techniques deposited excessive doses within the heart, increasing the frequency of myopathy

[74]. Clearly, all of these radiation parameters will influence the results of any drug–irradiation interactions.

The sequence and timing of drug and irradiation administration influences the frequency and intensity of toxicity. Steel has recently summarized a large volume of animal data on this point [41]. In general, when the modes are administered concurrently, deleterious normal tissue effects are most severe. The intensity decreases with greater intervals between the modes. This relationship is reasonably clear for acute reacting tissues such as the intestinal mucosa. Yet there is insufficient information to clearly determine the relevance of timing to chronic effects. If drugs are administered at a time when adverse effects due to radiation are just developing in some tissues, then interactions may occur which might not be seen if the drug had been given prior to this time. For example when the lung, due to the kinetics of cell repopulation in this organ, is experiencing its greatest irradiation-associated injury (around 100 days), treatment with certain chemotherapeutic agents such as cyclophosphamide may enhance the level of injury to a greater degree than if the drug had been administered at the time of irradiation [75]. This phenomenon has been rather euphemistically termed the 'recall' reaction when observed clinically [76].

Experimental data also exist on the relative difference in the biological effectiveness of administering a drug at the same time interval before as compared with after irradiation, with different degrees of apparent toxicity [77]. Yarnold has recently presented clinical data on patients with advanced testicular non-seminoma in which the gastrointestinal complications and subcutaneous fibrosis observed were dependent on the sequence and timing of drugs and irradiation [78]. When drugs and irradiation were administered in close proximity, complications were pronounced. The most severe hematopoietic damage occurred when drugs were given after irradiation to large volumes. Another example is provided by the experience from several clinical trials on the treatment of small cell lung cancer. When chemotherapy and radiotherapy are administered concomitantly, fatal pulmonary toxicity has a 25% incidence and esophageal stricture is encountered in 70% of patients. The incidence of life-threatening complications was less than 5% in patients treated by chemotherapy alone or by sequential or alternating chemotherapy and radiotherapy [79–81]. It appears that for most tissues therapy-related toxicity is greater when radiation is given prior to chemotherapy as compared with the opposite sequence, but exceptions exist and more information is needed.

Tumor factors relevant to the expression of normal tissue damage are suggested in Table 3.1 and are not appropriate for detailed discussion in this chapter. Yet some generalizations are of note. Certainly normal tissue effects can only be considered in the background of the goal of controlling the tumor. Devising the most effective combination of drugs and irradiation towards this end is accomplished only through improving therapeutic gain, which involves minimizing normal tissue effects. An obvious starting point is to select drugs which are independently active against the tumor but do not have overlapping toxicities with radiation on the critical normal tissues within the irradiated volume. This is complicated by the drug–radiation interactions which have been the subject of this chapter, and by recognition of the steepness of the dose-response curves for normal tissue toxicity as compared with tumor tissue. In general, a small increase in drug or radiation dose will have a relatively greater likelihood of increasing normal tissue toxicity than in controlling tumor, underscoring the importance of selecting agents whose toxicities are not overlapping (drug–drug or drug–radiation). The temporal sequencing of drugs and radiation is also relevant by virtue of the lack of evidence demonstrating an increased tumoricidal effect from concurrent administration of these modes, in contrast to sequential administration [82]. This suggests that optimizing the therapeutic ratio should at least include considerations for the sequential administration of chemotherapeutic agents which do not overlap in terms of their toxicity, and in terms of their interactions with radiotherapy. At a minimum, the radiation therapy technique (dose, volume, normal tissues treated) should be designed with a clear view of the potential interactions.

With a greater understanding of the interactions between chemotherapeutic agents and radiation therapy will come insights into enhancing the antitumor effects while minimizing normal tissue injury.

## References


1. Phillips, T. and Fu, K. The interaction of drug and radiation effects on normal tissues. *International Journal of Radiation Oncology, Biology, Physics*, **4**, 59–64 (1978)
2. Howes, A. Keynote address: Models of normal tissue injury following combined modality therapy. *National Cancer Institute Monograph*, **6**, 5–6 (1988)
3. Wara, W., Phillips, T., Margolis, L. and Smith, V. Radiation pneumonitis: a new approach to the derivation of time-dose factors. *Cancer*, **32**, 547–552 (1973)
4. Boal, D., Newburger, P. and Teele, R. Esophagitis induced by combined radiation and Adriamycin. *American Journal of Radiology*, **132**, 567–570 (1979)
5. Hoppe, R., Portlock, C., Glatstein, E. and Rosenberg, S. Alternating chemotherapy and irradiation in

the treatment of advanced Hodgkin's disease. *Cancer*, **43**, 472–481 (1979)

6. Coleman, C., Williams, C., Flint, A. *et al.* Hematologic neoplasia in patients treated for Hodgkin's disease. *New England Journal of Medicine*, **297**, 1249–1252 (1977)

7. Trask, C., Joannides, T., Harper, P. *et al.* Radiation-induced lung fibrosis after treatment of small cell carcinoma of the lung with very high-dose cyclophosphamide. *Cancer*, **55**, 57–60 (1985)

8. Von Hoff, D., Loyard, W., Basa, P. *et al.* Risk factors for doxorubicin-induced congestive heart failure. *Annals of Internal Medicine*, **91**, 710–717 (1979)

9. Brugieres, L., Hartmann, O., Travagli, J. *et al.* Hemorrhagic cystitis following high-dose chemotherapy and bone marrow transplantation in children with malignancies: incidence, clinical course, and outcome. *Journal of Clinical Oncology*, **7**, 194–199 (1989)

10. Bleyer, W. and Griffin, T. White matter necrosis, microangiopathy and intellectual abilities in survivors of childhood leukemia. Association with central nervous system irradiation and methotrexate therapy. In *Radiation Damage to the Nervous System* (eds H. Gilbert and A. Kagan), Raven Press, New York, pp. 155–174 (1980)

11. Kun, L. and Camitta, B. Hepatopathy following irradiation and Adriamycin. *Cancer*, **42**, 81–84 (1978)

12. Peters, L. and Ang, K. Unconventional fractionation schemes in radiotherapy. In *Important Advances in Oncology* (eds V. DeVita, S. Hellman and S. Rosenberg), J.B. Lippincott, Philadelphia, pp. 269–286 (1986)

13. Brady, L. (ed.). Long-term normal tissue effects of cancer treatment. *Cancer Clinical Trials*, **4**(Suppl. 7), 9–71 (1981)

14. Rubin, P. Radiation toxicology: quantitative radiation pathology for predicting effects. *Cancer*, **39** (Suppl. 2), 729–736 (1977)

15. Rubin, P. and Casarett, G. *Clinical Radiation Pathology*, Vols I and II, W.B. Saunders, Philadelphia (1968)

16. D'Angio, G., Farber, S. and Maddock, C. Potentiation of X-ray effects by actinomycin D. *Radiology*, **73**, 175–177 (1959)

17. Phillips, T. Tissue toxicity of radiation–drug interactions. In *Radiation–Drug Interactions in the Treatment of Cancer* (eds G. Sokol and R. Maickel), John Wiley and Sons, New York, pp. 175–200 (1980)

18. Jones, B., Brewslow, N. and Takashima, J. Toxic deaths in the second National Wilms' Tumor Study. *Journal of Clinical Oncology*, **2**, 1028–1033 (1984)

19. Ransom, J., Novak, R., Kumar, A. *et al.* Delayed gastrointestinal complications after combined modality therapy of childhood rhabdomyosarcoma. *International Journal of Radiation Oncology, Biology, Physics*, **5**, 1275–1279 (1979)

20. Rubin, P., Constine, L. and Van Ess, J. Special lecture: Scoring of late toxic effects – interaction of two modalities. *National Cancer Institute Monograph*, **6**, 9–18 (1988)

21. Creaven, P. and Mihich, E. The clinical toxicity of anti-cancer drugs and its prediction. *Seminars in Oncology*, **4**, 147–163 (1977)

22. Donaldson, S., Moskowitz, P., Canty, E. and Fajardo, L. Combination radiation–Adriamycin therapy: renoprival growth, functional and structural effects in the immature mouse. *International Journal of Radiation Oncology, Biology, Physics*, **6**, 851–859 (1980)

22a. Mitus, A., Tefft, M. and Fellers, F. Long-term follow-up of 108 children who underwent nephrectomy for malignant disease. *Pediatrics*, **44**, 912–921 (1969)

23. Steel, G. and Peckham, J. Exploitable mechanisms in combined radiotherapy–chemotherapy: the concept of additivity. *International Journal of Radiation Oncology, Biology, Physics*, **5**, 85–91 (1979)

24. Kun, L. and Moulder, J. General principles of radiation therapy. In *Principles and Practice of Pediatric Oncology* (eds P. Pizzo and D. Poplack), J.B. Lippincott, Philadelphia, pp. 233–262 (1988)

25. Valariote, F. and Edelstein, M. The role of cell kinetics in cancer chemotherapy. *Seminars in Oncology*, **4**, 217–226 (1977)

26. Bianchi, C., Bagnato, A. Paggi, M. and Floridi, A. Effect of Adriamycin on electron transport on rat, heart, liver and tumor mitochondria. *Experimental Molecular Pathology*, **48**, 123–135 (1987)

27. Botnik, L., Hannon, E. and Hellman, S. Late effects of cytotoxic agents on the normal tissue of mice. *Frontiers of Radiation Therapy and Oncology*, **13**, 36–47 (1979)

28. Wheldon, T., Michalowski, A. and Kirk, J. The effect of radiation on function in self renewing normal tissues with differing proliferative organisation. *British Journal of Radiology*, **55**, 759–764 (1982)

29. Trott, K-L. Radiation–chemotherapy interactions. *International Journal of Radiation Oncology, Biology, Physics*, **12**, 1409–1413 (1986)

30. Casarett, G. Aging. *Frontiers of Radiation Therapy and Oncology*, **6**, 479–485 (1972)

31. Hopewell, J. The importance of vascular damage in the development of late radiation effects in normal tissues. In *Radiation Biology in Cancer Research* (eds R. Meyn and H. Withers), Raven Press, New York, pp. 449–456 (1980)

32. Rubin, P. The Franz Buschke Lecture: Late effects of chemotherapy and radiation therapy: a new hypothesis. *International Journal of Radiation Oncology, Biology, Physics*, **10**, 5–34 (1984)

33. Fu, K. Biological basis for the interaction of chemotherapeutic agents and radiation therapy. *Cancer*, **55**, 2123–2130 (1985)

34. Brown, J. Drug or radiation changes to the host which would affect the outcome of combined modality therapy. *International Journal of Radiation Oncology, Biology, Physics*, **5**, 1151–1163 (1979)

35. Stanley, J., Shipley, W. and Steel, G. Influence of tumor size on hypoxic fraction and therapeutic sensi-

tivity of Lewis lung tumor. *British Journal of Cancer,* **36**, 105–113 (1977)

36. Siemann, D. Tumour size: a factor influencing the isoeffect analysis of tumour response to combined modalities. *British Journal of Cancer,* **41** (Suppl. IV), 294–298 (1980)

37. Griffen, T., Rasey, J. and Bleyer, W. The effect of photon irradiation on blood–brain barrier permeability to methotrexate in mice. *Cancer,* **40**, 1109–1111 (1977)

38. Hermens, A. and Barendsen, G. The proliferative status and clonogenic capacity of tumor cells in a transplantable rhabdomyosarcoma of the rat before and after irradiatiaon with 800 rad of X-ray. *Cell and Tissue Kinetics,* **11**, 83–100 (1978)

39. Banjamin, I., Xynos, F. and Rana, M. Effects of Adriamycin and hydroxyurea on human squamous cell carcinoma of cervix transplanted into nude mice. *Federation Proceedings,* **38**, 1319 (1979)

40. Hreshchyshyn, M., Aron, B., Boronow, R. *et al.* Hydroxyurea or placebo combined with radiation to treat stage IIIB and IV cervical cancer confined to the pelvis. *International Journal of Radiation Oncology, Biology, Physics,* **5**, 317–322 (1979)

41. Steel, G. The search for therapeutic gain in the combination of radiotherapy and chemotherapy. *Radiotherapy and Oncology,* **11**, 31–53 (1988)

42. Kelland, L. and Steel, G. Inhibition of recovery from damage induced by ionizing radiation in mammalian cells. *Radiotherapy and Oncology,* **13**, 285–299 (1988)

43. Bases, R. Modification of the radiation response determined by single cell techniques: Actinomycin D. *Cancer Research,* **19**, 1223–1229 (1959)

44. Dewit, L. Combined treatment of radiation and *cis*-diaminedichloroplatinum (II): a review of experimental and clinical data. *International Journal of Radiation Oncology, Biology, Physics,* **13**, 403–426 (1987)

45. Douple, E. and Richmond, R. Platinum complexes as radiosensitizers of hypoxic mammalian cells. *British Journal of Cancer,* **37** (Suppl.), 98–102 (1978)

46. D'Angio, G. Clinical and biological studies of actinomycin D and roentgen irradiation. *American Journal of Roentgenology,* **87**, 106–109 (1962)

47. Haselow, R., Adams, G., Oken, M. *et al.* Cis-platinum (DDP) with radiation therapy (RT) for locally advanced unresectable head and neck cancer. *Proceedings of the American Society of Clinical Oncology,* **2**, 160 (1983)

48. Begg, A. Additivity versus repair inhibition in fractionated treatments combining drugs and X-rays: a theoretical analysis. *International Journal of Radiation Oncology, Biology, Physics,* **13**, 921–929 (1987)

49. Elkind, M., Whitmore, B. and Alescio, T. Actinomycin D: suppression of recovery in X-irradiated mammalian cells. *Science,* **143**, 1454–1457 (1964)

50. Dritschilo, A., Piro, A. and Belli, J. Interaction between radiation and drug damage in mammalian cells: III. The effect of Adriamycin and actinomycin-D on the repair of potentially lethal radiation damage. *International Journal of Radiation Biology,* **35**, 549–560 (1979)

51. Tannock, I. Response of aerobic and hypoxic cells in a solid tumor to Adriamycin and cyclophosphamide and interaction of the drugs with radiation. *Cancer Research,* **42**, 4921–4926 (1982)

52. Belli, J. and Piro, A. The interaction between radiation and Adriamycin damage in mammalian cells. *Cancer Research,* **37**, 1624–1630 (1977)

53. Aristizabal, S., Manning, M., Miller, R. *et al.* Combined radiation–Adriamycin effect on human skin. *Frontiers of Radiation Therapy and Oncology,* **13**, 103–112 (1979)

54. Wu, D., Zhang, Y., Keng, P. *et al.* The interaction between bleomycin and radiation on cell survival and DNA damage in mammalian cell cultures. *International Journal of Radiation Oncology, Biology, Physics,* **11**, 2125–2131 (1985)

55. Tonkin, K., Kelland, L. and Steel, G. Chemotherapy-radiation interactions in human cervix carcinoma xenografts. *Br. J. Cancer,* **58**, 738–741 (1988)

56. Nicoll, J. Radiatiaon reaction enhanced by ifosfamide. *British Journal of Radiology,* **59**, 1039–1041 (1986)

57. Kovacs, C., Evans, M., Hooker, J. and Johnke, R. Long-term consequences of chemotherapeutic agents on hematopoiesis: development of altered radiation tolerance. *National Cancer Institute Monograph,* **6**, 45–49 (1988)

58. Thames, H., Jr., Withers, H., Peters, L. and Fletcher, G. Changes in early and late radiation responses with altered dose fractionation: Implications for dose-survival relationships. *International Journal of Radiation Oncology, Biology, Physics,* **8**, 219–226 (1982)

59. Jones, G. and Laukkanen, E. Tolerance revisited. *International Journal of Radiation Oncology, Biology, Physics,* **13**, 290–291 (1986)

60. Rubin, P., Van Houtte, P. and Constine, L. Radiation sensitivity and organ tolerances in pediatric oncology: a new hypothesis. *Frontiers of Radiation Therapy and Oncology,* **16**, 62–82

61. Phillips, T. and Fu, K. The interaction of drug and radiation effects on normal tissues. *International Journal of Radiation Oncology, Biology, Physics,* **4**, 59–64 (1978)

62. Eltringham, J., Fajardo, L. and Stewart, J. Adriamycin cardiomyopathy: enhanced cardiac damage in rabbits with combined drug and cardiac irradiation. *Radiology,* **115**, 471–472 (1975)

63. Steel, G., Adams, K. and Peckham, J. Lung damage in C57B1 mice following thoracic irradiation: enhancement by chemotherapy. *British Journal of Radiology,* **52**, 741–747 (1979)

64. Phillips, T. and Fu, K. Quantification of combined radiation therapy and chemotherapy effects on critical normal tissues. *Cancer,* **37**, 1186–1200 (1976)

65. Goldstein, L., Ross, G. and Phillips, T. The interaction of irradiation and BCNU in intestinal crypt cells. *International Journal of Radiation Oncology, Biology, Physics,* **5**, 1569–1571 (1979)

66. Lelieveld, P., Brown, J., Goffinet, D. *et al*. The effect of BCNU on mouse skin and spinal cord in single drug and radiation exposures. *International Journal of Radiation Oncology, Biology, Physics*, **5**, 1565–1568 (1979)

67. Fu, K., Lam, K. and Rayner, P. The influence of time sequence of *cis*-platinum administration and continuous low dose rate irradiation (CLDRI) on their combined effects on a murine squamous cell carcinoma. *International Journal of Radiation Oncology, Biology, Physics*, **11**, 2119–2124 (1985)

68. Legha, S., Benjamin, R., MacKay, B. *et al*. Reduction of doxorubicin cardiotoxicity by prolonged continuous intravenous infusion. *Annals of Internal Medicine*, **96**, 133–139 (1982)

69. Hall, E. *Radiobiology for the Radiologist*, 3rd edn, J.B. Lippincott, Philadelphia, pp. 107–136 (1988)

70. Sherman, D., Carabell, S., Belli, J. and Hellman, S. The effect of dose rate and adriamycin on the tolerance of thoracic radiation in mice. *International Journal of Radiation Oncology, Biology, Physics*, **8**, 45–51 (1982)

71. Clark, J., Schwartz, D., Flournoy, N. *et al*. Risk factors for airflow obstruction in recipients of bone marrow transplants. *Annals of Internal Medicine*, **107**, 648–656 (1987)

72. Rubin, P. Tolerance doses and volumes: the biology and pathophysiologic basis for radiation oncology dose/time/volume prescription. In *Syllabus: a Categorical Course in Radiation Therapy: Cure with Preservation of Function and Aesthetics* (ed. J. Wilson), Radiologic Society of North America, Illinois, pp. 93–102 (1988)

73. Austin-Seymour, M., Chen, G., Castro, J. *et al*. Dose volume histogram analysis of liver radiation tolerance. *International Journal of Radiation Oncology, Biology, Physics*, **12**, 31–35 (1986)

74. Applefeld, M.M. The late appearance of chronic pericardial disease in patients treated by radiotherapy for Hodgkin's disease. *Annals of Internal Medicine*, **94**, 338–341 (1984)

75. Collis, C. and Steel, G. Lung damage in mice from cyclophosphamide and thoracic irradiation: the effect of timing. *International Journal of Radiation Oncology, Biology, Physics*, **9**, 685–689 (1983)

76. Donaldson, S., Glick, J. and Wilbur, J. Adriamycin activating a recall phenomenon after radiation therapy. *Annals of Internal Medicine*, **81**, 407–408 (1974)

77. Phillips, T., Wharam, M. and Margolis, L. Modification of radiation injury to normal tissues by chemotherapeutic agents. *Cancer*, **35**, 1678–1684 (1975)

78. Yarnold, J., Horwich, A. and Duchesne, G. *et al*. Chemotherapy and radiotherapy for advanced testicular non-seminoma. 1. The influence of sequence and timing of drugs and radiation on the appearance of normal tissue damage. *Radiotherapy and Oncology* **1**, 91–99 (1983)

79. Tubiana, M. The 1987 Franz Buschke Lecture: the role of radiotherapy in the treatment of chemosensitive tumors. *International Journal of Radiation Oncology, Biology, Physics*, **16**, 763–774 (1989)

80. Brooks, B., Seifter, E., Walsh, T. *et al*. Pulmonary toxicity with combined modality therapy for limited stage small-cell lung cancer. *Journal of Clinical Oncology*, **4**, 200–209 (1986)

81. Arriagada, R., LeChevalier, T., Baldeyrou, P. *et al*. Alternating radiotherapy and chemotherapy schedules in small cell lung cancer, limited disease. *International Journal of Radiation Oncology, Biology, Physics*, **11**, 1461–1468 (1985)

82. Steel, G. Terminology of clinical combined radiotherapy–chemotherapy. *Radiotherapy and Oncology*, **14**, 315–316 (1989)

# 4

# Carcinogenic and genotoxic effects of antineoplastic agents

S. Venitt

Diseases desperate grown,
By desperate appliances are reliev'd,
Or not at all

The purpose of this chapter is to summarize the evidence for the mutagenicity and carcinogenicity of a range of agents used in the treatment of cancer. Space does not allow consideration of all agents in clinical use; instead, emphasis will be placed on classes of agent for which there are enough data to illuminate general principles and explore mechanisms. Although reference will be made to second tumours in patients treated with antineoplastic agents, this topic is covered in greater depth elsewhere in this volume and in references [1 8]. Effects on fertility and human germ cell mutation are considered in ref. [1] and Chapter 8. Connors [9] has reviewed the chemistry, metabolism and mutagenicity of individual antineoplastic drugs in relation to their carcinogenicity. Details of the mechanism of action of antitumour drugs are available in numerous texts [10–15]. Critical reviews of the carcinogenic and mutagenic properties of antitumour drugs are available in reference [1] and in monographs published by the International Agency for Research on Cancer (IARC) [16,17].

## Classifying agents as carcinogens

### Human data

The criteria adopted by IARC for classifying agents or exposures as carcinogenic to humans are summarized in Table 4.1. Of 51 agents or exposures for which there is unequivocal evidence for carcinogenicity in humans and which include smoking tobacco, smokeless tobacco and alcohol consumption, 11 are antineoplastic drugs or drug combinations [17,18]. Ionizing radiation brings the total to 12. Of 37 agents which are probably carcinogenic to humans, seven are antineoplastic drugs [17].

### Animal data

Although there are more physiological, biochemical and metabolic similarities between humans and other animals than there are differences, these may be critical in interpreting results of long-term carcinogenicity assays. Pharmacokinetics, metabolism and DNA repair capacity may differ between organs and tissues within the same species and between species. Laboratory animals (usually mice and rats) are highly inbred or are $F_1$ hybrids between inbred strains and may be unusually sensitive or resistant to the carcinogenic effects of a given chemical. Most human populations are outbred and individuals show great variability in their response to drugs and other xenobiotics. Numbers of animals used in long-term experiments are small compared with human populations likely to be exposed to a given substance. Therefore test substances (industrial chemicals, food and feed additives, cosmetics and other consumer products) are administered to animals, usually by feeding, at doses close to those which evince signs of toxicity, such as weight loss or tissue damage. Choice of an appropriate route of administration is often problematical, since human exposure is likely to be at low levels over long periods of time, conditions difficult or impossible to emulate in small rodents. High doses may overwhelm the normal metabolic and repair capacity of the species under test. These problems may be of lesser importance when testing antitumour drugs since most are given at high doses by

"

### Cell transformation

Strictly speaking, transformation of mammalian cells in culture is not a measure of genotoxicity since the mechanism by which it occurs is not known to be directly linked to genetic effects. Phenotypic alterations considered to be related to neoplastic transformation include altered morphology, focus formation on cell monolayers, indefinite lifespan ('immortalization'), growth in agar and altered growth on plastic surfaces. These are detected in cultured mammalian cells, either cell lines or early passage cultures from embryos.

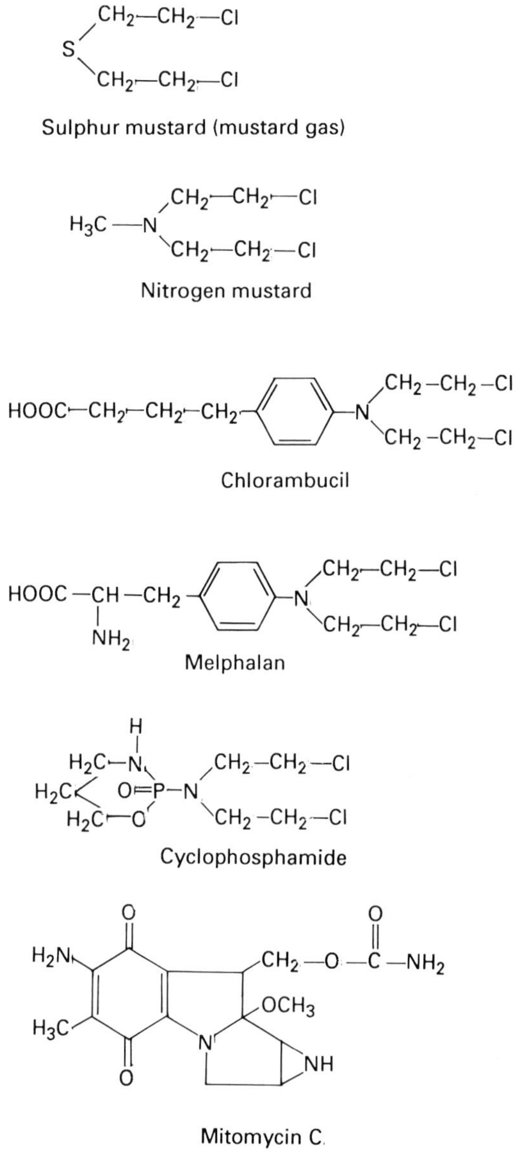

## Carcinogenicity and genotoxicity of antitumour agents

Table 4.1 summarizes the carcinogenicity and genotoxicity of major classes of drugs classified as carcinogenic or genotoxic by criteria adopted by IARC Working Groups [17].

### Alkylating agents

Table 4.1 reveals that of the 18 alkylating antitumour drugs listed, 11 are carcinogenic to animals and for four more there is limited evidence of carcinogenicity. All the drugs for which data are available possess genotoxic activity *in vivo* (several producing chromosomal anomalies in patients) or *in vitro*. Busulphan, chlorambucil, chlornaphazine, cyclophosphamide, melphalan, treosulphan and semustine are human carcinogens, whilst carmustine, lomustine, thiotepa and streptozotocin are probably carcinogenic to humans.

A common mechanism – the ability to react with DNA – determines both the antitumour properties of alkylating agents and their carcinogenicity and genotoxicity. The first chemical shown to be mutagenic was the alkylating agent mustard gas [41] (Figure 4.1), which was used as a chemical weapon in the 1914–1918 war. Soldiers killed by mustard gas were found to have very little bone marrow, whilst survivors showed marked leukopenia [42]. These findings stimulated research into chemical treatments for leukaemia, resulting in the development of nitrogen mustard which was first used in a patient in 1941. Cyclophosphamide (Figure 4.1), a pro-drug of *nor*-nitrogen mustard, was one of the first successful 'designer drugs' developed as a chemically and pharmacologically inactive transport form which became therapeutically active *in vivo* [43]. In 1960, Brookes and Lawley [44] demonstrated that mustard gas alkylated the N-7 position of guanine *in vitro* and nucleic acids of mice treated *in vivo*. Further studies showed that compounds with a single alkylating function ('monofunctional') tend to

**Figure 4.1** Chemical structure of alkylating agents

be both mutagenic and carcinogenic, whereas potent cytotoxic activity is associated only with those compounds which are difunctional or polyfunctional [31,45–47]. This supported the idea that the twin strands of the DNA helix could be cross-linked, thus preventing DNA replication. Such a mechanism would explain the extraordinary cytotoxicity of compounds such as mustard gas. Another line of evidence for cross-linking was target size. A DNA molecule appeared to be the only molecule large enough to sustain critical damage at the very low doses of mustard gas which inhibit DNA replication. At these doses RNA and protein synthesis are virtually unaffected [48]. Chemical and biophysical evidence for DNA cross-linking by a variety of cytotoxic di- and polyfunctional alkylating agents is now available [46,49].

As well as forming interstrand and intrastrand cross-links, these agents also form mono-adducts with DNA. It is likely that the mutagenic and carcinogenic properties of difunctional alkylating agents arise mainly from monofunctional alkylation of critical sites in DNA and that the balance between difunctional and monofunctional alkylation probably determines the mutagenic and carcinogenic potency of difunctional agents. A cell whose DNA contains pro-mutagenic mono-adducts but which cannot replicate its DNA because it is cross-linked is unable to produce mutant daughter cells. This explains the difficulty in demonstrating the mutagenicity of difunctional agents in mutant strains of bacteria which cannot excise DNA cross-links [50] and may account for the fact that multiple applications of low doses of these agents are often required to yield significant numbers of tumours in experimental animals [45].

Alkylating agents acquire electrons during chemical reactions and are said to be 'electrophilic', binding covalently to 'nucleophilic' atoms such as oxygen, nitrogen and sulphur which donate electrons. DNA is rich in nucleophilic centres by virtue of its high content of nitrogenous bases. Alkylating agents are archetypal carcinogens, inducing point mutation, chromosomal aberrations and neoplasia [31,45]. They can bind covalently to DNA at at least 20 different positions, depending, *inter alia*, on the nature of the agent, its reactivity and the stereochemistry and nucleophilicity of the particular DNA atom involved [31,34,45,51]. Of particular relevance to mutation and carcinogenesis is alkylation of DNA bases at atoms which participate in Watson–Crick base-pairing, the mechanism which ensures complementarity between opposite strands of the twin helix and accurate replication of the genetic code. Modification of base-pairing sites, for example by alkylation of the O-6 position of guanine or the O-4 position of thymine, may result in miscoding during DNA replication. For example, O-6-guanine will mis-pair with thymine instead of its correct complementary partner cytosine. At the next round of replication the strand containing thymine instead of cytosine will pair correctly with adenine, an error or mutation which will be perpetuated in succeeding cell generations. This is known as 'base-pair substitution' and is an example of how alkylating agents induce point mutations. The triplet code is changed so that one amino acid is substituted by another, resulting in a changed protein, or, by creation of a

chain-terminating triplet, a protein which is truncated. 'Frame-shift' mutation occurs by addition or deletion of bases during replication of adducted or intercalated DNA. This changes the reading frame of the genetic code, causing errors in the amino acid sequences of gene products. Base-pair substitution is characteristic of alkylating agents, whereas frame-shift mutation is typical of intercalating agents such as doxorubicin.

Mutation is not a passive event; in most cases enzymes involved in DNA repair or DNA processing intervene to convert 'pro-mutagenic lesions' such as DNA adducts into forms which can be expressed as mutations in daughter cells. The role of error-free and error-prone repair in mutagenesis and carcinogenesis has been reviewed by Friedberg [33].

The importance of point mutation in human cancer is illustrated by the discovery of a range of mutations of this type in activated transforming oncogenes (e.g. H-*ras*, N-*ras* and K-*ras*) from a variety of human tumours [24].

In addition to direct miscoding, alkylation of DNA leads to DNA strand breakage and chromosomal damage. Difunctional alkylating agents used in cancer chemotherapy are potent clastogens, suggesting that their carcinogenic properties may be attributable to chromosomal deletions and rearrangements as well as to point mutations. Single-strand DNA breaks following alkylation can occur by two mechanisms. In the first, alkylation of phosphate groups in the DNA backbone results in formation of phosphotriesters which may hydrolyse, resulting in a discontinuity in the affected strand. In the second, alkylation of DNA bases results in chemical or enzymatic loss of bases which leave holes – 'apurinic sites' (AP) – which are subsequently cleaved by specific AP-endonucleases, resulting in single-strand breaks [33,51].

Compounds like mustard gas, nitrogen mustard and nitrogen mustard analogues such as chlorambucil and melphalan (Figure 4.1) are intrinsically reactive, forming covalent bonds with pure DNA in solution or with cellular DNA in patients, and are thus 'directly-acting'. Other antitumour agents such as the nitrosoureas carmustine, lomustine and semustine release alkylating and carbamoylating moieties upon contact with aqueous media, whilst others, such as cyclophosphamide, dacarbazine and procarbazine are 'indirectly-acting', requiring metabolic activation by host tissues to release alkylating metabolites.

Mitomycin C (Figure 4.1) is a naturally occurring DNA cross-linking alkylating agent [52]. It alkylates DNA following reduction by enzymes, chemical reducing agents or mild acid. Metabolically reduced mitomycin C reacts with DNA to form an N-2-guanine mono-adduct which accounts for 90% of DNA alkylation. A bis-adduct is also formed which bridges the N-2 atoms of each of a pair of guanine moieties [53]. $^{32}$P-post-labelling revealed ten different DNA adducts in a variety of tissues of rats after injection of mitomycin C [54]. One adduct accounted for about 71% of the total. All adducts were chromatographically identical to those formed by the reaction of chemically reduced mitomycin C with DNA *in vitro*, demonstrating mitomycin C is activated by reduction. Adducts formed *in vivo* were predominantly monofunctional guanine derivatives (>90%), plus adenine, cytosine and thymine products. Thus, as in the case of difunctional alkylating agents of the nitrogen mustard family, mitomycin C reacts with DNA to yield both mono- and bis-adducts, the former predominating in amount and variety.

As well as modifying DNA by adduct formation, mitomycin C produces single-strand DNA breaks via free radicals, a property shared with several other natural products used as antitumour agents such as doxorubicin and bleomycin, but not associated with classical alkylating agents which induce single-strand breaks by phosphotriester formation or depurination.

Free radicals are atoms or molecules which contain an unpaired electron, and which seek out another electron to attain a more stable and less reactive state. Mitomycin C generates free radicals, such as the hydroxyl radical, by reaction of hydrogen peroxide with cellular iron complexed with protein or ATP [51]. The hydroxyl radical is the most reactive oxygen radical encountered in biological systems, degrading any molecule within diffusion distance, and is considered to be the ultimate species responsible for damaging DNA [51,55–59].

Mitomycin C is genotoxic. It induces mutation in bacteria, fungi and green plants; chromosomal aberrations and mutations in insects; specific locus mutations in mice; chromosomal aberrations in cultured human peripheral lymphocytes [60] and point mutations in cultured mammalian cells [61], chromosome aberrations in embryos from pregnant

mice treated *in vivo* [62], and micronuclei in lymphocytes of fetal mice and maternal bone marrow of mice treated in pregnancy [64]. Elevated levels of SCE were found in the peripheral lymphocytes from cancer patients treated with mitomycin C [65].

Mitomycin C is carcinogenic to animals, inducing sarcomas at the injection site in mice, peritoneal sarcomas in rats after intraperitoneal injection, and tumours at a variety of sites in rats following intravenous injection [60]. There are no data on the carcinogenicity of mitomycin C to humans, but in view of its potent genotoxicity and its carcinogenicity to animals, it should be regarded as a potential human carcinogen.

## Types of cancer caused by alkylating agents

Carcinogenicity tests in animals are useful for determining whether a given agent is carcinogenic *per se*, but can they predict the sites of tumours induced in patients? Table 4.2 compares the types of tumours induced by some of these drugs in laboratory animals with those found in patients and reveals a reasonable concordance between animal experiments and human data.

The commonest neoplasms resulting from treatment of patients with difunctional alkylating agents are rapidly fatal acute leukaemias [2]. It has been argued [66] that cancer caused by alkylating agents could represent a future public health problem of a size comparable to that of cancer caused by occupational exposure. For example, up to 75% of the 20 000 new cases of Hodgkin's disease which occur each year in Europe and North America may be treated with carcinogenic alkylating agents. Taking a conservative estimate of 5% incidence of acute leukaemia 10 years after treatment, there would be 750 new cases of rapidly fatal iatrogenic leukaemia per annual cohort [66].

Studies of patients treated with melphalan have consistently shown very large excesses of acute non-lymphocytic leukaemia in the decade following treatment. The relative risk of this malignancy was estimated to be in excess of 100; it increased with increasing dose and was not influenced to any extent by radiotherapy [17]. Cyclophosphamide appears to be less leukaemogenic than melphalan. For example, Greene *et al.* [67] found that women receiving melphalan for ovarian cancer were 2–3 times more likely to develop leukaemia than those treated with cyclophosphamide.

Squamous carcinoma of the skin accounts for about 5–10% of malignancies induced by cyclophosphamide or nitrogen mustard. The only other neoplasms which are consistently associated with alkylating agents are erythroleukaemias and lung tumours [2,4].

**Table 4.2 Principal sites of tumours induced by antitumour alkylating agents in laboratory animals and in patients. Compiled from data in ref. [17]**

| Agent | Laboratory animals | Patients |
|---|---|---|
| Busulphan | Leukaemia, lymphoma | Acute leukaemia |
| Chlorambucil | Lung; leukaemia, lymphoma | Lung; acute leukaemia |
| Cyclophosphamide | Bladder | Bladder; acute leukaemia |
| Melphalan | Lung; lymphoma | Acute leukaemia |
| Nitrogen mustard | Lung; lymphoma | Acute leukaemia(?) |

In 119 patients with rheumatoid arthritis treated with cyclophosphamide and 119 matched arthritics who were not so treated, 37 malignancies were detected in 29 cyclophosphamide-treated patients, compared with 16 malignancies in 16 controls ($P < 0.05$) during a mean follow-up of >11 years. Significant excesses of bladder cancer, haematological malignancies and skin cancer were also seen. The rate of development of malignancy in the cyclophosphamide-treated patients was significantly greater than in the control patients at 6 years following drug initiation, and this increased rate persisted even at 13 years [68].

As well as the direct carcinogenic effect exerted by alkylating agents, it has been suggested that immune suppression may play a part in the development of second cancers after cytotoxic chemotherapy. Activation of oncogenic viruses such as the Epstein–Barr virus (EBV) in immunosuppressed patients is another possibility. For example, treatment with alkylating agents of peripheral blood lymphocytes from healthy people or from patients with acquired immunodeficiency syndrome (AIDS) enhanced EBV transformation of these cells to immortalized lymphoblastoid cell lines. This was accompanied by alterations in the physical structure, organization and expression of the EBV genome [69].

## Reducing the risk of iatrogenic cancer

The usefulness of laboratory experiments in improving chemotherapy is illustrated by studies of the reduction by 2-mercaptoethane sulphonate ('mesna') of the carcinogenicity of cyclophosphamide to the rat bladder [70]. Cyclophosphamide is metabolized in the liver to aldophosphamide which decomposes spontaneously to yield reactive phosphoramide mustard and acrolein, believed to cause the acute haemorrhagic cystitis which can be a dose-limiting complication after high-dose cyclophosphamide therapy. Mesna prevents this by combining with cyclophosphamide metabolites in the urine. Petru and Schmähl [70] proposed that since the organ-specific carcinogenicity of cyclophosphamide is the same in rats as it is in humans, its carcinogenicity to the bladder could be prevented by mesna. They found that administration of cyclophosphamide with mesna reduced the cyclophosphamide-induced bladder tumours by a factor of 19. Mesna had no protective effect against other cyclophosphamide-induced tumours (nervous tissue, haematopoietic and lymphatic), confirming its specificity to the bladder. The authors suggest that treatment of patients with mesna may well protect them from developing bladder cancer following cyclophosphamide therapy. The same may also be true of other oxazaphosphorines such as ifosfamide

[43]. Prevention of acute toxicity to the bladder has allowed the use of higher doses of cyclophosphamide [43]. However, whilst it may protect humans from bladder cancer in the same way that it protects rats, there is nothing to suggest that mesna will protect the human bone marrow from cyclophosphamide-induced malignancy. In view of the positive link between cyclophosphamide dose and acute leukaemias [68] the use of the uroprotective agent mesna may well turn out to be a two-edged sword.

Another approach to reducing iatrogenic malignancy is to choose the drug which is the least carcinogenic when two or more drugs of equal therapeutic benefit are available. For example, using cyclophosphamide instead of melphalan may reduce the risk of acute leukaemia in women treated for ovarian cancer [67].

Further evidence for differences in leukaemogenic potency between different drugs has been presented by Kaldor *et al.* [71]. In an international collaborative study, these authors found 114 cases of leukaemia following ovarian cancer. The risk of leukaemia was greatest 4 or 5 years after chemotherapy began and was elevated for at least 8 years after its cessation. The relative risk for chemotherapy alone was 12 (4.4–32, 95% confidence interval). Cyclophosphamide, chlorambucil, melphalan, thiotepa and treosulfan, and the combination of doxorubicin and cisplatin, were independently associated with increased leukaemia risks. Chlorambucil and melphalan were the most potent leukaemogens, followed by thiotepa. Cyclophosphamide and treosulfan were weakest, the effect per gram of drug being substantially lower at high doses than at lower doses.

## Platinum compounds

Cisplatin (Figure 4.2), the first platinum antitumour drug, was discovered accidentally by Barnett Rosenberg, a biophysicist interested in the effects of electric fields on bacterial growth [72]. Using platinum electrodes and medium containing ammonium chloride he noticed that an alternating field caused the bacteria to form filaments. This was found to be due to formation of neutral platinum(II) and platinum(IV) salts, of which cisplatin (*cis*-diamminedichloroplatinum(II)) was one. Cisplatin induces filamentation and prophage production in lysogenic bacteria, phenomena characteristic of ultraviolet irradiation, X-irradiation and cytotoxic alkylating agents and indicative of DNA damage. Filamentation and formation of giant cells is caused by selective inhibition of DNA replication in cells which continue to synthesize RNA and protein. Therefore, cisplatin was tested for antitumour activity in animals and found to be active against a

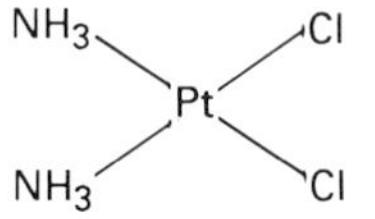

**Figure 4.2** Chemical structure of platinum agents

variety of tumours. Cisplatin entered phase I clinical trials in 1971–72 and is now established as an important drug, especially in the treatment of testicular and ovarian cancer.

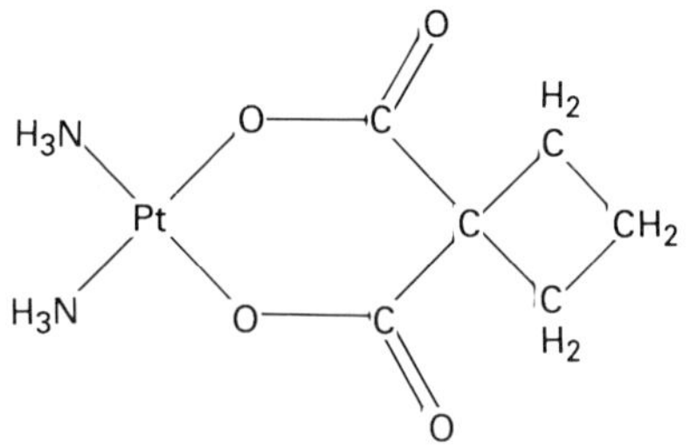

It was noted early on that antitumour activity was seen only in platinum salts which were difunctional and in which both reactive groups were on the same side of the square planar molecule (i.e. in the *cis* configuration) [72]. Moreover, *cis*-platinum(II) compounds were found to be markedly more mutagenic than *trans* isomers, on the basis of dose or of DNA binding [73]. Subsequent work has confirmed that the cytotoxic and antitumour activity of cisplatin results from its reaction with DNA [49,73]. Cisplatin reacts with DNA (or nucleophilic sites in other molecules such as proteins) only after one or more chloride ligands are replaced by water producing, at neutrality, positively charged aquo species which are electrophilic and reactive. The major reaction products are intrastrand cross-links between adjacent guanine residues on the same strand; interstrand cross-links between guanine residues on opposite strands are also formed, but to a much lower extent [74]. Reactions at a variety of other sites in DNA also occur [34]. These would be expected to promote point mutations by mechanisms similar to those associated with alkylating agents.

It is not surprising, therefore, that cisplatin is genotoxic. It induces DNA damage and point mutation in bacteria and fungi; point mutation and chromosomal damage in plants; aneuploidy and mutations in the fruit-fly; chromosomal aberrations, micronuclei and SCE in cultured rodent and human cells; transformation of Syrian hamster cells; structural chromosomal aberrations and SCE in rodents treated *in vivo*. Patients receiving cisplatin had cisplatin adducts in DNA and elevated levels of SCE in peripheral lymphocytes [29]. DNA adducts were present in tumour biopsies from patients treated with cisplatin or carboplatin [73].

Cisplatin is carcinogenic. Multiple intraperitoneal injections increased the incidence of lung adenomas in mice, and with the addition of the promoting agent croton oil to the skin, the incidence of skin papillomas. Cisplatin induced leukaemias when given as multiple intraperitoneal injections to rats [17]. Although there are case reports of tumours in patients treated with combination chemotherapy which included cisplatin, the clinical data are insufficient to classify cisplatin as a human carcinogen. However, it is categorized as 'probably carcinogenic to humans' because it is carcinogenic to animals, it is a potent genotoxin and because its pattern of genotoxic activity closely resembles that of difunctional alkylating agents, many of which are human carcinogens.

Although cisplatin is a useful drug, it is extremely toxic. This has led to a search for platinum compounds which are less toxic but possess antitumour activity at least equivalent to cisplatin. The most widely studied candidate is carboplatin which has now entered clinical use.

Carboplatin (Figure 4.2) possesses a single bidentate cyclobutane dicarboxylic acid ('CBDCA') ligand instead of the two *cis*-chloro ligands present in cisplatin. This makes carboplatin considerably less reactive with DNA than cisplatin, because the CBDCA moiety is more resistant to aquation than are the *cis*-chlorine atoms in cisplatin [74]. Extensive comparative studies of cisplatin and carboplatin in a variety of systems led Knox *et al.* [74] to conclude that equal binding of the two drugs to DNA *in vivo* results in equal toxicity; a much larger dose (20–40 times the cisplatin dose) of carboplatin is required to produce this level of DNA binding. However, once bound to DNA in equal amounts, cisplatin and carboplatin cause equal levels of difunctional DNA lesions, interstrand cross-links and cytotoxicity. The large differences in doses required to produce these effects are accounted for by the much faster aquation rate of cisplatin. It was argued that dissimilarity in antitumour effects between the two drugs was more likely to be due to differences in pharmacokinetics than to mechanistic differences between the two compounds at the molecular level. Although these studies addressed the cytotoxic and antitumour effects of these two drugs, this interpretation of the results may well hold good when considering the potential carcinogenicity of carboplatin.

There are no data on which to judge the carcinogenic potential of carboplatin in man or in experimental animals (Table 4.1). However, the evidence that carboplatin is genotoxic is sufficient to predict that this drug should be carcinogenic. Carboplatin induces mutation and DNA repair in bacteria, but to a significantly lower extent than cisplatin at equivalent doses [75]. Carboplatin induced dose-related increases in micronuclei and SCE in cultured Chinese hamster cells. On the basis of dose cisplatin was six times more potent in producing micronuclei and three times more potent in inducing SCE than carboplatin [76]. That carboplatin is markedly less clastogenic than cisplatin was confirmed in *in vitro* experiments with human peripheral lymphocytes which showed that carboplatin induced about the same frequency of SCE at 1 µg per ml as cisplatin did at 0.05 µg per ml. Carboplatin also produced a variety of chromosomal aberrations, again requiring higher doses than cisplatin to produce equivalent levels of aberrations. Elevated levels of SCE and chromosomal aberrations were observed in peripheral lymphocytes obtained from five patients who had received a single dose of carboplatin. In a patient followed for several weeks, the frequency of SCE returned to pretreatment levels 5 weeks after treatment [77].

Clearly, dose for dose, carboplatin is far less genotoxic than cisplatin, suggesting that if carboplatin were proved to be a carcinogen it would be less potent than cisplatin. Taking into account the overriding importance of DNA binding as the critical determinant of cytotoxicity [74], it is reasonable to argue that once bound to DNA in equal amounts both cisplatin and carboplatin might be equally carcinogenic.

## Intercalating agents

### *Doxorubicin and daunorubicin*

Doxorubicin and its close homologue daunorubicin (Figure 4.3) – archetypal anthracycline antibiotics – show a broad spectrum of antitumour activity and are widely used in cancer chemotherapy. Although there is little evidence on which to judge the carcinogenicity of doxorubicin to humans, there is sufficient evidence that this drug causes cancer in animals. In several independent experiments, doxorubicin produced mammary tumours following single intravenous injections to rats. Single or repeated subcutaneous injection caused local sarcomas and mammary tumours. Intravesicular instillation of doxorubicin in rats produced a low incidence of papillomas and enhanced the incidence of bladder tumours induced by a carcinogenic *N*-nitrosamine [17,60]. Single intravenous injections of doxorubicin into male and female rats, or repeated injections over 2 weeks, induced multiple mammary tumours

in females at significantly higher rates than in untreated animals. Mammary tumours were also seen in male rats treated with doxorubicin. Renal cell tumours were found in rats of the single-dose groups. Dysplastic foci in renal tubular epithelium occurred in the groups given single or repeated doses of doxorubicin. This study confirms that doxorubicin induces mammary neoplasms in rats and strongly suggests that systemic treatment may cause urothelial malignancy [78].

Daunomycin shows a similar pattern of carcinogenicity to animals, causing local sarcomas in mice following subcutaneous injection, and mammary and urothelial tumours in rats treated intravenously [60].

Doxorubicin is genotoxic; it causes chromosomal aberrations, SCE and DNA strand breaks in cells of treated patients. It is consistently positive at a variety of end points, including chromosomal aberrations, SCE and DNA damage in rodents treated *in vivo*, and in human and rodent cells treated *in vitro*. It induces point mutations in cultured rodent cells, in fungi and in bacteria and transmissible mutations in *Drosophila melanogaster* [29]. The evidence for the genotoxicity of daunorubicin is less extensive than for doxorubicin, but is sufficient to classify it as a broad-spectrum genotoxin [60,79,80]. Thus, doxorubicin and daunorubicin carry the stigmata of genotoxic carcinogens, and should be regarded as human carcinogens in the absence of evidence to the contrary.

Most of the work on the mode of action of doxorubicin has concentrated on its antineoplastic properties [81,82]. As in the case of alkylating and platinating agents, the carcinogenic and genotoxic activity of doxorubicin probably depends on one or more of the mechanisms which have been proposed for its cytotoxic effects. Three proposals have been made to explain the mode of action of doxorubicin: metabolic reduction and free radical formation; DNA intercalation; effects on membranes [81].

### *Metabolic reduction and free radical formation*

Metabolic reduction of doxorubicin to its semiquinone can occur via several enzymes, including xanthine oxidase, P450-reductase and NADH dehydrogenase. The semiquinone can react with oxygen to form superoxide radicals, which dismutate spontaneously or enzymatically (via superoxide dismutase) to hydrogen peroxide, which reacts with a variety of substrates, such as cellular Fe(II), to form the destructive hydroxyl radical which can induce DNA strand breaks [58,59,81]. As well as reduction by this one-electron mechanism, doxorubicin undergoes enzymatic two-electron reduction to its dihydroquinone via xanthine oxidase or ferridoxin reductase. Under anoxic conditions the dihydroquinone (and semiquinone) can rearrange and lose

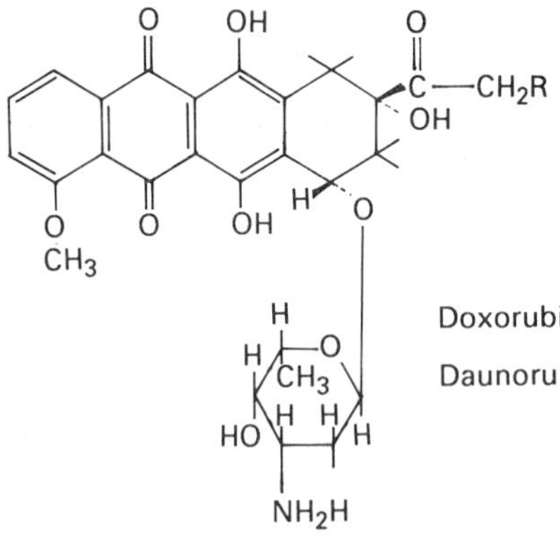

Doxorubicin (R = OH)

Daunorubicin (R = H)

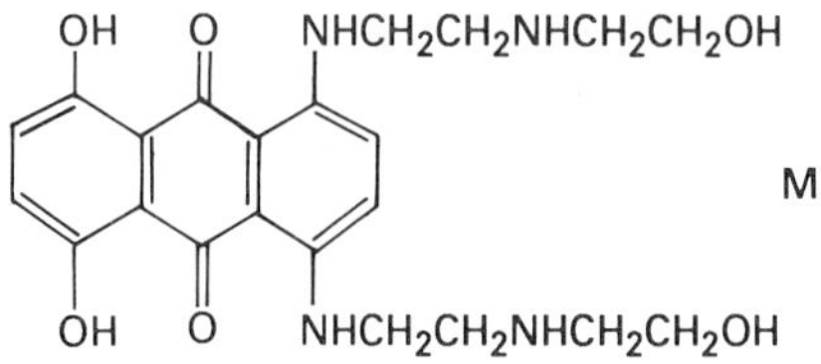

Mitoxantrone

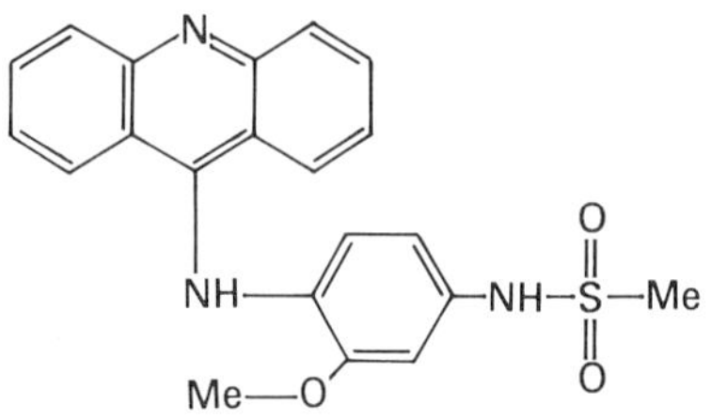

Amsacrine (*m*-AMSA)

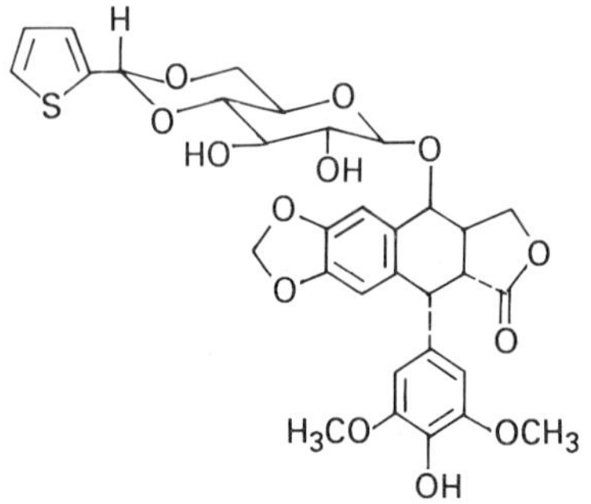

Teniposide (VM-26)

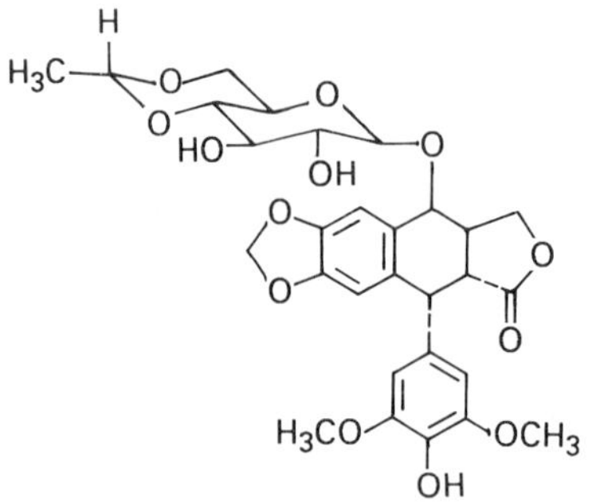

Etoposide (VP-16-213)

**Figure 4.3** Chemical structure of intercalating agents and epipodophyllotoxins their sugar moieties to yield the quinone methide, or a C-7 radical, both species capable of monofunctional DNA alkylation [81,82].

## Intercalation and topoisomerases

Intercalation is the physical binding of an agent such that it becomes wedged between the stacked bases of the DNA double helix. Doxorubicin in particular, and anthracyclines in general, are excellent intercalators. Intercalation alters a variety of DNA functions, e.g. doxorubicin at high concentrations ($\mu$M range) can inhibit DNA and RNA polymerases. However, it is the effect of intercalation on an enzyme known as topoisomerase II which is likely to be more relevant to the cytotoxic, genotoxic and carcinogenic properties of these drugs.

Topoisomerase II is one of several mammalian enzymes which control the degree of coiling adopted by DNA molecules over and above the primary double helical configuration of native DNA. The coiled-coil structure allows enormous lengths of DNA to be packed into very small volumes. For example, a single human somatic cell contains about half a metre of DNA packed into a nucleus whose diameter is measured in microns [83]. Clearly, a remarkable degree of topological management is necessary to ensure that such huge lengths of DNA are replicated accurately and that gene expression and regulation are controlled in an orderly manner. A few moments experimenting with a coiled telephone cable will illustrate some of the problems of accurately replicating an anti-parallel double-stranded helix which is attached at regular intervals to a nuclear matrix. At the end of DNA replication there are two interwound coiled coils of DNA which must be separated before mitosis can occur. Topoisomerases make transient cuts in DNA in order to relax coiled coils and allow replicated domains to separate or knots to untangle – a process known as decatenation.

Type I topoisomerases are monomeric, do not require ATP, cut single strands and become covalently bound to the break sites. Mammalian topoisomerase II is a homo-dimer, requires ATP and introduces a double-strand DNA cut staggered by four bases. Each subunit of the enzyme binds to the 5′ terminus of its respective DNA break point. After passage of one DNA duplex past the other, the breaks are rejoined and the enzyme dissociates from the DNA. Thus, strand breaks mediated by drugs which interfere with topoisomerase II are always associated with DNA fragments containing enzyme-protein bound to the 5′ ends [81,83]. Although the evidence that topoisomerase II is indeed a target for intercalating agents is compelling [83], the mechanism by which these drugs disrupt topoisomerase II activity has not been fully elucidated. Ross *et al.* [83] suggest that a stable 'cleavable complex' forms between the drug, the enzyme and DNA which accounts for the effects of intercalating agents and epipodophyllotoxins on the accumulation of strand breaks and the inhibition of strand passage which is peculiar to these drugs.

## Effects of anthracyclines on cell membranes

The cell membrane is another candidate for the site of action of anthracyclines such as doxorubicin. Doxorubicin changes a variety of membrane functions, including lectin-induced agglutination, ion transport, membrane fluidity and morphology, and lipid organization. For example, doxorubicin binds just as tightly to the membrane phospholipid cardiolipin as it does to DNA. There are parallels between the action of tumour promoters such as phorbol esters and anthracyclines such as aclacinomycin, marcellomycin and musettamycin in their ability to stimulate protein kinase C, which in turn is linked to the control of differentiation of tumour cells [81,84]. What contribution membrane-mediated effects make to the carcinogenicity of doxorubicin is unknown.

## Chromosomal aberrations and topoisomerase II

Drugs which produce DNA breaks by interfering with topoisomerase II induce chromosomal aberrations which are independent of cell cycle stage and are more typical of ionizing radiation than of alkylating agents. Most clastogens (including antitumour alkylating agents) are cell cycle specific. A round of DNA replication ('S phase' in the cell cycle) following drug exposure is necessary to allow processing of DNA lesions into visible damage, which is predominantly of the chromatid type. Chromosomal aberrations induced by ionizing radiation, on the other hand, are S-phase-independent, since ionizing radiation produces single or double-stranded DNA breaks directly without the need for DNA replication, processing or mis-repair. Discontinuities in DNA produced in unreplicated $G_1$ chromosomes will be duplicated during S phase and will appear as chromosome-type aberrations (involving both chromatids). DNA damage produced after S phase involves only one of the chromatids and will be manifested as chromatid-type aberrations [85,86]. Doxorubicin induces double-strand DNA breaks not only by effects on topoisomerase II but also by free radical formation. Moreover, doxorubicin or its metabolites appears to react covalently with DNA to some extent and the drug is a potent point mutagen in a variety of organisms. Thus, doxorubicin is an eclectic genotoxin which acts at several different targets.

Other antineoplastic drugs are cytotoxic and genotoxic via topoisomerase II but do not generate free radicals or bind covalently to DNA to any great extent. Mitoxantrone (Figure 4.3), a synthetic anthracenedione, is an example. It causes chromosomal damage *in vitro* and *in vivo* and is a weak frame-shift mutagen in bacteria at doses far higher than those which are clastogenic to mammalian cells. There are no data on its carcinogenicity to animals or man (Table 4.1). Far from generating free radicals, mitoxantrone is a powerful antioxidant and a potent inhibitor of lipid peroxidation [87]. It intercalates DNA and also binds to it electrostatically, probably to the anionic exterior of the DNA molecule so that the charged side arms of mitoxantrone link one stretch of DNA with another by 'inter-DNA linking'. Mitoxantrone at doses as low as 10 ng/ml inhibited topoisomerase II in human breast carcinoma cells in culture and produced protein-associated double- and single-strand DNA breaks in mouse leukaemia cells, indicating its effects on topoisomerase II. In addition, it induced single-strand breaks which were not associated with protein [88].

Amsacrine (Figure 4.3) is another intercalating drug which acts via topoisomerase II and is a potent clastogen in mammalian cells, producing both chromatid and chromosome-type damage [83,89,90]. Like mitoxantrone, amsacrine is a weak point mutagen to bacteria and mammalian cells [89,91–93], suggesting that covalent DNA binding plays little or no part in its genotoxic activity.

## Epipodophyllotoxins

Epipodophyllotoxins (etoposide, teniposide; Figure 4.3) are semisynthetic glucosides derived from podophyllotoxin, a product of the American mandrake *Podophyllum peltatum* and related plants [94]. Although there is no information on the carcinogenicity of these drugs (Table 4.1), they must be regarded with suspicion since they induce DNA strand breaks by interfering with topoisomerase II [83] and are potent genotoxins in mammalian cells [95–97]. Like amsacrine, etoposide and teniposide are very weak bacterial mutagens, inducing mutation only at very high doses [96,98], which suggests that these agents do not bind covalently to DNA. Although epipodophyllotoxins are not considered to be classical intercalating agents, etoposide has been shown to bind to DNA *in vitro* at pharmacologically relevant concentrations and computer modelling suggests that intercalation is possible [83].

## Bleomycins

Bleomycin is a mixture of glycopeptides extracted from the fungus *Streptomyces verticillus*. It is carcinogenic to laboratory animals, causing renal tumours and injection-site fibrosarcomas in rats following repeated injection [17]. Bleomycin is genotoxic to a wide variety of organisms, inducing chromosomal aberrations in lymphocytes of treated patients and human and rodent cells treated in culture. It causes a range of mutagenic effects in *D. melanogaster* and is positive in genotoxicity tests employing yeasts and bacteria [29]. As with the other antineoplastic antibiotics discussed in this chapter, the mode of action of bleomycin both as an antitumour agent and as a genotoxin depends on its remarkable chemistry and its effects on DNA. Bleomycin binds non-covalently to DNA, probably by intercalation [99]. In addition it chelates metals, especially iron and copper and behaves as a 'mini-enzyme', catalyzing free radical production by reduction of oxygen. The characteristic damage inflicted by bleomycin consists of single- and double-strand DNA breaks produced, it is thought, by cleavage of deoxyribose followed by liberation of DNA bases. Similar damage would be wrought by superoxide and hydroxyl free radicals, both of which are produced by the bleomycin–ferrous complex [100]. Bleomycin is another example of an S phase-independent clastogen ('liquid X-rays') which produces chromatid- and chromosome-type aberrations by inducing double-strand DNA breaks. Because it causes cancer in animals, and is a potent clastogen, bleomycin should be regarded as a potential human carcinogen.

## Spindle poisons

Vincristine and vinblastine (Figure 4.4) are dimeric indole-dihydroindole alkaloids extracted from the Madagascan periwinkle, *Catharanthus roseus*. Neither drug has been tested thoroughly for carcinogenicity in experimental animals, but what data exist do not suggest activity [17]. In a critical review of the genetic toxicology of vinca alkaloids, Degraeve [101] found no convincing evidence that vincristine or vinblastine was mutagenic, either to prokaryotes or eukaryotes. Vincristine sulphate gave negative results in a dominant lethal test and in a specific locus test in mice [102]. Vindesine sulphate, a semisynthetic vinca alkaloid, did not induce mutation in *S. typhimurium,* or sister chromatid exchange or chromosomal aberrations in bone marrow cells of Chinese hamsters treated *in vivo* [103].

The only chromosomal anomalies consistently associated with vinca alkaloids are aneuploidy and polyploidy [101,103,104]. The critical target of these spindle poisons is tubulin, the major protein component of microtubules which are the structural units of the mitotic and meiotic spindle. By binding to tubulin, spindle poisons prevent assembly of microtubules during metaphase. This results in the accumulation of mitotic figures, arrested metaphases, multipolar anaphases with lagging chromosomes

genotoxic effects. Incorporation of fraudulent bases into DNA may also account for some of the genetic activity of certain antimetabolites.

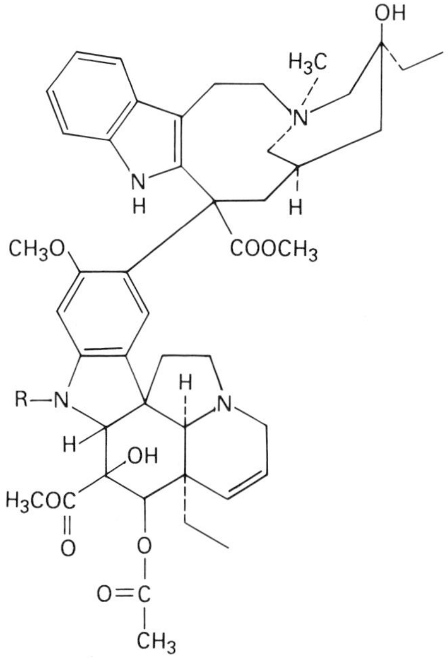

### *Folic acid antagonists: methotrexate*

Methotrexate (Figure 4.5) is a very widely used drug, not only in cancer chemotherapy but also in non-malignant conditions such as psoriasis and rheumatoid arthritis. Cohort studies of patients treated with methotrexate for trophoblastic tumours or psoriasis showed no increased risk of malignancy. A case control study of psoriasis patients was also negative [16,17]. Although several long-term carcinogenicity assays of methotrexate in rodents have

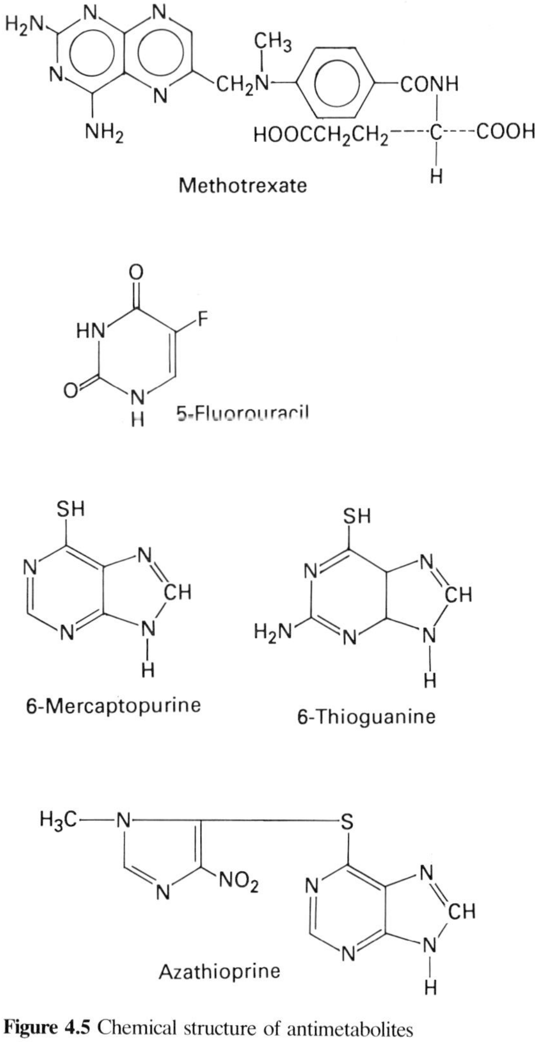

Vincristine (R = CHO)

Vinblastine (R = CH₃)

**Figure 4.4** Chemical structure of spindle poisons

Methotrexate

**Figure 4.5** Chemical structure of antimetabolites

5-Fluorouracil

6-Mercaptopurine

6-Thioguanine

Azathioprine

and polyploidy caused by doubling of chromosomes but failure of chromatid separation [105]. Aneuploidy (loss or addition of a few, usually one, chromosome) may play a role in carcinogenesis; for example, mitotic non-disjunction may lead to loss of a chromosome carrying a tumour-suppressor gene in a cell already carrying a defective recessive allele [26]. Constitutional aneuploidies are associated with an increased risk of cancer such as elevated risks of leukaemia in Down's syndrome, breast cancer in Klinefelter's syndrome and gonadoblastoma in XY/X0 individuals [106,107].

## Antimetabolites

Antimetabolites used in cancer chemotherapy block cell replication by interfering with the biochemical pathways for biosynthesis of nucleic acid precursors rather than by direct reaction with DNA. They fall into three main types: folic acid antagonists, pyrimidine antagonists, purine antagonists, all of which cause imbalances in intracellular deoxyribonucleotide pools, a mechanism associated with DNA damage and mutagenesis [108]. Thus, their mode of action as cytotoxic agents may well explain their

been reported to be negative, most of these studies were deficient in design or in reporting [16,17].

Methotrexate is clastogenic, producing chromosomal aberrations in bone marrow cells and sister chromatid exchanges in peripheral lymphocytes of patients. In mammalian cells treated *in vitro*, it produces sister chromatid exchange and chromosomal aberrations [29]. Methotrexate induces somatic and transmissible mutations in the fruit-fly *D. melanogaster* [17,109]. There is no convincing evidence that it is mutagenic to bacteria [29].

The primary target of methotrexate is dihydrofolate reductase, which reduces dihydrofolate to tetrahydrofolate, a precursor of several cofactors involved in the *de novo* synthesis of purines, methionine, glycine and thymidine monophosphate. Strong competitive binding of methotrexate to dihydrofolate reductase blocks synthesis of thymidine monophosphate, which prevents DNA and RNA synthesis and results in cell death. The cytotoxicity of methotrexate is therefore S phase-dependent. In addition, high concentrations of methotrexate can block uptake and enhance efflux of folate [110]. A direct inhibitory effect of methotrexate on thymidylate synthetase has also been implicated in its mode of action as a cytotoxin [110,111].

Precisely how methotrexate induces chromosomal aberrations is unknown. Mis-incorporation of uracil instead of thymine into DNA is a possible mechanism. The detection of significant amounts of deoxyuridine monosphosphate (dUMP) in DNA of cells of a human lymphoid cell line treated with methotrexate suggested that inhibition of thymidylate synthesis augments the biosynthesis of deoxyuridine triphosphate (dUTP) from deoxyuridine monosphosphate (dUMP), and that the large excess of dUTP over deoxythymidine triphosphate (dTTP) overwhelms enzymatic mechanisms which normally prevent incorporation of uracil into DNA [112]. Uracil incorporation is circumvented in mammalian cells by dUTPase which hydrolyses dUTP back to dUMP and by a uracil-DNA glycosylase which removes uracil from DNA [33]. Goulian *et al.* [112] suggested that methotrexate treatment produces DNA lesions by a self-defeating cyclic incorporation and removal of dUMP resulting from reinsertion of dUMP during gap repair at sites of uracil removal. Some support for this hypothesis was provided by experiments with another folate antagonist, piritrexim, which induced mis-incorporation of dUMP in several human cell lines. Biophysical studies indicated that DNA distributed into progressively smaller DNA fragment sizes in a dose-dependent manner, suggesting the presence of apurinic and apyrimidinic sites in DNA, lesions which would be expected during excision repair of mis-incorporated dUMP [113].

Mis-incorporation of dUMP following methotrexate treatment was not confirmed by Fraser and Pearson [114] who found no evidence for the presence of uracil in the DNA of human cells treated *in vitro* with methotrexate. However, these authors did not use the cell lines that were used by Goulian *et al.* [112] or Richards *et al.* [113]. Thus, mis-incorporation of dUMP as an explanation of the cytotoxic and clastogenic effects of methotrexate remains controversial.

## Pyrimidine antagonists: fluorinated pyrimidines

The most widely used fluorinated pyrimidine is the thymine analogue 5-fluorouracil (5-FU; Figure 4.5) which can be converted to its deoxyribonucleoside 5-fluoro-2′-deoxyuridine (5-FUdR) by thymidine phosphorylase. 5-FUdR is also used as a drug in its own right. There is little information upon which to judge the carcinogenicity of 5-FU or 5-FUdR. The only epidemiological study available revealed no increased risk of second cancers among 276 patients with colorectal cancer randomized to receive low-dose 5-FUdR adjuvant therapy, followed for 1774 person-years [17].

Experiments employing intravenous administration of 5-FU to mice and rats and oral administration to rats provided no evidence that this drug is carcinogenic, but the studies were judged to be limited with respect to duration and dose [17].

Neither chromosomal aberrations (in two patients) nor SCE (in three patients) were induced following administration of 5-FU. Two studies have shown that 5-FU induces micronuclei in the bone marrow of mice. In a single study it did not induce transmissible specific locus mutations in mice; it did not induce mutation in *D. melanogaster* but did cause mitotic crossing over in a fungus. Several studies show that 5-FU is clastogenic to Chinese hamster cells treated *in vitro* [29]. Studies in which cells were synchronized by mitotic selection showed that a peak of mutagenicity occurred in early S phase, suggesting that 5-FUdR acts at DNA growing points [115]. There is no decisive evidence that 5-FU is mutagenic to bacteria [29]. However, it is mutagenic to RNA viruses and is used extensively for producing viral mutants [116,117].

Both 5-FU and 5-FUdR are pro-drugs, i.e. they require metabolism to express their cytotoxic activity. The critical metabolites of both drugs are 5-fluorodeoxyuridine monophosphate (5-FdUMP) and 5-fluorouridine monophosphate (5-FUMP). In the presence of a tetrahydrofolate cofactor, 5-FdUMP binds to thymidylate synthetase and induces cell death by inhibition of *de novo* thymidylate synthesis (like methotrexate, see above) [118]. In addition, 5-FdUMP can be phosphorylated to the triphosphate (5-FdUTP) which could serve as a substrate for DNA polymerase, allowing incorporation of uracil instead of thymine.

Studies of the effects of fluorinated pyrimidines on human colon adenocarcinoma cells [119–123] and mouse bone marrow cells [111, 124–127] suggest that drugs such as 5-FU and 5-FUdR cause DNA damage by several mechanisms. These include the incorporation of 5-FU into DNA and the depletion of nucleotide pools, which would inhibit strand elongation and suppress DNA repair.

By analogy with 5-bromodeoxyuridine, the presence of 5-FU in DNA would also be expected to cause point mutation by GC to AT and AT to GC transitions by a tautomeric shift such that 5-FU would resemble cytosine rather than thymine [128,129]. However, because the fraudulent base is efficiently removed by uracil-DNA glycosylase and dUTP nucleotidohydrolase, the role of misincorporation of uracil into DNA by 5-FU and 5-FUdR in their cytotoxic and genotoxic properties remains uncertain.

Incorporation of 5-FUTP (the triphosphate of 5-FUMP) into RNA and the consequent derangement of RNA processing is well documented [111] and accounts for the mutagenicity of 5-FU to RNA viruses. To what extent the effects of fluorinated pyrimidines on RNA account for their genotoxic activity in mammalian cells is uncertain.

### *Purine antagonists*

With the exception of azathioprine, which is a human carcinogen and a broad-spectrum genotoxin, there are no data on which to judge the carcinogenicity of the antineoplastic purine antagonists listed in Table 4.1. Although it is used mainly as an immunosuppressive agent, azathioprine is of interest since one of its many metabolites is 6-mercaptopurine (6-MP) which is used in the treatment of leukaemia. This drug is genotoxic in its own right, inducing chromosomal aberrations in peripheral lymphocytes of patients, and in the bone marrow cells of several rodent species treated *in vivo*. It produces transmissible dominant lethal mutations in mice and rats and is clastogenic to human cells *in vitro*; it induces point mutation in bacteria [29]. A similar range of tests of 6-thioguanine (6-TG; Figure 4.5) has not been performed, but there are sufficient data to indicate that this drug is clastogenic and causes DNA damage in mammalian cells *in vitro* [130–133].

As in the case of methotrexate and 5-FU, the mechanisms underlying the cytotoxic effects of 6-MP and 6-TG are probably those which determine their genotoxicity. In both cases conversion of the thiopurine to its thionucleotide is necessary. Thionucleotides interfere with *de novo* purine biosynthesis and interconversions, inhibit RNA synthesis and, following incorporation into DNA, cause DNA strand breaks and chromosomal aberrations. Direct measurement of the incorporation of 6-TG into DNA of cultured Chinese hamster ovary cells, and analysis of the resulting DNA damage, showed that the predominant lesions were DNA strand breaks [131]. As 6-TG concentrations were increased, cytotoxicity (as measured by colony formation), DNA incorporation, and strand scission increased and reached a plateau. Alkali-labile sites were detected in the DNA of TG-treated cells, suggesting that depurination of TG residues by a glycosylase mechanism may occur [131].

## Ionizing radiation

Radiotherapy usually consists of high doses of low linear-energy-transfer (LET) radiation such as $\beta$-, $\gamma$- and X-rays. As well as being one of the earliest means of treating cancer – its use started at the end of the 19th century – ionizing radiation was the first mutagen to be discovered. Muller showed in 1927 that X-rays caused gene mutations and rearrangements of the linear order of genes in *D. melanogaster* [134]. Since then, abundant evidence has accumulated to confirm the mutagenicity of ionizing radiation [135,136] and to establish its carcinogenicity beyond peradventure [8,137–139].

Ionizing radiation is a broad-spectrum carcinogen; to a first approximation it causes cancer wherever sufficient exposure has occurred. The carcinogenicity of ionizing radiation depends on many variables including dose, dose rate, dose fractionation, the quality of the radiation and its uniformity, susceptibility of different tissues within a species and between different strains and different species, other genetic factors such as DNA repair capacity, immune status, gender, age at irradiation. The way these factors interact and the difficulties of establishing reliable dose-response relationships are discussed in depth by Fry and Storer [139].

A particularly striking feature of radiogenic neoplasms is their complex relationship with dose and with age at irradiation. A study of 14 111 patients treated for ankylosing spondylitis with a single course of partial body X-rays revealed a nearly five-fold excess of leukaemia, and a 1.6-fold increase in cancer at heavily irradiated sites close to the irradiation field. Radiogenic leukaemias reached a peak 3–5 years after treatment and by 18 years the excess risk was close to zero. In contrast, tumours at heavily irradiated sites did not increase until 9 years after irradiation, after which time the excess risk was maintained for a further 11 years [140]. In adult life susceptibility to radiogenic cancer increased with age at irradiation; patients irradiated at age 55 years or more suffered an excess leukaemia death rate more than 15 times that of patients treated at age 25 years or less, with similar differences for tumours at other sites. The increase in radiogenic leukaemia and other tumours with increasing age at irradiation suggests that radiation interacts multiplicatively with other exposures which are accumulated over time, and which predispose to development of cancer [140].

In some circumstances high doses appear to be proportionately less carcinogenic than low doses, presumably because the probability of killing target cells exceeds that of transforming them to malignancy [138–140]. This explanation is supported by the observation that on the basis of cell killing, ionizing radiation is a less effective mutagen than ultraviolet radiation and many chemical mutagens [135].

The way in which radiotherapy is given also determines the sites at which second cancers occur. For example, a study of data combined from 15 cancer registries showed that for all sites taken together, the risk of developing second cancers in women treated for cervical cancer with radiotherapy was only slightly greater than would have been expected in the general population, and that the large radiation doses did not substantially alter the risk of developing a second cancer. There was only a very slight increase in acute and myeloid leukaemias in these patients. Modest but significant increases in risks of solid tumours (bladder, rectum, bone, connective tissue, uterine corpus, ileum, kidney) and multiple myeloma at moderately and heavily irradiated sites ($>100\,$cGy) were apparent. Substantial doses to the stomach and colon did not increase the risk of cancer in those organs, and there were marked reductions in breast cancer risk which were attributed to irradiation of the ovaries [141].

Ionizing radiation is a broad-spectrum mutagen, inducing a variety of mutational events in mice, mammalian cells *in vitro*, insects, plants, fungi and bacteria and bacteriophage [135,136]. There are substantial data on the clastogenic effects of ionizing radiation on human chromosomes [142]. For example, in a study [143] of 190 patients treated with single doses or a course of ten doses of partial body X-irradiation for ankylosing spondylitis, chromosome damage in peripheral lymphocytes induced by a single dose increased as the square of the dose; each dose fraction increased chromosome damage cumulatively; after a total dose of 1500 cGy in ten fractions, the number of cells with unstable aberrations (e.g. breaks, dicentrics, acentrics) was four times greater than those with stable aberrations (transversions, translocations); the frequency of cells with unstable aberrations was greatly reduced 4 years after irradiation, but a small number of such aberrations persisted for many years after treatment; the frequency of cells with stable aberrations did not decline with time after treatment; there was no evidence that the chromosomal rearrangements

caused by X-irradiation reflected the specific rearrangements found in haematopoietic malignancies.

Ionizing radiation exerts its genotoxic and carcinogenic effects by damaging DNA. DNA damage may arise by direct interaction of the radiation energy with DNA, or indirectly from effects of reactive species – hydrogen peroxide, hydrogen atoms, hydrated electrons and hydroxyl radicals – formed from cellular constituents such as water, inorganic ions and a wide range of organic molecules [33,58]. Unlike the chemical agents already discussed, where the number of DNA adducts and other modifications induced by a given agent are limited to perhaps not more than ten or twenty, ionizing radiation may produce more than 100 different DNA modifications [55–57]. It modifies bases (products include hydroxylated purines and imidazole-ring opened purines), and induces single- and double-strand breaks and apurinic sites in DNA. Opportunities for deployment of the full repertoire of mutational events, ranging from base-pair substitutions to gross chromosomal anomalies, are therefore legion.

## Non-genotoxic carcinogens: tamoxifen

Most of the carcinogenic antineoplastic agents mentioned in this chapter are genotoxic and are probably carcinogenic *because* they are genotoxic. Many of the drugs which are genotoxic but unclassifiable as to their carcinogenicity may turn out to be carcinogens. However, there are agents and exposures which are carcinogenic or which enhance or promote tumour growth but which do not appear to be genotoxic [38]. Ethinyl oestradiol and tamoxifen (Table 4.1, Figure 4.6) fit this description and represent a class of carcinogens which depend on hormonal mechanisms. Tamoxifen (which has oestrogenic and anti-oestrogenic properties) reduces mortality of early breast cancer [144] and is now on trial as a prophylactic in women at high risk of breast cancer [145].

There is limited evidence that tamoxifen is not genotoxic – it was reported to be negative in the Ames test and in tests for dominant lethal mutations in mice [146,147].

The evidence that tamoxifen is carcinogenic is more substantial. Mice treated orally with tamoxifen at 5 or 50 mg/kg for a total of 15 months developed interstitial cell tumours of the testes and granulosa cell tumours of the ovary. These effects were attributed to the oestrogenic activity of tamoxifen, since similar lesions were seen in mice treated with synthetic steroidal oestrogens [146]. It has also been reported that tamoxifen caused liver tumours in rats [145,147]. In a study of new primary cancers in 1846

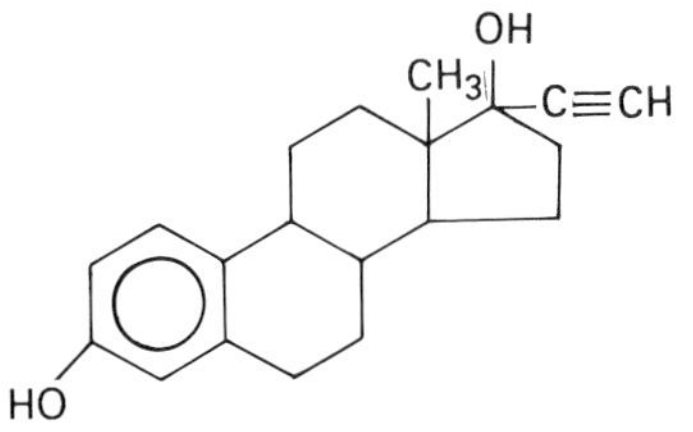

**Figure 4.6** Chemical structure of ethinyl oestradiol and tamoxifen

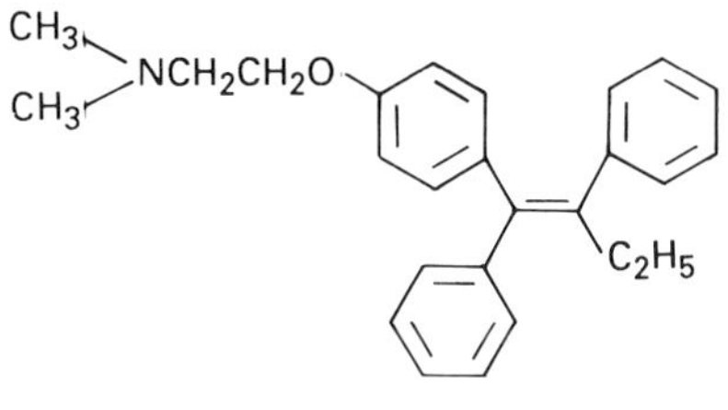

postmenopausal patients in a randomized trial of adjuvant tamoxifen following surgery for early breast cancer, the number of new cancers in the tamoxifen group did not differ significantly from that in the control group. However, in tamoxifen-treated patients second breast cancers occurred significantly less often than in the controls and endometrial cancer occurred significantly more often. The median follow-up was 4.5 years [148]. Simultaneous suppression of the growth of breast cancer and enhancement of endometrial cancer growth has been seen in mice which had been implanted with human tumours and treated with tamoxifen. A human endometrial tumour was stimulated to grow by tamoxifen given alone or when combined with oestradiol. This contrasted with the antagonistic action of tamoxifen on oestradiol-stimulated growth of a human breast tumour. These responses were seen even when the two tumour types were implanted on opposite sides of the same mouse, indicating that host metabolism of tamoxifen does not dictate tissue response [149].

The induction of genital tumours in women is consistent with the effects seen in mice and strongly supports the notion that tamoxifen owes its tumour-promoting activity to its oestrogenic properties. That steroidal oestrogens cause human endometrial cancer adds further weight to this idea [17].

Further evidence that tamoxifen and synthetic oestrogens are tumour promoters is available. For example, administration of low doses of synthetic oestrogens to rats previously given initiating doses of genotoxic carcinogens such as diethylnitrosamine (DEN) markedly enhance hepatocarcinogenesis [150,151], indicating tumour promotion rather than initiation. Using the appearance of γ-glutamyl transpeptidase-positive foci as an early marker of hepatocarcinogenesis in DEN-treated rats, Yager *et al.* [150] found that tamoxifen enhanced the appearance of these foci, suggesting that tamoxifen exerted a tumour-promoting effect on the rat liver.

## Conclusions

Many clinically useful antineoplastic drugs are carcinogenic to humans, and most are genotoxic. A rank-order of carcinogenic potency linked to a quantitative index of therapeutic efficacy would be a useful instrument for helping to deliver the most effective but least carcinogenic antineoplastic treatment. Unfortunately, such a listing is impossible for a variety of reasons, not the least being the paucity of dose-response data on which to base such an instrument. Nevertheless, a highly speculative qualitative ranking is presented below, based on earlier thoughts on the topic by Connors [9].

Of the types of drugs considered, those which bind covalently to DNA and which are powerful genotoxins – alkylating agents and platinum compounds – stand out as potent carcinogens. Anthracyclines such as doxorubicin are powerfully genotoxic via several mechanisms, including DNA intercalation, covalent binding, free radical formation and interference with topoisomerase II. These drugs, together with ionizing radiation, should probably be ranked close to alkylating and platinating agents. There is scant evidence on which to judge other intercalating and topoisomerase-dependent drugs such as mitoxantrone, amsacrine and the epipodophyllotoxins. However, it is tempting to rank them as less potent than doxorubicin-like drugs because they do not bind covalently to DNA, neither do they appear to generate free radicals. Bleomycins might also appear at this point – although they act by a free radical mechanism, they do not bind covalently to DNA. With the exception of azathioprine, most antimetabolites do not appear to be potent carcinogens and their genotoxic activity depends on indirect mechanisms rather than on covalent DNA binding. Non-genotoxic carcinogens or tumour promoters such as tamoxifen cannot be classified on the basis of genetic activity. However, in view of the proven efficacy of tamoxifen against breast cancer and the likelihood of its increasingly widespread use, note should be taken of its carcinogenicity to the endometrium.

## References


1. Sieber, S.M. and Adamson, R.H. Toxicity of antineoplastic agents in man: chromosomal aberrations, antifertility effects, congenital malformations, and carcinogenic potential. *Advances in Cancer Research*, **22**, 57–155 (1975)
2. Schmähl, D., Habs, M., Lorenz, M. and Wagner, I. Occurrence of second tumors in man after anticancer drug treatment. *Cancer Treatment Reviews*, **9**, 167–194 (1982)
3. Kyle, R.A. Second malignancies associated with chemotherapy. In *Toxicity of Chemotherapy* (eds M.C. Perry and J.W. Yarboro), Grune and Stratton, Orlando, pp. 479–506 (1984)
4. Henne, T. and Schmähl, D. Occurrence of second primary malignancies in man – a second look. *Cancer Treatment Reviews*, **12**, 77–94 (1985)
5. Rieche, K. Carcinogenicity of antineoplastic agents in man. *Cancer Treatment Reviews*, **11**, 39–67 (1984)
6. Young, D. and Canellos, G.P. Second malignancies and cancer therapy. *Clinics in Oncology*, **4**, 535–557 (1985)
7. Schmähl, D. and Kaldor, J.M. (eds). *Carcinogenicity of Alkylating Cytostatic Drugs*, IARC Scientific Publications No. 78, International Agency for Research on Cancer, Lyon, 338 pp. (1986)
8. Meadows, A.T. Second malignant neoplasms. *Clinics in Oncology*, **4**, 247–261 (1985)
9. Connors, T.A. Carcinogenicity of medicines. In *Chemical Carcinogens*, 2nd edn, Vol. 2, (ed. C.E. Searle), ACS Monograph 182, American Chemical Society, Washington DC, pp. 1241–1278 (1984)
10. Sartorelli, A.C., Lazo, J.S. and Bertino, J.R. (eds). *Molecular Actions and Targets for Cancer Chemotherapeutic Agents*, Academic Press, New York, 598 pp. (1981)
11. Crooke, S.T. and Prestayko, A.W. (eds) *Cancer and Chemotherapy. Volume III. Antineoplastic Agents*, Academic Press, New York, 398 pp. (1981)
12. Neidle, S. and Waring, M.J. (eds). *Molecular Aspects of Anti-Cancer Drug Action*, Macmillan, London, 404 pp. (1983)
13. Souhami, R. and Tobias, J. *Cancer and its Management*, Blackwell Scientific Publications, Oxford, 526 pp. (1986)
14. Pinedo, H.M. and Chabner, B.A. (eds). *Cancer Chemotherapy 8. The EORTC Cancer Chemotherapy Annual*, Elsevier, Amsterdam, 588 pp. (1986)
15. Pinedo, H.M., Longo, D.L. and Chabner, B.A. (eds). *Cancer Chemotherapy and Biological Response Modifiers Annual 9*, Elsevier, Amsterdam, 572 pp. (1987)
16. IARC. *IARC Monographs of the Evaluation of the Carcinogenic Risk of Chemicals to Humans. Some Antineoplastic and Immunosuppressive Drugs*, Vol. 26, International Agency for Research on Cancer, Lyon, 411 pp. (1981)
17. IARC. *IARC Monographs on the Evaluation of Carcinogenic Risks to Humans. Overall Evaluations of Carcinogenicity: An Updating of IARC Monographs, Vols 1 to 42*, International Agency for Research on Cancer, Lyon, 440 pp. (1987)
18. IARC. *IARC Monographs on the Evaluation of Carcinogenic Risks to Humans. Alcohol Drinking*, Vol. 44, International Agency for Research on Cancer, Lyon, 416 pp. (1988)
19. Rall, D.P. Laboratory animal toxicity and carcinogenesis testing. In *Living in a Chemical World. Occupational and Environmental Significance of Industrial Carcinogens*, (eds C. Maltoni and I.J. Selikoff), New York Academy of Sciences, New York, pp. 78–83 (1988)
20. Venitt, S. The aetiology of human cancers. In *Oncology for Nurses and Health Care Professionals, Vol. 1. Pathology, Diagnosis and Treatment*, 2nd edn (eds R. Tiffany and P. Pritchard), Harper and Row, London, pp. 29–68 (1988)
21. Moolgavkar, S.H. and Knudson, A.G. Mutation and cancer: a model for human carcinogenesis. *Journal of the National Cancer Institute*, **66**, 1037–1052 (1981)
22. Varmus, H.E. The molecular genetics of cellular oncogenes. *Annual Review of Genetics*, **18**, 553–612 (1984)
23. Weinberg, R.A. Finding the anti-oncogene. *Scientific American*, **259**, 34–41 (1988)
24. Nishimura, S. and Sekiya, T. Human cancer and cellular oncogenes. *Biochemical Journal*, **243**, 313–327 (1987)
25. Burck, K.B., Liu, E.T. and Larrick, J.W. *Oncogenes: An Introduction to the Concept of Cancer Genes*, Springer-Verlag, New York, 300 pp. (1988)
26. Ponder, B. Gene losses in human tumours. *Nature*, **335**, 400–402 (1988)
27. Bishop, J.M. The molecular genetics of cancer. *Science*, **235**, 305–311 (1987)
28. IARC. *Long-Term and Short-Term Assays for Carcinogens: A Critical Appraisal*. IARC Scientific Publications No. 83 (eds R. Montesano, H. Bartsch, H. Vainio *et al.*), International Agency for Research on Cancer, Lyon, 564 pp. (1986)
29. IARC. *IARC Monographs on the Evaluation of Carcinogenic Risks to Humans. Genetic and Related Effects: An Updating of Selected IARC Monographs from Volumes 1–42*, International Agency for Research on Cancer, Lyon, 729 pp. (1987)
30. Venitt, S. and Parry, J.M. (eds). *Mutagenicity Testing. A Practical Approach*, IRL Press, Oxford, 353 pp. (1984)
31. Singer, B. and Grunberger, D. *Molecular Biology of Mutagens and Carcinogens*, Plenum Press, New York, 347 pp. (1983)
32. Searle, C.E. (ed.), *Chemical Carcinogenesis*, 2nd edn, Vols 1 and 2, ACS Monograph 182, American Chemical Society, Washington DC, 1373 pp. (1984)
33. Friedberg, E.C. *DNA Repair*, W.H. Freeman, New York, 614 pp. (1984)

34. Hemminki, K. and Ludlum, D.B. Covalent modification of DNA by antineoplastic agents. *Journal of the National Cancer Institute*, **73**, 1021–1028 (1981)

35. Watson, W.P. Post-labelling for detecting DNA damage. *Mutagenesis*, **2**, 319–331 (1987)

36. Maron, D.M. and Ames, B.N. Revised methods for the Salmonella mutagenicity test. *Mutation Research*, **113**, 173–215 (1983)

37. Cole, J. and Arlett, C.F. The detection of gene mutations in cultured mammalian cells. In *Mutagenicity Testing – A Practical Approach* (eds S. Venitt and J.M. Parry), IRL Press, Oxford, pp. 233–273 (1984)

38. Cairns, J. The origin of human cancers. *Nature*, **289**, 353–357 (1981)

39. Mitelman, F. and Heim, S. Consistent involvement of only 71 of the 329 chromosomal bands of the human genome in primary neoplasia-associated rearrangements. *Cancer Research*, **48**, 7115–7119 (1988)

40. Chaganti, R.S.K. and German, J. (eds). *Genetics in Clinical Oncology*, Oxford University Press, New York, 280 pp. (1985)

41. Auerbach, C. and Robson, J.M. Chemical production of mutations. *Nature*, **302**, 157 (1946)

42. Krumbhaar, E.B. and Krumbhaar, H.D. The blood and bone marrow in yellow cross gas (mustard gas) poisoning. Changes produced in the bone marrow of fatal cases. *Journal of Medical Research*, **90**, 497–507 (1919)

43. Brock, N. Oxazaphosphorine cytostatics: past-present-future. Seventh Cain Memorial Award Lecture. *Cancer Research*, **49**, 1–7 (1989)

44. Brookes, P. and Lawley, P.D. The reaction of mustard gas with nucleic acids *in vitro* and *in vivo*. *Biochemical Journal*, **77**, 478–484 (1960)

45. Lawley, P.D. Carcinogenesis by alkylating agents. In *Chemical Carcinogenesis*, 2nd edn, Vol. 1, ACS Monograph 182, (ed. C.E. Searle), American Chemical Society, Washington DC, pp. 325–484 (1984)

46. Kohn, K.W. Molecular mechanisms of cross-linking by alkylating agents and platinum complexes. In *Molecular Actions and Targets for Cancer Chemotherapeutic Agents* (eds A.C. Sartorelli, J.S. Lazo and J.R. Bertino), Academic Press, New York, pp. 3–16 (1981)

47. Kohn, K.W. Biological aspects of DNA damage by cross-linking agents. In *Molecular Aspects of Anti-Cancer Drug Action*, (eds S. Neidle and M.J. Waring), Macmillan Press, London, pp. 315–361 (1983)

48. Venitt, S., Brookes, P. and Lawley, P.D. Effects of alkylating agents on the induced synthesis of beta-galactosidase by *Escherichia coli* B. *Biochimica Biophysica Acta*, **155**, 521–535 (1968)

49. Roberts, J.J. and Friedlos, F. Quantitative estimation of cisplatin-induced DNA interstrand cross-links and their repair in mammalian cells: relationship to toxicity. *Pharmacology and Therapeutics*, **34**, 215–246 (1987)

50. Green, M.H.L., Muriel, W.J. and Bridges, B.A. Use of a simplified fluctation test to detect low levels of mutagens. *Mutation Research*, **38**, 33–42 (1976)

51. Lown, J.W. The chemistry of DNA damage by antitumour drugs. In *Molecular Aspects of Anti-Cancer Drug Action* (eds S. Neidle and M.J. Waring), Macmillan Press, London, pp. 283–314 (1983)

52. Iyer, V.N. and Szybalski, W. A molecular mechanism of mitomycin C action: linking of complementary DNA strands. *Proceedings of the National Academy of Sciences of the USA*, **50**, 355–362 (1963)

53. Tomasz, M., Lipman, R., Chowdary, D. *et al.* Isolation and structure of a covalent cross-link adduct between mitomycin C and DNA. *Science*, **235**, 1204–1208 (1987)

54. Reddy, M.V. and Randerath, K. $^{32}$P-analysis of DNA adducts in somatic and reproductive tissues of rats treated with the anticancer antibiotic, mitomycin C. *Mutation Research*, **179**, 75–88 (1987)

55. Ward, J.F. Molecular mechanisms of radiation induced damage to nucleic acids. *Advances in Radiation Biology*, **5**, 181–239 (1975)

56. Bernhard, W.A. Solid-state radiation chemistry of DNA: the bases. *Advances in Radiation Biology*, **9**, 199–280 (1981)

57. Greenstock, C.L. Free-radical processes in radiation and chemical carcinogenesis. *Advances in Radiation Biology*, **11**, 269–293 (1984)

58. Vuillaume, M. Reduced oxygen species, mutation, induction and cancer initiation. *Mutation Research*, **186**, 43–72 (1987)

59. Meneghini, R. Genotoxicity of active oxygen species in mammalian cells. *Mutation Research*, **195**, 215–230 (1988)

60. IARC. *IARC Monographs on the Evaluation of the Carcinogenic Risk of Chemicals to Man. Some Naturally Occurring Substances*, Vol. 10, International Agency for Research on Cancer, Lyon, pp. 171–176 (1976)

61. Singh, B. and Gupta, R.S. Comparison of the mutagenic responses of 12 anticancer drugs at the hypoxanthine-guanine phosphoribosyl transferase and adenosine kinase loci in Chinese hamster ovary cells. *Environmental Mutagenesis*, **5**, 871–880 (1983)

62. Adler, I-D. New approaches to mutagenicity studies in animals for carcinogenic and mutagenic agents. II. Clastogenic effects determined in transplacentally treated mouse embryos. *Teratogenesis, Carcinogenesis and Mutagenesis*, **3**, 321–324 (1983)

63. Kram, D., Bynum, G.D., Senula, G.C. *et al. In utero* analysis of sister chromatid exchange: alterations in susceptibility to mutagenic damage as a function of fetal cell type and gestational age. *Proceedings of the National Academy of Sciences of the USA*, **77**, 4784–4787 (1980)

64. King, M.T. and Wild, D. Transplacental mutagenesis: the micronucleus test on fetal mouse blood. *Human Genetics*, **51**, 183–194 (1979)

65. Ohtsuru, M., Ishii, Y., Takai, S-I. *et al.* Sister

chromatid exchanges in lymphocytes of cancer patients receiving mitomycin-C treatment. *Cancer Research*, **40**, 477–480 (1980)

66. Kaldor, J. and Schmähl, D. Carcinogenicity of alkylating cytostatic drugs: conclusions and directions for future research. In *Carcinogenicity of Alkylating Cytostatic Drugs*, IARC Scientific Publications No. 78 (eds D. Schmähl and J.M. Kaldor), International Agency for Research on Cancer, Lyon, pp. 321–323 (1986)

67. Greene, M.H., Harris, E.L., Gershenson, D.M. *et al.* Melphalan may be a more potent leukemogen than cyclophosphamide. *Annals of Internal Medicine*, **105**, 360–367 (1986)

68. Baker, G.L., Kahl, L.E., Zee, B.C. *et al.* Malignancy following treatment of rheumatoid arthritis with cyclophosphamide. *American Journal of Medicine*, **83**, 1–9 (1987)

69. Henderson, E.E., Franks, C. and Fronko, G. Chemical carcinogen Epstein–Barr virus (EBV) synergism: EBV genome amplification and site-specific mutation during transformation. *International Journal of Cancer*, **43**, 72–79 (1989)

70. Petru, E. and Schmähl, D. Second malignancies – risk reduction. *Cancer Treatment Reviews*, **14**, 337–343 (1987)

71. Kaldor, J.M., Day, N.E., Pettersson, F. *et al.* Leukemia following chemotherapy for ovarian cancer. *New England Journal of Medicine*, **322**, 1–6 (1990)

72. Rosenberg, B. Cisplatin: its history and possible mechanisms of action. In *Cisplatin. Current Status and New Developments* (eds A.W. Prestayko, S.T. Crooke and S.K. Carter), Academic Press, New York, pp. 9–20 (1980)

73. Roberts, J.J. and Pera, M.F. Jr. DNA as a target for anticancer coordination compounds. In *Platinum, Gold and Other Metal Chemotherapeutic Agents: Chemistry and Biochemistry* (ed. S.J. Lippard), American Chemical Society, Washington, DC, pp. 1–25 (1983)

74. Knox, R.J., Friedlos, F., Lydall, D.A. and Roberts, J.J. Mechanism of cytotoxicity of anticancer platinum drugs: evidence that *cis*-diamminedichloroplatinum (II) and *cis*-diammine-(1,1- cyclobutanedicarboxylato-platinum(II) differ only in the kinetics of their interaction with DNA. *Cancer Research*, **46**, 1972–1979 (1986)

75. Venitt, S. and Crofton-Sleigh, C. Use of bacterial mutation assays and the SOS Chromotest in an investigation of the mode of action of four platinum anti-tumour drugs. *Mutagenesis*, **1**, 78 (1986)

76. Pleskova, I., Blasko, M. and Siracky, J. Chromosomal aberrations, sister chromatid exchange (SCEs) and micronuclei induction with three platinum compounds (*cis*-DDP, CHIP, CBDCA) in V79 cells *in vitro*. *Neoplasma*, **31**, 655–659 (1984)

77. Shinkai, T., Saijo, N., Eguchi, K. *et al.* Cytogenetic effect of carboplatin on human lymphocytes. *Cancer Chemotherapy and Pharmacology*, **21**, 203–207 (1988)

78. Jang, J.J., Takahashi, M., Hasegawa, R. *et al.* Mammary and renal tumor induction by low doses of adriamycin in Sprague-Dawley rats. *Carcinogenesis*, **8**, 1149–1153 (1987)

79. Marzin, D., Jasmin, C., Maral, R. and Mathe, G. Mutagenicity of eight anthracycline derivatives in five strains of *Salmonella typhimurium*. *European Journal of Cancer and Clinical Oncology*, **19**, 641–647 (1983)

80. Westendorf, J., Marquardt, H. and Marquardt, H. Structure-activity relationships of anthracycline-induced genotoxicity *in vitro*. *Cancer Research*, **44**, 5599–5604 (1984)

81. Myers, C.E., Mimnaugh, E.G., Yeh, G.C. and Sinha, B.K. Biochemical mechanisms of tumor cell kill by the anthracyclines. In *Bioactive Molecules Volume 6. Anthracycline and Anthracenedione-based Anticancer Agents* (ed. J.W. Lown), Elsevier, Amsterdam, pp. 527–569 (1988)

82. Myers, C. Anthracyclines. In *Cancer Chemotherapy 8. The EORTC Cancer Chemotherapy Annual* (eds H.M. Pinedo and B.A. Chabner), Elsevier, Amsterdam, pp. 52–64 (1986)

83. Ross, W.E., Sullivan, D.M. and Chow, K-C. Altered function of DNA topoisomerases as a basis for antineoplastic drug action. In *Important Advances in Oncology* (eds V.T. DeVita, S. Hellman and S.A. Rosenberg), J.B. Lippincott, Philadelphia, pp. 65–81 (1988)

84. Casazza, A.M. Anthracyclines as inducers of tumor cell differentiation. In *Anthracycline and Anthracenedione-based Anticancer Agents* (ed. J.W. Lown), Elsevier, Amsterdam, pp. 715–734 (1988)

85. Evans, H.J. and O'Riordan, M.L. Human peripheral blood lymphocytes for the analysis of chromosome aberrations in mutagen tests. In *Handbook of Mutagenicity Test Procedures* (eds B.J. Kilbey, M. Legator, W. Nichols and C. Ramel), Elsevier, Amsterdam, pp. 261–274 (1977)

86. Natarajan, A.T. Origin and significance of chromosomal alterations. In *Mutations in Man* (ed. G. Obe), Springer-Verlag, Berlin/Heidelberg, pp. 156–176 (1984)

87. Noval, R.F., Kharasch, E.D., Frank, P. and Runge-Morris, M. Anthracyclines, anthracenediones and anthrapyrazoles: comparison of redox cycling activity and effects on lipid peroxidation and prostaglandin production. In *Anthracycline and Anthracenedione-based Anticancer Agents* (ed. J.W. Lown), Elsevier, Amsterdam, pp. 475–526 (1988)

88. Durr, F.E. Biochemical pharmacology and tumor biology of mitoxantrone and ametantrone. In *Anthracycline and Anthracenedione-based Anticancer Agents* (ed. J.W. Lown), Elsevier, Amsterdam, pp. 163–200 (1988)

89. DeMarini, D.M., Doerr, C.L., Meyer, M.K. *et al.* Mutagenicity of *m*-AMSA and *o*-AMSA in mamma-

lian cells due to clastogenic mechanism: possible role of topoisomerase. *Mutagenesis*, **2**, 349–355 (1987)

90. Andersson, H.C. and Kihlman, B.A. The production of chromosomal alterations in human lymphocytes by drugs known to interfere with the activity of DNA topisomerase II. I. *m*-AMSA. *Carcinogenesis*, **10**, 123–130 (1989)

91. de la Iglesia, F.A., Fitzgerald, J.E., McGuire, E.J. *et al.* Bacterial and mammalian cell mutagenesis, sister-chromatid exchange, and mouse lung adenoma bioassay with the antineoplastic acridine derivative amsacrine. *Journal of Toxicology and Environmental Health*, **14**, 667–681 (1984)

92. Wilson, W.R., Harris, N.M. and Ferguson, L.R. Comparison of the mutagenic and clastogenic activity of amsacrine and other DNA-intercalating drugs in cultured V79 Chinese hamster cells. *Cancer Research*, **44**, 4420–4431 (1984)

93. Ferguson, L.R., Van Zilj, P. and Baguley, B.C. Comparison of the mutagenicity of amsacrine with that of a new clinical analogue, CI-921. *Mutation Research*, **204**, 207–217 (1988)

94. Issell, B.F., Rudolph, A.R. and Louie, A.C. Etoposide (VP-16-213): an overview. In *Etoposide (VP-16). Current Status and New Developments* (eds B.F. Issell, F.M. Muggia and S.K. Carter), Academic Press, Orlando, pp. 1–11 (1984)

95. Tominaga, K., Shinkai, T., Saijo, N. Cytogenetic effects of etoposide (VP-16) on human lymphocytes; with special reference to the relation between sister chromatid exchange and chromatid breakage. *Japanese Journal of Cancer Research (Gann)*, **77**, 385–391 (1986)

96. Gupta, R.S., Bromke, A., Bryant, D.W. *et al.* Etoposide (VP16) and teniposide (VM26): novel anticancer drugs, strongly mutagenic in mammalian but not in prokaryotic test systems. *Mutagenesis*, **2**, 179–186 (1987)

97. DeMarini, D.M., Brock, K.H., Doerr, C.L. and Moore, M.M. Mutagenicity and clastogenicity of teniposide (VM-26) in L5178Y TK+/−3.7.2C mouse lymphoma cella. *Mutation Research*, **187**, 141–149 (1987)

98. Nakanomyo, H., Hiraoka, M. and Shiraya, M. Mutagenicity tests of etoposide and teniposide. *Journal of Toxicological Sciences*, **11**, 301–310 (1986)

99. Muraoka, Y., Takita, T. and Umezawa, H. Bleomycin and peplomycin. In *Cancer Chemotherapy 8* (eds H.M. Pinedo and B.A. Chabner), Elsevier, Amsterdam, pp. 65–72 (1986)

100. Sikic, B.I. Clinical pharmacology of bleomycin. In *Bleomycin Chemotherapy* (eds B.I. Sikic, M. Rozencweig and S.K. Carter), Academic Press, Orlando, pp. 37–43 (1985)

101. Degraeve, N. Genetic and related effects of *Vinca rosea* alkaloids. *Mutation Research*, **55**, 31–42 (1978)

102. Ehling, U.H., Kratochvilova, J., Lehmacher, W. and Neuhauser-Klaus, A. Mutagenicity testing of vincris-tine sulfate in germ cells of male mice. *Mutation Research*, **209**, 107–113 (1988)

103. Röhrborn, G. and Basler, A. *In vitro* and *in vivo* studies on possible mutagenic effects of the Vinca alkaloid vindesine sulfate. In *Proceedings of the International Vinca Alkaloid Symposium – Vindesine*, (eds W. Brade, G.A. Nagel and S. Seeber), S. Karger, Basel, pp. 43–52 (1981)

104. Basler, A. Aneuploidy-inducing chemicals in yeast evaluated by the micronucleus test. *Mutation Research*, **174**, 11–13 (1986)

105. Önfelt, A. Mechanistic aspects on chemical induction of spindle disturbances and abnormal chromosome numbers. *Mutation Research*, **168**, 249–300 (1986)

106. Hook, E.B. ICPEMPC Working Paper 5/3. Perspectives in Mutation Epidemiology: 3. Contribution of chromosome abnormalities to human morbidity and mortality and some comments upon surveillance of chromosome mutation rates. *Mutation Research*, **114**, 389–423 (1983)

107. German, J. Heritable conditions that predispose to cancer. In *Genetics in Clinical Oncology* (eds R.S.K. Chaganti and J. German), Oxford University Press, New York, pp. 80–89 (1985)

108. Kunz, B.A. Mutagenesis and deoxyribonucleotide pool imbalance. *Mutation Research* **200**, 133–147 (1988)

109. Clements, J., Howe, D., Phillips, M. and Todd, N.K. The Drosophila wing test: a comparison of the sensitivity of different strains. *Mutation Research*, **203**, 117–123 (1988)

110. Bertino, J.R. Methotrexate: molecular pharmacology. In *Cancer and Chemotherapy. Volume III. Antineoplastic Agents* (eds S.T. Crooke and A.W. Prestayko), Academic Press, New York, pp. 311–322 (1981)

111. Allegra, C.J., Baram, J., Chabner, B.A. *et al.* Antimetabolites. In *Cancer Chemotherapy and Biological Response Modifiers Annual 9* (eds H.M. Pinedo, D.L. Longo, and B.A. Chabner), Elsevier, Amsterdam, pp. 1–22 (1987)

112. Goulian, M., Bleile, B. and Tseng, B.Y. Methotrexate-induced misincorporation of uracil into DNA. *Proceedings of the National Academy of Sciences of the USA*, **77**, 1956–1960 (1980)

113. Richards, R.G., Brown, O.E., Gillison, M.L. and Sedwick, W.D. Drug concentration-dependent DNA lesions are induced by the lipid soluble antifolate, piritrexim (BW301U). *Molecular Pharmacology*, **30**, 651–658 (1986)

114. Fraser, D.C. and Pearson, C.K. Is uracil misincorporation into DNA of mammalian cells a consequence of methotrexate treatment? *Biochemical and Biophysical Research Communications*, **135**, 886–893 (1986)

115. Aebersold, P.M. Mutation induction by 5-fluorodeoxyuridine in synchronous Chinese hamster cells. *Cancer Research*, **39**, 808–810 (1979)

116. McKay, E., Higgins, P., Tyrrell, D. and Pringle, C.

Immunogenicity and pathogenicity of temperature-sensitive modified respiratory syncytial virus in adult volunteers. *Journal of Medical Virology*, **25**, 411–421 (1988)

117. Rosenwirth, B., Ziegenhagen, D. and Eggers, H.J. Biochemistry and pathogenicity of echovirus 9. III. Thermosensitive mutants of echovirus 9, strain Barty, with reduced pathogenicity for newborn mice. *Medical Microbiology and Immunology*, **177**, 69–81 (1988)

118. Clendeninn, N.J. Curt, G.A., Allegra, C.J. *et al.* Antimetabolites. In *Cancer Chemotherapy 7. The EORTC Cancer Chemotherapy Annual* (eds H.M. Pinedo and B.A. Chabner), Elsevier, Amsterdam, pp. 1–30 (1985)

119. Lönn, U. and Lönn, S. Interaction between 5-fluorouracil and DNA of human colon adenocarcinoma. *Cancer Research*, **44**, 3414–3418 (1984)

120. Lönn, U. and Lönn, S. DNA lesions in human neoplastic cells and cytotoxicity of 5-fluoropyrimidines. *Cancer Research*, **46**, 3866–3870 (1986)

121. Lönn, U. and Lönn, S. Progressive formation of DNA lesions during treatment with anti-metabolites without incorporation of the drugs into DNA. *Mutation Research*, **200**, 243–247 (1988)

122. Lönn, U. and Lönn, S. Increased levels of DNA lesions induced by leucovorin-5-fluoropyrimidines in human colon adenocarcinoma. *Cancer Research*, **48**, 4153–4157 (1988)

123. Lönn, U. and Lönn, S. Increased growth inhibition and DNA lesions in human colon adenocarcinoma cells treated with methotrexate or 5-fluorodeoxyuridine followed by calmodulin inhibitors. *Cancer Research*, **48**, 3319–3323 (1988)

124. Schuetz, J.D., Wallace, H.J. and Diasio, R.B. 5-Fluorouracil incorporation into DNA of CF-1 mouse bone marrow cells as a possible mechanism of toxicity. *Cancer Research*, **44**, 1358–1363 (1984)

125. Schuetz, J.D. and Diasio, R.B. The effect of 5-fluorouracil on DNA chain elongation in intact bone marrow cells. *Biochemical and Biophysical Research Communications*, **133**, 361–367 (1985)

126. Schuetz, J.D., Collins, J.M., Wallace, H.J. and Diasio, R.B. Alteration of the secondary structure of newly synthesized DNA from murine bone marrow cells by 5-fluorouracil. *Cancer Research*, **46**, 119–123 (1986)

127. Schuetz, J.D., Wallace, H.J. and Diasio, R.B. DNA repair following incorporation of 5-fluorouracil into DNA of mouse bone marrow cells. *Cancer Chemotherapy and Pharmacology*, **21**, 208–210 (1988)

128. Goodenough, U. *Genetics*, Saunders College Publishing, Philadelphia, pp. 241–242 (1984)

129. Sowers, L.C., Eritja, R., Kaplan, B. *et al.* Equilibrium between a wobble and ionized base pair formed between fluorouracil and guanine in DNA as studied by proton and fluorine NMR. *Journal of Biological Chemistry*, **263**, 14794–14801 (1988)

130. Yajima, N., Kondo, K. and Morita, K. Reverse mutation tests in *Salmonella typhimurium* and chromosomal aberration tests in mammalian cells in culture on fluorinated pyrimidine derivatives. *Mutation Research*, **88**, 241–254 (1981)

131. Christie, N.T., Drake, S., Meyn, R.E. and Nelson, J.A. 6-Thioguanine-induced DNA damage as a determinant of cytotoxicity in cultured Chinese hamster ovary cells. *Cancer Research*, **44**, 3665–3671 (1984)

132. Maybaum, J., Hink, L.A., Roethel, W.M. and Mandel, H.G. Dissimilar actions of 6-mercaptopurine and 6-thioguanine in Chinese hamster ovary cells. *Biochemical Pharmacology*, **34**, 3677–3682 (1985)

133. Fairchild, C.R., Maybaum, J. and Kennedy, K.A. Concurrent unilateral chromatid damage and DNA strand breakage in response to 6-thioguanine treatment. *Biochemical Pharmacology*, **35**, 3533–3541 (1986)

134. Muller, H.J. Artificial transmutation of the gene. *Science*, **66**, 84–87 (1927)

135. Breimer, L.H. Ionizing radiation-induced mutagenesis. *British Journal of Cancer*, **57**, 6–18

136. DeMarini, D.M., Brockman, H.E., de Serres, F.J. *et al.* Specific-locus mutations induced in eukaryotes (especially mammalian cells) by radiation and chemicals: a perspective. *Mutation Research*, **220**, 11–29 (1989)

137. Boice, J.D. Cancer following medical irradiation. *Cancer*, **47**, 1081–1090 (1981)

138. Kohn, H.I. and Fry, R.J.M. Radiation carcinogenesis. *New England Journal of Medicine*, **310**, 504–511 (1984)

139. Fry, R.J.M. and Storer, J.B. External radiation carcinogenesis. *Advances in Radiation Biology*, **13**, 31–90 (1987)

140. Smith, P.G. and Doll, R. Mortality among patients with ankylosing spondylitis after a single treatment course with X-rays. *British Medical Journal*, **284**, 449–460 (1982)

141. IARC. *Second Cancer in Relation to Radiation Treatment for Cervical Cancer*, IARC Scientific Publications No. 52 (eds N.E. Day and J.D. Boice), International Agency for Research on Cancer, Lyon, pp. 207 (1983)

142. Ishihara, T. and Sasaki, M.S. (eds). *Radiation-Induced Chromosome Damage in Man*, Alan R. Liss, New York, 636 pp. (1983)

143. Buckton, K.E. Chromosome aberrations in patients treated with X-irradiation for ankylosing spondylitis. In *Radiation-Induced Chromosome Damage in Man* (eds T. Ishihara and M.S. Sasaki), Alan R. Liss, New York, pp. 491–511 (1983)

144. Early Breast Cancer Trialists' Collaborative Group. Effects of adjuvant tamoxifen and of cytotoxic therapy on mortality in early breast cancer. *New England Journal of Medicine*, **319**, 1681–1692 (1988)

145. Read, C. Breast cancer: drug ready to stand trial. *New Scientist*, 3 December, 36–37 (1988)

146. Tucker, M.J., Adam, H.K. and Patterson, J.S. Tamoxifen. In *Safety Testing of New Drugs. Laboratory Predictions and Clinical Performance* (eds D.R. Laurence, A.E.M. McClean and M. Weatherall), Academic Press, London, pp. 125–161 (1984)

147. Diver, J.M., Jackson, I.M. and Fitzgerald, J.D. Tamoxifen and non-malignant indications. *Lancet*, **i**, 733 (1986)

148. Fornander, T., Cedermark, B., Mattsson, A. *et al.* Adjuvant tamoxifen in early breast cancer: occurrence of new primary cancers. *Lancet*, **i**, 117–120 (1989)

149. Gottardis, M.M., Robinson, S.P., Satyaswaroop, P.G. and Jordan, V.C. Contrasting actions of tamoxifen on endometrial and breast tumor growth in the athymic mouse. *Cancer Research*, **48**, 812–815 (1988)

150. Yager, J.D., Roebuck, B.D., Paluszcyk, T.L. and Memoli, V.A. Effects of ethinyl estradiol and tamoxifen on liver DNA turnover and new synthesis and appearance of gamma glutamyl transpeptidase-positive foci in female rats. *Carcinogenesis*, **7**, 2007–2014 (1986)

151. Taylor, W. Risk factors associated with the use of sex hormones. *Anticancer Research*, **7**, 943–948 (1987)

152. Pak, K., Iwakasi, T., Miyakawa, M. and Yoshida, O. The mutagenic activity of anti-cancer drugs and the urine of rats given these drugs. *Urological Research*, **7**, 119–124 (1979)

153. Perrella, F.W. and Boutwell, R.K. Triethylenemelamine: an initiator of two-stage carcinogensis in mouse skin which lacks the potential of a complete carcinogen. *Cancer Letters*, **21**, 37–41 (1983)

154. Thompson, D.J., Dyke, I.L. and Molello, J.A. Reproduction and teratology studies on hexamethylmelamine in the rat and the rabbit. *Toxicology and Applied Pharmacology*, **72**, 245–254 (1984)

155. Zijlstra, J.A. and Vogel, E.W. The ratio of induced recessive lethals to ring-X loss has prognostic value in terms of functionality of chemical mutagens in *Drosophila melanogaster*. *Mutation Research*, **201**, 27–38 (1988)

156. Ashby, J., Callander, R.D. and Rose, F.L. Weak mutagenicity to *Salmonella* of the formaldehyde-releasing anti-tumour agent hexamethylmelamine. *Mutation Research*, **142**, 121–125 (1985)

157. Vyas, R.C., Adhvaryu, S.G. and Shah, V.C. Effects of CCNU therapy on human chromosomes. *Mutation Research*, **206**, 163–166 (1988)

158. IARC. *IARC Monographs on the Evaluation of the Carcinogenic Risk of Chemicals to Humans. Some N-nitroso Compounds. Volume 17*, International Agency for Research on Cancer, Lyon, 365 pp. (1978)

159. Manandhar, M., Cheng, M., Iatropoulos, M.J. and Noble, J.F. Genetic toxicology profile of the new antineoplastic drug mitoxantrone in the mammalian test systems. *Arzneimittelforschung*, **36**, 1375–1379 (1986)

160. Nishio, A., DeFeo, F., Cheng, C.C. and Uyeki, E.M. Sister-chromatid exchange and chromosomal aberrations by DHAQ and related anthraquinone derivatives in Chinese hamster ovary cells. *Mutation Research*, **101**, 77–86 (1982)

161. Turchini, M-F., Geneix, A., Perissel, B. *et al.* Typologie d'aberrations chromosomiques induites chez l'Homme par differentes antimitotiques. *Comptes Rendus de Société Biologique*, **179**, 331–339 (1985)

162. Raposa, T. Sister chromatid exchange studies for monitoring DNA damage and repair capacity after cytostatics *in vitro* and in lymphocytes of leukaemic patients under cytostatic therapy. *Mutation Research*, **57**, 241–251 (1978)

163. Pantelias, G.E. and Wolff, S. Cytosine arabinoside is a potent clastogen and does not affect the repair of X-ray-induced chromosome fragments in unstimulated human lymphocytes. *Mutation Research*, **151**, 65–72 (1985)

164. Reidy, J.A. Folate- and deoxyuridine-sensitive chromatid breakage may result from DNA repair during $G_2$. *Mutation Research*, **192**, 217–219 (1987)

165. Timson, J. Hydroxyurea. *Mutation Research*, **32**, 115–132 (1975)

166. Raposa, T. and Varkonyi, J. The relationship between sister chromatid exchange induction and leukemogenicity of different cytostatics. *Cancer Detection and Prevention*, **10**, 141–151 (1987)

167. Bruce, W.R. and Heddle, J.A. The mutagenic activity of 61 agents as determined by the micronucleus. *Salmonella*, and sperm abnormality assays. *Canadian Journal of Genetic Cytology*, **21**, 319–334 (1979)

168. Adams, M. and Warr, J.R. The mutagenic activity of hydroxyurea in *Chlamydomonas reinhardi*. *Mutation Research*, **41**, 217–224 (1976)

169. Zeigler-Skylakakis, K., Schwarz, L.R. and Andrae, U. Microsome- and hepatocyte-mediated mutagenicity of hydroxyurea and related aliphatic hydroxamic acids in V79 Chinese hamster cells. *Mutation Research*, **152**, 225–241 (1985)

170. Singh, H. and Newton, D. Mithramycin- and triethylene melamine-induced sperm abnormalities in Lakeview hamsters. *Environmental Mutagenesis*, **4**, 231–237 (1982)

171. Singh, B. and Gupta, R.S. Species-specific differences in the toxicity and mutagenicity of the anticancer drugs mithramycin, chromomycin A3, and olivomycin. *Cancer Research*, **45**, 2813–2820 (1985)

172. Horton, J.J., MacDonald, D.M. and Wells, R.S. Epitheliomas in patients receiving razoxane therapy for psoriasis. *British Journal of Dermatology*, **109**, 675–678 (1983)

173. Cerio, R., Wells, R.S. and MacDonald, D.M. The sequelae of razoxane therapy. *British Journal of Dermatology*, **113** (Suppl. 29), 27 (1985)

174. Albanese, R. and Watkins, P.A. The mutagenic activity of razoxane (ICRF 159): an anticancer agent. *British Journal of Cancer*, **52**, 725–731 (1985)

175. Witiak, D.T., Lee, H.J., Hart, R.W. and Gibson, R.E. Study of *trans*-cyclopropylbis(diketopiperazine) and chelating agents related to ICRF 159. Cytotoxicity, mutagenicity and effects on scheduled and unscheduled DNA synthesis. *Journal of Medicinal Chemistry*, **20**, 630–635 (1977)

176. Miller, E.G., Washington, V.H., Bowles, W.H. and Zimmermann, E.R. Mutagenic potential of some chemical components of dental materials. *Dental Materials*, **2**, 163–165 (1986)

# 5

# Acute complications of treating pediatric malignancy

C. DeLaat, M. Masterson, I.B. Lefkowitz and B.C. Lampkin

Acute complications of therapy for childhood cancer may occur at any time in the course of treatment and may be the result of any of the modalities of therapy, but most commonly are secondary to the effects of chemotherapeutic agents and/or radiation. Children under 1 year of age are more likely to have complications compared with older children, particularly if doses of chemotherapeutic agents and radiation are not decreased. Currently many children with cancer require intensive therapy to survive the disease. As a consequence, severe acute complications are occurring more frequently during the course of treatment. In this chapter we will discuss the most common severe acute complications and mention less common but significant complications.

Hematological, infectious, gastrointestinal, metabolic or renal and neurological complications are the most common complications which can be life-threatening or fatal. Other complications which may be fatal include cardiopulmonary and dermatological complications.

## Hematological and infectious complications

Hematological and infectious complications are by far the most common acute complications seen in children during the course of treatment. Bone marrow suppression is the most common hematological complication. Neutropenia is usually the first evidence of marrow suppression with thrombocytopenia and then anemia following. The degree of anemia, thrombocytopenia and neutropenia experienced is related to the life span of these cells, the mechanism of action and intensity of the radiation therapy or chemotherapeutic agent employed and

**Table 5.1 Common chemotherapeutic agents. From refs [1–4]**

| | Myelosuppressive nadir (days) | Myelosuppressive duration (days) |
|---|---|---|
| Cycle-specific agents: | | |
| Vincristine | 4 | 7 |
| Vinblastine | 5–9 | 14–21 |
| Bleomycin | N.A. | N.A. |
| Methotrexate | 7–14 | 14–21 |
| 6-Mercaptopurine | 7–14 | 14–21 |
| 6-Thioguanine | 7–14 | 14–21 |
| Cytosine arabinoside | 12–14 | 22–24 |
| Hydroxyurea | 7 | 14–21 |
| Epipodophyllo-toxins | 7–14 | 22–28 |
| | | |
| Cycle non-specific agents: | | |
| Cyclophosphamide | 8–14 | 18–25 |
| Nitrogen mustard | 7–14 | 28 |
| Actinomycin D | 7–15 | 22–25 |
| Anthracyclines | 10–14 | 21–28 |
| Cisplatin | 7–14 | 21–39 |
| Asparaginase | N.A. | N.A. |
| Steroid hormones | N.A. | N.A. |

N.A., not applicable

the amount of reserve marrow stem cells. Patients with a highly infiltrated marrow (leukemia patients or those with a large amount of metastatic tumor to the marrow) or patients with marrow compromised as a result of prior irradiation or chemotherapy will experience a greater degree of suppression in terms of nadir and duration. Agents that affect proliferating cells in all phases of the cell cycle (alkylating agents, anthracyclines) generally have a later onset of cell line suppression but a longer duration of cytopenia than cycle-specific agents (antimetabolites, vinca alkaloids) (Table 5.1) [1–4]. Finally, red blood cells and platelets remain in the circulation for 120 days and 9–12 days, respectively, and neutrophils for 6–8 h [5,6]. If their life span is shortened because of peripheral destruction, blood loss or sequestration, therapy-induced cytopenias are made more severe.

## Leukopenia

Leukopenia is one of the most serious complications of treatment. While the cancer patient also becomes lymphopenic during therapy, it is the duration and degree of granulocytopenia that is related directly to the risk of sepsis and infection [7]. Untreated infections in granulocytopenic patients are usually both rapidly fatal yet difficult to diagnose as the usual hallmarks of inflammation (erythema, swelling, tenderness) may not be apparent. Often fever alone is present and the approach to the febrile, granulocytopenic patient has been extensively reviewed [8–10]. From 55 to 70% of febrile granulocytopenic patients have an infection as an etiology of fever [10] so that the onset of fever (temperature $\geq 38.5\,°C$ or three temperatures $>38\,°C$ in a 24 h period) in a patient with an absolute neutrophil count of $<0.5 \times 10^9/l$ warrants empirical antibiotic therapy. Evaluation of such a patient should begin with an estimate of the degree of clinical toxicity and physical examination with particular emphasis on the common sites of infection in cancer patients (lung, perirectal area, periunguinal areas, all mucosal surfaces). A complete blood count, chest X-ray, blood cultures (from peripheral sites and central venous catheter if present) and other cultures such as throat, rectal, urine, etc. as indicated by examination are obtained. Empiric antibiotic therapy is selected to provide the patient with coverage against the life-threatening organisms that may be responsible for infection. In general this consists of a penicillinase-resistant penicillin or cephalosporin, coverage for Gram-negative organisms and an additional agent to provide two-drug therapy against *Pseudomonas* species is included. Bactericidal coverage is preferred. The best choice must be individualized to each treatment center according to the identification and sensitivities of the local pathogens.

Because of the short life span of neutrophils, complications associated with the administration of granulocytes and lack of efficacy except for Gram-negative infections, granulocyte transfusions are used only in patients with documented Gram-negative infections not improving on appropriate antibiotic therapy [11,12].

If both fever and granulocytopenia persist antibiotics should be continued, an aggressive search for occult foci of infection pursued and strong consideration given for antifungal coverage with amphotericin B.

## Hemostatic abnormalities

Thrombocytopenia is a frequent cause of hemostatic abnormalities in cancer patients. It is usually due to decreased platelet production, but may be due to or made worse by sequestration or enhanced platelet consumption. Although there is no absolute threshold level for platelet counts that will preclude serious hemorrhage, there is evidence that clinically significant bleeding is rare in patients with platelet counts $>20 \times 19^9/l$ [13]. Serious, life-threatening hemorrhage usually does not occur in the setting of thrombocytopenia alone, even with platelet counts $<20 \times 10^9/l$. However, since cancer patients usually have associated abnormalities of hemostasis (e.g. decreased vascular integrity with chemotherapy-induced mucositis, dysfunctional platelets or coagulopathy due to their underlying malignancy or treatment), it has been suggested [14] to transfuse platelets at $20 \times 19^9/l$ or with any degree of thrombocytopenia and active bleeding. Although prophylactic platelet transfusions at this level do decrease the incidence of bleeding in leukemic children, they have not been shown to influence mortality in leukemia [15,16] and their use is controversial. One unit per $m^2$ of body surface area should increase the platelet count by approximately $10 \times 10^9/l$. A general rule of thumb is to give infants 1–3 units, children 3–4 units and adolescents 4–8 units of platelets, with subsequent platelet transfusion requirements established by 1 h and 24 h post-transfusion counts and correlated with achievement of hemostasis.

Qualitative platelet defects can contribute to inadequate hemostasis in the face of normal platelet counts. Several semisynthetic penicillins often used in cancer patients (ticarcillin, carbenicillin and ampicillin among others) have been associated with platelet aggregation defects [17]. Uremia can also decrease platelet aggregation and this defect may be corrected by administering cryoprecipitate [18] or vasopressin [19]. Although these hemostatic defects are usually mild, in the face of thrombocytopenia they can contribute to significant hemorrhage.

Abnormalities of clotting factors in pediatric cancer patients are common and can lead to hemorrhage. Disseminated intravascular coagulation (DIC), characterized by both thrombosis and hemorrhage, disrupts all phases of the coagulation system. DIC in cancer patients can result from sepsis, the underlying malignancy or from chemotherapy. It exists in both acute, and subacute or chronic forms. In the acute form the patients may present with generalized bleeding and shock, whereas in the chronic form the patients have a more subtle presentation of spontaneous bruising, prolonged bleeding time and thrombosis. Patients with chronic DIC can readily evolve to the acute phase; this is sometimes heralded by an acute drop in the platelet count [20]. The laboratory diagnosis of DIC includes prolonged prothrombin time (PT) and partial thromboplastin time (PTT), decreased fibrinogen, increased fibrin degradation products (FDP) and microangiopathic changes on the blood smear. Factor levels are measured only to distinguish DIC from other acquired coagulopathies and to guide replacement therapy.

Management of acute DIC involves meticulous supportive care accompanying treatment of the underlying cause. Fibrinogen can be replaced with cryoprecipitate; 0.25 units/kg of cryoprecipitate will raise fibrinogen by about 125%. Platelets and clotting factors should be replaced as needed by following quantitative measures of platelets and procoagulants. Infants with DIC may require exchange transfusion to provide clotting factors without circulatory overload. The use of heparin remains controversial but is recommended for patients with large thromboses or with life-threatening hemorrhage who have not responded to treatment of the underlying cause [21]. An initial dose of 50–100 units/kg can be given with a continuous infusion maintenance dose of 10–15 units/kg/h and subsequent adjustment to maintain the PTT at 1.5–2 times normal.

Occasionally patients will present with a circulating inhibitor that prolongs the PT or PTT without symptoms of clinical bleeding. A mixed PT or PTT (50:50 with normal plasma) that does not correct will help distinguish these patients from those with chronic DIC. Management of chronic DIC consists entirely of treatment of the underlying cause, with replacement and anticoagulant therapy reserved for progression to clinically apparent hemorrhage or thrombosis.

Acute promyelocytic leukemia, a subtype of acute non-lymphocytic leukemia, is associated with a bleeding diathesis resembling DIC. Coagulation abnormalities include a prolonged PT, increased FDP and decreased fibrinogen. This coagulopathy, secondary to the release of procoagulants from the granules of the leukemic blasts, can progress to acute fulminant DIC [22,23]. Heparin has traditionally been used during induction chemotherapy of these patients to prevent or limit this tendency to develop DIC [24]. Recently [25] the use of routine heparinization for these patients has been questioned if aggressive supportive therapy with factor replacement and platelets is provided. Other subtypes of acute non-lymphoblastic leukemia, particularly those whose abnormal cells exhibit any degree of granularity, can also present with a similar clinical syndrome during induction therapy.

Of the chemotherapeutic agents used to treat childhood cancer, asparaginase has been most frequently associated with coagulation abnormalities. Asparaginase inhibits synthesis of a number of normal proteins including fibrinogen and other procoagulants; however, clinical bleeding is unusual. This is partly because production of antithrombin III and proteins C and S are also inhibited [26,27]. Hemostatic derangement during asparaginase therapy worsens progressively with frequency of administration and most thrombotic or hemorrhagic events occur in the third to fourth week after starting therapy with a typical schedule of 3 days/week administration. Overall, the incidence of hemorrhage or thrombosis associated with asparaginase is 1–2%. For reasons that are unclear, when bleeding or thrombosis occurs it has a predilection for intracranial sites leading to serious morbidity [28–30]. With this in mind, children on asparaginase should receive prompt laboratory investigation of any clinical symptoms suggestive of central nervous system hemorrhage or infarct. Replacement therapy consisting of cryoprecipitate or fresh frozen plasma, guided by factor quantitations, is given to correct the protein deficiencies. In the case of thrombosis, heparin may be indicated. It also is reasonable to provide close monitoring of the PT and fibrinogen of patients with an underlying hemostatic defect who require asparaginase and to treat this group prophylactically if significant abnormalities are detected. This group would include patients with hypercoaguable states such as those with pre-existing thrombus (superior vena cava syndrome) and those with marginal hepatic reserve (infants under 1 year).

## Anemia

Anemia secondary to bone marrow suppression may also be aggravated by blood loss or hemolysis. Hemolysis as a complication of lymphoma has been well described in adults, but occasionally occurs in the pediatric patient with Hodgkin's disease as well. The hemolytic anemia is Coomb's positive and responds to treatment of the underlying disease [31,32]. Cisplatin, an agent used as frontline therapy in several pediatric solid tumors, can be the cause of a severe Coomb's positive hemolytic anemia. The etiology is probably analogous to the hapten mechanism of penicillin-induced immune hemolysis and the hemolysis resolves on withdrawal of cisplatin [33,34]. Newer cisplatin analogues such as carboplatin also have caused this type of hemolysis. A microangiopathic hemolytic anemia has also been associated both with cisplatin and carboplatin therapy [35,36], as well as after therapy with alkylating agents or after bone marrow transplant in adults [37,38]. This anemia is seen in conjunction with thrombocytopenia and renal failure (the cancer-related hemolytic uremic syndrome). Examination of the peripheral smear shows fragmentation and schistocytes consistent with a microangiopathic process and renal involvement can be confirmed by kidney biopsy if necessary. Early recognition of this syndrome and removal of the offending agent is important since the usual supportive measures of anemia (red cell transfusion) and renal dysfunction (fluid therapy) may serve to accelerate the pathological process.

Anemia can be readily treated with transfusion of packed red blood cells to maintain cardiovascular stability and to provide an adequate oxygen-carrying capacity for delivery to tissues. Acute complications of red cell transfusion include immune-mediated transfusion reactions, circulatory overload, hemolysis without symptoms and transmission of endotoxin causing circulatory collapse and coagulopathy. The primary delayed complication of transfusions is the transmission of infectious diseases such as hepatitis, cytomegalovirus (CMV), human immunodeficiency virus and others. Since immunosuppressed CMV sero-negative recipients are at high risk of acquiring CMV infection from a CMV-positive donor, it is optimal to administer CMV-negative blood products to the patients if they undergo severely immunosuppressive chemotherapeutic regimens. A potentially fatal complication occurring in immunosuppressed patients is graft versus host disease from immunocompetent cells transfused into a recipient with impaired immunity [39]. This complication can be avoided by irradiating any blood product with 1500 rad prior to transfusion [40].

## Hyperleukocytosis

Hyperleukocytosis ($>100 \times 10^9$/l leukemic blast cells) is present in approximately 13% of children with acute lymphoblastic leukemia (ALL), 22% of children with acute non-lymphoblastic leukemia (ANLL) [41] and up to 80% of those with chronic myelogenous leukemia (CML) [42]. Complications of leukostasis can involve virtually any organ system, with the more severe morbidity resulting from pulmonary leukostasis, massive intracerebral hemorrhage or metabolic derangements from tumor lysis once chemotherapy is initiated. Risk of intracranial hemorrhage varies from approximately 1% of ALL patients to 11% of ANLL patients presenting with extreme leukocytosis [41]. The mechanism by which leukemic leukocytosis predisposes to an intracerebral bleed is unclear. Blast cell infiltration of vessel walls may lead to loss of vascular integrity and subsequent hemorrhage [43]; alternatively, leukostasis and leukemic thrombi may lead to ischemic microvascular damage and bleeding [44].

Therapeutic techniques for prophylaxis of intracerebral bleeding include cranial irradiation, exchange transfusion and leukopheresis. Of these therapies, exchange transfusion or leukopheresis may provide the best supportive measure since not only will there be protection against intracranial hemorrhage, but also the potential metabolic derangements will be treated by removing blast cells. If aggressive supportive care for metabolic derangements (hydration, alkalinization and allopurinol) is instituted, there is evidence that in ALL patients cranial radiation is not beneficial [45]. Cranial irradiation may have a role as prophylaxis against central nervous system hemorrhage if exchange transfusion cannot be instituted as an emergency, especially in ANLL and CML, or in patients who present with symptoms of intracranial hemorrhage in progress [46]. These symptoms and signs can include headache, stupor, dizziness, ataxia, visual blurring or papilledema. Other supportive measures, such as maintenance of the platelet count above $100 \times 10^9$/l and hemoglobin below 80 g/l (to decrease blood viscosity) should also be instituted.

## Specific infectious problems in leukopenic and immunosuppressed patients

### Pulmonary infiltrates

Most commonly, the cause of pulmonary infiltrates is infectious. Pulmonary infiltrates in non-neutropenic cancer patients can be due to any of the usual infectious pathogens that invade normal children and are generally lobar. Bilateral interstitial disease in the child receiving chemotherapy who is not neutropenic can be caused by mycoplasma, CMV or *Pneumocystis carinii*. Since *Pneumocystis carinii* pneumonia left untreated is usually fatal, these patients should be started on empiric therapy with trimethoprim/sulfamethoxazole (20 mg/kg/day) [10]. Failure to respond or worsening of disease should prompt an aggressive approach to diagnosis. Lung biopsy or bronchoalveolar lavage show the best yield for recovery of an infectious etiology [47,48]. Benefits of these procedures are the exclusion of other treatable infectious agents such as mycoplasma, herpes virus pneumonitis or influenza and possible confirmation of *Pneumocystis* pneumonia, thus allowing early change to pentamidine therapy (4 mg/kg/day) if the patient is unresponsive to trimethoprim/sulfamethoxazole. The use of steroids in patients with overwhelming *Pneumocystis* infection has shown promise, but should be reserved for histologically proven disease [49].

Interstitial pneumonia in neutropenic patients can include any of the usual bacterial pathogens that cause pneumonia (*Pneumococcus*, *Staphylococcus*,

*Hemophilus*) as lobar consolidation may not occur in the absence of leukocytes. These patients are also at high risk for Gram-negative infections including *Pseudomonas*. Prolonged neutropenia sets the stage for fungal superinfection (*Candida*, *Histoplasmosis*, *Aspergillus*). Clinical deterioration after 24–72 h of treatment in these patients warrants lung biopsy or lavage to identify the offending infectious agent if possible [50]. On the other hand, patients who respond to empiric therapy can be treated for 7–10 days after resolution of their neutropenia, thus avoiding the risks of invasive procedures.

### *Varicella zoster infections*

Varicella zoster infections can be fulminant in immunocompromised patients. Untreated primary varicella infections (chicken pox) are associated with a 7% mortality [51] caused by dissemination either to the lungs, central nervous system or gastrointestinal tract. Pediatric cancer patients especially at risk for varicella include those on steroids (most leukemic patients) and those with lymphoma, especially Hodgkin's disease. Recurrent herpes zoster (shingles) can also occur in these patients and cause significant morbidity in terms of neuralgias and the potential for dissemination.

Because of the severity of varicella zoster infections in children with cancer, immunoprophylaxis is given promptly with history of exposure to the virus. Since this virus is one of the most communicable, any exposure warrants the administration of zoster immune globulin (VZIG) and the interruption of chemotherapy. The administration of VZIG within 72 h effectively limits the course of the infection [52]. Chemotherapy may need to be interrupted for a short time after exposure, or withheld if the child develops overt disease until all the lesions are scabbed and no new lesions have appeared for 24 h. Patients who develop overt disease should also be treated with intravenous acyclovir (500 mg/m$^2$ every 8 hours) for 7 days or 2 days after the last day of new vesicle eruption [53]. Localized zoster infections (shingles) can also be treated with acyclovir, but if the patient is not lymphopenic this can be started as an outpatient and intravenous acyclovir reserved for dissemination of disease.

## Gastrointestinal complications

Gastrointestinal complications include nausea, vomiting, diarrhea, constipation, mucositis, esophagitis, typhlitis, pancreatitis, liver disease, and occasionally intestinal obstruction. Also, rarely, appendicitis, cholecystitis, or a ruptured viscus may develop during the course of treatment.

### Nausea, vomiting, diarrhea, constipation, mucositis, esophagitis

Nausea and vomiting are particular problems, especially in teenagers, and not infrequently these patients have anticipatory vomiting. Antiemetics are used in an attempt to decrease the vomiting with varying degrees of success. Hypnosis also may be of help. Constipation is most frequently seen in the patient who fails to take a stool softener while receiving vincristine. Occasionally, this complication causes severe abdominal pain, ileus and intestinal obstruction. Mucositis, and less commonly esophagitis, is a common side effect of chemotherapy, particularly with anthracyclines, methotrexate or cytosine arabinoside. Usually mucositis, pharyngitis and/or esophagitis are self-limited and clear within 1–2 weeks after stopping the drug or drugs. The combination of an anthracycline and cytosine arabinoside may produce severe mucositis and/or esophagitis in the patient with ANLL being induced into a remission. Severe mucositis and/or esophagitis may also occur in patients who receive radiation to the head, neck or mediastinum concomitantly with doxorubicin or actinomycin D [54,55] or can occur with the administration of either one of these drugs within months to years after the irradiation. Severe mucositis is commonly found after various preparative therapies for bone marrow transplantation with or without concomitant irradiation.

Diarrhea occasionally develops after chemotherapy without neutropenia but most commonly is associated with neutropenia, with or without documented sepsis. Not infrequently in the severely neutropenic patient there is mucositis, esophagitis, abdominal pain and multiple ulcers in the intestinal mucosa. These findings are particularly seen in patients undergoing bone marrow transplantation or patients with ANLL or other cancers receiving intensive chemotherapy and may herald severe enterocolitis and perforation of the bowel. Obviously the administration of the offending drugs should be halted and if they need to be continued these complications can usually be lessened by lowering their dosages. Treatment of diarrhea depends upon its etiology. Patients receiving very intensive chemotherapy or undergoing bone marrow transplantation may require supportive hyperalimentation.

Occasionally nausea and vomiting, abdominal pain, constipation or diarrhea may occur during the course of chemotherapy and/or radiotherapy and be the first indicator of a surgical complication not directly associated with therapy. Examples of such surgical complications are intestinal obstruction secondary to adhesions following abdominal surgery and appendicitis, which may develop in the patient whose white blood cell count is either low or normal.

## Typhlitis

This complication, a necrotizing inflammation of the cecum, has been seen particularly in children with acute leukemia and lymphoma who are receiving intensive chemotherapy and who are profoundly neutropenic. The presentation includes fever, abdominal pain (often localized to the right lower quadrant) and diarrhea in a patient with gastrointestinal mucositis. Diagnosis is difficult until the disease progresses to an acute abdomen, but by then mortality is high. Sepsis accompanies typhlitis as the inflamed cecum serves as a portal of entry to the blood, with Gram-negative bacteria and *Candida* being the most common organisms [56]. Surgical intervention, involving the resection of necrotic bowel, in combination with broad-spectrum antibiotic and blood component support, has been reported to improve outcome in these patients [57,58].

Thus, although most gastrointestinal symptoms are sequelae of chemotherapy and/or radiotherapy, a possible unassociated surgical abdomen must be kept in mind in evaluation of these patients.

## Hepatotoxicity

Hepatitis, as manifested by an increase in liver enzymes, is frequently seen during induction therapy in children with ALL or ANLL and during the post-induction intensification phase of therapy in children with ANLL. It also is seen, but less commonly, in children with solid tumors and occasionally in children with ALL during remission. During induction therapy of children with ALL, asparaginase is usually the offending drug and the most consistently abnormal liver function tests are lowered albumin levels and elevated SGOT levels [59,60]. In most cases the drug is continued without problems, but frequent monitoring of liver function studies is required. The offending agents in children with ANLL are usually cytosine arabinoside or 6-thioguanine [60]. In these patients withholding the drug is usually sufficient for the liver enzymes to return towards normal. Similarly, the occasional child with ALL will have elevation of transaminases while receiving 6-mercaptopurine and methotrexate for maintenance therapy. If the hepatitis is drug-related, the enzymes will decrease within days after stopping the drug or drugs. Hepatitis may not be drug-related and other causes should be excluded such as sepsis, hepatitis B, CMV, Epstein–Barr virus (EBV) and herpes simplex virus. If hepatitis persists, sepsis is excluded and the viral serological studies are normal, a liver biopsy may be indicated. The biopsy may demonstrate evidence of viral hepatitis or hepatotoxicity consistent with drugs or veno-occlusive disease. If the biopsy is equivocal, it may be necessary to use DNA hybridization techniques for detecting EBV, CMV and other viruses or immunohistology for detection of hepatitis B viral antigens. Hepatitis (non-A, non-B viral hepatitis), most likely secondary to blood transfusion, is a common etiology of hepatitis but is a diagnosis of exclusion.

Severe liver disease, which can be fatal, may occur when:

1. The liver receives high doses of radiation or when lesser doses of radiation are given in conjunction with drugs which potentiate radiation effects such as actinomycin D and doxorubicin;
2. Radiation or chemotherapy is given to the liver in a patient after a partial hepatectomy and the liver is regenerating; and
3. Very intensive chemotherapy with or without radiotherapy is given in association with either allogenic or autologous bone marrow transplantation.

The pathological findings after radiotherapy and/or chemotherapy in the regenerating liver consist principally of retardation or lack of regeneration [61,62]. In contrast, veno-occlusive disease (see below) is found most commonly after insult to the mature liver by radiotherapy and/or chemotherapy. Both radiation and chemotherapy have been found to retard regeneration of liver after partial hepatectomy by inhibiting both DNA and RNA synthesis [63]. To prevent abnormalities of liver regeneration in the patient who has had 50% or more liver parenchyma removed, chemotherapy or radiotherapy should be delayed for at least 2 weeks after surgery, or even longer if there is evidence of liver dysfunction. The dosage of the chemotherapy drugs to be given should also be decreased.

Children with right-sided Wilms' tumors who require radiotherapy to the tumor bed and chemotherapy may develop a special clinical entity characterized by liver dysfunction and transient leukopenia and thrombocytopenia [61]. Usually there is a modest increase in liver enzymes and alkaline phosphatase. The thrombocytopenia may be mild to severe but usually is more pronounced than the leukopenia. Obviously, drug therapy and radiotherapy need to be interrupted and an assessment of the liver damage made. A liver-spleen scan is helpful in outlining the extent of damage to the liver from irradiation [61]. Usually the thrombocytopenia and hepatic dysfunction lessen within days after stopping therapy. This complication of treatment of patients with right-sided Wilms' tumors is less common today than 10–20 years ago since lower doses of radiation are now given to the tumor bed. A liver biopsy in these patients in the past was consistent with veno-occlusive disease. The biopsy shown in Figure 5.1 was performed in 1970 in a 4-year-old girl with right-sided Wilms' tumor; at the time this clinical entity was just being recognized. This patient today is 23 years old but has evidence

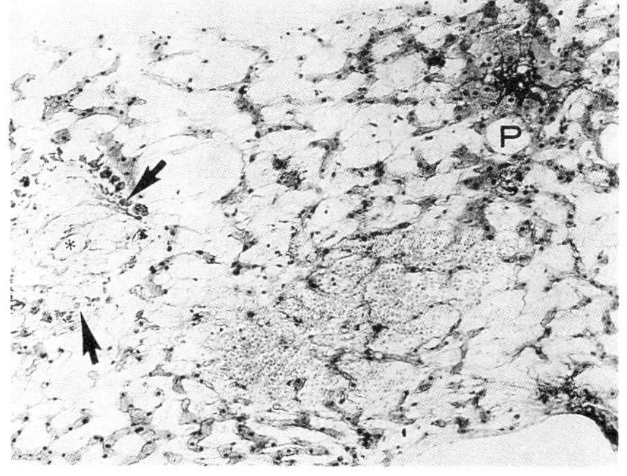

(a)

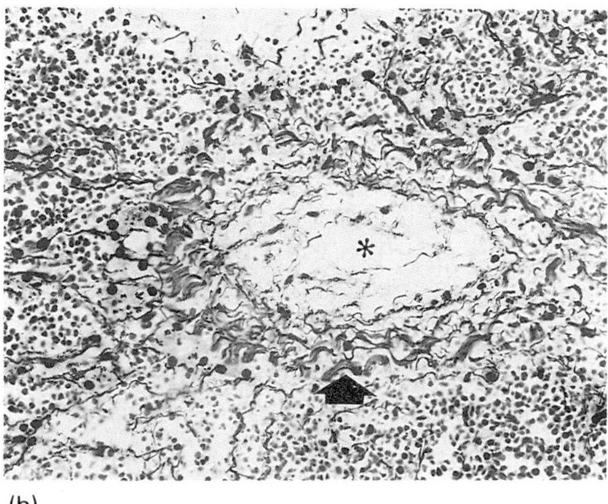

(b)

**Figure 5.1** Veno-occlusive disease post-biopsy. **a** Liver cell plates are atrophic and sinusoids are expanded and engorged. Central vein lumen (*) is markedly reduced by loose connective tissue. Original vein wall (arrows), P, portal area. Trichrome stain. ×200, reduced to 55% on reproduction. **b** Central vein lumen (*) almost completely occluded by new reticulin and loose collagen. Original central vein wall is indicated by arrow. Reticulin stain. ×400, reduced to 55% on reproduction

of portal hypertension and splenic sequestration. A liver biopsy is not indicated today since the clinical syndrome is well known and severe bleeding may occur secondary to thrombocytopenia and other coagulation abnormalities.

Today veno-occlusive disease (VOD) is most commonly seen in patients after bone marrow transplantation but has been reported after the administration of various chemotherapeutic agents, particularly 6-thioguanine and high-dose combination chemotherapy [64–67]. Jones and coworkers

reported an incidence of VOD of about 22% in 235 consecutive patients who underwent bone marrow transplantation [64]. Ninety-one of these patients were 19 years of age or less. In children under 10 years of age the incidence was 8% and was not significantly different from other age groups. The disease is characterized by specific clinical and pathological findings. Evidence of VOD usually develops by day 21 after transplantation and is characterized by hyperbilirubinemia (bilirubin >34 μmol/l) and usually modest elevations of SGOT and alkaline phosphatase. Other associated findings are ascites, hepatomegaly (which is usually painful) and weight gain greater than or equal to 5% over baseline. The diagnosis of VOD based on these clinical criteria was confirmed by histological examination in over 90% of cases; thus, this would therefore support no need for histological examination in a straightforward case. Of the transplant patients developing VOD, 47% died. The clinical presentation of VOD has not been so clearly defined after standard chemotherapy and the incidence is not known but may be increasing with intensive therapy.

The incidence of long-term consequences in children who have had severe liver disease secondary to therapy is unknown but these patients should be followed closely for development of cirrhosis and portal hypertension as they age.

## Pancreatitis

Overall acute pancreatitis is an uncommon complication of treatment of cancer in children but, when it occurs, it most commonly develops in children treated with asparaginase [68]. From 6.5 to 16.2% of children treated with asparaginase have been diagnosed as having acute pancreatitis [68,69]. The disease may develop as long as 16 weeks after treatment. Most of the patients treated with asparaginase also received prednisone and vincristine, but available evidence suggests that asparaginase is the offending agent.

The child presents with nausea, vomiting and abdominal pain and the diagnosis is made by finding elevated values of serum amylase, serum lipase, urinary amylase, an elevated amylase:creatinine clearance ratio or changes in the pancreatic sonogram consistent with pancreatitis. A strong clinical suspicion of pancreatitis must be maintained as serum lipase and amylase levels often remain normal. Usually the pancreatitis is mild and self-limiting but may be fatal [59]. Although very rare, acute pancreatitis also has been reported in a child in association with cytosine arabinoside treatment given in standard dosage and in several adults receiving high-dose cytosine arabinoside [70,71]. It has also been reported following cisplatin infusion in one child [72]. Obviously if pancreatitis is thought to be a toxic effect of a drug, the drug should be stopped. Acute pancreatitis also has been associated with tumor lysis of lymphomatous involvement of the pancreas following combination chemotherapy [73]; chemotherapy should not be stopped in these patients.

# Acute metabolic complications of treating pediatric malignancy

## Acute tumor lysis syndrome

The acute tumor lysis syndrome (ATLS) usually refers to the metabolic complications of hyperuricemia, hyperkalemia, hyperphosphatemia and hypocalcemia seen following treatment of certain malignancies with high growth fractions or exquisite sensitivity to chemotherapy [74–78]. Not all components of this syndrome always develop and these abnormalities may be exacerbated by other associated conditions such as dehydration or sepsis. Tumor lysis syndrome is most commonly seen in children with non-Hodgkin's lymphoma (NHL), particularly Burkitt's lymphoma and T cell lymphoblastic lymphoma, and B cell acute lymphoblastic leukemia (ALL).

Patients with massive tumor burdens such as large abdominal or mediastinal masses, organomegaly secondary to tumor infiltration and high leukocyte counts are at greatest risk of developing tumor lysis syndrome [74,75,79,80]. An elevated serum lactate dehydrogenase (LDH) level (>500 units/l) has also been demonstrated as a risk factor [74,75]. Patients with azotemia, oliguria, hyperuricemia, obstructive nephropathy secondary to a tumor mass, or evidence of other metabolic abnormalities, need to be identified as high risk for developing ATLS. Assessment of renal function should be made in all newly diagnosed patients with ALL or NHL and appropriate arrangements made early for possible intervention with renal supportive measures in those identified to be at high risk for ATLS.

Clinically there is an acute onset of renal dysfunction within the first 1–3 days following chemotherapy administration, although a small percentage of children can be in renal failure at presentation [74,79,81]. The degree of renal impairment can range from mild elevations of blood urea nitrogen (BUN) and creatinine to oliguria or complete renal failure. The initial symptoms in children are related to renal dysfunction and consist of lethargy, nausea, vomiting and occasionally flank pain secondary to uric acid calculi. Fatalities have resulted in this setting as a result of renal failure illustrating the need for proper assessment and management of these various metabolic disturbances which will be considered individually below.

## Hyperuricemia

The lysis of malignant cells produces a high purine load from destruction of nuclei which must be then degraded to uric acid. Uric acid is filtered by glomeruli and secreted in the renal tubules leading to precipitation in the distal nephron and obstruction. Several factors potentiate this:

1. Because of the excess serum concentration there is an increased secretion of uric acid.
2. Urine tends to be maximally concentrated in the distal tubules and collecting ducts.
3. In the increased acidity of the urine in the distal nephron (usual pH 5) uric acid exists predominantly as the less soluble, unionized form (p$K$ 5.4).

Often these patients will demonstrate uric acid crystals in their urine. An elevated serum uric acid out of proportion to elevation of BUN and creatinine suggests uric acid nephropathy [75]. A urine uric acid : creatinine ratio greater than 1 also appears specific to hyperuricemic nephropathy [75,82]. There is also evidence of higher excretion of uric acid, hypoxanthine and xanthine/dl of glomerular filtrate in patients who go on to develop acute renal failure [83].

## Treatment

Regardless of the initial uric acid level, all newly diagnosed patients with ALL or NHL, especially those with bulky disease, should receive treatment for existing or potential uric acid nephropathy prior to institution of cytotoxic therapy. This consists of promoting uric acid excretion and decreasing uric acid production.

Allopurinol is a competitive inhibitor of the enzyme xanthine oxidase which catalyzes two steps in the degradation of purines to uric acid; the conversion of hypoxanthine to xanthine and xanthine to uric acid. Allopurinol is effective in lowering the serum uric acid concentration when elevated at diagnosis and blunting the expected rise following the onset of therapy, thus preventing acute uric acid nephropathy. The standard dose of allopurinol used in children is 300 mg/m$^2$/day (or 10 mg/kg/day) but doses up to 500 mg/m$^2$/day for 2–3 days should be utilized in patients with massive tumor loads. The occurrence of nephrotoxicity secondary to increased urinary xanthine and xanthine stones has been reported in these patients with allopurinol use [84]. The most common side effects seen with allopurinol consist of an erythematous maculopapular rash (with increased incidence with concomitant ampicillin use), gastrointestinal upset, fever and hepatotoxicity. Allopurinol should be discontinued if rash develops because it can progress to a severe hypersensitivity reaction. Caution should be exercised in children requiring 6-mercaptopurine if still receiving allopurinol as 6-mercaptopurine is degraded by xanthine oxidase. If allopurinol is given concurrently, decreased clearance of 6-mercaptopurine administered at full dose can result in significant myelosuppression and other side effects.

Optimal hydration promotes increased excretion of uric acid by lowering the concentration of uric acid in the renal tubules with increased urine flow. Any underlying dehydration should be corrected and hydration fluids provided 1.5–2 times maintenance rate to keep the urine specific gravity less than 1.010. Alkalinization of the urine to achieve a urine pH of 7 or more increases the solubility of uric acid up to ten times that of acidic urine [85]. This can be accomplished by administering intravenous fluid of 5% dextrose at $3000\,ml/m^2/day$ with 150–200 mmol/$m^2$/day of $NaHCO_3$. It should be kept in mind that once uric acid has normalized, the allopurinol dose should be decreased and alkalinization stopped. Patients should receive these therapeutic or prophylactic measures for the first 24–48 h prior to administration of chemotherapy while the diagnostic workup is being completed. The overall fluid status of the patient must be monitored carefully (intake, urine output, weight, etc.) as some patients already in acute renal failure will not be able to excrete a high fluid intake and will develop volume overload. The following laboratory parameters should be monitored every 6 h at a minimum (and more frequently if problems develop): electrolytes, BUN, creatinine, calcium, phosphorus, magnesium, uric acid and urine pH.

If renal function deteriorates and urine output decreases, diuretic (furosemide 1 mg/kg by intravenous push) or mannitol (0.5–1.0 g/kg intravenously over 20 min) therapy should be tried to promote diuresis. Diuretics are preferred if the patient is oliguric because unexcreted mannitol will promote volume overload. If these measures fail or signs of renal failure develop, dialysis should be instituted (Table 5.2) [86].

Hemodialysis is preferred to peritoneal dialysis, if available, as it removes uric acid 10–20 times more efficiently [85,87]. These patients often also have bulky abdominal tumors which make peritoneal dialysis difficult. Continuous arteriovenous hemofiltration has been used in these children to alleviate fluid overload and azotemia [88,89]. We have recently used the technique of continuous arteriovenous hemodiafiltration (CAVHD) in three children with extensive Burkitt's lymphoma and B cell leukemia in renal failure at presentation [90].

**Table 5.2 Metabolic management of pediatric oncology patients. Adapted from ref. [86]**

1. Hydration:      $3000\,ml/m^2/day$

2. Alkalinization: 150–200 mEq/$m^2$/day $NaHCO_3$ (titrate to maintain urine pH >7.0)

3. Allopurinol:    $300\,mg/m^2/day$ or 10 mg/kg/day; increase to $500\,mg/m^2/day$ in patients with high risk of developing ATLS

4. Withhold chemotherapy until metabolic status stabilized

5. Monitor the following closely: electrolytes, BUN, creatinine, uric acid, calcium, phosphorus, magnesium, urine output

6. Indications for dialysis:
   serum $K^+$ $\geq 6.0$ mmol/l
   uric acid $\geq 600\,\mu$mol/l
   phosphorus $\geq 3.2$ mmol/l or rising rapidly
   symptomatic hypocalcemia, hyponatremia or hypomagnesemia
   volume overload or severe hypertension unresponsive to medical management

CAVHD has the efficiency of hemodialysis for removal of solutes and water but avoiding the more dangerous volume and osmolar shifts seen with hemodialysis in children. In all of these children, the metabolic complications of ATLS were easily managed with CAVHD and all recovered with normal renal function. Most patients will require dialysis or filtration for an average of 7 days. In almost all patients signs of diuresis and evidence of normalization of uric acid and renal function tests is evident by 48 h with eventual full recovery of renal function and no permanent renal damage. It is important to stress that there is a significant correlation between length of oliguria predialysis to length of recovery of renal function following institution of dialysis. One should not delay in initiating dialysis when oliguria is present and not improving with supportive care [87]. Early dialysis or hemodiafiltration may also facilitate management of other serious metabolic complications of ATLS. Radiation therapy if tumor infiltration of the kidneys is present can also improve renal function.

## *Hyperkalemia*

Massive tumor lysis can result in an early (within 12–48 h) and sudden elevation in serum potassium ($K^+$) that can be fatal [74,91]. Any underlying renal dysfunction will only accentuate the inability of the kidneys to excrete a high $K^+$ load. Acidosis, potassium-containing fluids or medications and $K^+$

**Table 6.4 (a) Risk factors for treatment-related infections and (b) prophylaxis against treatment-related infection**

(a)
Treatment-related factors:
 Degree of myelosuppression
 Duration of myelosuppression
 High-dose corticosteroids
 Use of indwelling central venous catheters
 Invasive procedures

Host factors:
 Disease-related immunodeficiencies (e.g. myeloma)
 Chronic infections, e.g. periodontal disease, chronic
 bronchitis, diverticular disease, old tuberculosis
 Asymptomatic carriage of specific organisms, e.g. *Staph.
 aureus*, *Aspergillus*
 Seropositivity to latent viruses (herpes simplex, CMV)
 Seronegativity to common viruses (e.g. CMV)

Environmental factors:
 Local pathogens, e.g. antibiotic-resistant organisms,
 *Aspergillus*
 Inadequate facilities

(b)
Host:
 Treatment of pre-existing infections
 Rigorous oral hygiene
 Bowel sterilization
 Prophylactic immunoglobulin
 Prophylaxis *versus* specific infections (e.g. *Pneumocystis
 carinii*)

Environment
 Cleanliness
 Handwashing
 Protected environment, e.g. side room, laminar flow
 and reverse-barrier measures (as appropriate)

## Host factors

As stated, the majority of neutropenic infections are caused by endogenous organisms. These line the skin and the mucosa of gastrointestinal and urogenital tracts. It follows that breaks in the skin or mucosal surface increase the incidence of infection. Thus invasive procedures such as venous cannulation, rectal examination or insertion of a urinary catheter can be hazardous, and mucositis or enteritis complicating cytotoxic or radiotherapy may be a portal for entry of bacteria [74].

Pre-existing foci of infection, such as periodontal disease or skin sepsis, predispose to systemic infection during neutropenia. Surveillance cultures can identify patients at risk of candidal and staphylococcal infection [75]. Patients who are seropositive for herpes simplex are at high risk of reactivation of the virus while immunosuppressed [76]. Although such reactivation is usually amenable to prompt specific therapy with acyclovir when it occurs, the associated

breach in the oral or perineal mucosa introduces further hazards from opportunistic infection [77]. Conversely, seronegativity to cytomegalovirus (CMV) is associated with a high incidence of infection with this organism in very intensively treated patients, unless a policy is adopted whereby screening effectively excludes transfusion of blood products collected from seropositive donors [78].

## *Prophylaxis against infection* (see Table 6.4b)

Reduction of the risk from infection during periods of neutropenia may be effected by the adoption of the following measures. Which steps are appropriate in a given situation will depend upon the predicted degree and duration of myelosuppression, and whether or not there are host or environmental factors which predispose to specific infections.

### *Bowel decontamination*

Neutropenic patients are at particular risk of Gram-negative septicaemia. Endogenous acquisition of the infection from the oral or gastrointestinal flora is the usual route. Gram-negative septicaemias have a high acute mortality even if broad-spectrum antibiotics are instituted early. The incidence of such infections can be reduced if the bowel is treated with oral antibiotics which will deplete the endogenous colonization of Gram-negative aerobic organisms such as *E. coli* and *Pseudomonas* spp. Co-trimoxazole [79] as well as the quinolones such as norfloxacin [80], has been shown to be effective at reducing the rate of Gram-negative infection, and does not appear to interfere with the resistance to colonization provided by the colonic anaerobic microflora. Co-trimoxazole has the disadvantage of delaying time to recovery of the granulocyte count, which may be of relevance at least in patients recovering from bone marrow transplantation [81].

Oral antifungals such as amphotericin [82] and possibly ketoconazole can reduce the incidence of infection from *Candida*, which is also acquired from the gastrointestinal tract.

### *Antiviral prophylaxis*

Acyclovir either orally or intravenously has been used as prophylaxis against reactivation of herpes simplex virus and herpes zoster infection in intensively treated patients. The cost and the small risk of development of resistant strains has discouraged some groups, and in patients with persisting immune incompetence, e.g. those who have undergone bone marrow transplantation, the risk of reactivation of virus returns when prophylaxis is discontinued [83]. At the authors' unit, oral acyclovir is continued for

1 year after bone marrow transplantation for recurrent leukaemia or non-Hodgkin's lymphoma as prophylaxis against zoster infection.

CMV is an important pathogen, particularly in recipients of allogeneic bone marrow who remain on immunosuppressive therapy, and others who have delayed immune reconstitution such as recipients of transplanted marrow that has been manipulated *in vitro* with the intention of depleting subsets of the normal lymphocyte population. The major sources of infection are transfused blood products in seronegative individuals and reactivation of latent virus in seropositives. The former group can be helped by exclusion of seropositive blood and platelet products by serological testing, such that 95% of patients can avoid acquisition of the virus [84]. CMV positive patients may benefit from attempts to suppress virus reactivation with an antiviral agent such as ganciclovir; encouraging results are available from a series of patients with AIDS who have been treated with this drug [85] although further information is required and there may be significant myelotoxicity.

## Prophylactic measures against specific organisms

*Pneumocystis carinii* is most frequently a problem in patients receiving regimens which include high doses of corticosteroid. The infection may occur in the absence of prolonged neutropenia. Effective prophylaxis has been documented in childhood acute lymphoblastic leukaemia with co-trimoxazole [86], and this agent is sometimes used, for example in the authors' unit, where moderately myelosuppressive treatment including a prolonged course of prednisolone is used in the treatment of non-Hodgkin's lymphoma.

Aspergillosis is an airborne infection and colonization of the upper respiratory tract can progress to invasive infections of the lung and systemic dissemination. Air filtration and laminar flow units may help to prevent acquisition of the organism, and local intranasal instillation of amphotericin has been used prophylactically in one unit with encouraging results [87]. The new oral antifungal itraconazole has activity against *Aspergillus* and it remains to be seen whether this agent will be of value in preventing this infection in high-risk units.

## The use of prophylactic immunoglobulin

A current UK Medical Research Council trial is assessing the value of gammaglobulin replacement in patients with myeloma undergoing intensive chemotherapy. This group are at high risk of serious bacterial sepsis and a high early death rate recently reported in patients receiving a chemotherapy regimen of moderate intensity comprising doxorubicin, vincristine and methylprednisolone underlines the need for effective augmentation of their defence against infection [88].

Prophylactic administration of intravenous hyperimmune globulin against CMV has reduced the incidence of infection in treated patients compared with untreated controls [89].

## Management of infection in neutropenic patients

### Unexplained fever

It is accepted that despite prophylactic measures, infections in granulocytopenic patients are frequently unavoidable. The majority of patients who are severely granulocytopenic for more than 1 week will develop fever due to presumed or microbiologically confirmed infection. Infection in the neutropenic host may present without local signs of sepsis; fever is the most important indicator which should prompt the institution of antibiotics even though the results of bacteriological investigations are not available, and an alternative explanation for the fever is considered, such as a drug reaction (e.g. the cytotoxic drugs bleomycin and cytosine arabinoside) or transfusion reaction. The importance of vigilant and experienced staff in observing and acting upon early signs cannot be overstated.

Antibiotics are not started before specimens are obtained for culture. Clinical examination to search for a source of infection is complemented by routine chest X-ray. This latter is performed because in neutropenic patients chest infection may be unaccompanied by signs or symptoms; however, even where the chest is the site of infection, the fever may precede the development of radiological abnormality. In the absence of symptoms, the frequency with which a diagnosis of pneumonia is made in a neutropenic patient with fever may be <5% [90].

There is considerable debate concerning the most appropriate therapy for the neutropenic host with significant fever (e.g. >38°C for 4 h or any fever in the presence of clinical signs). In the majority of centres a combination of an aminoglycoside and a broad-spectrum penicillin or cephalosporin is used. Some have argued in favour of monotherapy with ceftazidime [91], reducing the cost and nephrotoxicity of a combined approach, but although mortality has not been shown to be increased, other measurable end points such as resolution of fever without the use of further antibiotics are achieved less frequently.

With persisting neutropenia second infections occurring despite antibiotics are frequently encountered, and so continuing or recurrent fever should not necessarily be taken to indicate failure of the chosen combination [92]. If the fever resolves it has been said that the antibiotics should be continued until there has been recovery of the granulocyte count [93]. At the authors' unit antibiotics are continued for a minimum of 5 days and for at least 48 h after the lysis of fever.

Where positive cultures are obtained, an appropriate change from the empirical combination should be made. It has been shown that where two antibiotics selected empirically both have activity against the organism eventually isolated, the success rate is greater than if the organism is sensitive to only one of the pair [94,95]. This argues in favour of the use of two antibiotics in all but exceptional circumstances.

When fever fails to lyse, second line empirical therapy should be instituted, for example, after 48 h. In the absence of positive cultures and with no response to first or second line antibiotics, the likelihood of fungal infection increases significantly; it also increases with duration of neutropenia [96]. Fungal infection may be difficult to diagnose from serological tests and radiological investigation. Cultures are frequently negative even from biopsy tissue. The presence of fungal infection is widely underdiagnosed, as is apparent from the high rate of infection observed in cytopenic patients who come to post-mortem [97], although in this circumstance the importance of the fungal pathogen to the previous clinical state of the host is unclear. A low threshold for suspicion, and in some instances the empirical use of amphotericin B, is indicated [98]. Unfortunately amphotericin has low activity against *Aspergillus* and is toxic; newer antifungal agents such as itraconazole may have broader activity as well as lower toxicity, but at present cannot be regarded as effective alternatives.

CMV is the viral infection most important to consider in the neutropenic patient with unexplained fever. Since treatment for the major complication, CMV pneumonitis, is unsatisfactory once established, it is likely that early diagnosis of infection with the agent leads to more favourable outcome. The optimal management of infection is unclear, but there is some evidence that high-dose acyclovir may reduce the incidence of virus reactivation in seropositive patients [99], and established infection may respond to a combination of passive immunization with anti-CMV immunoglobulin and one of the new antiviral agents, ganciclovir or foscarnet [100].

## Gram-positive infection

Gram-negative septicaemia is the major life-threatening infection in neutropenic patients, and immediate treatment of fever is directed at this possibility. Gram-positive infections are, however, seen with increasing frequency [101,102]. This is a result of the use of powerful combinations of antibiotics with greatest activity against Gram-negative organisms, and the routine use of indwelling central venous catheters. In a recently reported series they accounted for 63% of all documented infections [103]. In some centres vancomycin is used routinely in first line antibiotic combinations for the febrile neutropenic patient as a means of providing broad-spectrum cover against Gram-positive organisms [104]. However it has been demonstrated that delay in treatment of Gram-positive infection until the organism has been isolated in culture is safe and effective [103]. Where the infection is associated with an indwelling catheter, diagnostic indicators of this are the isolation of coagulase-negative staphylococcus (*Staph. epidermidis*) and signs (e.g. local inflammation) or symptoms (e.g. pain) in the region of the catheter insertion point or its subcutaneous tunnel. The rate of infection of such catheters varies widely, but many units report the resolution of infection and successful conservation of a high proportion of catheters with vancomycin [105]. Since nephrotoxicity is a side effect of both vancomycin and the aminoglycosides, these agents should only be used in combination with care, at doses determined by nomogram.

## Management of localized infection

Where localized infection develops in the neutropenic individual, treatment will be directed against the likely infecting organism until cultures are available. Aspiration of seemingly minor skin lesions may be rewarded with the immediate identification of the organism by microscopy.

A specific problem relates to lower gastrointestinal infection presenting with abdominal pain or diarrhoea. Neutropenic patients who have received combination chemotherapy with or without radiotherapy may have diarrhoea as the result of one or more of several possible factors. Because the symptom is encountered so frequently, and because instrumentation and biopsy of the lower bowel is to be avoided in such patients, the diagnosis of *Clostridium difficile* infection is missed unless the possibility is actively entertained, and evidence for the presence of the organism and its associated toxin sought in repeated stool samples. Patients who may have received broad-spectrum antibiotics systemically and agents designed to decontaminate the intestinal tract orally are particularly at risk for this infection which can result in a severe necrotizing enterocolitis [106]. The treatment is with oral vancomycin or metronidazole, although the relapse rate is significant. Patients with toxin-producing diarrhoea should be isolated [107].

Sepsis and inflammation associated with discrete areas of the lower gastrointestinal tract are recognized in neutropenic patients, notably around the caecum (typhlitis) and the anorectal region. The typical localizing signs of an acute abdomen or abscess may be absent; recent reports suggest that a conservative approach to these apparently 'surgical' problems is rewarded with a lower mortality rate [108.109]. Surgical drainage procedures, where they have been undertaken, may fail to control the infection, and are associated with poor healing. The recommended management is therefore bowel rest and broad-spectrum antibiotics in an attempt to support the patient until the white cell count recovers.

## Complications and management of thrombocytopenia

Thrombocytopenia is predominantly a complication of patients receiving intensive treatment regimens or with leukaemia. It is rare in those receiving treatment of moderate intensity for solid tumours, Hodgkin's disease or non-Hodgkin's lymphoma (NHL) unless there is appreciable replacement of bone marrow with tumour, which is most frequently a finding in NHL. Bleeding, and in particular unheralded CNS or gastrointestinal haemorrhage, is the hazardous consequence which may result from a transient suppression of the platelet count. Bleeding as a cause of severe morbidity or mortality has declined considerably in importance for patients receiving such treatments over the past 10–15 years with improved conditions for the collection and storage of platelets [110], and widespread use of prophylactic transfusions.

The risk of bleeding is related to the circulating level of platelets which is influenced by rates of production and consumption. Coincident infection and non-therapy-related medications may depress the platelet count through an effect on both processes. The likelihood of bleeding at a particular count is also increased in the presence of infection, as well as by host-related factors such as age and the presence of hypertension and vascular disorders.

Most units adopt a policy of prophylactic support with platelet transfusion if the count drops below a minimum level, with the intention of minimizing the risk of serious bleeding. Even at higher levels, platelets should be given if there is evidence of minor bleeding, e.g. in the nose or mouth, or in the presence of increasing bruising or purpura. At the authors' unit prophylactic transfusions are given for counts of less than $20 \times 10^9/l$, though others have advocated a more conservative policy. The disadvantage of too vigorous platelet support is that there is a tendency to develop sensitization to a wide range of transfused foreign antigens, with the result that subsequent transfusions are ineffective; transfusion of HLA matched donor platelets may produce more favourable results in a patient who has

developed HLA antibodies [111], and the use of single donor transfusions has been shown to delay the development of antibody [112]. A small proportion of patients become refractory to all available platelet support. Bleeding in these individuals may be catastrophic. Improvement has been described after high-dose intravenous gammaglobulin, but this has not been universally confirmed [113].

After ablative treatment supported by bone marrow rescue, recovery of platelet counts to safe levels may take considerably longer than recovery of the granulocyte count, and may never return to normal levels. Risk factors are age and extent of prior myelotoxic therapy. The most likely consequence of this is prolonged hospital stay and the inconvenience of continued dependence on platelet transfusional support, but clearly also carries a chronic risk of bleeding complications.

## Mucositis

Mucositis occurs as a manifestation of cytotoxic-induced failure of mucosal repair mechanisms, and local mucosal infection during the leucocyte nadir. In the majority of cases these processes are linked and occur simultaneously. The results are stomatitis and gastrointestinal disturbance, which can contribute significantly to the overall toxicity of moderately intensive chemotherapy regimens.

### *Stomatitis*

The likelihood of a patient suffering from stomatitis during a course of chemotherapy depends upon the drugs being used (see Table 6.5), and also on a variety of host factors. Methotrexate, 5-fluorouracil and doxorubicin are particularly associated with this complication [114]. Very severe mucositis may be

**Table 6.5 Chemotherapy agents particularly associated with mucositis**

| Drug | Comments |
| --- | --- |
| Methotrexate | Toxicity enhanced in presence of impaired renal function. Prevented by adequate folinic acid rescue |
| Doxorubicin | Severity markedly increased by recent or simultaneous radiotherapy. Dose-limiting in recent studies using haemopoietic growth factors to reduce myelotoxicity |
| 5-Fluorouracil | Dose-related. Allopurinol mouth washes may reduce severity [127] |
| Actinomycin D | Severity increased by radiotherapy |

seen in patients who receive doxorubicin after radiotherapy to the head and neck, and where escalated doses of this drug have been given (for example in association with haemopoietic growth factors to reduce the degree of myelosuppression), mucositis becomes the dose-limiting toxicity (M. Bronchud, 1989, personal communication). That individual factors are important is suggested by the observation that there is a tendency for certain patients to develop severe stomatitis recurrently during successive courses of treatment [114]. Periodontal disease is widespread in a chronic subclinical form in the general population, and this can exacerbate during periods of neutropenia [115]. Apart from causing often severe local discomfort, the tissue damage can provide a portal for entry of pathogens such as Gram-negative bacteria to the systemic circulation. If the underlying disease is acute leukaemia, infiltration of the oral mucosa before the start of therapy may predispose to later ulceration.

The normal flora of the mouth may be altered by the hospital environment [116] and by the use of broad-spectrum antibiotics. Overgrowth with *Candida* and reactivation of herpes simplex are the most frequent specific local infections encountered. The latter may result in florid ulceration without vesicle formation in myelosuppressed individuals, and clinical diagnosis may be difficult.

Folinic acid, given orally or intravenously starting 24 h after methotrexate, can reduce the incidence and degree of mucositis from that drug. There are no other specific remedies, and management depends upon vigorous prophylaxis against oral infection and appropriate treatment should this develop. Careful attention should be paid to oral and dental hygiene, with an examination by an oral surgeon ideally being performed before intensive treatment is started. Regular use of antiseptic mouthwashes and topical antifungals such as nystatin and amphotericin (available in lozenge form outside the USA) should be continued throughout the treatment period. It is important that staff provide continued encouragement for what can become a very tedious ritual. Prophylaxis against herpes simplex reactivation with acyclovir is used by some groups for seropositive individuals. When severe stomatitis occurs despite prophylaxis, adequate analgesia is required as well as, for example, systemic antibiotics if there is evidence of bacterial infection, or systemic antifungals if topical agents are ineffective or poorly tolerated.

Abnormalities which occur in the oral mucosa can also develop in the pharynx and the oesophagus, as a result of the same mechanisms. The typical presenting symptom is dysphagia, though some patients may complain of heartburn or epigastric pain, and candidal infection in the oesophagus can result in minor haematemesis [117]. Oesophageal candidiasis is frequently found in the absence of oral infection, and may require barium swallow or endoscopy for a diagnosis to be made. Confirmed oesophageal candidiasis should be treated with oral ketoconazole or intravenous amphotericin. In a prospective study of patients who had undergone intensive therapy supported by allogeneic transplant and had unexplained vomiting at least 2 weeks after therapy, over 40% had unsuspected viral infection of the oesophagus (predominantly herpes simplex and CMV) diagnosed by endoscopic biopsy [118].

## Acute intestinal complications of therapy

Intestinal mucosa, having a high cell turnover rate, is also a site for primary damage as a result of both chemotherapy and radiotherapy. In intensive treatment regimens the relevance of this is unclear. Sequential changes in the intestinal mucosa have been documented in patients receiving combination chemotherapy for solid tumours, but the importance of this in terms of reduction in absorptive capacity did not appear to be great [119].

Cyclophosphamide alone does not appear to cause significant damage. However, when high-dose cyclophosphamide was given together with total body irradiation, extensive changes were seen on sequential rectal biopsies over the initial 20 days, which were thought to correlate with the patient's symptoms of abdominal pain and diarrhoea [120].

Cytosine arabinoside was assumed to be the agent responsible for widespread changes in the intestinal mucosa seen in a series of patients with leukaemia at post-mortem, and these changes in turn were thought to correlate with the high incidence of systemic infection in these patients, as a result of a breakdown in the normal mucosal barrier [121]. It is general experience that patients with leukaemia and lymphoma receiving high doses of cytosine arabinoside are prone to episodes of intestinal dilatation, usually accompanied by profuse diarrhoea which may be difficult to treat.

Gastrointestinal motility can be affected by the acute neurotoxic effects of vincristine on the autonomic nerve supply to the bowel. This is most prominent in older patients and most commonly presents with constipation (in 30% of treated patients) or, in occasional instances, with paralytic ileus. Where lymphoma involves the small bowel, cytotoxic therapy may predispose to perforation and bleeding as the tumour recedes. In one series, however, perforation usually indicated progressive lymphoma rather than response to treatment [122].

### Effect of therapy on nutrition

All the above complications have an additional significance in that their presence tends to interfere to some degree with the maintenance of a normal oral dietary intake. Intensive therapy regimens in which significant gastrointestinal toxicity is expected often include the use of intravenous feeding to limit the catabolic effect of treatment. Despite improved nutritional parameters in treated patients, there is no consistent evidence to date from the small number of randomized trials that have been performed that such measures can improve either the response to antineoplastic therapy or survival [123,124]. There may, however, be some psychological benefit to be gained from the arrest or reversal of weight loss associated with the underlying tumour or cytotoxic therapy, and this may also result in improved performance status and functional capacity after treatment is completed. Against this should be set the cost of intravenous nutrition which may need to be continued for several weeks, and the increased risk of sepsis from intravenous feeding administered through an indwelling central intravenous catheter. In patients with an intact gastrointestinal tract but who are at risk of nutritional deficiency as a result of poor appetite, nausea or debility, enteral feeding through a fine bore nasogastric tube is an alternative which is relatively free from complications.

# Early psychological effects of treatment

Psychological morbidity associated with cancer treatment is dealt with in depth elsewhere in this volume. It is appropriate here to consider briefly the aspects which affect the patient's early adjustment to a course of chemotherapy, and also to his perception of the side effects of treatment.

At the start of a course of therapy, the acceptance of the diagnosis of cancer is the most difficult problem facing the patient. In a study of newly diagnosed cancer patients attending three US treatment centres, 40% were found to be suffering from anxiety and depression; in the majority of these psychological morbidity was felt to be due to a failure to adapt to the implications of diagnosis and treatment [125]. Other studies concentrating on patients receiving chemotherapy have found a higher incidence of these problems. Treatment-related side effects predispose to development of conditioned responses such as anticipatory anxiety or anticipatory nausea and vomiting [126]. These might be provoked by anything associated with the experience of treatment. Management depends upon early recognition, so that appropriate discussion, counselling, behavioural therapy or drug treatment can be prescribed as appropriate. Failure to diagnose the problem may lead to disruption of specific anticancer treatment.

# Conclusions

The first few weeks after the delivery of cancer chemotherapy are frequently hazardous and uncomfortable for the patient. Recognition of the potential problems and the way in which they may be avoided or ameliorated can render the treatment more tolerable and so improve the chances of its success. Over the past decade, during which the drug treatment of cancer has gone through a phase of consolidation rather than rapid advancement, some of the most important developments have been in the treatments which are available to support the patient through this initial period. These include improvements in antiemetic therapy, transfusion facilities, antimicrobial agents and psychosocial support. In the near future use of haemopoietic growth factors might be expected to lessen the incidence and duration of myelosuppression; 'biological' and other new approaches to cancer treatment may well have broadly lower toxicity than currently established agents. It is appropriate to be cautiously optimistic that the acute consequences of cancer treatment will come to be feared significantly less than they have been up to the present time.

# References


1. Rudnick, S.A. and Feinstein, A.R. An analysis of the reporting of results in lung cancer drug trials. *Journal of the National Cancer Institute*, **64**, 1337–1343 (1980)
2. Price, C.G.A. and Slevin, M.L. Difficult decisions: chemotherapy in lung cancer. *Postgraduate Medical Journal*, **65**, 291–298 (1989)
3. Coates, A., Abrahan, S., Kaye, S.D. *et al*. On the receiving end – patient perception of the side-effects of cancer chemotherapy. *European Journal of Cancer and Clinical Oncology*, **19**, 203–208 (1983)
4. Love, R.R., Leventhal, H., Easterling, M.A. and Nerenz, D.R. Side effects and emotional distress during cancer chemotherapy. *Cancer*, **63**, 604–612 (1989)
5. Nerenz, D.R., Leventhal, H. and Love, R.R. Factors contributing to emotional distress during cancer chemotherapy. *Cancer*, **50**, 1020–1027 (1982)
6. Slevin, M.L., Plant, H., Stubbs, L. *et al.* Balancing the possible benefits against the risk of cytotoxic chemotherapy – patients' and doctors' decisions. *British Journal of Cancer*, **58**, 266 (1988)
7. Richardson, J.L., Marks, G. and Levine, A. The influence of symptoms of disease and side effects of treatment on compliance with cancer therapy. *Journal of Clinical Oncology*, **6**, 1746–1752 (1988)
8. Peroutka, S.J. and Snyder, S.H. Antiemetics: neurotransmitter receptor binding predicts therapeutic actions. *Lancet*, **i**, 658–659 (1982)
9. Miner, W.D. and Sanger, G.H. Inhibition of cisplatin-induced vomiting by selective 5-

hydroxytryptamine *m*-receptor antagonism. *British Journal of Pharmacology*, **88**, 497–499 (1986)

10. Jordan, N.S., Shauer, P.K., Shauer, A. *et al*. The effect of administration rate on cisplatin-induced emesis. *Journal of Clinical Oncology*, **3**, 559–561 (1985)

11. Kessler, J.F., Alberts, D.S., Pleiza, P.M. *et al*. An effective five-drug antiemetic combination for prevention of chemotherapy-related nausea and vomiting. Experience in 84 patients. *Cancer Chemotherapy and Pharmacology*, **16**, 282–286 (1986)

12. Westbrook, C., Glaholm, JN. and Barrett, A. Vomiting associated with whole body irradiation. *Clinical Radiology*, **38**, 263–266 (1987)

13. Stefanek, M.E., Sheidler, R.V. and Fetting, J.H. Anticipatory nausea and vomiting. Does it remain a significant clinical problem? *Cancer*, **62**, 2654–2657 (1988)

14. Morrow, G.R. Prevalence and correlates of anticipatory nausea and vomiting in chemotherapy patients. *Journal of National Cancer Institute*, **68**, 585–588 (1982)

15. Gralla, R.J., Tyson, L.B., Bordin, L.A. *et al*. Antiemetic therapy: a review of recent studies and a report of a random assignment trial comparing metoclopramide and delta-9-tetra-hydrocannabinol. *Cancer Treatment Reports*, **68**, 163–172 (1984)

16. Allen, S.G., Cornbleet, M.A., Warrington, P. *et al*. Trial of dexamethasone and high dose metoclopramide versus placebo and high dose metoclopramide in cisplatin-induced emesis. *Proceedings of the American Society of Clinical Oncology*, **3**, 89 (1984)

17. Soukop, M. and Cunningham, D. Nausea and vomiting induced by cytotoxic drugs. In *Baillière's Clinical Oncology*, Vol. 1, No. 2 (ed. T.D. Bates), Baillière Tindall, London (1987)

18. Kris, M.G., Tyson, L.B., Gralla, R.J. *et al*. Extrapyramidal reactions with high-dose metoclopramide. *New England Journal of Medicine*, **309**, 433–434 (1983)

19. Cunningham, D., Bradley, C.J., Forrest, G.J. *et al*. Comparison of antiemetic efficacy of domperidone, metoclopramide and dexamethasone in patients receiving outpatient chemotherapy regimens. *British Medical Journal*, **295**, 250 (1987)

20. Cunningham, D., Hawthorn, J., Pople, A. *et al*. Prevention of emesis in patients receiving cytotoxic drugs by GR38032F, a selective 5-HT$_3$ receptor antagonist. *Lancet*, **i**, 1461–1463 (1987)

21. Laszlo, J., Clark, R.A., Hanson, D.C. *et al*. Lorazepam in cancer patients treated with cisplatin: a drug having antiemetic, amnesic and anxiolytic effects. *Journal of Clinical Oncology*, **3**, 864–869 (1985)

22. Slevin, M.L. Quality of life in cancer patients. In *Clinics in Oncology*, Vol. 3, No. 2 (eds P.F.M. Wrigley and A.R. Timothy), W.B. Saunders, London (1984)

23. Wiltshaw, E. Ovarian trials at the Royal Marsden. *Cancer Treatment Reviews*, **12**, (Suppl A), 67–72 (1985)

24. Smith, I.E., Evans, B.D., Gore, M.E. *et al*. Carboplatin and etoposide as first line combination therapy for small-cell lung cancer. *Journal of Clinical Oncology*, **5**, 185–189 (1987)

25. McElwain, T.J., Toy, J. and Smith, M.J. A combination of chlorambucil, vinblastine, procarbazine and prednisolone for treatment of Hodgkin's disease. *British Journal of Cancer*, **36**, 276–280 (1977)

26. Hickman, R.O., Buckner, C.D., Clift, R.A. *et al*. A modified right atrial catheter for access to the venous system in marrow transplant recipients. *Surgery, Gynecology and Obstetrics*, **148**, 871–875 (1979)

27. Larson, D.L. What is the appropriate management of tissue extravasation by anti-tumour agents? *Plastic and Reconstructive Surgery*, **75**, 397–405 (1985)

28. Ignoffo, R.J. and Friedman, M.A. Therapy of local toxicities caused by extravasation of cancer chemotherapeutic drugs. *Cancer Treatment Reviews*, **7**, 17–73 (1980)

29. Olver, I.N., Aisner, J., Hament, A. *et al*. A prospective study of topical dimethyl sulfoxide for treating anthracycline extravasation. *Journal of Clinical Oncology*, **6**, 1732–1735 (1988)

30. Chait, L.A. and Dinner, M.I. Ulceration caused by cytotoxic drugs. *South African Medical Journal*, **49**, 1935–1936 (1975)

31. Sells, R.A., Owen, R.R., New, R.R. and Gilmore, I.T. Reduction in toxicity of doxorubicin by liposomal entrapment. *Lancet*, **ii**, 624–625 (1988)

32. Balazsovits, J.A.E., Mayer, L.D., Bally, M.B. *et al*. Analysis of the effect of liposome encapsulation on the vesicant properties, acute cardiac toxicities and antitumour efficacy of doxorubicin. *Cancer Chemotherapy and Pharmacology*, **23**, 81–86 (1989)

33. Weiss, R.B. and Bruno, S. Hypersensitivity reactions to cancer chemotherapeutic agents. *Annals of Internal Medicine*, **94**, 66–72 (1982)

34. Evan, W.E., Tsiatis, A., Rivera, G. *et al*. Anaphylactoid reactions to *Escherichia coli* and *Erwinia* asparaginase in children with leukaemia and lymphoma. *Cancer*, **49**, 1378–1383 (1982)

35. Nesbit, M., Chard, R. and Evans, A. Evaluation of intramuscular *versus* intravenous administration of L-asparaginase in childhood leukaemia. *American Journal of Pediatric Hematology and Oncology*, **1**, 9–13 (1979)

35a. Blackledge, G., Lawton, F., Buckley, H. and Crowther, D. Phase II evaluation of bleomycin in patients with advanced epithelial ovarian cancer. *Cancer Treatment Reports*, **68**, 549–550 (1984)

36. Dinarello, C.A., Ward, S.B. and Wolff, S.M. Pyrogenic properties of bleomycin. *Cancer Chemotherapy Reports*, **57**, 393–398 (1973)

37. Carter, J.J., McLaughlin, M.L. and Benn, M.M. Bleomycin-induced fatal hyperpyrexia. *American Journal of Medicine*, **74**, 523 (1983)

38. Von Hoff, D.D., Layard, M.W., Basa, P. *et al.* Risk factors for doxorubicin-induced congestive cardiac failure. *Annals of Internal Medicine*, **91**, 710–717 (1979)

39. Signori, E. and Guevara, D. Evaluation of cardiac arrhythmias by 24 hour Holter monitoring during adriamycin administration. *Proceedings of the American Association for Cancer Research*, **22**, 355 (1981)

40. Ganina, F., DiPetro, N. and Magni, O. Clinical toxicity of 4-epi-doxorubicin (epirubicin). *Tumori*, **71**, 233 (1985)

41. Villani, F., Comazzi, R., Genitoni, V. *et al.* Preliminary evaluation of myocardial toxicity of 4-deoxydoxorubicin: experimental and clinical results. *Drugs and Experimental Clinical Research*, **11**, 223–231 (1985)

42. Weiss, R.B., Grillo-Lopez, A.J., Marsoni, S. *et al.* Amsacrine-associated cardiotoxicity: an analysis of 82 cases. *Journal of Clinical Oncology*, **4**, 159–163 (1986)

43. Piotti, P., Villani, F., Comazzi, R. *et al.* Cardiac function evaluation in AMSA-treated patients. *Tumori*, **71**, 59–61 (1984)

44. Goldberg, M.A., Antin, J.H., Guinan, E.C. and Rappeport, J.M. Cyclophosphamide cardiotoxicity: an analysis of dosing as a risk factor. *Blood*, **68**, 1114–1118 (1986)

45. Gottdiener, J.S., Applebaum, F.R., Ferrans, V.J. *et al.* Cardiotoxicity associated with high-dose cyclophosphamide therapy. *Archives of Internal Medicine*, **141**, 758–763 (1981)

46. Weiss, H.D., Walker, M.D. and Wiernik, P. Neurotoxicity of commonly used antineoplastic agents. *New England Journal of Medicine*, **291**, 75–81 (1974)

47. Meanwell, C.A., Blake, A.E., Kelly, K.A. *et al.* Prediction of ifosfamide/mesna associated encephalopathy. *European Journal of Cancer and Clinical Oncology*, **22**, 815–820 (1986)

48. Barnett, M.J., Richards, M.A., Ganesan, T.S. *et al.* Central nervous system toxicity of high-dose cytosine arabinoside. *Seminars in Oncology*, **12**(Suppl. 3), 227–232 (1985)

49. Hwang, T.L., Yung, A., Estey, E.H. and Fields, W.S. Central nervous system toxicity with high dose Ara-C. *Neurology*, **35**, 1475–1479 (1985)

50. Willox, J.C., Corr, J., Shaw, J. *et al.* Prednisolone as an appetite stimulant in patients with cancer. *British Medical Journal*, **288**, 27 (1984)

51. Cohen, L.F., Barlow, J.E., Magrath, I.T. *et al.* Acute tumour lysis syndrome: a review of 37 patients with Burkitt's lymphoma. *American Journal of Medicine*, **68**, 486–491 (1980)

52. Slevin, M.L., Bell, R., Cotterill, A.M. and Lister, T.A. The 'tumour overkill syndrome'. A potentially lethal complication of cancer chemotherapy. *Postgraduate Medical Journal*, **57**, 727–729 (1981)

53. DeConti, R.C. and Calabresi, P. Use of allopurinol for prevention and control of hyperuricemia in patients with neoplastic disease. *New England Journal of Medicine*, **274**, 481–486 (1966)

54. Groth, S., Nielson, H., Sorensen, J.B. *et al.* Acute and long term nephrotoxicity of *cis*-platinum in man. *Cancer Chemotherapy and Pharmacology*, **17**, 191–196 (1986)

55. Kelsen, D.P., Alcock, N. and Young, C.W. Cisplatin nephrotoxicity: correlation with plasma platinum concentrations. *American Journal of Clinical Oncology*, **8**, 77–80 (1985)

56. Campbell, A.B., Kalman, S.M. and Jacobs, C. Plasma platinum levels: relationship to cisplatin dose and nephrotoxicity. *Cancer Treatment Reports*, **67**, 169–172 (1983)

57. Hayes, D.M., Cvitkovic, E., Goldbery, R.B. *et al.* High-dose cisplatinum diammine-dichloride: amelioration of renal toxicity by mannitol diuresis. *Cancer*, **39**, 1372–1381 (1977)

58. Gonalez-Vitule, J.C., Hayes, D.M., Cvitkovic, E. and Sternberg, S.S. Acute renal failure after *cis*-dichloro-diammine platinum(II) and gentamicin-cephalothin therapies. *Cancer Treatment Reports*, **62**, 693–698 (1978)

59. Lam, M. and Adelstein, D.J. Hypomagnesaemia and renal magnesium wasting in patients treated with cisplatin. *American Journal of Kidney Disease*, **8**, 164–169 (1986)

60. Pitman, S.W. and Frei, E. Weekly methotrexate-calcium leucovorin rescue: effects of alkalinsation on nephrotoxicity; pharmacokinetics in the CNS; and use in CNS non-Hodgkin's lymphoma. *Cancer Treatment Reports*, **61**, 695–701 (1977)

61. Scheef, W., Klein, H.O., Brock, N. *et al.* Controlled clinical studies with an antidote against the urotoxicity of oxazaphophorines: preliminary results. *Cancer Treatment Reports*, **63**, 501–505 (1979)

62. Bryant, B.M., Jarman, M., Ford, H.T. and Smith, I.E. Prevention of isophosphamide-induced urothelial toxicity with 2-mercaptoethane sulphonate sodium (mesnum) in patients with advanced carcinoma. *Lancet*, **ii**, 657–659 (1980)

63. Cutting, H.O. Inappropriate secretion of antidiuretic hormone secondary to vincristine therapy. *American Journal of Medicine*, **51**, 269–271 (1971)

64. DeFronzo, R.A., Braine, H. and Colvin, Water intoxication in man after cyclophosphamide therapy. *Annals of Internal Medicine*, **178**, 861–869 (1973)

65. Ohnuma, T., Holland, J.F., Freeman, A. and Sinks, L.F. Biochemical and pharmacological studies with L-asparaginase in man. *Cancer Research*, **30**, 2297–2305 (1970)

66. Bronchud, M., Scarffe, J.H., Thatcher, N. *et al.* Phase I/II study of recombinant human granulocyte colony stimulating factor in patients receiving intensive chemotherapy for small cell lung cancer. *British Journal of Cancer*, **56**, 809–813 (1987)

67. Gabrilove, J.L., Jakubowski, A., Scher, H. *et al.* Effect of granulocyte colony-stimulating factor on

neutropenia and associated morbidity due to chemotherapy for transitional-cell carcinoma of the urothelium. *New England Journal of Medicine*, **318**, 1414–1422 (1988)

68. Schimpff, S.C., Young, V.M., Green, W.H. *et al.* Origin of infection in acute non-lymphocytic leukaemia: significance of hospital acquisition of potential pathogens. *Annals of Internal Medicine*, **77**, 707–714 (1972)

69. Johanson, W.G., Pierce, A.K. and Sanford, J.P. Changing pharyngeal flora of hospitalized patients: emergence of gram-negative bacilli. *New England Journal of Medicine*, **281**, 1137–1140 (1969)

70. Ribas-Mundo, M., Granena, A. and Roxman, C. Evaluation of a protective environment in the management of granulocytopenic patients. A comparative study. *Cancer*, **48**, 419–424 (1981)

71. Armstrong, D. Protected environments are discomforting and expensive and do not offer meaningful protection. *American Journal of Medicine*, **76**, 685–689 (1984)

72. Aisner, J., Schimpff, S.C., Bennett, J.E. *et al.* Aspergillus infections in cancer patients: association with fire proofing materials in a new hospital. *Journal of the American Medical Association*, **235**, 411–412 (1976)

73. Stephenson, J.R., Heard, S.R., Richards, M.A. and Tabaqchali, S. Gastrointestinal colonisation and septicaemia with *Pseudomonas aeruginosa* due to contaminated thymol mouthwash in immune compromised patients. *Journal of Hospital Infection*, **6**, 369–78 (1986)

74. Prentice, H.G., Hann, I.M. and Grob, J.P. The prophylaxis of infection in patients with malignant disease. In *Clinics in Oncology*, Vol. 4, No. 3 (eds J.M.A. Whitehouse and G.M. Mead), W.B. Saunders, London (1985)

75. Sande, M.A. and Mandell, G.L. Effect of rifampicin on nasal carriage of *Staphylococcus aureus*. *Antimicrobial Agents and Chemotherapy*, **7**, 294–297 (1975)

76. Saral, R., Burns, W.H. and Prentice, H.G. Herpes virus infections: clinical manifestations and therapeutic strategies in immunocompromised patients. *Clinics in Haematology*, **13**, 645–660 (1984)

77. Saral, R. Management of mucocutaneous herpes simplex virus infections in immunocompromised patients. *American Journal of Medicine*, **85**(Suppl. 2A), 57–60 (1988)

78. Hersman, J., Meyers, J.D., Thomas, E.D. *et al.* The effect of granulocyte transfusions upon the incidence of cytomegalovirus infection after allogeneic marrow transplantation. *Annals of Internal Medicine*, **96**, 149–152 (1982)

79. Gurwith, M.J., Brunton, J.L., Lank, B.A. *et al.* A prospective controlled investigation of prophylactic trimethoprim/sulfamethoxazole in hospitalized granulocytopenic patients. *American Journal of Medicine*. **66**, 248–256 (1979)

80. Karp, J.E., Merz, W., Hendricksen, C. *et al.* Oral norfloxacin for prevention of gram-negative bacterial infections in patients with acute leukaemia and granulocytopenia. *Annals of Internal Medicine*, **106**, 1–6 (1987)

81. Watson, J.G., Jameson, B., Powles, R. *et al.* Cotrimoxazole *versus* non-absorbable antibiotics in acute leukaemia. *Lancet*, **i**, 6–9 (1982)

82. Ezdinli, E.Z., O'Sullivan, D.D., Wasser, L.P. *et al.* Oral amphotericin for candidiasis in patients with haematological neoplasms. *Journal of the American Medical Association*, **242**, 258–260 (1979)

83. Perren, T.J., Powles, R.L., Easton, D. *et al.* Prevention of herpes zoster in patients by long-term oral acyclovir after allogeneic bone marrow transplantation. *American Journal of Medicine*, **85**(Suppl. 2A), 99–101 (1988)

84. Bowden, R.A., Sayers, M., Gleaves, C.A. *et al.* Cytomegalovirus-seronegative blood components for the prevention of primary cytomegalovirus infection following marrow transplantation: considerations for blood banks. *Transfusion*, **27**, 478–481 (1987)

85. Laskin, O.L., Cederberg, D.M., Mills, J. *et al.* Gancyclovir for the treatment and suppression of serious infections caused by cytomegalovirus. *American Journal of Medicine*, **83**, 201–207 (1987)

86. Hughes, W.T., Kuhn, S., Subhash, C. *et al.* Successful chemoprophylaxis for *Pneumocystis carinii* pneumonitis. *New England Journal of Medicine*, **297**, 1419–1426 (1977)

87. Meurier-Carpenter, F., Snoeck, R., Gerain, J. *et al.* Amphotericin B nasal spray as prophylaxis against aspergillosis in patients with neutropenia. *New England Journal of Medicine*, **311**, 1056 (1984)

88. Forgeson, G., Selby, P., Lakhani, S. *et al.* Infused vincristine and adriamycin with high dose methylprednisolone (VAMP) in advanced previously treated multiple myeloma patients. *British Journal of Cancer*, **58**, 469–473 (1988)

89. Winston, D.J., How, G., Lin, C.H. *et al.* Intravenous immune globulin for prevention of cytomegalovirus infection and interstitial pneumonia after bone marrow transplantation. *Annals of Internal Medicine*, **106**, 12–18 (1987)

90. Jochelson, M.S., Altschuler, J. and Stomper, P.C. The yield of chest radiography in febrile and neutropenic patients. *Annals of Internal Medicine*, **105**, 708–709 (1986)

91. Pizzo, P.A., Hathorn, J.W., Hiemen, Z. *et al.* A randomized trial comparing ceftazidime alone with combination antibiotic therapy in cancer patients with fever and neutropenia. *New England Journal of Medicine*, **315**, 552–558 (1986)

92. Pizzo, P.A., Practical considerations for the management of fever and infections in neutropenic patients. In *Clinics in Oncology*, Vol. 4, No. 3 (eds J.M.A. Whitehouse and G.M. Mead), W.B. Saunders, London (1985)

93. Pizzo, P.A., Robichaud, K.J., Gill, F.A. *et al.*

Duration of empiric antibiotic therapy in granulocytopenic patients with cancer. *American Journal of Medicine*, **67**, 194–200 (1979)

94. Klasterksy, J., Cappel, R. and Daneau, D. Clinical significance of *in vitro*, synergism between antibiotics in Gram-negative infections. *Antimicrobial Agents and Chemotherapy*, **2**, 470–475 (1972)

95. DeTongh, C.A., Joshin, J.H., Thompson, B.W. *et al.* Antibiotic synergism and response in gram negative bacteremia in granulocytopenic cancer patients. *American Journal of Medicine*, **80**, 96–100 (1986)

96. Gerson, S.L., Talbot, G.H., Lusk, E. *et al.* Invasive pulmonary aspergillosis in adult acute leukaemia: clinical clues to its diagnosis. *Journal of Clinical Oncology*, **3**, 1109–1116 (1985)

97. DeGregorio, M.W., Lee, W.M.F., Linker, C.A. *et al.* Fungal infections in patients with acute leukaemia. *American Journal of Medicine*, **73**, 861–869 (1973)

98. Pizzo, P.A., Robichaud, K.T., Gill, T.A. and Witebsky, F.B. Empiric antibiotic and antifungal therapy for cancer patients with prolonged fever and granulocytopenia. *American Journal of Medicine*, **72**, 181–211 (1982)

99. Meyers, J.D., Reed, E.C., Shepp, D.H. *et al.* Acyclovir for prevention of cytomegalovirus infection and disease after allogeneic marrow transplantation. *New England Journal of Medicine*, **318**, 70–75 (1988)

100. Reed, E.C., Bowden, R.A., Dandliker, P.S. *et al.* Treatment of cytomegalovirus pneumonia in bone marrow transplant patients with gancyclovir and anti-CMV immunoglobulin. *Blood*, **70**(Suppl. 1), 313 (1987)

101. Wade, J.C., Schimpff, S.C., Newman, K.A. and Wiernik, P.H. *Staphylococcus epidermis*: an increasing cause of infection in patients with granulocytopenia. *Annals of Internal Medicine*, **97**, 503–508 (1982)

102. Kilton, L.J., Fossieck, B.E., Cohen, M.H. and Parker, R.H. Bacteraemia due to Gram-positive cocci in patients with neoplastic disease. *American Journal of Medicine*, **66**, 596–602 (1979)

103. Rubin, M., Hathorn, J.W., Marshall, D. *et al.* Gram-positive infections and the use of vancomycin in 550 episodes of fever and neutropenia. *Annals of Internal Medicine*, **108**, 30–35 (1988)

104. Karp, J.E., Dick, J.D., Angelopulos, C. *et al.* Empiric use of vancomycin during prolonged treatment induced granulocytopenia: randomized, double-blind, placebo-controlled clinical trial in patients with acute leukaemia. *American Journal of Medicine*, **81**, 237–242 (1986)

105. Hiemenz, J., Skelton, J. and Pizzo, P.A. Perspective on the management of catheter-related infections in cancer patients. *Pediatric Infectious Diseases*, **5**, 6–11 (1986)

106. Warson, H.E., Price, A.B., Honour, P. and Borriello, S.P. *Clostridium difficile* and the aetiology of pseudomembranous colitis. *Lancet*, **i**, 1063–1066 (1978)

107. Kim, K.H., Fekety, R., Batts, D.H. *et al.* Isolation of *Clostridium difficile* from environment and contacts of patients with antibiotic-associated colitis. *Journal of Infectious Diseases*, **143**, 42–50 (1981)

108. Shaked, A., Shinar, E. and Freind, H. Neutropenic typhlitis; a plan for conservation. *Diseases of Colon and Rectum*, **26**, 351–352 (1983)

109. Shaked, A., Shinar, E. and Freind, H. Managing the granulocytopenic patient with acute perianal inflammatory disease. *American Journal of Surgery*, **152**, 510–512 (1986)

110. Murphy, S. Platelet storage for transfusion. *Seminars in Hematology*, **22**, 165–177 (1985)

111. Duquesnoy, R.J. Filip, D.J., Rodey, G.E. *et al.* Successful transfusion of platelets mismatched for HLA antigens to alloimmunized thrombocytopenic patients. *American Journal of Hematology*, **2**, 219–226 (1977)

112. Sintnicolaas, K., Vriesendorp, H.M., Sizoo, W. *et al.* Delayed alloimmunization by random single donor platelet transfusions. *Lancet*, **i**, 750–754 (1981)

113. Schiffer, C.A., Hogge, D.S., Aisner, J. *et al.* High dose intravenous gammaglobulin in alloimmunized platelet transfusion recipients. *Blood*, **64**, 937–9-J (1984)

114. Peterson, D.E. Oral lesions. In *Toxicity of Chemotherapy* (eds M.C. Perry and M.D. Yarbro), Grune and Stratton, Orlando, Florida (1984)

115. Overholser, C.D., Peterson, D.S., Williams, L.T. and Schimpff, S.C. Periodontal infection in patients with acute non-lymphocytic leukaemias: prevalence of acute exacerbations. *Archives of Internal Medicine*, **142**, 551–554 (1982)

116. Fainstain, V., Rodriguez, W., Turck, M. *et al.* Patterns of oropharyngeal and fecal flora in patients with leukaemia. *Journal of Infectious Diseases*, **144**, 10–18 (1981)

117. Regnard, C.F.B. Dysphagia. In *Baillière's Clinical Oncology*, Vol. 1, No. 2 (ed. T.D. Bates), Baillière Tindall, London (1987)

118. Spencer, G.D., Hackman, R.C., McDonald, G.B. *et al.* A prospective study of unexplained nausea and vomiting after marrow transplantation. *Transplantation*, **42**, 602–607 (1986)

119. Shaw, M.T., Spector, M.H. and Ladman, A.J. Effects of cancer, radiotherapy and cytoxic drugs on intestinal structure and function. *Cancer Treatment Reviews*, **6**, 141–152 (1979)

120. Epstein, R.J., McDonald, G.B., Sale, G.E. *et al.* The diagnostic accuracy of rectal biopsy in acute graft versus host disease: a prospective study of thirteen patients. *Gastroenterology*, **78**, 764–771 (1980)

121. Slavin, R.E., Dias, M.A. and Saral, R. Cytosine arabinoside induced gastrointestinal toxic alterations in sequential chemotherapeutic protocols. A clinical pathological study of 33 patients. *Cancer*, **42**, 1747–1759 (1978)

122. Lundy, J., Sherlock, P., Kurtz, R. *et al.* Spontaneous perforation of the gastrointestinal tract in patients

with cancer. *American Journal of Gastroenterology*, **63**, 447–450 (1975)

123. Popp, M.B., Fisher, R.I., Wesley, R. *et al.* A prospective randomised study of adjuvant parenteral nutrition in the treatment of advanced diffuse lymphoma: influence on survival. *Surgery*, **90**, 195–203 (1981)

124. Samuels, M.L., Selig, D.E., Ogden, S. *et al.* Intravenous hyperalimentation and chemotherapy for stage III testicular cancer. A randomized study. *Cancer Treatment Reports*, **65**, 615–627 (1981)

125. Derogatis, L.R., Morrow, G.R., Fetting, J. *et al.* The prevalence of psychiatric disorders among cancer patients. *Journal of the American Medical Association*, **249**, 751–757 (1983)

126. Moher, D., Arthur, A.Z. and Pater, J.C. Anticipating nausea and/or vomiting. *Cancer Treatment Reviews*, **11**, 257–264 (1984)

127. Clark, P.I. and Slevin, M.L. Allopurinol mouthwashes and 5-fluorouracil induced oral toxicity. *European Journal of Surgical Oncology*, **II**, 267 (1985)

# 7

# Late effects of childhood cancer therapy

## D.O. Walterhouse and A.T. Meadows

This chapter deals with the delayed, and perhaps long-lasting, effects of pediatric cancer and its treatment. Only time will enable us to appreciate the full range of these effects and their relative permanence. In the past decade, delayed toxicities have been the subject of numerous investigations and their results have been reviewed [1–3]. Despite the proliferation of such material, few reports address the overall magnitude of chronic long-term disability faced by survivors of childhood cancer [4]. It has only been since the early 1970s that children have been cured in large enough numbers with modern therapy (e.g. combined modality and multiple drugs) to permit a systematic study of late consequences; most survivors are, therefore, only now entering young adulthood.

Limitations of large numbers and long follow-up times notwithstanding, we have attempted to present a balanced view of the problems likely to be encountered by practitioners who treat children and provide ongoing care to those who are cured. Newer therapies and approaches to treatment will undoubtedly result from the study of acceptable and prohibitive toxicities now being observed. We have organized this material by general diagnostic categories (leukemia, lymphoma, solid tumors and central nervous system tumors), and included second neoplasms separately; more detailed consequences of specific treatment modalities and effects on particular organs can be found elsewhere in this volume.

## Leukemia

Acute leukemia accounts for about 30% of childhood cancer; with current therapy approximately 60–70% of these children will be cured. Lymphoblastic leukemia (ALL) is the major subtype but the data presented are applicable to non-lymphocytic leukemia (ANLL) as well. This group represents the largest group of survivors of childhood cancer and their late effects of cancer therapy are, therefore, of considerable importance. Children surviving ALL have been the subjects of several studies. In a series of 77 ALL patients examined in a systematic fashion in our late follow-up clinic, 41% were found to have some long-term disability [4]. The majority of these, however, are mild and it can be expected that many of the more severe disabilities will not be observed in the future as therapies change. The effects of newer treatments, however, remain unknown. Questions concerning growth, gonadal function, intelligence and second malignancies often arise and what is currently known will be presented.

## Growth

Growth retardation in ALL can result from the local effects of radiation therapy on growing bones, effects of cranial irradiation on the hypothalamic–pituitary axis leading to growth hormone deficiency, effects of radiation therapy on thyroid or gonadal function, prolonged steroid therapy, effects of chronic illness, or psychosocial factors.

Several studies have indicated that patients treated for ALL with combination chemotherapy without cranial radiation therapy have normal linear growth, although bone age may be retarded [5–7]. Cranial or craniospinal radiation is reported to produce blunting of growth in long-term survivors of ALL, but overall loss of height is small and rarely of clinical importance [7–9]. Zurlo *et al.* [7] reported that pubertal girls were most severely affected although the population included a proportion of patients who had received abdominal radiation in addition to cranial radiation. Kirk *et al.* [9] reported that younger children and those tall for age at diagnosis were more severely affected.

Some ALL survivors develop growth hormone deficiency following cranial irradiation. In Kirk *et al.*'s series partial or complete growth hormone deficiency was seen in response to standard provocative tests in 30 of 46 patients [9]. Costin reported growth hormone deficiency after 18–24 Gy cranial irradiation, although in some patients a subtle dysregulation in spontaneous peaks in growth hormone secretion resulted despite a normal growth hormone response to provocative testing [10]. Blatt *et al.* [11] and Moell *et al.* [12] have separately reported blunting of spontaneous growth hormone secretion in survivors of ALL who received 24 Gy cranial irradiation, occurring in the latter report during puberty in girls. These abnormalities in spontaneous growth hormone secretion contribute to the rare growth retardation seen in children with ALL.

Craniospinal irradiation has also been reported to affect sitting height by local effects on the vertebral bodies. The overall effect, however, is small when doses up to 24 Gy are used but may be compounded by other reasons for growth retardation.

Hypothyroidism can contribute to short stature. Robison *et al.* reported thyroid function abnormalities in 10% of ALL patients treated with chemotherapy and 18 or 24 Gy cranial or craniospinal radiation [13]. Only 3%, however, showed primary hypothyroidism with the remaining patients demonstrating compensated hypothyroidism.

Growth failure is a known complication of prolonged steroid therapy. Studies of children with asthma and nephrotic syndrome indicate that children treated for less than 6 months with doses less than $3\,mg/m^2/day$ of prednisone, however, do not suffer from substantial growth suppression [14]. Treatment for longer than 6 months in children may show a permanent decrease in growth and final adult height [15]. Although ALL doses are high, children rarely receive steroid therapy continuously for more than 6 weeks at a time and the overall effect on growth would be expected to be small.

Although the cause is uncertain, obesity has frequently been reported following treatment for ALL. Meadows and Hobbie reported obesity in 21 of the 77 children with ALL followed long-term [4]. Obesity was significantly associated with severe learning problems. All of these children received 24 Gy cranial irradiation, perhaps suggesting a central, hypothalamic effect leading to both sequelae.

## Gonadal function

The majority of boys receiving or who have received therapy for ALL undergo puberty normally, and there are reports of successful fatherhood both during and following chemotherapy for ALL [16,17]. In general, it is felt that chemotherapy without alkylating agents is unlikely to cause testicular damage. Blatt *et al.* reported a series of 14 boys with ALL treated with combination chemotherapy (prednisone, vincristine, methotrexate and 6-mercaptopurine) [18]. Nine patients were prepubertal, four were intrapubertal, and one was sexually mature at the start of therapy. Throughout the follow-up period (mean of 5.5 years) all patients had normal testicular function as determined by Tanner staging and by serum gonadotropin and testosterone levels. Semen samples from six patients were unremarkable except for one sperm count that fell in the low–normal range. These results indicate that the administration of antileukemic chemotherapy can be compatible with normal gonadal development.

Following 18–24 Gy testicular irradiation for testicular leukemia, permanent sterility results. Testosterone levels may remain normal, although follicle-stimulating hormone and luteinizing hormone (LH) levels may be elevated. In other cases testosterone levels may be low. Brauner *et al.* reported that 10 of 12 children who received 24 Gy to both testes showed insufficient Leydig cell function as expressed by a low response of plasma testosterone to human chorionic gonadotropin or an increased basal LH or both [19]. In another series, Shalet *et al.* reported abnormalities in gonadotropin secretion consistent with testicular damage in nine of 11 boys treated with testicular irradiation, with the majority of these patients requiring androgen replacement therapy [20].

Most girls treated for ALL seem to undergo normal sexual maturation and there are now many young women treated for ALL who have subsequently given birth to normal children. Siris, Leventhal and Vaitukaitis reported normal ovarian function in 28 out of 35 females treated for ALL [21]. In the remaining seven, four had hypothalamic dysfunction and three had primary ovarian dysfunction which was reversible in two. Normal sexual development correlated best with pubertal status at the onset of leukemia with only one of 17 patients diagnosed before puberty experiencing altered pubertal progression, whereas six of 18 with onset during puberty or after menarche experienced abnormalities. Shalet *et al.* found biochemical evidence of ovarian dysfunction in three of seven prepubertal girls treated with combination chemotherapy for leukemia. All three subjects with ovarian failure received cyclophosphamide in varying doses [22].

Incidental irradiation of the ovaries during therapy with 24 Gy craniospinal irradiation as central nervous system prophylaxis has been reported to cause delayed menarche and perhaps gonadal failure in half of the girls so treated [23]. Precocious and premature puberty have also been reported in about 13% of girls and 3% of boys treated for ALL before the age of eight with 18–24 Gy prophylactic cranial or craniospinal irradiation [24]. It has been suggested that premature activation of the hypothalamic–pituitary–gonadal axis may occur as a consequence of hypothalamic dysfunction due to cranial irradiation. Irradiation to the cranium may result in premature thelarche or menarche secondary to activation of the hypothalamic–pituitary–gonadal axis, while spinal irradiation may produce end-organ damage and result in delayed menarche.

## Central nervous system (CNS) effects

The combination of chemotherapy and cranial irradiation has clearly been associated with significant CNS damage in patients treated for ALL. Necrotizing leukoencephalopathy presenting with developmental regression, dementia, spasticity, ataxia, seizures, hemiplegia, pseudobulbar paresis, obtundation, or most severely as coma and death, has been reported most frequently 4–12 months following radiotherapy [25,26]. Almost all children who have developed this complication have received more than 20 Gy cranial irradiation, although intrathecal and intravenous methotrexate also play a role. In one series 55% of patients treated with 24 Gy cranial irradiation, intrathecal methotrexate and intravenous methotrexate (doses of 40–80 mg/m$^2$ intravenously, weekly) developed leukoencephalopathy [27]. The incidence of leukoencephalopathy after radiation therapy alone, intrathecal methotrexate alone, or intravenous methotrexate alone is much lower, ranging between 0.5% and 2% of children at risk. There is no known effective treatment for leukoencephalopathy, although once present rehabilitation efforts should be vigorous, as some patients make significant recoveries [28].

Mineralizing microangiopathy has rarely been reported following radiation doses below 20 Gy and an inconsistent relationship between computed tomographic scan findings and neuropsychological outcome has been reported, with some patients with extensive calcifications showing little in the way of cognitive impairment [29].

Evidence for neuropsychological sequelae of a less severe nature than those described above in children with leukemia who have received central nervous system prophylaxis has accumulated over the past decade. In the series of 77 patients treated for ALL who were seen in our late follow-up clinic, the most common effect of treatment, seen in 35% of patients, was severe learning problems necessitating special education [4]. Eiser and others subsequently have shown intelligence quotient (IQ) deficits in the range of 10–20 IQ points among children who have received 24 Gy cranial irradiation [30]. Meadows *et al.* and Peckham *et al.* reported declines in IQ and learning deficits in 61% of survivors of leukemia who had been treated with 24 Gy cranial irradiation and intrathecal methotrexate [31,32]. Children aged between 2 and 5 years and children who had a higher IQ at the time of initial evaluation showed the most severe changes. Moderate to severe impairment was seen most commonly in visual motor integration, problem solving, and general memory. Moss, Nannis and Poplack reported the cognitive areas that showed the greatest differences between children with leukemia and their siblings were associative thinking, remote memory, abstract ability, and perceptual abilities with children who were treated when they were less than 5 years of age being more likely to have greater neuropsychological dysfunction [33]. These changes may not appear for 3–5 years after therapy. In that study, children who had received methotrexate but no irradiation did not differ from their siblings.

It is now possible to achieve the same therapeutic success as was achieved with 24 Gy CNS prophylaxis with 18 Gy or with intrathecal chemotherapy. In a prospective study comparing a group treated with 18 Gy with one having received chemoprophylaxis, significant differences in post-therapy freedom from distractibility was observed with the former group performing less well on this composite score (A.T. Meadows, personal communication). Recently, Mulhern *et al.* compared children treated with irradiation, intrathecal methotrexate and intensive systemic chemotherapy with children treated with intrathecal and high-dose intravenous methotrexate and found similar difficulties, primarily related to memory, in both groups [34].

## Other systems and problems (lens, teeth, bones and liver)

Cataracts can result from the use of steroid hormones or from irradiation of the lens with doses between 4 and 20 Gy [35]. The estimated radiation dose to the lens for children receiving 24 Gy cranial irradiation is 5 Gy [36], and children treated with prophylactic irradiation are rarely affected [37]. Steroid therapy can cause subcapsular cataracts, the incidence of which increases with higher dosage and longer duration of therapy.

Dental abnormalities have been described in children who have undergone therapy for ALL. About 40% of children treated with 18–24 Gy show root or crown abnormalities of the first maxillary molars [38]. Chemotherapy for ALL, without radiation therapy, has also been shown to cause shortening and thinning of the premolar roots in children treated for ALL before the age of 10 years [39].

Careful dental follow-up with meticulous oral hygiene is recommended as patients with shorter roots can be expected to lose teeth earlier than if roots are normal.

Use of corticosteroids or methotrexate in children with ALL can cause skeletal undermineralization (osteoporosis) leading to bony fractures [40,41].

Chronic hepatotoxicity can result from therapy with methotrexate and 6-mercaptopurine. Methotrexate-related hepatic damage is insidious, but progressive hepatic cell damage may lead to hepatic fibrosis and cirrhosis. The incidence of hepatic injury secondary to 6-mercaptopurine has been reported to be between 10% and 40% [42]. Prolonged administration may lead to intrahepatic cholestasis and hepatocellular necrosis with biochemical elevation of serum bilirubin and elevation of serum transaminases. After cessation of therapy, hepatotoxicity secondary to chemotherapy is usually reversible but may progress to chronic liver disease. The incidence of chronic liver disease varies. Despite abnormal liver function tests during treatment, fewer than 1% of survivors of ALL have evidence of chronic liver disease. Infectious hepatitis acquired during therapy for leukemia may also lead to chronic liver disease [43].

# Lymphoma

Lymphoma (Hodgkin's disease and non-Hodgkin's lymphoma) accounts for approximately 12–15% of childhood cancer. Many long-term survivors of Hodgkin's disease have been evaluated for late effects of therapy since excellent cure rates have been achieved for many years. In view of these excellent cure rates, efforts are now frequently directed at alternative treatment regimens or dose reductions in an attempt to reduce long-term effects of therapy. Some of the important late effects of therapy will be reviewed including risks of infection following splenectomy, gonadal dysfunction, thyroid abnormalities, cardiac complications, pulmonary complications and musculoskeletal abnormalities.

## Overwhelming bacterial infection

Staging laparotomy with splenectomy has been a part of the staging evaluation for many Hodgkin's disease patients since the early 1970s. Spontaneous sepsis is a serious risk in asplenic patients, and in 1979 Chilcote *et al.* reported the development of overwhelming bacterial infection in 20 of 200 asplenic children with Hodgkin's disease, ten of whom later died [44]. More recent studies have demonstrated a considerably lower incidence of postsplenectomy sepsis, although the risk probably

ranges from 3 to 10% [45–47]. Most cases of overwhelming sepsis occur within 2 years after splenectomy, but isolated episodes have been reported up to 12 years later [48–50]. Splenic irradiation to 40 Gy can ablate splenic function to the same extent as surgery and, therefore, also increases the risk of overwhelming bacterial infection [51]. There have been no case reports of typical overwhelming sepsis among patients treated with less than 20 Gy [52]. In order to try to prevent this life-threatening late effect of therapy for Hodgkin's disease, pneumococcal vaccine and possibly *H. influenzae* B vaccine should be given, ideally a week before splenectomy [53,54]. Penicillin prophylaxis is recommended indefinitely in patients who have had surgical or irradiation-induced splenectomy.

## Gonadal function

Byrne *et al.* recently reported in a retrospective cohort study of long-term survivors of childhood cancer, including 253 male and female Hodgkin's disease patients, a significant depression of fertility in married survivors of only two types of cancer: Hodgkin's disease and male genital cancer [55]. Irradiation, MOPP (mechlorethamine, vincristine (Oncovin), procarbazine and prednisone), and MOPP analogues all may damage the gonads in children undergoing therapy for Hodgkin's disease. ABVD (doxorubicin (Adriamycin), bleomycin, vinblastine and dacarbazine), in contrast, does not appear to cause gonadal damage [56].

The relative radiosensitivity of the prepubertal and pubertal testis is not known. Incidental irradiation, however, to the testis from an inverted-Y field can cause transient or, less commonly, permanent oligospermia or azospermia [57]. Perdick and Hoppe showed that 27.5–45 Gy pelvic irradiation caused temporary azospermia in the majority of men, with 88% showing normal sperm counts after 26 months [58]. Donaldson and Kaplan found three of five irradiated boys capable of fathering normal children [57]. The remaining two had reduced sperm counts. Many attempts have been made to protect spermatogenesis from radiotherapy utilizing hormonal pretreatment and van Alphen *et al.* have recently demonstrated a substantial protective effect to radiation-induced testicular damage in monkeys using a 16-day pretreatment course of follicle-stimulating hormone (FSH) [59].

Alkylating agents cause some gonadal injury to males. There are rare cases in which young men have fathered children 8 years or more after MOPP. However, testicular injury following MOPP chemotherapy is generally more complete than that following irradiation, with less likelihood of recovery [60]. The probability of recovery of spermatogenic function and fertility appears low or absent among postpubertal adolescent and adult males. Insufficient numbers of boys who were prepubertal at the time of treatment have been followed for long enough periods to determine whether the effects on fertility for this subgroup will be different from those for postpubertal males. It appears that the prepubertal testis, compared with the postpubertal testis, is relatively insensitive to the cytotoxic effects of alkylating agents; Sherins *et al.* found elevated FSH and germinal aplasia in males treated with MOPP therapy for Hodgkin's disease during puberty but not in boys who received the same therapy in the prepubertal period [61]. These males had normal FSH, LH and testosterone levels. Rivkees and Crawford studied the hypothesis that chemotherapy-induced gonadal damage is proportional to the degree of gonadal activity during treatment [62]. The data suggest that damage is more likely to occur in patients who were treated when sexually mature compared with those who were treated when prepubertal. Whitehead *et al.* also demonstrated that severe testicular damage is common after treatment with MOPP with nine of ten late pubertal or adult subjects showing gonadal dysfunction, while all four prepubertal patients showed normal gonadal function [63]. Pubertal development was normal in all patients in this series. In the series from Stanford, five postpubertal males who received six cycles of MOPP chemotherapy and in whom semen analyses were performed showed absolute azospermia 4–11 years after chemotherapy [57]. Further efforts are needed to test whether induced gonadal quiescence during chemotherapy, perhaps with an analogue of gonadotropin releasing hormone, will reduce the high incidence of gonadal failure following chemotherapy [64].

Ovarian function is also compromised by irradiation and chemotherapy for Hodgkin's disease during childhood. The ovaries of women over 40 years of age appear to be more sensitive to radiation effects than those of younger women, and women who receive both combination chemotherapy and pelvic radiation have a greater chance of ovarian failure compared with those who receive only one treatment modality. Oophoropexy is now a standard procedure in young girls undergoing staging laparotomy for Hodkin's disease, and fertility may be retained despite temporary amenorrhea [65,66]. In a review of females treated for Hodgkin's disease at Stanford, all 11 girls aged less than 13 years treated with upper abdominal radiation and all seven treated to the pelvis with midline ovarian blocking retained ovarian function [57]. Among women between the ages of 13 and 40 years who were treated with pelvic radiation, 18 of 19 retained ovarian function. Thirteen (68%) did have temporary amenorrhea lasting up to 4 years and six (32%) had menopausal symptoms. Of 20 patients in the older age group who had the potential for becoming

pregnant, seven women had 11 pregnancies with nine normal births and two therapeutic abortions.

Chemotherapy damages the ovary less than the testis. The age of the patient, the doses of specific agents and the combined use of irradiation all contribute to the potential for ovarian injury. Combination chemotherapy, in particular MOPP for Hodgkin's disease, is known to cause persistent amenorrhea in 25–65% of adults treated [67,68]. Chapman *et al.* documented chemotherapy-induced ovarian failure in 84% of women older than 30 years compared with 31% under that age at the time of therapy [68]. In the study by Rivkees and Crawford, 71% of pubertal females, 7% of midpubertal females, and none of the prepubertal females developed gonadal dysfunction following chemotherapy for Hodgkin's disease [62]. Although the addition of pelvic irradiation to chemotherapy for Hodgkin's disease may increase ovarian dysfunction, Kaplan and Donaldson reported that eight of ten girls treated with chemotherapy and 14 of 15 girls treated with combined modality therapy had normal menses [57]. In contrast, Horning *et al.* found that 56% of young women treated with MOPP had normal menses, while 15% had no menses [66]. Addition of pelvic irradiation to MOPP increased the gonadal toxicity with only 20% having normal menses and 55% being amenorrheic. In this series, young age at the time of treatment was associated with less gonadal damage. There were seven pregnancies among 13 patients treated with chemotherapy and five among 11 combined modality patients. Meadows *et al.* recently reported that most adolescents receiving alkylating agent therapy and pelvic radiation developed ovarian failure [69]. In a postmenarchal group four of five who had pelvic radiation with 6–9 months of alkylating agents were amenorrheic, as were five of 22 who received alkylating agents alone or alkylating agents with radiation therapy outside the pelvis. In the premenarchal group, all four who had pelvic radiation with 6–9 months of alkylating agents failed to achieve menarche while all nine who received alkylating agents for 6 months without pelvic radiation achieved normal menarche.

## Thyroid

Cancer curative doses of neck irradiation can damage the thyroid. The incidence of hypothyroidism following radiation therapy varies considerably in different reports depending on the criteria used to establish the diagnosis. As many as 80% of patients may develop some form of thyroid dysfunction, most commonly chemical hypothyroidism. Clinical hypothyroidism is less common [70–80]. Factors that predispose patients to hypothyroidism are high doses of irradiation, pre-irradiation lymphangiogram, and perhaps young age [75,77]. Constine reported thyroid abnormalities in 17% of children who received 26 Gy or less and in 78% of those who received more than 26 Gy to the cervical region for treatment of Hodgkin's disease [78]. The interval between irradiation and development of hypothyroidism ranges from 3 months to 6 years [79]. If overt hypothyroidism develops, the patients should be treated with hormone replacement. Some investigators recommend that children with elevated thyroid stimulating hormone (TSH) levels after neck irradiation should be given thyroid replacement therapy to reduce thyroid stimulation from prolonged TSH elevation [80]. Benign thyroid nodules, thyroid cancer, and Graves' hyperthyroidism have rarely been reported following radiation therapy [71–79].

## Cardiac complications

Since treatment for Hodgkin's disease often involves radiotherapy to the heart, and current chemotherapeutic regimens include anthracyclines, we should consider long-term cardiac toxicity in this section. The overall incidence of cardiac damage in 120 pediatric Hodgkin's disease patients at Stanford was 13%. The incidence was dose-dependent; while 19% of 85 patients treated with greater than 36 Gy were affected, none of 35 patients treated with less than 25 Gy was affected [57]. In general, irradiation in the 36–44 Gy dose range induces cardiac disease in some Hodgkin's disease patients.

Pericarditis is the most common complication following radiation therapy to the mediastinum. Up to 30% of patients who receive radiation therapy to the pericardium in doses greater than 35 Gy may develop pericarditis, although less than 11% are symptomatic. With equally weighted anterior and posterior fields and the use of subcarinal blocking, the frequency decreases to 2.5% [81]. Symptoms may not develop until many years after radiation therapy, and a spectrum from asymptomatic pericardial effusions which usually resolve spontaneously, to effusions causing tamponade requiring pericardiocentesis, to constrictive pericarditis, a potential life-threatening emergency, can be seen.

Of particular concern in the pediatric population is the small but real incidence of arterial vascular injury following high-dose, mantle-field irradiation, with subsequent development of premature coronary artery disease. The frequency of this complication is not known. In the Stanford series of 120 pediatric patients, two cases of coronary artery disease were reported [57]. Dunsmore, LoPonte and Dunsmore reported three patients who developed myocardial infarction at an untimely age (ages 28, 31 and 36) 4–12 years after radiation therapy for Hodgkin's disease, and in a second series of 545

patients irradiated between birth and 44 years of age, there were five deaths from coronary artery disease as compared with no deaths among 106 patients who had no irradiation [82]. Of particular note are deaths at 18, 20 and 25 years of age, 2–11 years after irradiation. Boivin and Hutchison, however, reported no statistically significant increase in coronary artery disease as compared with the general population in a series of 957 long-term survivors of Hodgkin's disease [83].

It does not appear that MOPP chemotherapy increases cardiac morbidity. Treatment with low-dose mediastinal irradiation (20 Gy) with MOPP/ABVD (median cumulative dose of doxorubicin 176 mg/m$^2$) resulted in a low risk for cardiac complications [84]. Santoro *et al.* also failed to detect significant cardiac damage in patients treated with either ABVD-RT-ABVD or MOPP-RT-MOPP [56]. Longer follow-up, however, may reveal an increased frequency of cardiac complications in patients receiving anthracyclines in addition to mediastinal irradiation.

## Pulmonary

Both chemotherapy and radiation therapy for Hodgkin's disease have been associated with long-term pulmonary toxicity. Mediastinal or whole lung irradiation may cause acute or chronic pneumonitis in up to 20% of patients 2–6 months after irradiation. Clinically the patients present with dyspnea, cough and sometimes fever, and chest X-ray may show a widened mediastinum with shaggy borders around mediastinal structures. This effect is dose-dependent. Pneumonitis was documented in 5% of patients receiving 35–40 Gy mantle irradiation for Hodgkin's disease: however, lowering the radiation dose to 15–25 Gy essentially eliminated this complication [57,81]. Acute radiation pneumonitis generally resolves within weeks to months and rarely may result in chronic restrictive disease. Steroid therapy appears to benefit some patients but must be withdrawn slowly. Chronic pleural effusions, asymptomatic paramediastinal and apical fibrosis, and restriction of lung volume have all been reported following mediastinal irradiation for Hodgkin's disease [57,70,85].

Chemotherapeutic agents when given alone are not frequently associated with pneumonitis or pulmonary fibrosis, except for the well-known effect of bleomycin. Chronic restrictive disease does not occur with less than 200 units/m$^2$ and is more likely to occur in older patients. More than 10% of adults treated with bleomycin developed pulmonary fibrosis following treatment with doses of greater than 400 units [86]. The radiomimetic effect of doxorubicin or bleomycin may contribute to radiation pneumonitis in patients receiving ABVD.

Late pulmonary complications may also result from serious infection such as *Pneumocystis carinii*, varicella and measles.

## Musculoskeletal

The standard doses and fields of radiation used to treat Hodgkin's disease impair growth of bones and soft tissues. These abnormalities are particularly marked in young children and are proportional to the bone growth remaining [86]. Donaldson and Kaplan found reduction in sitting height in 17 of 30 patients treated with 36 Gy [57]. In contrast, among 44 children given less than 25 Gy and chemotherapy, there were none with abnormal standing height and only six with abnormal sitting height.

Shortening of the interclavicular distance, small clavicles, sternal deformities and atrophy of the soft tissues of the neck are often apparent following mantle irradiation. Scoliosis and kyphosis were reported by Probert and Parker in four of 29 patients treated for Hodgkin's disease or medulloblastoma following doses exceeding 35 Gy to the spine or flank [87]. Retroperitoneal fibrosis has been reported following 44 Gy to the abdomen for Hodgkin's disease [88].

Chemotherapy alone does not appear to cause long-term growth retardation or soft tissue damage. However, the radiomimetic effects of anthracyclines may increase radiation injury to soft tissues and bone, and prednisone with or without radiotherapy may contribute to avascular necrosis of the femoral or humeral heads, slipped femoral capital epiphysis, and osteonecrosis [89].

## Solid tumors

As with other types of childhood cancer, patients with solid tumors are showing steady improvements in survival rates. As a group these tumors account for approximately one-third of childhood cancer. The most common types include rhabdomyosarcoma, osteogenic sarcoma, Ewing's sarcoma, Wilms' tumor and neuroblastoma. These tumors are treated with combinations of surgery, chemotherapy and radiation therapy. Some, such as advanced stage rhabdomyosarcoma and neuroblastoma, require particularly aggressive therapy and, although there are few survivors, the late effects of such therapy are often severe. Others, such as Wilms' tumor and low stage neuroblastoma, show excellent responses with less intensive therapy and current therapeutic strategies are aimed at reducing the long-term toxicity. Solid tumors can occur in the head and neck area, trunk and extremities, and therapy with local as well as systemic modalities may result in a wide spectrum of disability. In this section those effects involving the heart, lungs, kidneys, organs of the head and neck area, and musculoskeletal systems will be reviewed. Although other complications occur, we have chosen to review the most representative and important ones here.

## Cardiac

Complications regarding the cardiovascular system are among the most serious of cancer treatment, and acute cardiomyopathy following therapy with anthracyclines such as doxorubicin (Adriamycin) and daunorubicin (Daunomycin) has been well described. These agents are used in the therapy of childhood sarcomas, neuroblastoma, Wilms' tumor, as well as leukemia and lymphoma. Risk factors have been identified that affect the incidence of cardiotoxicity, the most important being the total cumulative dose. The incidence in patients who receive a total dose of less than $550\,mg/m^2$ of doxorubicin is 1–5%, but increases sharply with higher doses, approaching 30% in patients who have received doses greater than $600\,mg/m^2$. Factors which may enhance anthracycline-induced cardiomyopathy include prior radiation therapy and young age, with children under 5 years of age at greater risk [90–92]. Other chemotherapeutic agents such as cyclophosphamide and actinomycin D have been reported to increase the frequency and severity of anthracycline-induced cardiotoxicity [93–95]. Less toxicity has been reported with low-dose weekly administration or with continuous infusions, but these schedules may also differ in antitumor efficacy [96–100]. Radionuclide angiography has been found to be a reliable method of evaluating left ventricular function in patients receiving doxorubicin [101], and sequential testing with resting and exercise studies is recommended during therapy [102–104]. Systolic time intervals and echocardiography lack both sensitivity and specificity [105–107], while endomyocardial biopsy seems to be a reliable means of predicting cardiotoxicity, although it has the disadvantage of being an invasive study [108,109].

The prognosis of children who develop cardiotoxicity from anthracycline therapy is poor with overall mortality rates between 20 and 83% [110]. If cardiomyopathy develops, the drug should be discontinued and supportive care should be given. Development of doxorubicin cardiotoxicity may have a long latency period with cases in the literature reported many years following therapy [111,112]. Reversibility of anthracycline-induced cardiotoxicity with time has also been reported [113].

Patients treated with anthracyclines should be counselled concerning limitation of activities which increase cardiac afterload, such as weight lifting and childbirth. Sudden death has also been reported without antecedent cardiac failure and may be related to strenuous physical activity and also to the use of other cardiac toxins such as cocaine. It has been suggested that fatal dysrhythmias may arise from damage to the conduction system or from an ectopic focus of myocardial irritability [112–114].

## Pulmonary

Both chemotherapy and radiation therapy have been associated with pulmonary toxicity in patients with solid tumors. Following whole lung irradiation with 20 Gy along with chemotherapy including actinomycin D for Wilms' tumor, a reduction in lung volume and dynamic compliance have been reported as early as a few months following therapy. Failure of alveolar multiplication may explain the reduced lung volume, and failure of chest wall growth may contribute to the restrictive impairment. Few such patients are symptomatic, however, as only two of 48 were in the series reported by Benoist *et al.* [115]. Most of the patients, however, were not disabled and most experienced no dyspnea on moderate exertion. Littman *et al.* reported reduced lung volumes and obstruction of small airways in Wilms' tumor patients treated with 14 Gy pulmonary irradiation for pulmonary metastases [116]. Only two of 15 patients were symptomatic. Concomitant chemotherapy with actinomycin D or doxorubicin may enhance the effects. Radiation pneumonitis presenting as pulmonary nodules on chest X-ray has been reported following whole lung irradiation for Ewing's sarcoma [117]. These nodular changes are important to recognize since they may be confused with tumor metastases and may respond to steroid therapy.

## Renal

Unilateral nephrectomy is part of the current therapy for primary renal tumors of childhood including Wilms' tumor and mesoblastic nephroma. Long-term follow-up of these patients has shown compensatory changes occurring in the remaining kidney. Structural hypertrophy develops during the first 3 years following nephrectomy, with the remaining kidney becoming 35–65% larger than normal, and has been shown to be most pronounced in patients who have undergone nephrectomy before 3 years of age [118]. Most studies show that renal function as determined by serum creatinine and creatinine clearance does not show significant impairment with follow-up as long as 23 years after unilateral nephrectomy [119]. Mild proteinuria and hypertension, both more commonly seen in males, have been reported following unilateral nephrectomy in childhood, but are rarely of clinical significance [120]. In

patients with Wilms' tumor, however, the remaining kidney may be exposed to radiation scatter which has been reported to cause hypertension more than 10 years after therapy [121].

Abdominal and pelvic irradiation have been associated with renal damage. Patients who receive doses of radiotherapy of more than 23 Gy to both kidneys are at increased risk of radiation nephritis. Use of radiomimetic chemotherapeutic agents, such as doxorubicin, actinomycin D, and possibly ifosfamide may increase this risk. Radiation nephritis can occur months to years after treatment and is characterized by proteinuria, hypertension, anemia and progressive renal failure [122–124].

Chemotherapeutic regimens for pediatric solid tumors often include cisplatin, cyclophosphamide, and ifosfamide. Cisplatin (*cis*-platinum) has acute effects on renal tubules, but long-term effects on the kidneys remain uncertain. Heptatic metabolites of cyclophosphamide, which are excreted in the urine, may potentially damage the bladder mucosa causing hemorrhagic cystitis. Excellent hydration with periodic voiding reduces this long-term complication. Ifosfamide has recently been shown to cause a Fanconi-like syndrome of renal tubular damage leading to rickets in some patients, specifically those less than 6 years of age at the time of therapy and those having only one kidney [125].

## Head and neck

Children treated for soft tissue sarcomas of the head and neck with combined modality therapy including radiation enhancing drugs show a variety of treatment-related effects which may involve the eyes, ears, teeth, salivary glands, pituitary gland, facial soft tissues or bones.

Radiation-induced cataracts are well known. The latent period between exposure and cataract appearance ranges from 6 months to 35 years, with an approximate average of 2–3 years [126]. Single doses to the lens of 6–7.5 Gy or fractionated doses to the lens of less than 16 Gy have been reported to cause cataracts. Cataracts were essentially universal in patients treated on the Intergroup Rhabdomyosarcoma Study (IRS) I for orbital rhabdomyosarcoma, occurring within 12–18 months after therapy [127]. Patients received 50–60 Gy to the primary tumor site in 5–6 weeks using 0.2 Gy fractions of supervoltage irradiation. Fromm *et al.* reported in a series of 20 children with soft tissue sarcomas of the head and neck that all but one lens receiving 28 Gy or more developed cataracts [128].

Whole orbit radiation doses of less than 40 Gy rarely cause severe xerophthalmia, whereas doses greater than 57 Gy usually lead to loss of vision within 1 year. Fromm *et al.* reported dry eyes developing in six patients given doses of at least 28 Gy [128]. Four were symptomatic.

Retinal changes after radiation may appear with doses as low as 10 Gy in 1 week. In the study reported above only three of 11 irradiated eyes showed retinal changes following doses of 40–51 Gy to the lens but all of them were considered clinically insignificant. With a median follow-up of 6 years, 10 of 11 eyes treated had vision that could be corrected to 20/40 acuity or better [128].

Hearing problems are uncommon following radiation therapy to the head and neck. However, radiation doses of 40–60 Gy in 4–6 weeks to the middle ear have been reported to cause transient acute middle ear effusion which generally clears spontaneously with no significant hearing loss [129]. In the Children's Hospital of Philadelphia study only one child showed mild to moderate conductive loss due to a thickened tympanic membrane and middle ear mucosa after receiving 53 Gy middle ear dose [128].

Ototoxicity is a known complication of therapy with cisplatin. The ototoxicity appears to be dose-related, although it is not yet clear whether a modifying effect is achieved through specific variations in schedule of administration (bolus or infusion), in the amount and type of hydration, or in the concurrent use of osmotic diuretics such as mannitol. Dini *et al.* reported that all six children who received more than three courses (600 mg/m$^2$ cumulative dose) of high-dose cisplatin (40 mg/m$^2$ daily for five consecutive days as a 1 h infusion) had high frequency hearing loss, with two children also showing significant hearing loss for low frequencies. The hearing loss increased after each course [130]. Brock *et al.* reported that 12 of 14 children developed high frequency hearing loss following high-dose cisplatin (cumulative dose of at least 200 mg/m$^2$). No child was recognized at the time to have clinically significant hearing loss, but of the eight surviving children three now require hearing aids [131]. Brock has also reported moderate to severe high frequency hearing loss in 50% of children who were more than 2 years off treatment and had received cisplatin for germ-cell tumors (nine patients), neuroblastoma (19 patients) or osteosarcoma (two patients) [132]. One-third of the children needed bilateral high frequency hearing aids. No correlation, however, in this study could be found between the severity of the hearing loss and the total cumulative dose of cisplatin. Children who receive cranial irradiation simultaneously with cisplatin or prior to cisplatin experience more significant hearing losses at all frequencies, including the areas for speech perception [133]. The mechanism for this enhanced toxicity of cisplatin with simultaneous or prior cranial irradiation is unknown. Detection of hearing loss is difficult in children but it is very important in an age group which is actively developing language skills.

Numerous human case reports have shown that radiation to developing teeth may cause maldevelopment of roots and crowns. The severity of these developmental abnormalities is dependent on the stage of development of the irradiated tooth and the radiation dose. Developing dental structures are quite sensitive to radiation, with any developing tooth in a treated field receiving a dose as low as 4 Gy showing some developmental abnormality [128]. Jaffe *et al.* reported foreshortening and blunting of roots, incomplete calcification, premature closure of apices, delayed or arrested tooth development, and caries following combined modality therapy including radiation to the head and neck [38]. Again, the abnormalities were more severe in those patients who received radiation at an earlier age and at higher dosages.

Salivary gland irradiation may cause transient or permanent quantitative and qualitative changes in saliva. Decreased flow as well as increased acidity and viscosity may occur. This may lead to excessive caries. Severely reduced parotid secretory activity has been shown following radiation doses of at least 45 Gy to 50% or more of the parotid gland volume [128].

Growth hormone deficiency and growth failure after incidental irradiation to the hypothalamic–pituitary region for head and neck tumors has also been reported [134]. Marked deceleration of statural growth occurred in 61% of the children treated for orbital rhabdomyosarcoma in IRS I and was thought to be related to incidental irradiation to the pituitary gland [127]. Growth failure with documented growth hormone deficiency occurred in five of 15 prepubertal patients after incidental pituitary irradiation. All five had received pituitary doses of at least 44 Gy [128]. Other studies of hypothalamic–pituitary function in patients receiving incidental irradiation to the region for head and neck tumors have shown deterioration of pituitary and hypothalamic function as late as 6–10 years after therapy [135].

Hypoplasia of the facial bones of children treated for head and neck tumors has been described [136]. One-half of the children with orbital rhabdomyosarcoma reported in IRS I had evidence of limited bone growth of the orbit [127]. This effect was related to age. Retarded growth of irradiated soft tissue also contributes to facial deformity. Growing soft tissues may in fact be more sensitive to radiation than bone. All children in the Children's Hospital of Philadelphia study received tumor doses of greater than or equal to 40 Gy and, as expected, some degree of bony or soft tissue deformity was found in all who were 9 years of age at diagnosis or younger. Severe deformity, however, was reported only in those patients who received a tumor dose greater than 50 Gy [128].

Children treated for soft tissue sarcomas of the head and neck should have close follow-up since appropriate prophylactic and symptomatic management may minimize these late effects of treatment. For example, careful dental hygiene may prevent caries, treatment of xerophthalmia may prevent corneal damage, and cataract removal may prevent amblyopia in susceptible children.

## Musculoskeletal

Following abdominal irradiation for neuroblastoma, Wilms' tumor or sarcomas, patients are at risk of developing kyphosis and scoliosis especially during the adolescent growth spurt. Up to 1967, with the use of orthovoltage radiation and doses greater than 32 Gy to bone, King and Stowe reported that seven of 150 children (4.7%) with neuroblastoma and six of 183 children (3.3%) with Wilms' tumor developed kyphosis or scoliosis [137]. More recently, Mayfield *et al.* reported that 76% of 74 children with neuroblastoma who received radiation therapy had residual spinal deformity after a mean follow-up of 12.9 years [138]. Treatment deformities were more commonly seen following orthovoltage doses exceeding 30 Gy and asymmetrical radiation of the spine. In another series, Thomas *et al.* reported that scoliosis with or without kyphosis was the most common late effect encountered following combined modality therapy for Wilms' tumor. While 14 of 29 5-year survivors had scoliosis, only two of the 14 had received less than 20 Gy [139]. The chance that these deformities will continue to occur is much less now, owing to a decreased dose for Wilms' tumor and the general use of supervoltage rather than orthovoltage radiation.

There may be an increased frequency of slipped femoral capital epiphysis in pediatric patients who have received radiation to the pelvis along with chemotherapy. There are reports in the literature of patients with pelvic neuroblastoma, rhabdomyosarcoma, and Hodgkin's disease developing slipped femoral capital epiphysis following pelvic radiation therapy and prolonged combination chemotherapy [140–142]. Ryan and Walters suggest that by exposing the proliferating cells of the femoral head to radiation and chemotherapy, a weakened plate results which slips, either directly related to the damage or indirectly because of inability to sustain the normal stress encountered. It is recommended that the femoral heads and acetabula be shielded when radiation to this area is not crucial to the therapy of the underlying disease [140]. Radiographs of the pelvis should be obtained periodically in patients at risk in order to diagnose this condition prior to symptoms and thus allow for early treatment [143].

## Central nervous system tumors

Brain tumors represent the second most common neoplasm of childhood and account for 20% of all childhood malignant disease. Overall, approximately 50% of these patients survive long-term. Surgery, radiation therapy and chemotherapy, including most commonly vincristine, carmustine (BCNU), lomustine (CCNU), methotrexate, cisplatin and carboplatin are used in the treatment of childhood brain tumors. Late effects of the disease and its therapy may have a major impact on the lives of these children affecting the central and peripheral nervous systems as well as other systems. Neuropsychological effects, effects on endocrine function, and effects on pulmonary function will be reviewed in this section. Previous sections referring to irradiation of the head and neck area, ototoxicity, and use of cisplatin and methotrexate also apply.

## Neuropsychological

When compared with children with other malignancies, it has been suggested that children with brain tumors fare less well in terms of physical ability, education and employment. In a questionnaire study by Li and Stone and a subsequent report, moderate or severe disabilities were reported by 24 of 102 brain tumor survivors (24%) as compared with five of 142 patients with other cancers (4%) [144,145]. Brain tumor patients also attained slightly lower academic and occupational levels. LeBaron *et al.* reported that at least 50% of such children experience serious problems, including motor, sensory, cognitive, academic and emotional problems [146]. All but two children in that series were reported by teachers to be 'slow workers' and only four of 15 patients were able to maintain their school work in regular classes [146]. In the study by Li *et al.*, however, of 102 brain tumor patients 78 patients had mild or no disabilities, whereas 24 patients had moderate or severe functional impairments [145]. Several other studies report that 60–90% of brain tumor patients have mild or no functional deficits and generally perform well in school and at work [146–152]. The proportion of patients with below average IQ scores ranges from 40 to 90% and behavioral disorders, including immaturity, depression, antisocial behavior, aggressive behavior, and fearful behavior have been reported to be similar in frequency.

Differences in the frequency of neuropsychological, academic and social problems which are reported in the literature are in part due to patient selection, treatment methods and method of performance status assessment. Several factors, however, have been identified which affect outcome. Hirsch *et al.* reported that non-irradiated children with astrocytoma generally functioned better than irradiated patients, although a proportion of the non-irradiated patients also had serious intellectual, academic or behavioral deficits [152]. Brain tumor patients are in general treated with more irradiation than children with leukemia, and fare worse intellectually than patients surviving leukemia. This suggests that there may be a relationship between the dose of radiation therapy and the degree of sequelae. However, the effects of the brain tumor itself, of surgery, and of postoperative complications may also play a significant role. Mental retardation has been reported more commonly in patients under 2–5 years of age when treated, in those with cerebral astrocytomas, in those with tumors that encroach upon the hypothalamus and/or thalamus, and in those with untreated panhypopituitarism. The effects of increased intracranial pressure and hydrocephalus on outcome remain unknown.

Reducing the neuropsychological late effects of brain tumors and therapy in childhood will depend on early diagnosis, avoidance of irradiation in young children when possible, and close follow-up. Children with intellectual impairments may be able to learn if material is presented in an appropriate fashion, and special methods of education need to be explored for this population.

## Endocrine

The detrimental effects of treatment on endocrine function in children with brain tumors have been related primarily to cranial irradiation and those children who are less than 10 years of age at the time of diagnosis seem most likely to show the most severe deficits [153]. Chemotherapeutic agents used for brain tumors may have effects on the gonads.

Growth hormone deficiency is the most common endocrine abnormality following radiation therapy for childhood brain tumors. Most observers have found that the responses of growth hormone to provocative tests are abnormal in the majority (67–100%) of such patients, and decreased growth velocity is reported in 30–100% of patients. Following doses to the whole brain of 36–60 Gy, or 46–54 Gy to the posterior fossa, Duffner *et al.* reported growth hormone deficiency developing as early as 3 months following completion of radiation therapy and progressing over time [154]. Six months after therapy 80% of patients had growth hormone deficiency. Pasqualini *et al.* reported decreased height in 11 of 13 children (85%) treated with surgery, radiotherapy and chemotherapy for medulloblastoma, and growth hormone deficiency in nine of the 13 patients (69%) [155]. A radiation dose of 30–36 Gy was given to the whole cerebrospinal axis followed by 20–26 Gy to the posterior fossa. In a second report by Duffner *et al.*, abnormal responses to growth hormone stimulation were seen in 10 of 12 (83%) children with brain tumors. All prepubertal patients showed deceleration of linear growth [156]. Replacement with recombinant growth hormone is recommended in these patients, although

Lustig *et al.* demonstrated the effectiveness of growth hormone releasing factor for growth hormone deficiency secondary to cranial irradiation [157]. Their results support the hypothesis that cranial irradiation in children can lead to hypothalamic growth hormone releasing factor deficiency secondary to radiation injury.

Children with brain tumors treated with craniospinal irradiation may develop chemical or clinical hypothyroidism. Duffner *et al.* reported abnormal thyroid function tests in four of 14 patients (28%) with brain tumors [156]. Two patients had primary hypothyroidism and two had secondary or tertiary hypothyroidism. In the Pasqualini series of 13 children with medulloblastoma, nine patients showed elevated TSH secretion [155]. Concentrations of thyroxine ($T_4$) and tri-iodothyronine ($T_3$) were normal in all patients. The patients received doses of thyroid irradiation in the range of 12–14 Gy. This is a higher rate of thyroid dysfunction than appears in most reports of patients with medulloblastoma.

Gonadal function is less commonly affected by radiation therapy alone for brain tumors; however, chemotherapy with nitrosoureas alone or in combination with procarbazine has been reported to have long-term effects on the gonad [158]. Clayton *et al.* reported testicular damage following therapy with these agents for childhood brain tumors [159]. The patients usually had small testes and an elevated basal FSH level, indicating that they were likely to be azoospermic or severely oligospermic. Pubertal development, however, appeared normal. These gonadal effects are felt to be irreversible in the male. This same group has also reported a series of 21 girls treated with neuraxis irradiation followed by adjuvant chemotherapy with carmustine or lomustine and procarbazine for brain tumors [160]. The majority of girls showed evidence of primary ovarian dysfunction including elevated basal FSH levels or exaggerated FSH responses to GnRH. Pubertal development or timing of menarche was not affected. In contrast to the male, the ovarian dysfunction caused by nitrosoureas and procarbazine may be reversible with normalization of FSH levels. Effects on fertility and on the timing of menopause remain unknown.

## Pulmonary

Carmustine (BCNU) is used in the treatment of childhood brain tumors, and pulmonary toxicity following treatment with this agent is well established [161–165]. Ryan and Walters reported the development of pulmonary toxicity 2.5 years after therapy with carmustine (cumulative dosage 1720 mg/m$^2$) in a 4-year-old child with medulloblastoma [166]. Cough, tachypnea and fatigue developed followed by progressive pulmonary insufficiency. Pulmonary pathological findings included interstitial fibrosis and alveolar dysplasia. Bailey *et al.* reported the case of a 22-month-old with medulloblastoma who developed fatal pulmonary fibrosis following carmustine therapy (cumulative dose equivalent to 1550 mg/m$^2$) [161]. Additional reports include adults who developed fatal, progressive, fibrosing alveolitis after receiving cumulative doses of carmustine in the 2–4 g range [162–164]. Symptoms included non-productive cough and increasing dyspnea. Chest radiographs demonstrated decreased lung volume and bilateral apical thickening. Pulmonary function tests showed decreased vital capacity. Pathological findings included extensive interstitial and pleural fibrosis without evidence of infection or malignancy.

Aronin *et al.* has suggested limiting the total carmustine dosage to 1400 mg/m$^2$ since the probability of pulmonary toxicity following doses above 1500 mg/m$^2$ approaches 50% [165]. There have, however, been reports of pulmonary toxicity developing in pediatric patients following considerably lower doses (800–1100 mg/m$^2$) [167]. In the series reported by Aronin *et al.*, patients who developed pulmonary toxicity had a significantly higher prevalence of pre-existing lung diseases such as asthma and recurrent pneumonias in the pediatric age group [165]. Pulmonary function should be followed closely in these patients, and carmustine therapy should be discontinued in patients with symptoms or laboratory abnormalities. The efficacy of corticosteroids in treating carmustine toxicity has not been established.

# Second malignant neoplasms

When a child is cured of cancer in the early years of life, there is probably nothing more devastating to both the child and the family than to be faced with a second malignant neoplasm (SMN). The magnitude of the risk of new neoplasms in such cured children is estimated to be 10–15 times greater than the cancer incidence among age-matched individuals [168–170]. This is an early estimate and does not consider the entire lifetime of such cured patients; there have been too few individuals who have attained the ages at which many of the adult cancers would normally become manifest. The risk to survivors of childhood cancer is not uniform; fortunately, some have a small risk of developing new tumors while in others host characteristics (either single genes or susceptibility characteristics) or treatment greatly increase susceptibility to additional cancers.

Differences in risk for SMN among survivors is well illustrated by the data from two large pediatric groups in which retinoblastoma, a cancer with a prominent genetic fraction, is the first neoplasm in

a disproportionately large number of cases [171,172]. That therapeutic interventions can also spuriously increase the risk is illustrated by Hodgkin's disease. Although rare in childhood, it is the second most common first neoplasm in the Late Effects Study Group registry with excess risk for leukemia attributable to alkylating agent chemotherapy and, for solid tumors, to irradiation [173,174].

The importance of studying SMN in children is three-fold: predisposed individuals need to be counselled in advance regarding their risks and followed expectantly; selection of therapy should be based, at least in part, on experience gained from observing such children for second neoplasms; and an understanding of the mechanisms by which new cancers are produced as a result of specific genes, of host susceptibilities such as in neurofibromatosis, or because of treatment, can be gained by their study.

## Predisposing conditions

Retinoblastoma is the prototypic embryonal neoplasm associated with an increased risk of SMN. Although approximately 90% of patients give a negative history, epidemiological evidence leads to the conclusion that all with bilateral disease (25%) and some with unilateral disease (10%) carry the gene [175]. While the location of the gene is known, the characteristic finding, a deletion of chromosome 13*q*14, is visible in only 6% of patients [176]. It is those with the gene who are predisposed to SMN, particularly bone and soft tissue sarcomas, with 10% of survivors being affected within 20 years [177].

Whether or not children with the genetic forms of Wilms' tumor and neuroblastoma will also have an increased SMN risk is not yet known [178]. The goal of research in this area would be to develop the technology for identifying susceptible children with all embryonal neoplasms so that they can be encouraged to adopt behaviors which will lead to early diagnosis and treatment of subsequent malignant neoplasms.

Predisposing conditions such as neurofibromatosis, xeroderma pigmentosum, the nevoid basal cell carcinoma syndrome and Turcot's syndrome are known to occur excessively in children with second malignant neoplasms [171]. The actual risk, however, in excess of that experienced by unaffected children is not known. Perhaps these children are more susceptible than others to some of the therapeutic modalities utilized in the treatment of their initial tumor. We know that those with ataxia telangiectasia are more sensitive to the killing effects of radiation, but whether or not they are also susceptible to new tumors is not yet known. It is also possible that some children who survive a first cancer are more susceptible to environmental carcinogens. It would be of great interest to determine whether such individuals have a heightened ability to form mutagens following exposure to carcinogens such as cigarette smoke.

That certain cancers occur more commonly in families is well known. The multiple endocrine neoplasia syndromes do not often affect children, but the associations noted between sarcomas of soft tissue and bone in young children and breast cancer at an early age in female relatives has been reported by Li and Fraumeni and recently by Birch and colleagues and Williams and Strong [179–181]. Others have reported an association between tumors of the central nervous system and the lymphohematopoietic system [182]. The Late Effects Study Group also observed that, in families in which these two tumors occurred as double primaries, there was also a tendency for them to occur in more than one family member as single primaries.

## Therapeutic effects

Both radiation and chemotherapy are known to be associated with new cancers. The earliest reports appearing in the literature were those in which radiation appeared to play an active role in the development of both leukemias and solid tumors, the former occurring after lower doses and the latter after higher doses. It is possible that children are more sensitive to the effects of radiation at certain periods in their lives. For example, doses sustained by young children to growing bone are more likely to result in bone cancer during periods of rapid growth 10–15 years later than similar doses given to fully grown individuals [183]. The Late Effects Study Group found a 100-fold excess risk of bone cancer following treatment with doses exceeding 40 Gy in children [184].

Chemotherapy has also been implicated in increasing SMN risk but, thus far, there is scant evidence for its relationship to solid tumors. Cyclophosphamide has been associated with a small excess risk for bone sarcomas in irradiated children [177,184] but the principal effects of alkylating agents have been exerted on bone marrow precursor cells. In the Late Effects Study Group registry, analysis demonstrated a dose-response relationship between alkylating agents and acute non-lymphocytic leukemia [173]. A subsequent cohort study of almost 1000 children with Hodgkin's disease confirmed that relationship and also showed that splenectomy increased that risk, independently [174]. There is recent evidence to suggest an epipodophyllotoxin/T cell leukemia interaction in the etiology of non-lymphocytic leukemias [185].

More extensive discussion of the factors associated with genetic and therapeutic risk factors can be found in recent reviews [186].

Unlike the typical adult who is 60 years old when cured of cancer, the average child is 10 years old and has a life time ahead. If one considers that 4000 children annually in the United States can now look forward to this increased life span, the number of potentially productive years is great. It is of considerable concern to pediatric oncologists that newer and more aggressive therapies now used for children with diseases resistant to conventional treatment have unknown long-term toxicities. Since few children receive such treatment, and the expectation is that fewer still will survive for long periods, pediatric oncologists and others who care for survivors should remain alert to deleterious consequences of new treatment and should collaborate with others in reporting such effects promptly.

## References


1. Meadows, A.T. and Silber, J.H. Delayed consequences of therapy. In *Cancer in Children, Clinical Management*, 2nd edn (eds J. Bloom, J. Lemerle, P.A. Voute and A. Barrett) Springer-Verlag, Heidelberg, pp. 70–81 (1986)
2. Byrd, R. Late effects of treatment of cancer in children. *Pediatric Clinics of North America*, **32**, 835–857 (1985)
3. Nesbit, M.E. Jr. *Clinics in Oncology: Late Effects in Successfully Treated Children with Cancer*, London, W.B. Saunders (1985)
4. Meadows, A.T. and Hobbie, W.L. The medical consequences of cure. *Cancer*, **58**, 524–528 (1986)
5. Sunderman, C.R. and Pearson, H.A. Growth effects of long-term antileukemia therapy. *Journal of Pediatrics*, **75**, 1058–1062 (1969)
6. Wells, R.J., Foster, M.B., D'Ercole, J. and McMillan, C.W. The impact of cranial irradiation on the growth of children with acute lymphocytic leukemia. *American Journal of Diseases in Children*, **137**, 37–39 (1983)
7. Zurlo, M.G., Senesi, E., Terracini, B. *et al.* Height of children off therapy after acute lymphoblastic leukemia. *Pediatric Hematology and Oncology*, **5**, 187–195 (1988)
8. Moell, C., Garwicz, S., Westgren, U. *et al.* Height, weight, and growth hormone secretion in children treated for acute leukemia. *European Paediatric Haematology and Oncology*, **1**, 167–172 (1984)
9. Kirk, J.A., Stevens, M.M., Menser, M.A. *et al.* Growth failure and growth-hormone deficiency after treatment for acute lymphoblastic leukaemia. *Lancet*, **i**, 190–193 (1987)
10. Costin, G. Effects of low-dose cranial radiation on growth hormone secretory dynamics and hypothalamic–pituitary function. *American Journal of Diseases in Children*, **142**, 847–852 (1988)
11. Blatt, J., Bercu, B.B., Gillin, J.C. *et al.* Reduced

pulsatile growth hormone secretion in children after therapy for acute lymphoblastic leukemia. *Journal of Pediatrics*, **104**, 182–186 (1984)

12. Moell, C., Garwicz, S., Westgren, U. and Wiebe, T. Disturbed pubertal growth in girls treated for acute lymphoblastic leukemia. *Pediatric Hematology and Oncology*, **4**, 1–5 (1987)

13. Robison, L.L., Nesbit, M.E., Sather, H.N. *et al.* Thyroid abnormalities in long-term survivors of childhood acute lymphoblastic leukemia (ALL) (abstract). *Pediatric Research*, **19**, 266 (1985)

14. Kerrebijn, K.F. and Kroon, J.P. Effect on height of corticosteroid therapy in asthmatic children. *Archives of Diseases in Children*, **43**, 556–561 (1968)

15. Lam, L.N. and Arneil, G.C. Long-term dwarfing effects of corticosteroid treatment for childhood nephrosis. *Archives of Diseases in Children*, **43**, 589–594 (1968)

16. Lilleyman, J.S. Male fertility after successful chemotherapy for lymphoblastic leukaemia (letter). *Lancet*, **ii**, 1125 (1979)

17. Matthews, J.H. and Wood, J.K. Male fertility during chemotherapy for acute leukemia (letter). *New England Journal of Medicine*, **303**, 1235 (1980)

18. Blatt, J., Poplack, D.G. and Sherins, R.J. Testicular function in boys after chemotherapy for acute lymphoblastic leukemia. *New England Journal of Medicine*, **304**, 1121–1124 (1981)

19. Brauner, R., Czernichow, P., Cramer, P.H. *et al.* Leydig-cell function in children after direct testicular irradiation for acute lymphoblastic leukemia. *New England Journal of Medicine*, **309**, 25–28 (1983)

20. Shalet, S.M., Horner, A., Ahmed, S.R. and Morris-Jones, P.H. Leydig cell damage after testicular irradiation for lymphoblastic leukaemia. *Medical and Pediatric Oncology*, **13**, 65–68 (1985)

21. Siris, E.S., Leventhal, B.G and Vaitukaitis, J.L. Effects of childhood leukemia and chemotherapy on puberty and reproductive function in girls. *New England Journal of Medicine*, **294**, 1143–1146 (1976)

22. Shalet, S.M., Beardwell, C.G., Twomey, J.A. *et al.* Endocrine function following the treatment of acute leukemia in childhood. *Journal of Pediatrics*, **90**, 920–923 (1977)

23. Hamre, M.R., Robison, L.L., Nesbit, M.E. *et al.* Effects of radiation on ovarian function in long-term survivors of childhood acute leukemia: a report from the Childrens Cancer Study Group. *Journal of Clinical Oncology*, **5**, 1759–1765 (1987)

24. Leiper, A.D., Stanhope, R., Kitching, P. and Chessels, J.M. Precocious and premature puberty associated with treatment of acute lymphoblastic leukaemia. *Archives of Diseases in Children*, **62**, 1107–1112 (1987)

25. Bleyer, W.A. and Griffin, T.W. White matter necrosis, mineralizing microangiopathy, and intellectual abilities in survivors of childhood leukemia: associations with central nervous system irradiation and methotrexate therapy. In *Radiation Damage to the Nervous System* (eds H.A. Gilbert and A.R. Kagan), Raven Press, New York, pp. 155–174 (1980)

26. Price, R.A. and Jamieson, P.A. The central nervous system in childhood leukemia. II: Subacute leukoencephalopathy. *Cancer*, **35**, 306–318 (1975)

27. Mauer, A.M. and Simone, J.V. The current status of the treatment of childhood acute lymphoblastic leukemia. *Cancer Treatment Reviews*, **3**, 17–41 (1976)

28. Packer, R.J., Meadows, A.T., Rorke, L.B. *et al.* Long-term sequelae of cancer treatment on the central nervous system in childhood. *Medical and Pediatric Oncology*, **15**, 241–253 (1987)

29. Brouwers, P., Riccardi, R., Fedio, P. and Poplack, D.G. Long-term neuropsychologic sequelae of childhood leukemia: correlation with CT brain scan abnormalities. *Journal of Psychiatry*, **106**, 723–728 (1985)

30. Eiser, C. Intellectual abilities among survivors of childhood leukemia as a function of CNS irradiation. *Archives of Diseases in Children*, **53**, 391–395 (1978)

31. Meadows, A.T., Gordon, J., Massari, D.J. *et al.* Declines in IQ scores and cognitive dysfunction in children with acute lymphocytic leukaemia treated with cranial irradiation. *Lancet*, **ii**, 1015–1018 (1981)

32. Peckham, V.C., Meadows, A.T., Bartel, N. and Marrero, O. Educational late effects in long-term survivors of childhood acute lymphocytic leukemia. *Pediatrics*, **81**, 127–133 (1988)

33. Moss, H.A., Nannis, E.D. and Poplack, D.G. The effects of prophylactic treatment of the central nervous system on the intellectual functioning of children with acute lymphocytic leukemia. *American Journal of Medicine*, **71**, 47–52 (1981)

34. Mulhern, R.K., Wasserman, A.L., Fairclough, D. and Ochs, J. Memory function in disease-free survivors of childhood acute lymphocytic leukemia given CNS prophylaxis with or without 1800 cGy cranial irradiation. *Journal of Clinical Oncology*, **6**, 315–320 (1988)

35. Britten, M., Halnan, K. and Meredith, W. Radiation cataract – new evidence on radiation dosage to the lens. *British Journal of Radiology*, **39**, 612–617 (1966)

36. Kline, R.W., Gerlin, M.T. and Kun, L.E. Cranial irradiation in acute leukemia: dose estimate in the lens. *International Journal of Radiation Oncology, Biology, Physics*, **5**, 117–121 (1979)

37. Weaver, G., Chauvenet, A., Smith, T. and Schwartz, A. Ophthalmic evaluation of long-term survivors of childhood acute lymphoblastic leukemia. *Cancer*, **58**, 963–968 (1986)

38. Jaffe, N., Toth, B., Hoar, R. *et al.* Dental and maxillofacial abnormalities in long-term survivors of childhood cancer: effects of treatment with chemotherapy and radiation to the head and neck. *Pediatrics*, **73**, 816–823 (1984)

39. Rosenberg, S.W., Kolodney, H., Wong, G.Y. and Murphy, M.L. Altered dental root development in long-term survivors of pediatric acute lymphoblastic leukemia. *Cancer*, **59**, 1640–1648 (1987)

40. Nesbit, M., Krivit, W. and Heyn, R. Acute and chronic effects of methotrexate on hepatic, pulmonary and skeletal systems. *Cancer*, **37**, 1048 (1976)

41. Rimsza, M.E. Complications of corticosteroid therapy. *American Journal of Diseases in Children*, **132**, 806–810 (1978)

42. Einhorn, M. and Davidson, I. Hepatotoxicity of mercaptopurine. *Journal of the American Medical Association*, **188**, 802–806 (1964)

43. Locasciulli, A., Vergani, G.M., Uderzo, G. *et al.* Chronic liver disease in children with leukemia in long-term remission. *Cancer*, **52**, 1008–1087 (1983)

44. Chilcote, R.R., Baehner, R.L. and Hammond, G.D. Septicemia and meningitis in children splenectomized for Hodgkin's disease. *New England Journal of Medicine*, **295**, 798–800 (1976)

45. Weitzman, S. and Aisenberg, A.C. Fulminant sepsis after the successful treatment of Hodgkin's disease. *American Journal of Medicine*, **62**, 47–50 (1977)

46. Ertel, I.J., Boles, E.T. Jr and Newton, W.A. Jr. Infection after splenectomy. *New England Journal of Medicine*, **296**, 1174 (1977)

47. Donaldson, S.S., Glatstein, E. and Vosti, K.L. Bacterial infections in pediatric Hodgkin's disease: relationship to radiotherapy, chemotherapy and splenectomy. *Cancer*, **41**, 1949–1958 (1978)

48. Hays, D.M., Ternberg, J., Chen, T.T. *et al.* Complications related to 234 staging laparotomies performed in the intergroup Hodgkin's disease in childhood study. *Surgery*, **96**, 471–478 (1984)

49. Green, D.M., Stutzman, L., Blumenson, L.E. *et al.* The incidence of post-splenectomy sepsis and herpes zoster in children and adolescents with Hodgkin's disease. *Medical and Pediatric Oncology*, **7**, 285–297 (1979)

50. Rosner, F. and Zarrabi, M.H. Late infections following splenectomy in Hodgkin's disease. *Cancer Investigation*, **1**, 57–65 (1983)

51. Dailey, M.O., Coleman, C.N. and Kaplan, H.S. Radiation-induced splenic atrophy in patients with Hodgkin's disease and non-Hodgkin's lymphoma. *New England Journal of Medicine*, **302**, 215–217 (1980)

52. Stevens, M., Brown, E. and Zipursky, A. The effect of abdominal radiation on spleen function: a study in children with Wilms' tumor. *Pediatric Hematology and Oncology*, **3**, 69–72 (1986)

53. Minor, D.R., Schiffman, G. and McIntosh, L.S. Response of patients with Hodgkin's disease to pneumococcal vaccine. *Annals of Internal Medicine*, **90**, 887–892 (1979)

54. Levine, A.M., Overturf, G.D., Field, R.F. *et al.* Use and efficacy of pneumococcal vaccine in patients with Hodgkin's disease. *Blood*, **54**, 1171–1175 (1979)

55. Byrne, J., Mulvihill, J.J., Myers, M.H. *et al.* Effects of treatment on fertility in long-term survivors of childhood or adolescent cancer. *New England Journal of Medicine*, **317**, 1315–1321 (1987)

56. Santoro, A., Viviani, S., Zucali, G. *et al.* Comparative results and toxicity of MOPP *versus* AVBD combined with radiotherapy (RT) in PS IIB, III(A,B) Hodgkin's disease. *Proceedings of the American Society of Clinical Oncology*, **2**, 223 (C-872) (1983)

57. Donaldson, S.S. and Kaplan, H.S. Complications of treatment of Hodgkin's disease in children. *Cancer Treatment Reports*, **66**, 977–989 (1982)

58. Perdick, T.J. and Hoppe, R.T. Recovery of spermatogenesis following pelvic irradiation for Hodgkin's disease. *International Journal of Radiation Oncology, Biology, Physics*, **12**, 117–121 (1986)

59. van Alphen, M.M.A., van de Kant, H.J.G. and de Rooij, D.G. Protection from radiation-induced damage of spermatogenesis in the Rhesus monkey (*Macaca mulatta*) by follicle-stimulating hormone. *Cancer Research*, **49**, 533–536 (1989)

60. Stricker, S., Crosby, K. and Carey, R.W. Paternity after chemotherapy-induced sterility in Hodgkin's disease. *New England Journal of Medicine*, **304**, 1175 (1981)

61. Sherins, R.J., Olivery, C.L.M. and Ziegler, J.L. Gynecomastia and gonadal function in adolescent boys treated with combination therapy for Hodgkin's disease. *New England Journal of Medicine*, **299**, 12–16 (1978)

62. Rivkees, S.A. and Crawford, J.D. The relationship of gonadal activity and chemotherapy-induced gonadal damage. *Journal of the American Medical Association*, **259**, 2123–2125 (1988)

63. Whitehead, E., Shalet, S.M., Morris-Jones, P.H. *et al.* Gonadal function after combination chemotherapy for Hodgkin's disease in childhood. *Archives of Diseases in Childhood*, **47**, 287–291 (1982)

64. Glode, L.M., Robinson, J. and Gould, S.F. Protection from cyclophosphamide-induced testicular damage with an analogue of gonadotropin-releasing hormone. *Lancet*, **i**, 1132 (1981)

65. LeFloch, O., Donaldson, S.S. and Kaplan, H.S. Pregnancy following oophoropexy and total nodal irradiation in women with Hodgkin's disease. *Cancer*, **38**, 2263–2268 (1976)

66. Horning, S.J., Hoppe, R.T., Kaplan, H.S. and Rosenberg, S.A. Female reproductive potential after treatment for Hodgkin's disease. *New England Journal of Medicine*, **304**, 1377–1382 (1981)

67. Schilsky, R.L., Sherins, R.J., Hubbard, S.M. *et al.* Long-term follow-up of ovarian function in women treated with MOPP chemotherapy for Hodgkin's disease. *American Journal of Medicine*, **71**, 522–526 (1981)

68. Chapman, R.M., Sutcliffe, S.B. and Malpas, J.S. Cytotoxic-induced ovarian failure in women with Hodgkin's disease. I. Hormone function. *Journal of the American Medical Association*, **242**, 1877–1881 (1979)

69. Meadows, A.T., Gallagher, J.A., Jarrett, P. *et al.* Ovarian function following therapy for childhood Hodgkin's disease (HD). *Medical and Pediatric Oncology*, **17**, 345, Abstract 257 (1989)

70. Morgan, G.W., Freeman, A.P., McLean, R.G. *et al.* Late cardiac, thyroid and pulmonary sequelae of mantle radiotherapy for Hodgkin's disease. *International Journal of Radiation Oncology, Biology, Physics*, **11**, 1925–1931 (1985)

71. Kaplan, M.M., Garnick, M.B., Gelber, R. *et al.* Risk factors for thyroid abnormalities after neck irradiation for childhood cancer. *American Journal of Medicine*, **74**, 272 (1983)

72. Green, D.M., Brecher, M.L., Yakar, D. *et al.* Thyroid function in pediatric patients after neck irradiation for Hodgkin's disease. *Medical and Pediatric Oncology*, **8**, 127–136 (1980)

73. Devney, R.B., Sklar, C.A., Nesbit, M.E. *et al.* Serial thyroid function measurements in children with Hodgkin's disease. *Journal of Pediatrics*, **105**, 223 (1984)

74. Sullivan, M., Reid, H., Broin, H. and Lewis, E. Noninvasive (ultrasound) screening for thyroid abnormalities in 21 survivors of Hodgkin's disease (HD) of childhood. *Proceedings of the American Society of Clinical Oncology*, **5**, 196 (1986)

75. Smith, R.E., Adler, R.A., Clark, P. *et al.* Thyroid function after mantle irradiation in Hodgkin's disease. *Journal of the American Medical Association*, **245**, 46–49 (1981)

76. Shalet, S.M., Rosenstock, J.D., Beardwell, C.G. *et al.* Thyroid function following external irradiation to the neck for Hodgkin's disease in childhood. *Radiology*, **28**, 511–515 (1977)

77. Glatstein, E., McHardy-Young, S., Brast, N. *et al.* Alterations in serum thyrotropin (TSH) and thyroid function following radiotherapy in patients with malignant lymphoma. *Journal of Clinical Endocrinology and Metabolism*, **32**, 833–841 (1971)

78. Constine, L.S., Donaldson, S.S., McDougall, R. *et al.* Thyroid dysfunction after radiotherapy in children with Hodgkin's disease. *Cancer*, **53**, 878–883 (1984)

79. Schimpff, S.C., Diggs, C.H., Wiswell, J.G. *et al.* Radiation-related thyroid dysfunction: implications for the treatment of Hodgkin's disease. *Annals of Internal Medicine*, **92**, 91–98 (1980)

80. Lange, B.J. and Meadows, A.T. Late effects of Hodgkin's disease treatment in children. In *Hodgkin's Disease in Children* (ed. W.A. Kamps), Kluwer Academic Publishers, Boston, pp. 195–220 (1989)

81. Carmel, R. and Kaplan, H. Mantle irradiation in Hodgkin's disease. An analysis of technique, tumor eradication and complications. *Cancer*, **37**, 2813–2825 (1976)

82. Dunsmore, L.D., LoPonte, M.A. and Dunsmore, R.A. Radiation-induced coronary artery disease. *Journal of the American College of Cardiology*, **8**, 239–244 (1986)

83. Boivin, J.F. and Hutchison, G.B. Coronary heart disease mortality after irradiation for Hodgkin's disease. *Cancer*, **49**, 2470–2475 (1982)

84. LaMonte, C.S., Yeh, S.D.J. and Straus, D.J. Long-term follow-up of cardiac function in patients with Hodgkin's disease treated with mediastinal irradiation and combination chemotherapy including doxorubicin. *Cancer Treatment Reports*, **70**, 439–444 (1986)

85. Comis, R.L. Bleomycin pulmonary toxicity. In *Bleomycin: Current Status and New Developments* (eds S.K. Carter, S.T. Crooke and H. Umezawa), Academic Press, New York, pp. 279–291 (1978)

86. Silber, J.H., Littman, P.S. and Meadows, A.T. Stature loss following skeletal irradiation for childhood cancer. *Journal of Clinical Oncology*, **8**, 304–312 (1990)

87. Probert, J.C. and Parker, B.P. The effects of radiation therapy on bone growth. *Radiology*, **114**, 155–162 (1975)

88. Chao, N., Levine, J. and Horning, S.J. Retroperitoneal fibrosis following treatment for Hodgkin's disease. *Journal of Clinical Oncology*, **5**, 231–232 (1987)

89. Blijham, G.H., Vermeulen, A. and Mendes de Leon, D.E. Osteonecrosis of sternum and rib in a patient treated for Hodgkin's disease. *Cancer*, **56**, 2292–2294 (1985)

90. Sallan, S.E. and Clavell, L.A. Cardiac effects of anthracyclines used in the treatment of childhood acute lymphoblastic leukemia: a 10-year experience. *Seminars in Oncology*, **11**, 19–21 (1984)

91. Pratt, C.B., Ransom, J.L. and Evans, W.E. Age-related adriamycin cardiotoxicity in children. *Cancer Treatment Reports*, **62**, 1381–1384 (1978)

92. Von Hoff, D.D. and Layard, M.W. Risk factors for development of daunorubicin cardiotoxicity. *Cancer Treatment Reports*, **65**(Suppl 4), 19–23 (1981)

93. Gilladoga, A.C., Manuel, C., Tan, C.T.C. *et al.* The cardiotoxicity of adriamycin and daunomycin in children. *Cancer*, **37**, 1070–1078 (1976)

94. Kushner, J.R., Hansen, V.L. and Hammer, S.P. Cardiomyopathy after widely separated courses of adriamycin exacerbated by actinomycin D and mithramycin. *Cancer*, **36**, 1577–1584 (1975)

95. Minow, R.A., Benjamin, R.S. and Gottlieb, J.A. Adriamycin (NSC-123127) cardiomyopathy: an overview with determination of risk factors. *Cancer Chemotherapy Reports*, **6**, 195–201 (1975)

96. Weiss, A.J. and Manthel, R.W. Experience with the use of adriamycin in combination with other anticancer agents using a weekly schedule, with particular reference to lack of cardiac toxicity. *Cancer*, **40**, 2046–2052 (1977)

97. Legha, S.S., Benjamin, R.S., Mackay, B. *et al.* Reduction of doxorubicin cardiotoxicity by prolonged continuous intravenous infusion. *Annals of Internal Medicine*, **96**, 133–139 (1982)

98. Torti, F.M., Bristow, M.R., Howes, A.E. *et al.* Reduced cardiotoxicity of doxorubicin delivered on a weekly schedule: assessment by endomyocardial biopsy. *Annals of Internal Medicine*, **99**, 745–749 (1983)

99. Weiss, A.J., Metter, G.E., Fletcher, W.S. *et al.* Studies on adriamycin using a weekly regimen

demonstrating its clinical effectiveness and lack of cardiac toxicity. *Cancer Treatment Reports*, **60**, 813–822 (1976)

100. Chlebowski, R.T., Paroly, W.S., Pugh, R.P. *et al.* Adriamycin given as weekly schedule without a loading course: clinically effective with a reduced incidence of cardiotoxicity. *Cancer Treatment Reports*, **60**, 47–51 (1980)

101. Druck, M.N., Gulenchyn, K.Y., Evans, W.K. *et al.* Radionuclide angiography and endomyocardial biopsy in the assessment of doxorubicin cardiotoxicity. *Cancer*, **53**, 1666–1674 (1984)

102. Schwartz, R.G., McKenzie, W.B., Alexander, J. *et al.* Congestive heart failure and left ventricular dysfunction: a complication of doxorubicin therapy: seven-year experience using serial radionuclide angiocardiography. *American Journal of Medicine*, **82**, 1109–1118 (1987)

103. Almeri, S.T., Bonow, R.O., Myers, C.E. *et al.* Prospective evaluation of doxorubicin cardiotoxicity by rest and exercise radionuclide angiography. *American Journal of Cardiology*, **58**, 607–613 (1986)

104. Alexander, J., Dainiak, N., Berger, H.J. *et al.* Serial assessment of doxorubicin cardiotoxicity with quantitative radionuclide angiocardiography. *New England Journal of Medicine*, **300**, 278–283 (1979)

105. Bristow, M.R., Mason, J.W., Billingham, M.E. and Daniels, J.R. Doxorubicin cardiomyopathy: evaluation by phonocardiography, endomyocardial biopsy, and cardiac catheterization. *Annals of Internal Medicine*, **88**, 168–175 (1978)

106. Bloom, K.R., Bini, R.M., Constance, M.W. *et al.* Echocardiography in adriamycin cardiotoxicity. *Cancer*, **41**, 1265–1269 (1978)

107. Ramos, A., Meyer, R.A., Korfhazen, J. *et al.* Echocardiographic evaluation of adriamycin cardiotoxicity in children. *Cancer Treatment Reports*, **60**, 1281–1284 (1976)

108. Friedman, M.A., Bozdech, M.J., Billingham, M.E. and Rider, A.K. Doxorubicin cardiotoxicity: serial endomyocardial biopsies and systolic time intervals. *Journal of the American Medical Association*, **240**, 1603–1606 (1978)

109. Pegelow, C.H., Popper, R.W., de Wit, S.A. *et al.* Endomyocardial biopsy to monitor anthracycline therapy in children. *Journal of Clinical Oncology*, **2**, 443–446 (1984)

110. Goorin, A.M., Borow, K.M., Goldman, A. *et al.* Congestive heart failure due to adriamycin cardiotoxicity: its natural history in children. *Cancer*, **47**, 2810–2816 (1981)

111. Freter, C.E., Lee, T.C., Billingham, M.E. *et al.* Doxorubicin cardiac toxicity manifesting seven years after treatment: case report and review. *American Journal of Medicine*, **80**, 483–485 (1986)

112. Steinherz, L., Steinherz, P., Tan, C. and Murphy, L. Cardiac toxicity 4–20 years after completing anthracycline therapy. *Proceedings of the American Society of Clinical Oncology*, **8**, 296 (Abstract 1151) (1989)

113. Lewis, A.B., Crouse, V.L., Evans, W. *et al.* Recovery of left ventricular function following discontinuation of anthracycline chemotherapy in children. *Pediatrics*, **68**, 67–72 (1981)

114. Couch, R.D., Loh, K.K. and Sugino, J. Sudden cardiac death following adriamycin therapy. *Cancer*, **48**, 38–39 (1981)

115. Benoist, M.R., Lemerle, J., Jean, R. *et al.* Effects on pulmonary function of whole lung irradiation for Wilms' tumour in children. *Thorax*, **37**, 175–180 (1982)

116. Littman, P., Meadows, A.T., Polgar, G. *et al.* Pulmonary function in survivors of Wilms' tumor: patterns of impairment. *Cancer*, **32**, 2773–2776 (1976)

117. Cohen, M.D., Mirkin, D.L., Provisor, A. *et al.* Lung nodules after whole lung radiation. *American Journal of Pediatric Hematology and Oncology*, **5**, 283–286 (1983)

118. Aperia, A., Broberger, O., Wikstad, I. and Wilton, P. Renal growth and function in patients nephrectomized in childhood. *Acta Paediatrica Scandinavica*, **66**, 185–192 (1977)

119. Robitaille, P., Lortie, L., Mongeau, J-G. and Sinnassansy, P. Long-term follow-up of patients who underwent unilateral nephrectomy in childhood. *Lancet*, **i**, 1297–1299 (1985)

120. Hakim, R.M., Goldszer, R.C. and Brenner, B.M. Hypertension and proteinuria: long-term sequelae of uninephrectomy in humans. *Kidney International*, **25**, 930–936 (1984

121. Koskimies, O. Arterial hypertension developing 10 years after radiotherapy for Wilms' tumour. *British Medical Journal*, **285**, 996–998 (1982)

122. Arneil, G.C., Emmanuel, I.G. and Flatman, G.E. Nephritis in two children after irradiation and chemotherapy for nephroblastoma. *Lancet*, **i**, 960–963 (1974)

123. Cassady, J.R., Tefft, M., Feller, R.M. *et al.* Considerations in the radiation therapy of Wilms' tumor. *Cancer*, **32**, 598–608 (1973)

124. Madrazo, A., Schwarz, G. and Churg, J. Radiation nephritis: a review. *Journal of Urology*, **124**, 822–827 (1975)

125. Burk, C.D., Restaino, I., Kaplan, B. and Meadows, A.T. Ifosfamide-induced renal tubular dysfunction and rickets in children with Wilms' tumor. *Journal of Pediatrics*, **117**, 331–335 (1990)

126. Merriam, G.R., Szechter, A. and Focht, E.F. The effects of ionizing radiations on the eye. *Frontiers of Radiation Therapy and Oncology*, **6**, 346–385 (1972)

127. Heyn, R., Ragab, A., Raney, R.B. Jr *et al.* Late effects of therapy in orbital rhabdomyosarcoma in children: a report from the Intergroup Rhabdomyosarcoma Study. *Cancer*, **57**, 1738–1743 (1986)

128. Fromm, M., Littman, P., Raney, R.B. *et al.* Late effects after treatment of twenty children with soft tissue sarcoma of the head and neck. *Cancer*, **57**, 2070–2076 (1986)

129. Dias, A. Effects on the hearing of patients treated by irradiation in the head and neck area. *Journal of Laryngology*, **80**, 276–287 (1966)

130. Dini, G., Lanino, E., Rogers, D. *et al.* Resistant and relapsing neuroblastoma: improved response rate with a new multiagent regimen (OC-HDP) including high-dose *cis*-platinum. *Medical and Pediatric Oncology*, **15**, 18–23 (1987)

131. Brock, P., Pritchard, J., Bellman, S. and Pinkerton, C.R. Ototoxicity of high-dose *cis*-platinum in children (letter). *Medical and Pediatric Oncology*, **16**, 368–369 (1988)

132. Brock, P., Yeomans, E., Bellman, S. and Pritchard, J. Ototoxicity in children treated with *cis*-platinum for germ cell and other tumours (abstract). *Medical and Pediatric Oncology*, **15**, 327 (1987)

133. Walker, D.A., Pillow, J., Waters, K.D. and Keir, E. Enhanced *cis*-platinum ototoxicity in children with brain tumours who have received simultaneous or prior cranial irradiation. *Medical and Pediatric Oncology*, **17**, 48–52 (1989)

134. Samaan, N.A., Vieto, R., Schultz, P.N. *et al.* Hypothalamic, pituitary and thyroid dysfunction after radiotherapy to the head and neck. *International Journal of Radiation Oncology, Biology, Physics*, **8**, 1857–1867 (1982)

135. Dawson, W.B. Growth impairment following radiotherapy in childhood. *Clinical Radiology*, **19**, 241–256 (1968)

136. Guyuron, B., Dagys, A.P., Munro, I.R. and Ross, R.B. Effect of irradiation on facial growth: a 7–25 year follow-up. *Annals of Plastic Surgery*, **11**, 423–427 (1983)

137. King, J. and Stowe, S. Results of spinal fusion for radiation scoliosis. *Spine*, **7**, 574–585 (1982)

138. Mayfield, J.K., Riseborough, E.J., Jaffe, N. and Nehme, M.E. Spinal deformity in children treated for neuroblastoma: the effect of radiation and other forms of treatment. *Journal of Bone and Joint Surgery*, **63A**, 183–193 (1981)

139. Thomas, P.R.M., Griffith, K.D., Fineberg, B.B. *et al.* Late effects of treatment for Wilms' tumor. *International Journal of Radiation Oncology, Biology, Physics*, **9**, 651–657 (1983)

140. Ryan, B.R. and Walters, T.R. Slipped capital femoral epiphysis following radiotherapy and chemotherapy. *Medical and Pediatric Oncology*, **6**, 279–283 (1979)

141. Rubin, P. and Casarett, G.W. *Clinical Radiation Pathology*, W.B. Saunders, Philadelphia, pp. 519–521 (1968)

142. Botnick, E.B., Goodman, R., Jaffe, N. *et al.* Stages I–III Hodgkin's disease in children: results of staging and treatment. *Cancer*, **39**, 599–603 (1977)

143. Dickerman, J.D., Newberg, A.H. and Moreland, M.D. Slipped capital femoral epiphysis (SCFE) following pelvic irradiation for rhabdomyosarcoma. *Cancer*, **44**, 480–482 (1979)

144. Li, F.P. and Stone, R. Survivors of cancer in childhood. *Annals of Internal Medicine*, **84**, 551–553 (1976)

145. Li, F.P., Winston, K.R. and Gimbrere, K. Follow-up of children with brain tumors. *Cancer*, **54**, 135–138 (1984)

146. LeBaron, S., Zeltzer, P.M., Zeltzer, L.K. *et al.* Assessment of quality of survival in children with medulloblastoma and cerebellar astrocytoma. *Cancer*, **62**, 1215–1222 (1988)

147. Bloom, H.J.G., Wallace, E.N.K. and Henk, J.M. The treatment and prognosis of medulloblastoma in children. *American Journal of Roentgenology*, **105**, 43–62 (1969)

148. Danoff, B.F., Cowchock, F.S., Marquette, C. *et al.* Assessment of the long-term effects of primary radiation therapy for brain tumors in children. *Cancer*, **49**, 1580–1586 (1982)

149. Spunberg, J.J., Chang, C.H., Goldman, M. *et al.* Quality of long-term survival following irradiation for intracranial tumors in children under the age of two. *International Journal of Radiation Oncology, Biology, Physics*, **7**, 727–736 (1981)

150. Eiser, C. Psychological sequelae of brain tumours in childhood: a retrospective study. *British Journal of Clinical Psychology*, **20**, 35–38 (1981)

151. Bamford, F.N., Morris-Jones, P., Pearson, D. *et al.* Residual disabilities in children treated for intracranial space-occupying lesions. *Cancer*, **37**, 1149–1151 (1976)

152. Hirsch, J.F., Reiner, D., Czerichow, P. *et al.* Medulloblastoma in childhood: survival and functional results. *Acta Neurochirurgica*, **48**, 1–15 (1979)

153. Voorhess, M.L., Brecker, M.L., MacGillivaray, M.H. *et al.* Hypothalamus–pituitary function of children with acute lymphocytic leukemia after three forms of central nervous system prophylaxis. *Cancer*, **57**, 1287–1291 (1986)

154. Duffner, P.K., Cohen, M.E., Voorhess, M.L. *et al.* Long-term effects of cranial irradiation on endocrine function in children with brain tumors: a prospective study. *Cancer*, **56**, 2189–2193 (1985)

155. Pasqualini, T., Diez, B., Domene, H. *et al.* Long-term endocrine sequelae after surgery, radiotherapy, and chemotherapy in children with medulloblastoma. *Cancer*, **59**, 801–806 (1987)

156. Duffner, P.K., Cohen, M.E., Anderson, S.W. *et al.* Long-term effects of treatment on endocrine function in children with brain tumors. *Annals of Neurology*, **14**, 528–532 (1983)

157. Lustig, R.H., Schriock, E.A., Kaplan, S.L. and Grumbach, M.M. Effect of growth hormone-releasing factor on growth hormone release in children with radiation-induced growth hormone deficiency. *Pediatrics*, **76**, 274–279 (1985)

158. Ahmed, S.R., Shalet, S.M., Campbell, R.H.A. and Deaxin, D.P. Primary gonadal damage following treatment of brain tumors in childhood. *Journal of Pediatrics*, **103**, 562–565 (1983)

159. Clayton, P.E., Shalet, S.M., Price, D.A. and Morris-

Jones, P.H. Testicular damage after chemotherapy for childhood brain tumours. *Journal of Pediatrics*, **112**, 922–926 (1988)

160. Clayton, P.E., Shalet, S.M., Price, D.A. and Morris-Jones, P.H. Ovarian function following chemotherapy for childhood brain tumours. *Medical and Pediatric Oncology*, **17**, 92–96 (1989)

161. Bailey, C.C., Marsden, H.B. and Morris-Jones, P.H. Fatal pulmonary fibrosis following 1,3-bis(2-chloroethyl)-1-nitrosourea (BCNU) therapy. *Cancer*, **42**, 74–76 (1978)

162. Richter, J.E., Hastedt, R., Dalton, J.F. *et al.* Pulmonary toxicity of bischloroethylnitrosourea: report of a case with transient response to corticosteroid therapy. *Cancer*, **43**, 1607–1612 (1979)

163. Pridgen, D.B., Aiken, S.C., Speir, W.A. *et al.* Progressive fibrosing alveolitis complicating prolonged therapy with 1,3-bis(2-chloroethyl)-1-nitrosourea (BCNU). *American Review of Respiratory Diseases*, **115**, 153 (1977)

164. Crittenden, D., Tranum, B.L. and Haut, A. Pulmonary fibrosis after prolonged therapy with 1,3-bis(2-chloroethyl)-1-nitrosourea. *Chest*, **72**, 372–373 (1977)

165. Aronin, P.A., Makaley, M.S. Jr, Rudnick, S.A. *et al.* Prediction of BCNU pulmonary toxicity in patients with malignant gliomas: an assessment of risk factors. *New England Journal of Medicine*, **303**, 183–188 (1980)

166. Ryan, B.R. and Walters, T.R. Pulmonary fibrosis: a complication of 1,3-bis(2-chloroethyl)-1-nitrosourea (BCNU) therapy. *Cancer*, **48**, 909–911 (1981)

167. Durant, J.R., Norgard, M.J., Murad, T.M. *et al.* Pulmonary toxicity associated with bischloroethylnitrosourea (BCNU). *Annals of Internal Medicine*, **90**, 191–194 (1979)

168. Mike, V., Meadows, A.T. and D'Angio, G.J. Incidence of second malignant neoplasms in children: results of an international study. *Lancet*, **ii**, 1326–1331 (1982)

169. Tucker, M.A., Meadows, A.T., Boice, J.D. *et al.* Cancer risk following treatment of childhood cancer. In *Radiation Carcinogenesis: Epidemiology and Biological Significance* (eds J.D. Boice and J.F. Fraumeni), Raven Press, New York, pp. 211–224 (1984)

170. Hawkins, M.M., Draper, G.J. and Kingston, J.L. Incidence of second primary tumours among childhood cancer survivors. *British Journal of Cancer*, **56**, 339–347 (1987)

171. Meadows, A.T., Baum, E., Fossati-Bellani, F. *et al.* Second malignant neoplasms in children: an update from the Late Effects Study Group. *Journal of Clinical Oncology*, **3**, 532–538 (1985)

172. Kingston, J.E., Hawkins, M.M., Draper, G.J. *et al.* Patterns of multiple primary tumours in patients treated for cancer during childhood. *British Journal of Cancer*, **56**, 331–338 (1987)

173. Tucker, M.A., Meadows, A.T., Boice, J.D. Jr *et al.* Leukemia after therapy with alkylating agents for childhood cancer. *Journal of the National Cancer Institute*, **78**, 459–464 (1987)

174. Meadows, A.T., Obringer, A.C., Marrero, O. *et al.* Second malignant neoplasms following childhood Hodgkin's disease: treatment and splenectomy as risk factors. *Medical and Pediatric Oncology*, **17**, 477–484 (1989)

175. Knudson, A.G. Mutation and cancer: a statistical study of retinoblastoma. *Proceedings of the National Academy of Sciences of the USA*, **68**, 820–823 (1971)

176. Bunin, G.R., Emanuel, B.S., Meadows, A.T. *et al.* Frequency of 13q abnormalities among 203 patients with retinoblastoma. *Journal of the National Cancer Institute*, **81**, 370–374 (1989)

177. Draper, G.J., Sanders, B.M. and Kingston, J.E. Second primary neoplasms in patients with retinoblastoma. *British Journal of Cancer*, **53**, 661–671 (1986)

178. Knudson, A.G. Jr. Genetics and the child cured of cancer. In *Status of the Curability of Childhood Cancers* (eds J. van Eys and M.P. Sullivan), Raven Press, New York, pp. 295–305 (1980)

179. Li, F.P. and Fraumeni, J.F. Jr. Prospective study of a family cancer syndrome. *Journal of the American Medical Association*, **247**, 2692–2694 (1982)

180. Birch, J.M., Hartley, A.L., Marsden, H.B. *et al.* Excess risk of breast cancer in the mothers of children with soft tissue sarcomas. *British Journal of Cancer*, **49**, 325–331 (1984)

181. Williams, W.R. and Strong, L.C. Genetic epidemiology of soft tissue sarcomas in children. In *Familial Cancer. First International Research Conference, Basel* (ed. W. Muller), Karger, Basel, Switzerland, pp. 151–153 (1985)

182. Farwell, J. and Flannery, J.T. Cancer in relatives of children with central nervous system neoplasms. *New England Journal of Medicine*, **311**, 749–753 (1984)

183. Meadows, A.T., Strong, L.C., Li, F.P. *et al.* Bone sarcoma as a second malignant neoplasm in children: influence of radiation and genetic predisposition. *Cancer*, **46**, 2603–2606 (1980)

184. Tucker, M.A., D'Angio, G.J., Boice, J.D. Jr *et al.* Bone sarcomas linked to radiotherapy and chemotherapy in children. *New England Journal of Medicine*, **317**, 588–593 (1987)

185. Pui, C-H., Behm, F.G., Raimondi, S.C. *et al.* Secondary acute myeloid leukemia in children treated for acute lymphoid leukemia. *New England Journal of Medicine*, **321**, 136–142 (1989)

186. Meadows, A.T. Second malignant neoplasms. In *Clinics in Oncology Vol. 4: Late Effects in Successfully Treated Children with Cancer* (ed. M.E. Nesbit Jr), W.B. Saunders, London, pp. 247–261 (1985)

# 8

# Long-term survivors of childhood and adolescent cancer: their fertility and the health of their offspring

**J. Byrne and J.J. Mulvihill**

Improved survival rates after treatment for childhood and adolescent cancer is the great success story of modern cancer medicine. However, increased longevity and cure allow recognition of late complications of treatment that can persist or emerge years after all therapy has ceased. As the gain in years of life increases, these late effects become more important. The prospect of impaired fertility is one of the most difficult of these late complications for former patients and clinicians to deal with. The need to balance precise information about future reproductive performance against the possibility of raising needless fears in the patient and family is further complicated by the lack of accurate information for counselling. Even when fertility appears to be preserved, there may be difficulties in conceiving or fathering a child and anxiety about the health of children is frequent.

In this chapter we discuss what is known about the effects of treatment on proven fertility in long-term survivors of childhood and adolescent cancer, what is known about the course of pregnancy and about its outcome, including the health of children of survivors. We mention briefly the effects of cancer therapy administered during pregnancy and conclude with guidelines for genetic and reproductive counselling of cancer patients and their families, as well as long-term survivors.

## Studies of fertility and offspring

Studies of proven fertility in survivors of childhood and adolescent cancer have been infrequent, partly because cancer in childhood is rare and also because long-term observations, into the third decade, are needed before reproduction is tested. For these reasons studies of long-term survivors of childhood cancer are often confined to clinical investigations at single institutions with good patient follow-up, which in turn limits the numbers of survivors enrolled, and restricts the analysis to simple descriptive statistics. Unfortunately, reproductive events are too complicated to be adequately treated in a descriptive manner. Simon [1] has pointed out several potential difficulties with analyses of these kinds of data, such as considering as equivalent the outcomes of multiple pregnancies to the same individual and single pregnancies to multiple individuals, and the implications of clustering of abnormal pregnancies in one woman.

Late effects of cancer treatment on fertility as measured by endocrine status have been studied for some time and are fairly well understood. Some generalizations can be made about the effects of therapy on gonadal functioning. The nature and dose of chemotherapy and the site and dose of radiotherapy are of crucial importance in determining the degree of fertility impairment. Treatment with alkylating agents such as cyclophosphamide is very much more gonadotoxic than treatment with non-alkylating agents such as doxorubicin [2] and damage is dose-dependent [3,4]. The damage associated with radiotherapy can be directly related to distance from the gonads, shown for instance by Hamre *et al.* [5] for elevated gonadotropins and by Byrne *et al.* [6] for proven fertility. Host characteristics also determine response; for instance after chemotherapy prepubertal children are less affected than children treated during or after puberty; girls are less severely affected than boys; in fact, girls treated before puberty have fewer ill effects [4,6]. Figure 8.1, adapted from Rivkees and Crawford [4], illustrates some of these effects.

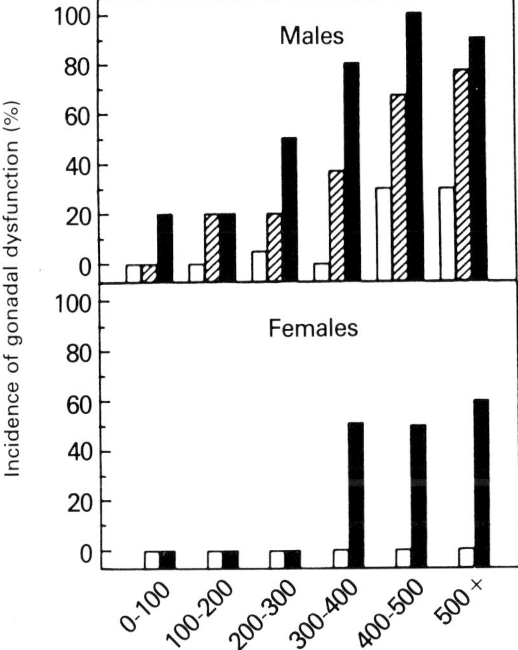


**Figure 8.1** Incidence of cyclophosphamide-induced gonadal dysfunction as related to pubertal stage during therapy and total dose of cyclophosphamide administered for treatment of renal disease: □, prepubertal; ▨, midpubertal; ■, sexually mature. Midpubertal females not included due to small numbers. Adapted from Rivkees and Crawford [4] with permission

However, the direct effects of radiation which lead to cell death are quite different from the long-term systemic effects seen after chemotherapy. Direct radiation damage to the gonads and organs of the pelvis may result in aplasia and loss of function, whereas chemotherapy has both systemic and targeted effects. Moreover, the site of the cancer and the type of directed treatment will determine the nature and severity of lasting defects. The sex of the survivor, the age at diagnosis, the location of the cancer and the type of treatment all lead to different kinds of late complications.

## Why study the offspring of survivors?

### *To provide clinical counselling*

Survivors, their physicians and families need information about the risk of problem pregnancies. Current advice to couples ranges from specific instructions not to have children to reassurance that there is nothing to worry about, or no advice at all. Some centers recommend that the survivor's chromosomes be studied before starting a family; others advise that prenatal diagnosis be performed.

Every couple undertaking a pregnancy faces some risk of an adverse outcome. As with fertility itself, any excess risk theoretically due to the parent's cancer or its treatment, would depend on a number of other factors such as the age of the parent when cancer was diagnosed, the type of cancer, the interval since diagnosis and treatment, and the type, duration and dose of treatment received. It is likely, too, that any risk will differ for males and females. A potential difficulty in using information currently available for counselling (Table 8.1) is that patients diagnosed and treated today will receive different therapeutic agents, doses or combinations from those used in the past.

### *To search for mutagenicity*

A mutagen is a chemical or other agent that causes sudden and permanent change in the human genetic material. In theory there is good reason for concern about the mutagenic effects of cancer treatments. Cancer patients constitute a cohort of people exposed to immense doses of chemicals and ionizing radiation which are specifically designed to interfere with the normal function of DNA. Thus, it would not be surprising if cancer survivors had a high rate of spontaneous abortions with chromosomal anomalies, especially in the first trimester, or stillbirths, or children with congenital malformations, or other conditions arising from a single gene defect. All of these could be interpreted as being the result of the action of a mutagen [7].

X-rays and alkylating agents were the first agents shown to cause mutations in experimental systems. Many cancer treatments are mutagenic *in vitro*, as in the salmonella assay (the Ames test). In tests conducted *in vitro* in human tissues, cancer drugs have been shown to cause mutations at the hypoxanthine-guanine phosphoribosyltransferase locus (HGPRT), the mutant gene which causes the Lesch-Nyhan syndrome. Cancer drugs can also cause temporary elevations in sister chromatid exchanges and long lasting chromosome changes of other types.

The search for *in vivo* genetic effects in offspring of Japanese survivors of atomic bombs has not shown a significant germ-cell effect due to a single dose of radiation [8]. Germ-cell alteration after chronic, fractionated and high-dose exposure, such as that given for cancer therapy, cannot be ruled out. Hence, the study of offspring of cancer survivors is one way of gaining some knowledge about

**Table 8.1 Pregnancy outcomes in twelve large series of childhood cancer survivors**

| Authors | Dates of diagnosis | Types of cancer | No. pregnant subjects | Total no. of pregnancies | Total fetal deaths | | | | Livebirth outcomes | | | | | | Malformations |
|---|---|---|---|---|---|---|---|---|---|---|---|---|---|---|---|
| | | | | | Ectopic | Miscarriage | Elective abortion | Stillbirth | Live births | Normal | Malformed | Infant deaths | SGA/ preterm | Cancer in off-spring | |
| Li et al., 1979[a] [53] | ?–1978 | Various | 146 | 287 | 0 | 25 | 19 | 1 | 242 | 213 | 20 | 7 | | 2 | 16 minor; 4 major (Marfan's syndrome, deafness, Hirschsprung's disease, pyloric stenosis) |
| Blatt et al., 1980 [54] | ?–1980 | Various | 30 | 42 | 0 | 2 | 10 | 0 | 28 | 27? | 1 | | | | No major defects; congenital hip dysplasia |
| Horning et al., 1981 [30] | 1968–79 | Hodgkin's disease | 20 | 28 | 0 | 0 | 5 | 0 | 24 | 21 | 0 | | 3 | | None |
| Marradi et al., 1982 [55] | | Leukemia | 14 | –[b] | –[b] | –[b] | –[b] | –[b] | 23 | 21 | 2 | | | 0 | Multiple congenital anomalies; gastroschisis |
| Bundey and Evans 1982 [56] | | | 24 | 48 | 0 | 3 | 0 | 0 | 44 | 43 | 1 | 0 | 0 | 0 | Pyloric stenosis |
| Andrieu et al., 1983 [57] | 1972–76 | Hodgkin's disease | 22 | 34 | 1 | 4 | 7 | 0 | 22 | 21 | 1 | 0 | 0 | 0 | Hip dysplasia |
| Senturia et al., 1985 [58] | 1964–83 | Testicular cancer | 27 | –[b] | –[b] | –[b] | –[b] | –[b] | 40 | 33 | 7 | 0 | 0 | 0 | Strabismus, cryptorchidism, dental enamel hypoplasia, total anomalous pulmonary venous return, clubfoot and cryptorchidism, inguinal hernia, Marfan's syndrome |

| | | | | | | | | | | | | | | |
|---|---|---|---|---|---|---|---|---|---|---|---|---|---|---|
| NCI study<br>Mulvihill *et al.*, 1945–74, 1989 [48] | Various | —[b] | —[b] | —[b] | —[b] | —[b] | —[b] | (2308) | —[b] | —[b] | —[b] | —[b] | 7 | 3 major |
| Byrne *et al.*, 1945–69, 1988 [33] | Wilms' tumor | 27 | 59 | 0 | 15 | 7 | 0 | 37 | 21 | 6 | 1 | 9 | 1 | 3 minor; 3 major |
| Mulvihill *et al.*, 1957–77, 1987 [23] | Various | 40 | 55 | 0 | 5 | 5 | 2 | 43 | 30 | 6 | | 7 | 0 | 3 minor; 3 major (hydrocephalus, tracheomalacia, pelvic asymmetry) |
| Li *et al.*, 1931–79, 1987c [44] | Wilms' tumor | 118 | 244 | 0 | 32 | 32 | 0 | 180 | 155 | 0 | 1 | 24 | 0 | None |
| Greene and Hall, 1960–81, 1988 [59] | Hodgkin's disease | 22 | 47 | 0 | 7 | 3 | 1 | 33 | 30 | 2 | | 1 | | Ventricular septal defect, hydrocele |
| Hawkins and Smith, 1940–77, 1989 [18] | Various ART | —[b] | —[b] | 9/40 | | | | | | | | | | |
| | NART | | | 11/174 | | —[b] | —[b] | 1348 | —[b] | —[b] | —[b] | —[b] | 25 | —[b] |
| Approximate total[d] | No. | | 490 | 844 | 1 | 93 | 88 | 4 | 716 | 615 | 45 | 9 | 44 | 34 |
| | % | | | | 12.3 | 10.4 | | (4359) | | 6.3 | | 6.1 | (0.8) | |

[a]Includes data published previously in Li and Jaffe [17] and in Holmes and Holmes [60].
[b]Data not reported.
[c]Includes data published in Green *et al.*, 1982 [61].
[d]Totals do not add up and percentages are approximate because of overlap between studies and differing data reporting practices.
SGA, small for gestational age; ART, abdominal radiotherapy; NART, no abdominal radiotherapy

of January 1989 there were 214 cases entered, mostly of women who were treated for Hodgkin's disease or leukemia. No pregnancies fathered by men who were in treatment were collected, partly because they are rarely reported, and partly because of the remoteness of the risk.

## Treatment during pregnancy

The existence of individual case reports of malformations after exposure to cancer therapy in the first trimester might be taken as support for the teratogenic potential of chemotherapeutic agents, convincingly demonstrated in animal studies [10]. However, technical problems with these reports prevent firm establishment of a causal relationship in many instances. For example, relatively few pregnancies have been studied, only 214 in the NCI cancer registry to date. Close examination of the individual case reports (i.e. malformed ear, bowed tibia, cerebral hemorrhage, grooves in the hard palate, retinal defects) raises the possibility of over-diagnosis in at least some instances. Other known causes such as chromosomal syndromes or amniotic band syndrome should be ruled out before assigning causality. Dysmorphology evaluations of liveborn children should be done by experienced personnel. In the case of elective abortions after known exposures, autopsies should be carried out by experienced pathologists who are unaware of the circumstances of the termination. For some substances, chiefly the antimetabolite aminopterin, teratogenicity seems established.

The possibility that exposure to chemotherapeutic agents during pregnancy might cause miscarriage was suggested by a Finnish study which found an excess of fetal loss to oncology nurses who were dispensing chemotherapeutic agents [20]. The records of the Reproductive Registry were searched for supporting data without success [19]. This association awaits confirmation.

Excessive rates of low birth weight and preterm delivery were found in some studies of women who developed leukemia and were treated during pregnancy [21–23], but not in all [24]. Since these women were critically ill during their pregnancies, and were treated with a variety of chemotherapeutic agents, it is not yet clear what degree of risk to assign.

## Complications in long-term survivors

### Marriage

Earlier investigations of quality of life after childhood cancer suggested that survivors marry at about the same rate as the general population [25–27]. However, Koocher and O'Malley [27] found an association between severity of physical impairment as a result of cancer treatment during childhood and unmarried status in women in their study, but not in men.

In the NCI study of childhood cancer survivors and sibling controls we asked about numbers and dates of marriages and live-in relationships. Insofar as marriage stability measures psychological well-being, it seems that most groups of survivors do quite well in coping with the cancer experience. Overall rates of marriage were somewhat reduced in survivors, with most of the difference due to males, who were about 20% less likely than male controls to marry [28]. Marriage was considerably less likely for men who had survived tumors of the brain or

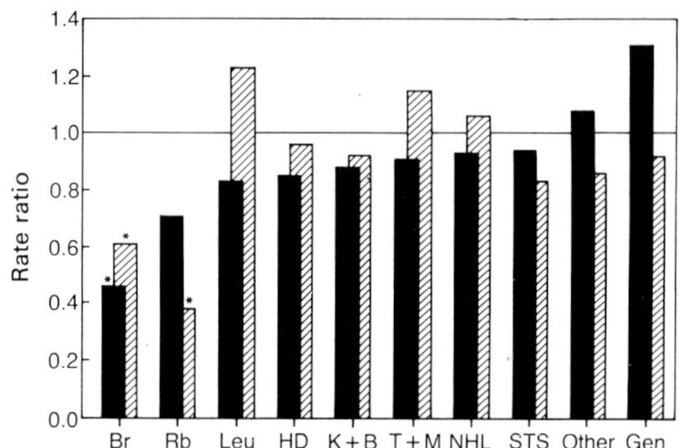


**Figure 8.2** Marriage in long-term survivors of childhood and adolescent cancer (the NCI study). Adjusted rate ratios were derived from proportional hazards models that controlled for income and education, age at follow-up and vital status. Br, brain and central nervous system tumours; Rb, retinoblastoma; Leu, leukemia; HD, Hodgkin's disease; K+B, kidney + bone cancer; T+M, thyroid cancer + melanoma; NHL, non-Hodgkin's lymphoma; STS, soft tissue sarcoma; Other, all other cancers; Gen, genital cancers. Asterisks indicate rate ratios significantly less than one (*P*<0.05). From ref. [28]

central nervous system compared with controls (adjusted rate ratio (RR) = 0.48) with a tendency for men younger at diagnosis to do even worse (RR = 0.34 for those diagnosed before age 10 compared with 0.60 for diagnosis at older ages). Women with brain tumors were also less likely to marry than female controls, but more so than men (Figure 8.2). It seems probable that the major functional problems arising from brain surgery and radiation to the brain make these survivors poor candidates for marriage [29].

## Divorce

In the NCI study of divorce after marriage men who had survived brain tumors were once again more likely to divorce, but only if they were diagnosed before the age of 10 years. Men who were survivors of retinoblastoma were also more likely to be divorced than controls. However, divorce was not more likely for any other group of men; no group of women was more likely than controls to be divorced (Figure 8.3).

## Fertility

Proven fertility after childhood or adolescent cancer has been examined on two large series, one limited to women who had been treated for Hodgkin's disease [30] and the other the NCI study [6] which covered a variety of sites and treatments. In the women who had previously had Hodgkin's disease diagnosed between the ages of 13 and 40 years, 20 of 103 women reported pregnancies [30]. The effect of different treatments was evident in the proportion of women who still had regular menses (Figure 8.4),

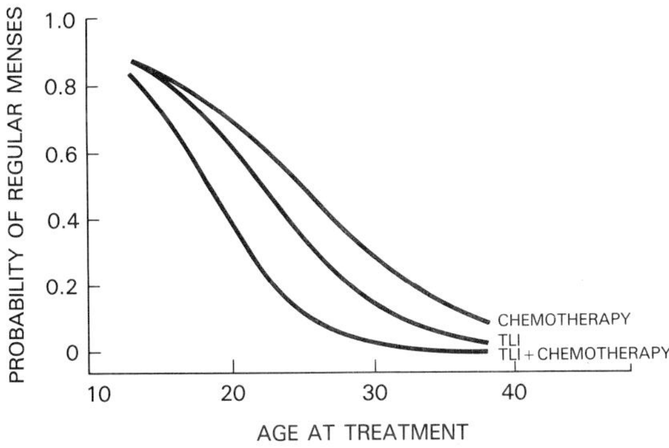


**Figure 8.4** Probability of regular menses after chemotherapy, total lymphoid irradiation (TLI), and total lymphoid irradiation and chemotherapy, according to the age at time of treatment. Reproduced from ref. [30] with permission

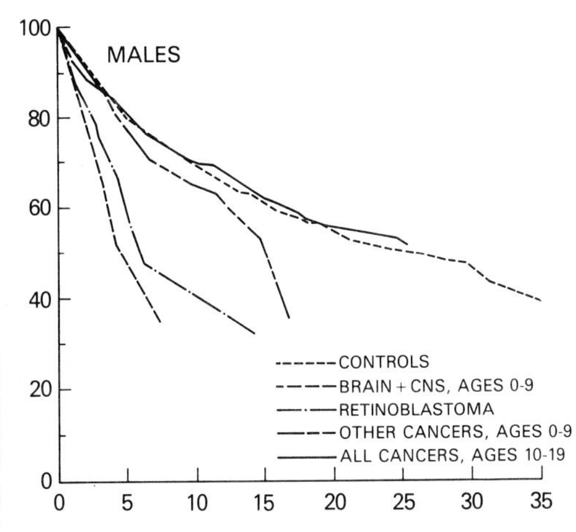


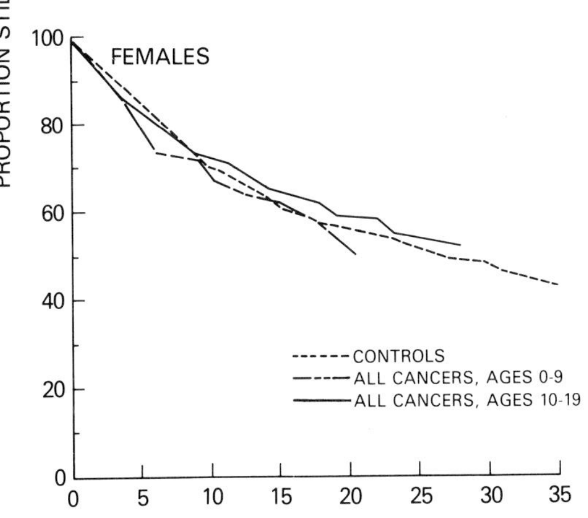


**Figure 8.3** NCI study of long−term survivors of childhood and adolescent cancer. Percentage of cancer survivors and controls who were still married at the time of follow−up, by sex, tumor type and age at diagnosis (Kaplan–Meier curves). From ref. [28]

and the percentage reporting pregnancies. For both outcomes, women who were treated with total lymphoid irradiation (TLI) did better than those treated with combination chemotherapy (MOPP, i.e. mechlorethamine, vincristine (Oncovin) procarbazine and prednisone, or PAVe, i.e. procarbazine, melphalan and vinblastine), who did better than those who received both. Of the 37 women who were treated with TLI, 37% reported pregnancies, compared with 24% of women treated with combination chemotherapy and only 10% of 50 women who received both types of therapy.

In the large NCI study of 2283 survivors of both sexes treated with a variety of agents [6] we noted a 15% fertility deficit overall among survivors who had no known reason for infertility; men were less likely than women to become parents (RR = 0.76 *versus* 0.93, respectively). In our study fertility was defined as ever or never pregnant or fathered a pregnancy. Fertility was depressed chiefly in survivors of Hodgkin's disease and male genital cancer, and only slightly in survivors of other types of

**Table 8.3 Adjusted relative fertility of survivors of cancer, according to type of cancer[a]. From ref. [6]**

| Type of cancer | No. of survivors | Adjusted relative fertility[b] (95% confidence interval) |
|---|---|---|
| Hodgkin's disease | 253 | 0.77 (0.64–0.92) |
| Soft tissue sarcoma | 177 | 0.82 (0.66–1.02) |
| Brain and central nervous system tumor | 142 | 0.90 (0.72–1.11) |
| Thyroid carcinoma | 140 | 0.85 (0.68–1.07) |
| Bone cancer | 90 | 0.85 (0.63–1.15) |
| Non-Hodgkin's lymphoma | 71 | 0.81 (0.56–1.16) |
| Melanoma | 64 | 0.98 (0.70–1.38) |
| Male genital cancer | 37 | 0.45 (0.26–0.78) |
| Retinoblastoma | 31 | 0.73 (0.43–1.25) |
| Wilms' tumor | 29 | 1.47 (0.81–2.65) |
| Female genital cancer | 26 | 1.04 (0.62–1.76) |

[a]Includes pregnancies of wives of male subjects and excludes subjects presumed not to be at risk of pregnancy. Values were derived from Cox regression models after adjustment for age at marriage and year of marriage and stratification according to sex.

[b]The relative fertility indicates the probability of pregnancy among survivors as compared with that among the controls.

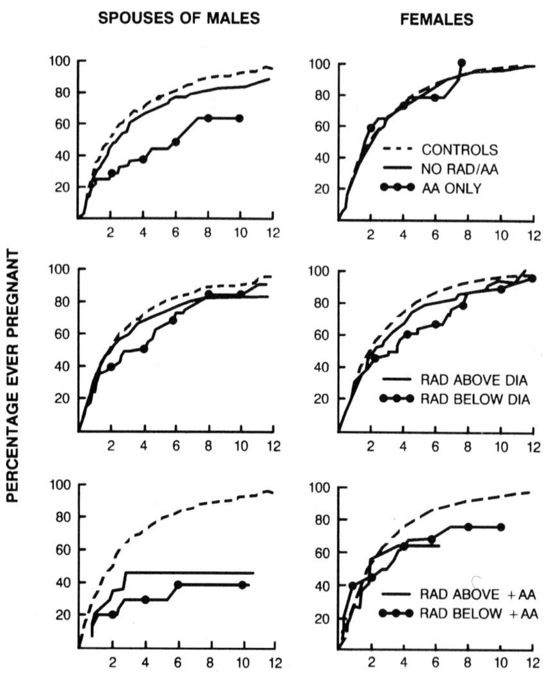


**Figure 8.5** NCI study of long-term survivors of childhood and adolescent cancer. Effects of different treatments on fertility, expressed as percentage ever pregnant or fathered a pregnancy (Kaplan–Meier curves), by sex. RAD, radiation; AA, alkylating agents; DIA, diaphragm. From ref. [6]

tumors (Table 8.3). Treatment effects were pronounced (Figure 8.5), and in the same direction as in Horning's study, with survivors who had a combination of radiotherapy and alkylating agents least likely to be fertile. Men were more susceptible to the effects of alkylating agent therapy than women, whose fertility remained relatively intact after treatment with alkylating agents without radiation.

## Primary amenorrhea and early menopause

Girls treated with alkylating agents or with radiation to the abdomen or pelvis before puberty are known to be at risk for primary amenorrhea, both from clinical evidence and from pathological studies [3,31–34]. Studies of prepubertal girls found evidence of ovarian failure [35–37] which may be reversible, although the possibility of early menopause cannot be ruled out. In fact, because the young ovary seems to resist damage from cancer therapy [4], suggestions have been advanced that temporary cessation of ovarian function by administration of gonadal hormone analogs might preserve gonadal function [38]. To date there have been no reports of successful therapy.

Studies in the late 1970s and early 1980s in women who had been treated for Hodgkin's disease indicated a considerable risk for early menopause or secondary amenorrhea, which increased with the age of the woman at treatment [39]. Stillman *et al.* [40] found that 68% of girls who had both ovaries within the radiation fields developed ovarian failure; most of these survivors were treated with combined chemotherapy and radiation. However, alkylating agent chemotherapy alone as adjuvant treatment for poor prognosis brain tumors has been followed by biochemical evidence of primary ovarian failure in some girls treated before the age of 11 years; however, all progressed normally to puberty, indicating some potential for recovery [37]. In the NCI study we found that some women who had been treated for brain tumors and other types of malignancies before puberty never started menarche [34]. Long-term follow-up studies are needed to determine the entire range of risk associated with different treatments. Although recovery may occur and fertility be demonstrated, the possibility of depletion of germ-cells may lead to early menopause.

Few studies have examined early menopause after childhood cancer therapy. In Horning's study [30] the probability of regular menses fell off sharply as age at treatment advanced, and combined treatment with TLI and chemotherapy with alkylating agents was more strongly associated with early menopause than either of these separately. In unpublished data from our NCI study we found that women treated with a combination of alkylating agents and radiation below the diaphragm for childhood cancer had rates of early menopause four times higher than controls [34].

As the offspring of survivors age, another concern may appear. Fetuses *in utero* exposed to chemotherapeutic agents may have escaped teratogenesis, but their gonads are very sensitive to cytotoxic agents. At the fourth month of development the ovaries contain many millions of follicles, which undergo rapid atresia during prenatal life leaving only a few million at birth [41]. Parental exposure to chemotherapeutic agents may speed up this process, which could lead to early menopause.

## Outcome of pregnancy

Twelve large series have documented the outcomes of pregnancies and the health of offspring of survivors of cancer in childhood or adolescence (Table 8.1). This summary includes only pregnancies begun after cancer therapy had ceased and excludes pregnancies in progress during cancer therapy. The experience of women treated for gestational trophoblastic tumors is omitted in order to focus on the particular problems faced by survivors of cancers that occur in children and adolescents. We use this table in the following sections to discuss what is known at this date about various untoward outcomes of pregnancy, i.e. fetal death, birth defects, and cancer in offspring. Conclusions drawn from this summary must be treated cautiously, since the studies varied in their aims and in their methods of collecting and presenting data, and few had enough subjects to pursue detailed analyses.

### Fetal deaths and low birthweight

In the cumulated series (Table 8.1), the proportion of recognized conceptions that ended in fetal loss (defined as miscarriage, ectopic pregnancy or stillbirth) was about 13%, after exclusion of elective abortions. The proportion of recognized pregnancies ending in miscarriage is usually estimated to be 15% [42]. Hence, there is no suggestion here of an increased risk for spontaneous fetal loss or miscarriage after cancer treatment. However, the effects of particular treatments or specific tumor types may be obscured by this summarized information. Too few studies listed pregnancy outcomes according to the type of cancer treatment they received to allow any statements to be made on this issue.

Many sources of error are possible in estimating miscarriage rates. The proportion of miscarriages differs according to the trimester of pregnancy, being less in the second trimester than in the first

[43]; if an environmental exposure is thought to be the cause then recall bias may operate; many so-called miscarriages that occurred in a time before legalized abortion became widespread in the United States may not, in fact, have been spontaneous. Of the series listed in Table 8.1, some counted only pregnancies that lasted longer than 20 weeks, and reporting practices may differ from place to place. Only two reports in this series compared observed rates to a comparison group, which is especially valuable when collecting data on events as difficult to quantify as miscarriages. The large series of pregnancies to cancer survivors in the Oxford study [18] revealed that, among the first pregnancies after treatment, women treated with direct abdominal radiation had significantly more miscarriages than women not so treated (22% *versus* 6% respectively). In one controlled study, Li and Stone [25] reported no difference in the rate of fetal loss after treatment for a variety of tumors of childhood. In another study [23] a statistically significant increased risk of fetal wastage was linked to increasing duration of therapy with alkylating agents (statistically significant trend test, $P < 0.001$); however, direct radiation effects and other confounding variables were not ruled out.

The reproductive experiences of survivors of Wilms' tumor have received particular attention since Li *et al.* [44] reported an eight-fold relative risk for perinatal mortality and a four-fold excess risk for low birthweight in the offspring of women treated with abdominal radiotherapy for this malignancy. This finding stimulated two other reports (to date); both have confirmed and extended the earlier finding. Byrne *et al.* [33] found that the wives of male survivors were not at risk for abnormal pregnancies, whereas female survivors had four times more abnormal pregnancies than female controls; the numbers were too small to examine the proportion of miscarriages separately, but apart from one woman with a bicornuate uterus, there was no suggestion of an excess rate of miscarriages. All five pregnancies of this woman ended in miscarriage, presumably due to her malformed uterus, probably one of a spectrum of birth defects associated with Wilms' tumor. In this study there was a suggestion of an increase in malformations, compatible either with the spectrum of malformations seen in Wilms' tumor, or with radiation-induced intrauterine constraint ('no room in the womb'). Hawkins and Smith [18] reported that the first children born to women treated for Wilms' tumor with abdominal radiation were on average 500 g lighter than similar children born to women treated without abdominal radiation, or to children of all male survivors of Wilms' tumor; no other tumor type carried a high risk for low birthweight in offspring. Damage to the vasculature and elastic properties of the uterus may impair adequate expansion and lead to positional deformities and early delivery.

Apart from the special problems of women who have been treated with abdominal radiation, there has not yet been convincing evidence of excess rates of fetal loss in survivors. In theory, mutagenic therapy could cause heritable defects, which if lethal could lead to early miscarriages; however, this remains to be shown.

These studies highlight the problems involved in separating out the correlates of cancer from the effects of treatment in some cases, making it difficult to establish causal relationships. Recent analyses of fetal wastage have demonstrated the phenomenon of selective fertility, i.e. the tendency for a couple to rapidly replace a perinatal death. In studies of reproductive loss after cancer treatment, the effect of selective fertility could be reduced by analyzing only the first pregnancy after exposure [45]. In short, pregnancies occurring after therapy for childhood and adolescent cancer do not seem to be at increased risk for miscarriage. However, more detailed studies are still needed to examine the specific effects of individual treatments.

Of the 844 pregnancies to survivors in the cumulated series (Table 8.1) about 10% were electively aborted, many for maternal anxiety related to the cancer history.

## *Birth defects in offspring of cancer survivors*

Among all the children who were examined in the 12 series (Table 8.1), the overall rate of malformations (3%) is similar to expected rates in the general population [46,47]. Preliminary analysis of data from the NCI series of offspring born to survivors of childhood and adolescent cancer showed that the rate of birth defects was 4%, again similar to the general population and similar to the rate in the sibling controls [48].

## *Cancer in offspring of cancer survivors*

Fears about the risk of cancer in their offspring are common among cancer survivors and arise, at least in part, because of the hereditary nature of some childhood cancers. Among the 12 large series which reported on the offspring of survivors, three reported on offspring with cancer (Table 8.1). Among 242 live births Li and Stone [25] described two children with cancer, one with retinoblastoma whose father had retinoblastoma previously; the other a girl with acute myelocytic leukemia whose mother had survived a brain tumor at age 10. The first is certainly a single gene disorder; the second resembles clusters of familial cancer of unknown cause. A similar pattern was seen in the Oxford

study where 25 cancers arose among 1348 offspring of survivors; 23 were in offspring of survivors of heritable retinoblastoma known to be transmitted to offspring as an autosomal dominant characteristic, and the other two conformed to a previously described pattern of familial aggregation of cancer. In the NCI study of cancer survivors the overall risk of cancer in the offspring was not statistically higher than expected values based on either sibling controls or the general population [49]. The single significant raised risk (RR = 2.9; Table 8.4) in survivors under

**Table 8.4 Cancer in offspring of childhood cancer survivors. From ref. [49]**

| Age at follow-up (years) | Offspring of | | | | | | | |
|---|---|---|---|---|---|---|---|---|
| | Survivors (2308 offspring) | | | | Controls (4719 offspring) | | | |
| | *OBS* | *EXP* | *PY* | *RR* | *OBS* | *EXP* | *PY* | *RR* |
| 0–4 | 5 | 1.7 | 9935 | 2.8[a] | 2 | 3.5 | 20297 | 0.6 |
| 5–9 | 1 | 0.8 | 7122 | 1.3 | 2 | 1.6 | 14736 | 1.3 |
| 10–14 | 1 | 0.5 | 4503 | 2.2 | 3 | 1.0 | 9608 | 3.1 |
| 15–19 | 0 | 0.4 | 2404 | 0.0 | 3 | 1.0 | 5479 | 3.0 |
| 20+ | 0 | 0.4 | 1082 | 0.0 | 1 | 1.5 | 3835 | 0.7 |
| Total | 7 | 3.8 | 25046 | 1.9 | 11 | 8.5 | 53954 | 1.3 |

[a]90% confidence interval = 1.1–6.0. OBS, observed numbers; EXP, expected numbers based on data from the Connecticut Tumor Registry compared by life-table methods; PY, person-years at risk; RR, rate ratio of OBS/EXP.

4 years of age was probably due to the occurrence of retinoblastoma and Wilms' tumor. Our data had good statistical power to detect an effect during childhood. However, since the offspring of survivors were only 11 years old on average when we questioned their parents, our study cannot rule out an excess of cancer in the older childhood years, or even later.

# Advice to the patient and clinician

Survivors of childhood or adolescent cancer, or their parents if the child is very young, should be informed of the long-term consequences of cancer and its therapy, even if they do not ask. Survivors and their families should have as much information as possible about their diagnosis and therapy so that the causes of late effects might be understood. This information should be given both verbally and in writing. In our study we were surprised to find that a substantial proportion of our survivors, who were on average 32 years old at interview, said 'No' when asked if a doctor had told them that they had cancer

[50]. Studies of long-term survivors have shown that they may not be as concerned about their health as they ought to be; for instance, they smoke only slightly less often their brothers and sisters [51]. As a group of people who may be at increased risk for another cancer both because of their previous history and also because of the carcinogenic agents with which they were treated, cancer survivors especially should not smoke.

Most patients and their families will readily accept a life-saving treatment at the cost of infertility in years to come. The option of sperm banking should be discussed with older males, and possibly the freezing of ova with older females. But not all treatments cause infertility, and not all apparently infertile patients are really unable to have children. Some patients recover fertility years after treatment has ceased [52], and one woman in our study conceived and bore a healthy child without ever having menstruated after she was treated for a brain tumor at age 18. Use of birth control is probably advisable even if fertility seems unlikely if the couple really does not want a family.

However, when fertility is maintained and pregnancy is sought there may be considerable anxiety generated by the fear of having an unhealthy baby. As a first step, the advisor should make every effort to understand the etiology of the survivor's cancer, since the same cause may still be operating and may result in an excess risk of cancer in the next generation. Although an explanation is not often evident, the environmental and family histories should be reviewed to rule out the presence of some familial form of cancer. A similar survey of the medical and family history of the spouse is also indicated.

Should chromosomes be studied when pregnancy is contemplated? Karyotyping of peripheral blood cells is likely to show chromosome breakage in survivors who had radiotherapy. The health consequences of this finding are uncertain. In our opinion the test is not indicated unless a specific structural anomaly is sought, such as $13q-$ in retinoblastoma, or $11p-$ in Wilms' tumor.

Should prenatal diagnosis be done during pregnancy? If no predisposing condition or etiological factor is uncovered, the survivor who has been treated prior to pregnancy should be told that although there are *theoretical* concerns about possible genetic damage the results of the studies to date are reassuring. From Table 8.1 it can be seen that the risk of miscarriage and birth defects is no more than expected in the general population. This information should be presented with the caveat that subgroups exposed to specific agents may have increased risks, and we have not yet accumulated enough information to provide more precise advice. We consider that, aside from the customary indications which may well include parental anxiety,

prenatal diagnosis is not indicated in pregnancies of survivors whose cancer treatment occurred well before the pregnancy began.

If cancer arises in one member of a couple contemplating pregnancy, birth control should be used assiduously. We have very little information about the consequences to a pregnancy where one of the parents is undergoing cancer treatment at conception, and many theoretical concerns remain. Also, a serious situation exists when a woman needs cancer treatment during her pregnancy, especially in the first trimester. Many successful pregnancies have been reported under these circumstances, but infants exposed to either radiation or chemotherapy have been born with birth defects [10]. Current experience is mainly represented by case reports which do not allow firm conclusions to be drawn as to outcome or management. Such pregnancies should be closely monitored at a high-risk clinic with ultrasound examinations, in part to provide reassurance to parents, and in part to accumulate larger case series for more secure counselling.

# Acknowledgements

We thank Dilys Parry, Patricia Siraganian and Robert Miller for careful reading of the manuscript, and Sadie Holmes for manuscript preparation.

# References

1. Simon, R. Statistical methods for evaluating pregnancy outcomes in patients with Hodgkin's disease. *Cancer*, **45**, 2890–2892 (1980)
2. Viviani, S., Santoro, A., Ragni, G. *et al.* Gonadal toxicity after combination chemotherapy for Hodgkin's disease. Comparative results of MOPP vs ABVD. *European Journal of Clinical Oncology*, **21**, 601–605 (1985)
3. Himelstein-Braw, R., Peters, H. and Faber, M. Morphological study of the ovaries of leukaemic children. *British Journal of Cancer*, **38**, 82–87 (1978)
4. Rivkees, S.A. and Crawford, J.D. The relationship of gonadal activity and chemotherapy-induced gonadal damage. *Journal of the American Medical Association*, **259**, 2123–2125 (1988)
5. Hamre, M.R., Robison, L.L., Nesbit, M.E. *et al.* Effects of radiation on ovarian function in long-term survivors of childhood acute lymphoblastic leukemia: a report from the Children's Cancer Study Group. *Journal of Clinical Oncology*, **5**, 1759–1765 (1987)
6. Byrne, J., Mulvihill, J.J., Myers, M.H. *et al.* Effects of treatment on fertility in long-term survivors of childhood or adolescent cancer. *New England Journal of Medicine*, **317**, 1315–1321 (1987)
7. Mulvihill, J.J. and Miller, J.R. Mutation epidemiology

and its prospects for detecting human germinal mutagens. *Handbook of Mutagenicity Test Procedures*, 2nd edn, Elsevier Science Publishers, New York, pp. 841–851 (1984)

8. Neel, J.V., Satoh, C., Goriki, K. *et al.* Search for mutations altering protein charge and/or function in children of atomic bomb survivors: final report. *American Journal of Human Genetics*, **42**, 663–676 (1988)

9. Jablon, S. Epidemiologic perspectives in radiation carcinogenesis. In *Radiation Carcinogenesis: Epidemiology and Biological Significance* (eds J.D. Boice and J.F. Fraumeni), Raven Press, New York, pp. 1–8 (1984)

10. Schardein, J.L. *Chemically Induced Birth Defects*, Marcel Dekker, New York and Basel (1985)

11. Goldstein, L. and Murphy, D.P. Amenorrhea during serial roentgen exposures due to intervening pregnancy. *American Journal of Obstetrics and Gynecology*, **18**, 696–698 (1929)

12. Miller, R.W. and Mulvihill, J.J. Small head size after atomic irradiation. *Teratology*, **14**, 355–358 (1976)

13. Otake, M. and Schull, W.J. *In utero* exposure to A-bomb radiation and mental retardation; a reassessment. *British Journal of Radiology*, **57**, 409–414 (1984)

14. Li, F.P. Host factors in the development of childhood cancers. *Seminars in Oncology*, **5**, 17–23 (1978)

15. Li, F.P., Dreyfus, M.G. and Antman, K.H. Asbestos-contaminated nappies and familial mesothelioma. *Lancet*, **i**, 908–909 (1989)

16. Li, F.P., Fraumeni, J.F. Jr, Mulvihill, J.J. *et al.* A cancer family syndrome in twenty-four kindreds. *Cancer Research*, **48**, 5358–5362 (1988)

17. Li, F.P. and Jaffe, N. Progeny of childhood cancer survivors. *Lancet*, **ii**, 707–709 (1974)

18. Hawkins, M.M. and Smith, R.A. Pregnancy outcomes in childhood cancer survivors: probable effects of abdominal irradiation. *International Journal of Cancer*, **43**, 399–402 (1989)

19. Mulvihill, J.J. and Stewart, K.R. Outcomes of 99 pregnancies among women exposed to antineoplastic drugs in the first trimester. *New England Journal of Medicine*, **314**, 1049 (1986)

20. Selevan, S.G., Lindbohm, M., Hornung, R.W. and Hemminki, K. A study of occupational exposure to antineoplastic drugs and fetal loss in nurses. *New England Journal of Medicine*, **313**, 1173–1178 (1985)

21. Feliu, J., Juarez, S., Ordonez, A. *et al.* Acute leukemia and pregnancy. *Cancer*, **61**, 580–584 (1988)

22. Reynoso, E.E., Shepherd, F.A., Messner, H.A. *et al.* Acute leukemia during pregnancy: the Toronto Leukemia Study Group experience with long-term follow-up of children exposed *in utero* to chemotherapeutic agents. *Journal of Clinical Oncology*, **5**, 1098–1106 (1987)

23. Mulvihill, J.J., McKeen, E.A., Rosner, F. and Zarrabi, M.H. Pregnancy outcome in cancer patients: experience in a large cooperative group. *Cancer*, **60**, 1143–1150 (1987)

24. Avilés, A. and Niz, J. Long-term follow-up of children born to mothers with acute leukemia during pregnancy. *Medical and Pediatric Oncology*, **16**, 3–6 (1988)

25. Li, F.P. and Stone, R. Survivors of cancer in childhood. *Journal of Internal Medicine*, **84**, 551–553 (1976)

26. Holmes, H.A. and Holmes, F.F. After ten years, what are the handicaps and life styles of children treated for cancer? *Clinical Pediatrics*, **14**, 819–832 (1976)

27. Koocher, G.P. and O'Malley, J.E. *The Damocles Syndrome*, McGraw-Hill, New York (1981)

28. Byrne, J., Fears, T.R., Steinhorn, S.C. *et al.* Marriage and divorce after childhood and adolescent cancer. *Journal of the American Medical Association*, **262**, 2693–2699 (1989)

29. Chin, H.W. and Maruyama, Y. Age at treatment and long-term performance results with medulloblastoma. *Cancer*, **53**, 1952–1958 (1984)

30. Horning, S.J., Hoppe, R.T., Kaplan, H.S. and Rosenberg, S.A. Female reproductive potential after treatment for Hodgkin's disease. *New England Journal of Medicine*, **304**, 1377–1382 (1981)

31. Ahmed, S.R., Shalet, S.M., Campbell, R.H.A. and Deakin, D.P. Primary gonadal damage following treatment of brain tumors in childhood. *Journal of Pediatrics*, **103**, 562–565 (1983)

32. Nicosia, S.V., Matus-Ridley, M. and Meadows, A.T. Gonadal effects of cancer therapy in girls. *Cancer*, **55**, 2364–2372 (1985)

33. Byrne, J., Mulvihill, J.J. Connelly, R.R. *et al.* Reproductive problems and birth defects in survivors of Wilms' tumor and their relatives. *Medical and Pediatric Oncology*, **16**, 233–240 (1988)

34. Byrne, J., Fears, T.R., Gail, M.H. *et al.* Early menopause after treatment for childhood or adolescent cancer. Submitted for publication (1990)

35. Siris, E.S., Leventhal, B.G. and Vaitukaitis, J.L. Effects of childhood leukemia and chemotherapy on puberty and reproductive function in girls. *New England Journal of Medicine*, **294**, 1143–1146 (1976)

36. Whitehead, E., Shalet, S.M., Morris Jones, P. *et al.* Gonadal function after combination chemotherapy for Hodgkin's disease in childhood. *Archives of Disease in Childhood*, **47**, 287–291 (1982)

37. Clayton, P.E., Shalet, S.M., Price, D.A. and Morris Jones, P. Ovarian function following chemotherapy for childhood brain tumours. *Medical and Pediatric Oncology*, **17**, 92–96 (1989)

38. Redman, J.R. and Bajorunas, D.R. Gonadal activity and chemotherapy-induced gonadal damage. *Journal of the American Medical Association*, **260**, 2064–2065 (1988)

39. Chapman, R.M., Sutcliffe, S.B. and Malpas, J.S. Cytotoxic-induced ovarian failure in women with Hodgkin's disease. *Journal of the American Medical Association*, **242**, 1877–1881 (1979)

40. Stillman, R.J., Schinfeld, J.S., Schiff, I. *et al.* Ovarian failure in long-term survivors of childhood malig-

nancy. *American Journal of Obstetrics Gynecology*, **139**, 62–66 (1981)

41. Baker, T.G. A quantitative and cytological study of germ cells in human ovaries. *Proceedings of the Royal Society of London, Series B*, **158**, 417–433 (1963)

42. Warburton, D. and Fraser, F.C. Spontaneous abortion risks in man: data from reproductive histories collected in a medical genetics unit. *Human Genetics*, **16**, 1–25 (1964)

43. Boué, J., Philippe, E., Giroud, A. and Boué, A. Phenotypic expression of lethal chromosomal anomalies in human abortuses. *Teratology*, **14**, 3–20 (1976)

44. Li, F.P., Gimbrere, K., Gelber, R.D. *et al.* Outcome of pregnancy in survivors of Wilms' tumor. *Journal of the American Medical Association*, **257**, 216–219 (1987)

45. Skjaerven, R., Wilcox, A.J., Lie, R.T. and Irgens, L.M. Selective fertility and the distortion of perinatal mortality. *American Journal of Epidemiology*, **128**, 1352–1363 (1988)

46. Kalter, H. and Warkany, J. Congenital malformations. *New England Journal of Medicine*, **308**, 424–431, 491–497 (1983)

47. Nelson, K. and Holmes, L.B. Malformations due to presumed spontaneous mutations in newborn infants. *New England Journal of Medicine*, **320**, 19–23 (1989)

48. Mulvihill, J.J., Byrne, J., Steinhorn, S.A. *et al.* Genetic disease in offspring of survivors of cancer in the young. *American Journal of Human Genetics*, **39**, A72 (1986)

49. Mulvihill, J.J., Myers, M.H., Connelly, R.R. *et al.* Cancer in offspring of long-term survivors of childhood and adolescent cancer. *Lancet*, **ii**, 814–817 (1987)

50. Byrne, J., Lewis, M.E., Halamek, L. *et al.* Childhood cancer survivors' knowledge of their diagnosis and treatment. *Annals of Internal Medicine*, **110**, 400–403 (1989)

51. Haupt, R., Byrne, J., Mostow, E. and Mulvihill, J.J. Smoking habits in survivors of childhood and adolescent cancer. Submitted for publication (1990)

52. Shalet, S.M., Williams, C.A.V. and Whitehead, E. Pregnancy after chemotherapy-induced ovarian failure. *British Medical Journal*, **290**, 898 (1985)

53. Li, F.P., Fine, W., Jaffe, H. *et al.* Offspring of patients treated for cancer in childhood. *Journal of National Cancer Institute,* **62**, 1193–1197 (1979)

54. Blatt, J., Mulvihill, J.J., Ziegler, J.L. *et al.* Pregnancy outcome following cancer chemotherapy. *American Journal of Medicine,* **69**, 828–832 (1980)

55. Marradi, P., Schaison, F., Alby, N. *et al.* Les enfants nés de parents leucémiques. *Nouvelle Revue Française d'Hématologie,* **124**, 75–80 (1982)

56. Bundey, S. and Evans, K. Survivors of neuroblastoma and ganglioneuroma and their families. *Journal of Medical Genetics,* **19**, 16–21 (1982)

57. Andrieu, J.M. and Ochoa-Molina, M.E. Menstrual cycle, pregnancies and offspring before and after MOPP therapy for Hodgkin's disease. *Cancer,* **52**, 435–438 (1983)

58. Senturia, Y.D., Peckham, C.S. and Peckham, M.J. Children fathered by men treated for testicular cancer. *Lancet,* **ii**, 766–769 (1985)

59. Green, D.M. and Hall, B. Pregnancy outcome following treatment during childhood or adolescence for Hodgkin's disease. *Pediatric Hematology and Oncology,* **5**, 269–277 (1988)

60. Holmes, G.E. and Holmes, F.F. Pregnancy outcome of patients treated for Hodgkin's disease. A controlled study. *Cancer,* **41**, 1317–1322 (1987)

61. Green, D.M., Fine, W.E. and Li, F.P. Offspring of patients treated for unilateral Wilms' tumor in childhood. *Cancer,* **49**, 2285–2288 (1982)

62. Mulvihill, J.J. Genetic repertory of human neoplasia. In *Genetics of Human Cancer* (eds J.J. Mulvihill, R.W. Miller and J.F. Fraumeni Jr), Raven Press, New York, pp. 137–143 (1977)

# 9

# Late complications of cured adult malignancy

**M. Langer and C.N. Coleman**

## Introduction

Consequences of cancer treatment appearing months to years following therapy are termed 'late'. It is convenient to distinguish between those delayed consequences which are infrequently seen, known as late complications, and those more commonly expected, often referred to as late effects. For a treatment regimen to be practical, the more likely effects should be less serious. Some effects nevertheless remain far from trivial, e.g. infertility following chemotherapy for lymphoma or xerostomia following radiation to the salivary glands, and anticipating their appearance must be an integral part of the therapeutic program.

Although cancer recurrence may be catastrophic, the delayed consequences of curative therapy should guide treatment choice and research design. It is desirable to know the likelihoods of possible complications and effects, how they may be reduced and what may be done to treat or compensate for those outcomes which remain unavoidable. These goals are less easily achieved when the adverse outcomes are delayed than when they appear in tandem with treatment. Time lags confound the identification of causes of complications. Since acute toxicity does not usually predict late toxicity, changes in drug or radiation doses in response to early signs of normal tissue stress will not necessarily affect treatment outcome. Furthermore, latent complications may be unveiled by the addition of a treatment which does not add to the late toxicity but rather acts only to permit long-term survival to be seen [1].

Nevertheless, progress has been made in defining complications and effects for the standard treatments of some diseases. Recognition of organ sensitivities to radiation and particular drugs has guided the design of new treatment strategies. For example, improved dose-delivery techniques have allowed radiotherapists to literally 'get around' dose-limiting normal structures [2] while identification of agents responsible for leukemogenesis and sterility has led to the construction of more favorable drug regimens for lymphomas.

The specific organ system toxicities of radiation, chemotherapy and surgery are discussed elsewhere in this volume. Here we review the descriptors of treatment delivery for radiation and chemotherapy, and test how well they predict measures of treatment effect. The concept of dose intensity has been utilized for the description of acute toxicity and efficacy of some chemotherapeutic regimens [3]. Although the means of calculating dose intensity and validity of this concept have been debated [4], it nevertheless serves as a descriptor of chemotherapeutic regimens ranging from standard regimens to bone marrow transplantation. While the data correlating treatment intensity with late effects are limited, we will describe some of the data available for three important categories of late damage – namely, second malignancies, and pulmonary and neuropsychiatric damage.

## Treatment measures
### Radiation treatment

The effect of a course of conventional (megavoltage photon) treatment delivered to an individual patient depends upon the distribution of radiation dose within organ volumes of interest and the schedule of treatment delivery. The dose delivered to any point within tissue is a measure of the energy lost to molecular ionization or excitation in a small mass of tissue about that point. For a fixed number of

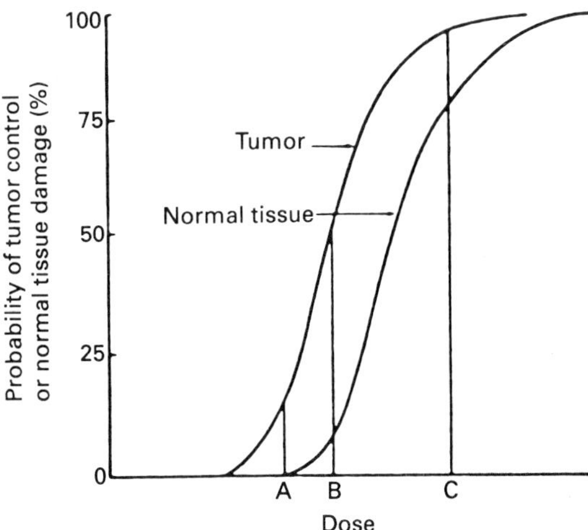

**Figure 9.1** Idealization of sigmoidal dose-response curves. The probability of response sharply increases with dose over a small range of dose. It is desirable that the probability of tumor control exceeds that of normal tissue destruction. In the figure the dose-response curves for tumor and normal tissues bear the same shape, but are displaced relative to each other. The true shape of the curves for doses given as part of a fractionated program of clinical treatments are not known. Points A, B and C show that even if two dose-response curves bear the same shape, the relative likelihood of observing the monitored effects (here, for example, tumor control and normal tissue damage) will depend on the administered dose. Reproduced with permission from ref. [79]

treatment sessions and relative spatial distribution of dose, the likelihood of organ damage is often drawn to be sigmoidal [5] (Figure 9.1), with the dose triggering a toxic reaction taken as distributed normally or log-normally within a population. The unit of dose is the Gray (Gy) defined as 1 joule of energy lost to molecular ionization and excitation per kilogram of tissue. In older nomenclature, dose was expressed in rad (r) where 1 Gy = 100 r or 1 rad = 1 centigray (cGy).

In general, the distribution of dose over sensitive normal structures will not be uniform. The probability of complications in an organ depends on the doses given to fractional amounts of its volume. This volume dependence has been qualitatively recognized for heart [5], lung [6], liver [7] and bowel [8] in reviews of radiation complications, and has been incorporated into an international protocol (ICRU 38) for the description of gynecological treatments. Advances in computer planning and imaging have more recently allowed the dose distributed within fractional amounts of an organ to be quantified [9]. Such a compilation is known as a dose-volume

histogram (Figures 9.2 and 9.3). Relations between organ complications and fractional volume irradiated to beyond critical doses have been quantified in clinical studies of lung [10], liver [11] and soft tissue of the breast [12]. Confirmation of the significance for late rectal complications of the tissue volume irradiated to $>60$ Gy has been obtained in a large series of patients with cervix cancers [13,14]. Complication probability was found to depend jointly on the dose to the rectal point closest to the implant source (a surrogate for the maximal rectal dose) and on the overall treatment volume treated to $>60$ Gy. Theoretical models of volume effect have been developed [15–17] and parameters given for skin tolerance [18].

The number of treatments into which the total administered dose is divided, known as fractions, and the time spanning the first to last treatment which is typically of the order of several weeks, further modifies the biological tissue effect. The dose necessary to produce a given effect seems to vary as the product of powers of the fraction number and time. This formalism, initially based on acute skin toxicities but since extended to late appearing injuries in other tissues, may be written as:

$$D^* = D \times N^{-\nu} \times T^{-\tau} \tag{9.1}$$

where $D$ is dose, $N$ is the fraction number, $T$ is the treatment span time (in days), $\nu$ and $\tau$ are tissue-specific exponents which are small positive numbers less than one, and $D^*$ is a factor which standardizes the biological effect produced by different combinations of dose and fraction schedule satisfying the equation. Acute skin reactions appear to be governed by the power-law relation for fractionation changes with exponents of $\nu = 0.24$ and $\tau = 0.11$; the standardization factor $(D^*)$ associated with normal skin tolerance to orthovoltage X-rays is known as the nominal standard dose [19] and is about 1760. Thus 30 fractions of 200 cGy over 42 days or 21 fractions of 253.6 cGy over 31 days provide similar 'isoeffects' or expectations of approaching the limits of skin tolerance. Modern treatments, using higher energy beams which spare skin, may be prescribed to higher doses. Clinical and experimental data have yielded fractionation exponents which are larger and time exponents which are smaller for late appearing and usually irreversible tissue changes (e.g. pulmonary fibrosis, CNS deterioration and nephritis) than for those reactions appearing earlier and which may be reversed (e.g. mucositis). Differences in the fractionation exponent are dominant so that it is possible to produce effects in late reacting tissues which are relatively larger than those in early reacting tissue by decreasing the fraction number. For example, the threshold for partially treated brain injury would be crossed by a substantial margin if a program of 30 fractions of 200 cGy were replaced by 21 treatments of

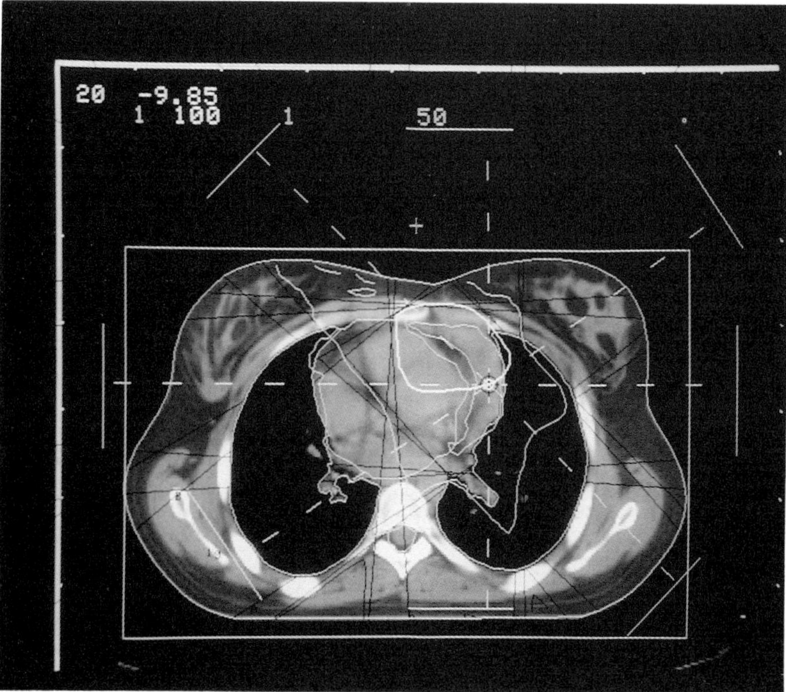





**Figure 9.2** Illustration of the distribution of radiation deposition within a body. Distributions may be considered directly or else analyzed as histograms of the volume distribution of dose across normal and tumor structures of interest. A computer tomographic image in transverse section through the thorax is shown within the rectangular box. In this example, four pairs of opposed beams (anteroposterior, lateral, 45° RAO/LPO, 45° LAO/RPO) are designed so that their central axes converge at a common point, the isocenter. The direction of the central axis of each beam is shown in heavy white dotted lines; rays off this axis will be slightly divergent. Each beam may be shaped so that within each transverse plane its field edges enclose the projection of the tumor outline (with a small margin) onto the beam direction. In this schematic, the width of each field edge relative to the central axis of the beam is shown by the heavy white perpendicular at the end of each dotted line. Critical structures of interest may be identified on the transverse image. The right and left lungs, the heart, the spinal cord and the tumor are shown here outlined along with the external patient contour. The isocenter is seen to lie approximately at the center of the tumor situated at the anterolateral border of the heart on the left. The amount of radiation directed through each beam may be independently chosen, and the relative amounts (or beam weights) will then determine the resulting dose distribution. Sophisticated algorithms, considering radiation scatter, beam divergence, and possibly inhomogeneity of beam attenuation by structures of different composition, permit accurate determination of dose at any point within the treatment volume. Points of common dose may be smoothly connected on isodose lines. Two such lines, one of 50% and the other forming a small circle of 100% are illustrated here for some arbitrary set of beam weights. The 50% line dips about halfway into the left lung and avoids the right lung; the 100% line is situated over the anterior portion of the tumor and adjacent heart and is shown in bold white. (Illustration courtesy of Dr Peter Kijewski, Harvard Joint Center for Radiation Therapy)

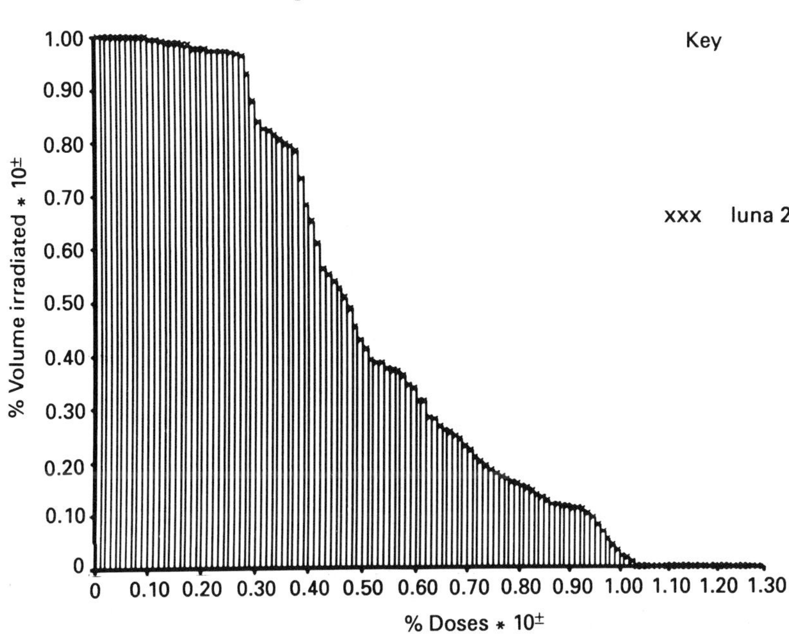


**Figure 9.3** The distribution of dose across organ volumes of interest in one transverse plane may be roughly estimated by visual inspection. It is possible to more accurately present this information as histograms of the cumulative volume distribution of dose. Such a histogram has been prepared for the left lung (lung2) in the thoracic plan illustrated in Figure 9.2. The vertical axis shows that part of the structure's volume irradiated to at least that fractional dose indicated at the corresponding point on the horizontal axis. The axes are labelled at 10% intervals of increasing volume (vertical) or dose (horizontal). The graph shows that about 42% of the lung receives greater than 50% of the dose, and <5% of the lung receives more than 100% of the dose. Inspection of the two isodose lines, superimposed on the transverse image of the treatment volume in Figure 9.2 verifies these numbers. If an actual dose of 40 Gy were prescribed to a point receiving 100% relative dose in the illustrated plan, then about 42% of the lung would receive more than a 20 Gy threshold dose for local pulmonary dysfunction. In this example, the lung volume was considered on only one transverse slice but such histograms may be generated for organ volumes defined in three dimensions. The dose-volume histogram is a new tool available to radiation therapists which allows better estimation of the likely toxicity of therapy and the potential of constructing less morbid plans. It is a consequence of advances in computer imaging and data manipulation. (Illustration courtesy of Dr Peter Kijewski, Harvard Joint Center for Radiation Therapy)

253 cGy, even though the total dose is reduced from 6000 cGy to 5313 cGy and the condition of the overlying skin is maintained at the margin of tolerance. Tumor response to fractionation and time span changes are unclear. A review by Beck-Bornholdt of experimental data suggests that tumor control may be quite insensitive to fractionation number [20]. He found in his own work that R1H rat rhabdomyosarcoma irradiated in schedules of 3–10 fractions/week in doses of 1–12 Gy show a surviving proportion of cell clonogens that is independent of fraction number, suggesting a potential therapeutic benefit to treating with smaller fractions, particularly when late effects which are sensitive to fraction number and size are dose-limiting. Optimal treatment schedules for human tumor control, however, are not known.

The power-law relation provides a simple mechanism for predicting tolerance limits from sparse clinical data on organ toxicities. Models

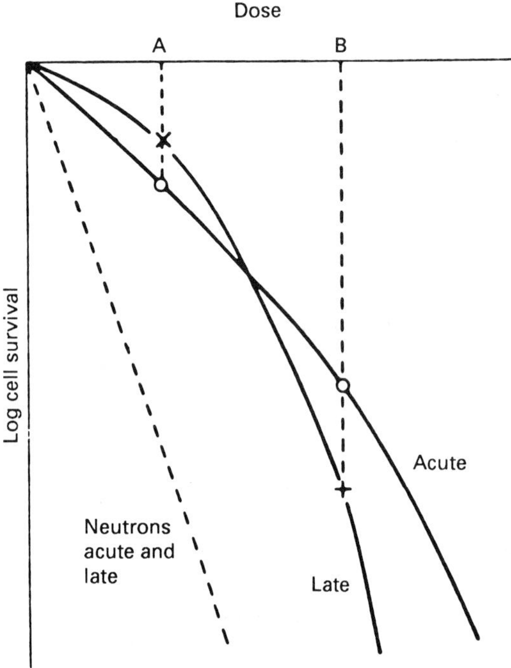



**Figure 9.4** Idealized cellular survival function curves for single fraction radiation treatment. The solid curves satisfy the linear quadratic model, in which the logarithm of survival is a quadratic function of the administered dose. They are labelled so as to also illustrate the hypothesis that the ratio of the coefficients of the linear and quadratic terms ($\alpha/\beta$) is smaller for cells of late responding tissues than for those of acute responding tissues. It is thought that the quadratic term may vanish for some kinds of non-conventional radiations, such as neutrons, as illustrated by the dashed curve which could apply to cells of either late or acutely responding tissues. Reproduced with permission from ref. [24]

which develop isoeffect relations for tissues from the recursive application of the single fraction cellular survival function from *in vitro* assays, for which the logarithm of the surviving proportion of cells may be taken to be quadratic in dose ($-\ln S \sim \alpha d + \beta d^2$), have more recently been described both without [21] and with [22] adjustments for repopulation over the treatment course. In such models, the ratio of the coefficients of the linear and quadratic dose terms ($\alpha/\beta$) in the cell survival function determine the sensitivity of the tolerance dose in tissue to fractionation. Figure 9.4 illustrates that, for single treatments, cells of both acute and late reacting tissues are thought to become increasingly sensitive to dose changes with larger administered doses, but that a curve of the logarithm of cell survival ($\ln S$) as a function of dose bends more sharply for late than for acute reacting tissues; the dose response of

tumors may perhaps be considered to be like that of the acute reacting tissues (see above). This difference could permit greater cell kill in acute than in late reacting tissues if a small dose is given in a single treatment, but a reversal in the relative cell kill between the two tissue types if the single administered dose is made large. If the effect in tissue of a course of treatment were dependent on the surviving proportion of cells whose population was reduced repeatedly by a fixed percentage in each treatment session according to the quadratic relation illustrated in Figure 9.4 – i.e. if isoeffect was maintained by constancy in the expression $n(\alpha d + \beta d^2)$ where $n$ is the fraction number and $d$ is the dose per fraction – then the reciprocal of the total cumulative dose required to preserve an effect (the 'isoeffect' dose) should vary linearly with the dose per fraction. Such a plot is known as a $F_e$ curve. Alternatively, a plot of the logarithm of the total isoeffect dose ($\ln D$) against the logarithm of the dose per fraction ($\ln d$) will yield a curve whose slope at any value of $\ln d$ gives the change in the logarithm of the total dose necessary to maintain a particular effect following a small change in the logarithm of the dose per fraction ($\ln d$). Curves of this sort collected for a series of normal tissue reactions are shown in Figure 9.5. It may be observed that at any level of ln dose per fraction ($\ln d$), late effect curves are steeper than curves of acute appearing effects, illustrating the greater sensitivity of late reacting tissues to fraction size; additional interpretation of the slope is given in the legend [23,24].

There are non-standard kinds of ionizing radiation which exhibit very different dose and dose schedule effects from those seen with conventional photons (X-rays or gamma rays) and electrons. These have the physical characteristics of producing more dense ionizations than do conventional treatments. The predicted biological effects of these treatments (such as the neutrons illustrated in Figure 9.4) and their dependency on treatment schedules are not worked out, and they remain the subject of investigation.

## Chemotherapy

The toxicity of chemotherapy programs may depend on the particular drugs used, how they are sequenced or combined with radiation, the dose schedule and method of drug administration, and for some effects, at least, the cumulative cyclic and lifetime levels of drug exposure. Drug reactions may be separated into those which are idiosyncratic, for which there is an indefinite relation of the severity or probability of complications to dose, and those for which a dose-response relation can be more clearly established. Methotrexate-precipitated pneumonitis provides an example of an idiosyncratic

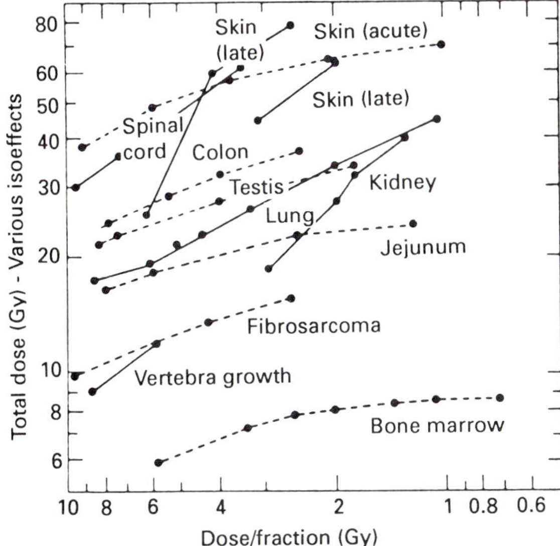


**Figure 9.5** Isoeffect plots constructed to test application of the linear quadratic model to fractionation effects in tissues. Predicted tissue effects may be derived by assuming their appearance to depend on cell survival and by taking the surviving proportion of cells to be that resulting from the recursive application of the quadratic log cell survival function upon that dose used in each treatment session. Under these assumptions, the model predicts a linear graph of the reciprocal of the total dose against dose per fraction with a treatment schedule producing a particular biological effect. Alternatively, a plot of log total dose ($\ln D$) preserving an effect against $-$dose/fraction ($-\ln d$) will yield a curve whose slope is given by $\{(\beta/\alpha)d/[1 + (\beta/\alpha)d]\}$ [23,24]. Such a curve will be steeper at a given dose/fraction level if the $\alpha/\beta$ ratio is smaller for the cells in the system being examined. A series of experiments with different tissues are plotted in just this way, and appear to satisfy the predictions of the model. Early responses are plotted on dashed curves and late responses on solid curves. At any value of dose/fraction, the slope of the isoeffect curve plotted this way may also be interpreted as giving the change in the logarithm of the ratio of the isoeffect dose of the system under study to that of a system not exhibiting fractionation dependency, which results from a small disturbance in the logarithm of dose/fraction applied to the two systems [24]. As illustrated in Figure 9.4, it is thought that the survival of cells irradiated with neutrons may exemplify a system dependent only on cumulative dose, and not on the dose/fraction, i.e. one for which $-\ln S \sim \alpha d$. Reproduced with permission from ref. [80]

reaction, while the cardiomyopathy of doxorubicin (Adriamycin) shows a dose-response relationship. Even among those reactions which are dose-dependent, there may be great variations among individuals in the dose response. Explanations for this include differences in the metabolism of the drug and in organ exposure to drug-produced toxins, pre-existing subclinical organ dysfunction, and the ability to repair or compensate for specific tissue injuries. The large variety of factors modulating drug effects makes it difficult to predict injuries from elementary principles. Some information is nevertheless available on the long-term risks of particular chemotherapies that have been given to large enough groups of survivors of certain diseases. Additional understanding, albeit qualitative, of the potential risks of drug combinations have emerged from the classification of drugs by their biochemical actions.

Administered dose may be described by the amount prescribed and by the timing and route of administration, or the amount given per unit weight or per body surface area. Measured or derived values for weight or surface area may be modified or not by height and body-build factors to correct for changes from the ideal brought about by illness. It is unclear which of these measures best relates to expectations of cure and injury, so that no universal definition of chemotherapy dose exists. Normalizing by body surface area may allow better correlation of dose with acute hematopoietic toxicity across different animal species, but this correction may not be optimally suited for the observation of a dose response in late reacting tissues within humans [25]. Tolerance may be increased by giving a drug as an infusion over several days instead of as a bolus, and larger doses may be given to select patients in whom interval testing shows relative resistance of dose-limiting tissues to the agent being titrated.

This principle has been applied to the use of doxorubicin in combination with 5-fluorouracil (5-FU) and cyclophosphamide in the treatment of breast cancer. Patients receiving doxorubicin as a 48 or 96 h infusion and in whom cardiac function is monitored by non-invasive testing at 450 mg/m$^2$ and by endomyocardial biopsy at 600 mg/m$^2$ may safely receive higher total doses of this drug than the 450 mg/m$^2$ cut-off traditionally applied when bolus delivery without cardiac monitoring is used. A prospective study showed no worse rates of response, response duration or survival with the infusion plus monitoring method compared with bolus delivery, with lessened rates of cardiac toxicities along with some worsening in the rates of acute and usually reversible mucositis [26].

This kind of change in method of drug delivery might be viewed in analogy to altered fractionation schemes in radiotherapy. Means exist for increasing total dose without compromise in late tissue tolerance, with the possible aggravation of reversible acute toxicities, but the benefit of dose changes so produced on tumor control is uncertain. Proposals for standardizing the reporting of chemotherapy administration are available [27] but as yet no system has become commonly accepted.

Creasey has classed drugs by their biochemical

chemotherapy [35]. No new leukemias were seen at > 11 years with over 35 patients still at risk. Final estimates of the leukemogenic risk cannot be made until large numbers of patients have been followed for some time after the hazard rate returns to that of the general population.

Age at primary treatment may also determine risk of subsequent leukemogenesis. The Stanford report found that although a significant difference existed in the *actuarial incidence* of leukemia among Hodgkin's disease patients under 50 years at initial treatment from a larger incidence in older patients, the *relative risk* of leukemia compared with a matched general population was not statistically different in the two age groups [31]. Time to appearance of leukemia could not be shown by other workers to be related to age [34]. Other reports have cited significant increases in leukemogenic risk, perhaps by a factor of three [36] or greater [37,39] in patients older than 40 years at initial treatment, and a statistically larger relative risk among patients aged 40–60 years [33].

Salvage treatments may carry different risks than similar treatments initially applied and sequencing of initial treatment modalities may determine the leukemogenic risk. The Finsen Institute found an increased leukemogenic risk in those treated with salvage chemotherapy over those who received chemotherapy as part of the initial therapy plan [37], but a difference between initial and salvage combined modality treatment was not found to be significant by the Milan group [36]. Initial and salvage chemotherapies were not found to carry different risks of second leukemias by two groups [31,39], but the NCI found a significantly increased risk in patients who received both chemotherapy and radiation as a consequence of salvage measures over those who had initial treatment with radiation or chemotherapy alone [34]. In an update, Blayney *et al.* from the NCI [35] suggest that the leukemogenic risk is small in patients who can be treated with six or less cycles of MOPP alone. As noted below, the prolonged use of alkylating agents in other diseases such as ovarian, breast and colon cancers does increase the risk. However, some patients who received only six cycles of MOPP or MOPP-like therapy have developed leukemia, although the risk for developing leukemia with only six cycles of MOPP has not been clearly defined. It is possible that initial treatment changes the susceptibility to induction of leukemia by subsequent salvage treatment, perhaps as a result of impaired immune surveillance, but it is also possible that the difference, if any, in susceptibility is related to the disease recurrence.

It would be desirable to identify the particular drugs responsible for leukemogenesis, so that a search for substitutions could be profitably undertaken, but etiological mechanisms are obscured by retrospective data from studies designed to answer questions very different from carcinogenesis. Comparison of MOPP with some non-MOPP alkylating regimens show larger risks in the MOPP treated group. Use of PAVe (procarbazine, melphalan, vinblastine) was found to be associated with a significantly reduced risk of leukemia in comparison with MOPP in another study [31]. Regimens containing nitrosoureas or mustard were found to carry similar late leukemia risks in one study [37], but another series found a three-fold increase in relative risk of second leukemias for four-drug regimens containing mustard over those with nitrosoureas instead [33]. With 8-year median follow-up, no leukemias have been observed in 180 patients with Hodgkin's disease treated with ABVD (doxorubicin, vinblastine, bleomycin and dacarbazine) and radiation compared with the 2.4 expected according to rates of leukemia seen with any treatment in a larger group of 1329 patients [36]. Freedom from disease progression appears to be as good with ABVD as with the MOPP standard, and indeed was found to be statistically superior in a randomized trial of combined modality treatment for moderately advanced Hodgkin's disease [40], so that secondary leukemias may be avoidable, but unfortunately other late effects due to different drugs may ensue.

Solid tumors have also been seen in larger than expected numbers in Hodgkin's disease series (Table 9.2). Most series of patients treated with chemotherapy alone show a small risk of subsequent cancers at 10–15 years, with a relative risk that may not be greater than unity [31]. Among patients treated with radiation alone, it has not been possible to associate solid tumor risk with treatment volumes [31]; indeed one study found the relative risk of second malignancy of any kind to be significantly greater than 1.0 in patients treated with less than extended field irradiation but not in those treated with larger fields [32]. Attempts to demonstrate such correlations may be confounded by association of treatment volumes with other factors, such as disease stage, chemotherapy use and disease or treatment-related immunosuppression, which may influence the carcinogenic potential.

The hazard rate for solid tumors in patients treated with radiation or chemotherapy (mostly radiation) alone was found to increase with time in one study [31], but no such time-dependent change could be shown among patients treated with combined modality therapy [34]. Stage at primary disease presentation could not be related to subsequent risk of solid tumors [33], and the same study found that, in contrast to leukemogenic potential, the risk of solid tumors was not disproportionately larger in older than younger patients.

Observations of second solid tumors in Hodgkin's disease patients have shown a median time to appearance of 70 months, but all excess tumors may not have been as yet observed. Epidemiological studies have shown a significant association of radiation with an excess risk of late second solid tumors but strategies to reduce this risk remain uncertain. Despite the inability to demonstrate field size dependency of carcinogenic risk, the simplest explanation of radiation carcinogenesis – cellular transformation through ionization – would imply that a relation of volume with carcinogenesis would exist. If so, identification of patients who might be safely treated with smaller than presently conventional fields could allow a reduced risk of second solid tumors.

Separate tabulations of late non-Hodgkin's lymphomas have shown these malignancies to appear in 1–2% of cases at 10–15 years, carrying a relative risk of about 20, with a median time to appearance of 50–120 months [31]. There is concern that the hazard rate for lymphoma is constant in the first decade subsequent to diagnosis of the Hodgkin's disease, but then rises [31]. Further analysis shows that the increased lymphoma incidence is maintained among patients treated with radiation alone, and to a varying extent among patients treated with combined modality therapy (Table 9.4), but is not yet found among those treated with chemotherapy alone. It is known that suppression of cellular immunity may allow development of lymphomas, but whether this is the mechanism through which the lymphoma association with Hodgkin's disease treatments appears is hypothetical.

In pediatric populations, it is known that patients with certain malignancies have a genetic defect that predisposes them to developing other malignancies, the classic example being retinoblastoma and osteosarcoma [41]. As yet there are no pretreatment markers in adults that will indicate an increased susceptibility to a treatment-related complication. However, there are indicators that do appear very early in the course of some treatment-related malignancies that may antedate the overt clinical disease by months or years. It is known that second leukemias in Hodgkin's disease patients are often preceded by a preleukemic phase characterized by pancytopenia and myelodysplasias; indeed, such dysplasias may themselves be fatal [41]. In 39 cases of acute non-lymphocytic leukemia, preleukemia, or myeloproliferative syndrome in which cytogenetic banding could be completed, there were 35 cases for which abnormalities in chromosomes 5 or 7 were discovered. All but one of the 35 cases of chromosome 5 or 7 changes were associated with partial or total loss of a long arm. Such work may yield assays for determining the contribution of treatment components to leukemogenesis and may permit the early treatment of these treatment-induced neoplasms.

Hodgkin's disease provides the best studied example of the carcinogenic and leukemogenic risks of antineoplastic therapy. However, the numbers of patients with this disease are small compared with the populations developing solid tumors. Long-term risk of carcinogenesis in the solid tumor populations is becoming increasingly important as survival rates improve and as adjuvant treatments with potentially toxic long-term effects are adopted because of modest improvements effected in short-term survival. The US National Cancer Institute has initiated a late cancer surveillance program of patients enrolled in institute-funded randomized treatment trials. Completed studies have shown no excess

**Table 9.4 Hodgkin's disease: late non-Hodgkin's lymphoma (NHL) selected by treatment**

| *Study* | *% Actuarial risk* | | | *Relative risk* | *Median time to NHL observation (months)* |
|---|---|---|---|---|---|
| | *5 year* | *10 year* | *11–15 year* | | |
| Unselected patients: | | | | | |
| Stanford [31] | 1.0 | 1.0 | 2.0 | 18 | ~48 |
| Milan [36] | | | 1.3 | | |
| Combined treatment: | | | | | |
| Yale [38] | 1.2 | 3.5 | | | 120 |
| Stanford [31] | | | 0.9 | 22 | |
| Milan [36] | | | 0–1.4 | | |
| Chemotherapy only: | | | | | |
| Stanford [31] | | | 0.0 | 21 | |
| Milan [36] | | | 0.0 | | |
| Radiation only: | | | | | |
| Stanford [31] | | | 3.5 | | |
| Milan [36] | | | 1.9 | | |

leukemia in Veteran's Administration trials of adjuvant thiotepa or 5-fluorodeoxyuridine (floxuridine) for colorectal cancers, but a significant leukemogenic risk to adjuvant methyl-CCNU (semustine) for gastrointestinal malignancies at high cumulative doses [43,44]. A dose-response relation for the leukemogenic risk was demonstrated, with an increase in the relative risk from 8.7 if methyl-CCNU in doses of $<500\,\text{mg/m}^2$ was prescribed to 36.7 if $>1000\,\text{mg/m}^2$ of the drug was given [45]. The NSABP has shown a modest increase in the relative risk of leukemias in breast cancer patients treated with adjuvant L-phenylalanine mustard chemotherapy or adjuvant locoregional radiation following mastectomy, but no significantly increased incidence in patients treated with radiation to the breast only after lumpectomy [46]. Study of five ovarian cancer series showed large (50–100) relative risks of leukemias in patients treated with chemotherapy alone or in combination with radiation, particularly when alkylating agents were employed. The risk is particularly high for patients given prolonged treatment who receive a high cumulative dose of alkylating agent. Radiation alone was not associated with leukemia [47]. A survey of several studies showed no increased risk of leukemias in women treated by radiation for cervix cancer [48]. Combined radiation and chemotherapy for small cell cancer was associated in two studies with a very high risk of subsequent leukemias [49,75].

More detailed reviews of second malignancies in cancer treatment may be found in the references, and elsewhere in this volume. Work in this field has shown that measures of the intensity of radiation or drug treatment are useful in defining risks of second malignancies and in suggesting less carcinogenic strategies of cancer treatment.

## Pulmonary dysfunction

Treatment for intrathoracic tumors entails a risk of producing early and late lung damage. Poor oxygenation, labored breathing, dyspnea, and reduced exercise tolerance may develop months to years after treatment. It would be desirable to have a standard set of measures by which the clinical observations could be described, but no such standard exists. Without common descriptors of damage, it will not be possible to make good predictions of treatment effect. The range of complications reported after definitive radiation for lung cancer include:

1. An 87% risk of radiographic pneumonitis (including changes of 'lung shrinkage' which might otherwise be described as fibrosis) [50].
2. A 29–38% risk of any of a group of recorded clinical sequelae (severe dyspnea, fever, dysphagia or postradiologic lung disease) [51].

3. A 6% risk of pneumonitis, pneumothorax or fibrosis reported in a large multi-institutional series [52], a sixth of which were fatal.

Even if reproducible measures of dysfunction were available, it would still not necessarily follow that they would be good measures of treatment effect, as poor breathing and increased lung density may be consequent to local recurrence as well as local complications. Results of treatment may be estimated by relating full descriptions of initial patient condition and of treatment applied to good measures of quality of late survival. There has been work towards establishing these relations, but results remain incomplete.

## *Breast cancer: uniform volumes, no intrathoracic disease*

Radiation for breast cancer provides a relatively simple problem for the analysis of late treatment effect since the lungs themselves are not affected by the cancer or related conditions, as they are for intrathoracic malignancies. Standard techniques for primary and postoperative irradiation are available, and it has been shown that estimates of lung area in at least one plane can be obtained with simple measurements taken of patient anatomy and simulation radiographs [10]. Chemotherapy, when used as an adjuvant, typically consists of one of a few recognized treatment regimens whose included drugs show only modest radiation interactions. Nevertheless, there are still enough possible permutations of treatment parameters to make it difficult to relate outcome to treatment delivered. For example, treatments may differ in their choice of fraction size, in whether they are used postoperatively or definitively, in whether the target is the breast alone or also the regional lymphatics and whether these include the internal mammary chain or do not. Nevertheless, a relation between lung volume included within the 70% isodose line and pneumonitis has been exhibited in women treated postoperatively with either tangential fields or these supplemented by nodal fields [10]. In a separate study, a 5% diminishment of $FEV_1$ was found in 18 women 0.25–6.5 years after completion of adjuvant postoperative breast irradiation compared with unmatched controls [53]. Fraction size and volumes were large in this series; tangential fields and en face internal mammary ports received 40 Gy in 2.5 Gy fractions and an anterior supraclavicular field, anterior axillary port, and a posterior axillary boost field were used to give the remaining regional nodes 40 Gy in 5 Gy fractions. Nine women were recorded to suffer clinical symptoms but no correlation could be made between the presence of symptoms or radiographic changes on the one hand and a battery of spirometric and blood gas measurements on the other. Although the lack of correlation has been explained by the small volumes of lung which were irradiated [53], it appears that these volumes were still sufficiently large to produce symptomatology, illustrating the inadequacy of pulmonary function tests in describing post-treatment dysfunction. The $FEV_1$ was found in this study to have been reduced to 54% and 57% of predicted in two of 19 patients in whom this measurement was made and in the remainder was maintained at $\geqslant 85\%$, while none of 20 unmatched controls were found with an $FEV_1$ below 88%, suggesting that marked flow changes can be found in a small number of patients treated with this technique for postoperative breast cancer. No irradiated patient smoked more than half a pack per day. It appears that lungs may be damaged by large fraction treatments given postoperatively to the chest wall and the draining lymphatics, but patients reporting symptoms are not necessarily identifiable by spirometry and blood gas testing.

## Hodgkin's disease: uniform fields, intrathoracic disease

The analysis of pulmonary damage from mantle irradiation of Hodgkin's disease is complicated by differences in lung volume included within portals whose shape needs conform to disease extent, and by the use of chemotherapy regimens some of which may be pulmonary toxic. Nevertheless, there is far greater uniformity in the amounts of functional lung irradiated and in the selection of added chemotherapies than is the case with primary cancer of the lung. Furthermore, local disease control is far more likely for Hodgkin's disease than for lung cancer.

Mantle fields for Hodgkin's disease produce an 8–10% reduction in total lung capacity [54,55]. Small differences in $FEV_1$ of about this magnitude may also be found [55], but few, if any, treated patients will show $FEV_1$ levels <80% of predicted [56], even when extensive mediastinal adenopathy (greater than one-third the diameter of chest on a PA film) is included, along with treatment of an entire lung to low dose (16 Gy) in small fractions (about 0.6 Gy). A small number of patients will show moderately severe respiratory or obstructive lung disease (5%) and about a quarter will show some mild restrictive or obstructive damage on spirometry. Depending on the volume treated, 40–65% of patients will admit to mild dyspnea on exertion, compared with one of a small group of seven patients identified with Hodgkin's disease but with neither thoracic disease nor thoracic irradiation. About 21% of irradiated patients show abnormal peak oxygen consumption of <80% predicted, with this fraction being twice as large (30%) in cases of extensive mediastinal adenopathy treated also with

chemotherapy as in other irradiated cases (13%). An additional 24% of irradiated patients show borderline abnormalities with reductions of 10–20% in oxygen consumption, compared with 29% in non-irradiated patients without chest disease.

Separately, electrocardiography shows abnormalities in 13% of patients, mostly right bundle branch block, but a significant difference in the percentage of patients showing these or other borderline abnormalities from that expected in the general population may not be seen. The significant numbers of patients, 50%, in an irradiated series who reported dyspnea on exertion in comparison with 14% among patients who were not irradiated was not matched by like numbers scoring abnormalities on respiratory and ventilation testing or on electrocardiography, indicating again that available testing may yield only a partial picture of clinical disabilities.

The addition of potentially pulmonary toxic chemotherapy may further confound estimates of expected lung damage following standard mantle irradiation for Hodgkin's disease. A randomized trial of MOPP *versus* ABVD chemotherapy in addition to radiation for moderately advanced Hodgkin's disease [40] showed a non-significant difference in the deterioration of vital capacity and $FEV_1$ among patients tested more than 5 years after therapy, and a significantly larger fraction of late radiographic abnormalities (59%) in ABVD-treated patients over those treated with MOPP (30%). Four ABVD patients of 57 who showed chest X-ray changes suffered from dyspnea on exertion up to 3 years post-treatment [40].

Extensive work with irradiated Hodgkin's disease patients, then, indicates a 10% reduction in total lung capacity and probably $FEV_1$ following mantle treatment. Most patients show a 10–15% risk of developing abnormal peak oxygen consumption of <80% predicted, and this risk is doubled in those who receive chemotherapy and radiation for extensive mediastinal adenopathy. Depending, perhaps, on how patients are questioned, fewer or greater numbers of patients will admit to dyspnea on exertion. A battery of laboratory tests which can robustly identify patients admitting to dyspnea on exertion has yet to be demonstrated. ABVD chemotherapy used in conjunction with radiation may double the chances of observing late chest X-ray changes and is associated with a small number of patients admitting to significant dyspnea on exertion in contrast to almost none treated with MOPP alone who so reply.

## Lung cancer: non-uniform field, intrathoracic disease

Predicting late effects of radiotherapy for lung cancer demands not only that cases with like amounts of treated lung be observed, with similar initial tumor burdens, but also that initial compromise of lung function by tumor and comorbid disease be similar within groups whose late effects are to be registered. These criteria are difficult to satisfy and considerable uncertainty remains in our ability to predict late pulmonary damage, and to know the magnitude of importance of measures of treatment volume and pretreatment function.

A consequence of this uncertainty is that clinical studies of pulmonary effects of radiation may prove not to be robust. This might be contrasted with pulmonary studies in Hodgkin's disease, e.g. where fairly stable decrements of about 10% in total lung capacity and similarly modest decrements in maximum oxygen consumption are reported in several studies. Failure to produce similar results for lung cancer is particularly frustrating as large numbers of people suffer from this disease, a realistic object of treatment is often only palliation and concern about the significant probability of producing lung damage can compromise treatment volumes and doses. Treatment failure and complications may result in individual distress as well as considerable economic costs.

Various abnormalities may be found in serial pulmonary function measurements revealing ill-defined connections to initial and comorbid disease and to the delivered treatment. Early workers sought to relate lung effects to the volume integral of dose, which is a measure of the amount of energy made available for ionization within tissue by a course of treatment. This quantity has, though, proved to be too compact a description of the radiation delivered to be a useful indicator of late lung damage. A preliminary study of pulmonary functions and gas exchange 4 weeks after treatment in 15 patients treated with megavoltage or multiple field orthovoltage techniques found no significant difference in lung volumes and gas tensions, but a decrease in diffusion capacity. This decrease was found to be related to the volume integral of dose given to the chest [57]. An extension of this study to include regular testing up to 1 year after treatment showed significant late decreases in vital capacity and residual volume [58] which could then not be correlated with integral dose. Stabilization of early deterioration in diffusion capacity was found and this decrease, too, could no longer be correlated with the volume integral of dose. Gas tensions did not appear to be affected by treatment. Scintigrams showed that regions of lung which were larger than those appearing involved with tumor on standard radiography showed diminished perfusion, and this diminution worsened after treatment.

Regional analysis of the radiation delivered may provide a better correlation with delayed pulmonary damage than the integral of dose over the whole lung volume. Quantitative ventilation and perfusion scans have been used to predict the volume of functioning lung capacity destroyed by treatment and its relation to deterioration in pulmonary function test performance. A study of 115 patients tested before undergoing definitive radiation therapy for lung cancer found 49 available for repeat testing at a median interval of 1 year following treatment [59]. Reductions in $FEV_1$ in the repeat tested group could not be predicted from estimates of the amount of functional lung treated to beyond a particular dose (of 40 Gy). However, if patients were grouped according to their pretreatment pulmonary functions, among those with the fewest pretreatment abnormalities, good correlations could be found between fractions of lung volume irradiated to >40 Gy and the magnitude of subsequent loss in $FEV_1$. Among 19 patients with no greater than 10% shift of ventilation or perfusion to the uninvolved lung and with pretreatment $FEV_1$ of >50% of predicted, two-thirds showed a reduction in $FEV_1$ proportionate to within 25% of the estimated functioning lung receiving >40 Gy. Proportionate decreases in test values were not found among the remaining patients who had substantial pretreatment compromises in $FEV_1$ or in the normal distribution of blood and air-flow between the two lungs before treatment. All patients suffered an increase in airway resistance of 31–34%. A 10% decrease in total lung capacity and a borderline statistically significant decrease in diffusing capacity of the lung for carbon monoxide ($D_LCO$) of 28% was found only among patients who had minimal abnormalities in the distribution of ventilation or perfusion between treatments and whose initial $FEV_1$ was >50% of predicted. No significant differences in blood gases were found in any of the patients. These results point to the confounding influences of the effects of cancer and comorbid disease on predictions of treatment damage. Even the directions of change in dose or volume likely to maintain acceptable function in an organ affected by cancer may be difficult to predict.

## Neuropsychiatric damage

Late neuropsychiatric abnormalities following elective whole brain irradiation present a problem in treatment design for which qualitative solutions are available. Among the largest number of adult patients affected by this problem are those with small cell lung cancer. Whether the qualitative solutions for reducing the risk of brain abnormalities are good enough to justify continuation of elective brain irradiation remains controversial.

Elective brain irradiation has been shown in randomized [60] and non-randomized [61] studies to reduce the incidence of clinically evident brain metastases by about a factor of three, from about 20–30% [61–64] to about 5–10%. Although this reduction in brain metastases does not provide an improvement in survival, it is nevertheless important as reviews of the efficacy of cranial radiation in controlling brain metastases once clinically evident show it to control symptoms in only 50–60% of cases [65].

Demonstration of the efficacy of radiation in reducing the appearance of brain metastases was repeated in a number of randomized and non-randomized studies. Treatment protocols, by and large, included whole brain radiotherapy given in large fractions of 2.5–3.0 Gy each to a dose of about 30 Gy; treated patients also often received combination chemotherapy containing high-dose intravenous methotrexate or nitrosoureas which are known to be able to penetrate the blood–brain barrier. The radiation fraction sizes were larger than those used for most adjuvant and curative programs of treatment; they were similar to those employed in palliation of cases for which survival is usually short. For example, a review of seven randomized trials [61] of elective brain irradiation included four in which CCNU (lomustine) was part of the prescribed treatment given to all patients. Four of these seven studies also utilized 3.0 Gy fractions in the radiation arm.

Observations of the small numbers of late survivors of small cell lung cancer treated with elective brain irradiation and combination chemotherapy showed many to have either neuroradiological abnormalities or symptoms or signs of neurological deficit (Table 9.5). Various proportions of patients were found affected depending, perhaps, on whether a deliberate inquiry for functional deficits was made, and on the thresholds for neuroradiological and neuropsychiatric test abnormalities. Changes were found both among those receiving nitrosoureas and those who did not.

In the light of these findings, workers have sought to modify the treatment protocols in ways which might attenuate undesirable effects of therapy. Nitrosoureas have been removed from many treatment protocols in which elective brain irradiation is to be used. The dose per radiation treatment has been reduced to exploit presumed differences in the fractionation sensitivities of normal brain and tumor. It has not yet been shown, though, that late survivors of small cell cancer of the lung treated electively to the brain with the revised regimens exhibit less severe and more infrequent neurological abnormalities, so that the optimal approach to the problem of subclinical brain metastases is uncertain. The ability of schedule changes to eliminate late neurological effects is further complicated by the possibility that chemotherapy and subclinical metastases contribute to the observed deterioration in

**Table 9.5 Morbidity of elective brain irradiation (EBI) in small cell cancer of the lung**

| Reference | Dose (Gy) | Fractions | Time (days) | No. of patients | Chemotherapy | % Incidence of neurological effect | | |
|---|---|---|---|---|---|---|---|---|
| | | | | | | Symptomatic | With signs | With radiologic abnormalities |
| Chak *et al.* [68] | 30 | 10 | 12 | 49 | PbCVL;CAE;EAM | 14 | | |
| Lee *et al.* [69] | 30 | 10 | 12 | 20 | (ECHV + PbIM;VIA-CEM; VIA-CEV;EIV; CAV;PbCM) ± auto | 15 | | 70 |
| | None | – | – | 5 | CAV;CV;CMV | 0 | | 0 |
| Perez in [67] | 30 | 10 | 12 | 15 | | 33 | | |
| Craig *et al.* [70] | 30 | 10 | 12 | 13 | CAV;CAVE | 66 | | 70–100 |
| Johnson *et al.* [71] | 20–27 | 8–10 | 11–38 | 9 | Low doses CML; ACE-EA;PbAV | | 55 | 66 |
| | 20–30 | 5–15 | 5–19 | 6 | High doses CAV;CML; CM | | 100 | 33 |
| Komaki *et al.* [61] | 25–30 | 10 | 12 | 16 | CAV;CMV | | 0 | |
| Ellison *et al.* [72] | 24 | 8 | 12 | 10 | CMVL | 40 | | 0 |
| Sher *et al.* [73] | 30 | 8–10 | 12 | 9 | CAV-PE;CAV-PE-CE ± (L-Pb-C-A-P-E) | 44 | | |
| Licciardello *et al.* [74] | 30 | 10 | 12 | 15 | CAV;CEV | 13 | | |
| Volk *et al.* [75] | 30 | N/a | N/a | 8 | AMEPbVCL;CAV; CAVM | 12 | | |
| Looper *et al.* [76] | 36 | N/a | N/a | 18 | CAV ± nitrosourea | | 78 | |
| Catane *et al.* [77] | 20–30 | 10–15 | 10–21 | 13 | CAV ± itM | 0 | 23 (mild) | 62 |
| Livingston *et al.* [78] | 30 | 10 | 17 | | CAV-CE-CM | ?12 | | |

N/a, not available; Pb, procarbazine; C, cyclophosphamide; A, doxorubicin (Adriamycin); V, vincristine; P, cisplatin; E, etoposide; M, methotrexate; H, hydroxydaunorubicin; I, ifosfamide; auto, autologous bone marrow transplant; itM, intrathecal methotrexate; L, CCNU

## Growth retardation

The growth of the limbs can be significantly retarded by cancer treatment, particularly radiotherapy in the area of the epiphyseal plate or if an epiphysis has to be resected as part of the tumour resection. The 'growing' prosthesis described by Scales is one answer to this problem. The other is to consider leg lengthening once treatment of the tumour has been completed and there has been a reasonable disease-free interval. Unfortunately the commonest sites for bone tumours are often the most rapidly growing parts of the child's skeleton, particularly around the knee and the shoulder. Damage to the epiphysis at these sites will cause maximal growth retardation. However, modern advances in limb-lengthening techniques have made this method of treatment much more widely applicable and less demanding on the patient, particularly as much of it can be done as an outpatient.

It should be stressed that limb-lengthening still remains an exacting technique which requires great care and attention to detail and is not without its complications, both minor and major. The recent advances have evolved from the much greater use of external fixation devices for the management of fractures. Leaders in this field have been Wagner in Germany, Ilizarov in Russia and the Italian School of de Bastiani in Verona and Montecelli in Rome. An excellent review article of these methods was published by Paley in 1988 [17]. The technique of 'intraosseous lengthening' where a segment of bone has been removed or lost and a segment of the same bone can be moved into the gap allowing bone to reform behind it, using the Ilizarov or Montecelli type of frame, is undoubtedly a possibility for bridging large gaps which have been resected. This method is an alternative to the custom-made prosthesis or allograft. The basis of all these methods is that the bone is held with pins attached either to a unilateral bar in the dynamic axial fixation (DAF) favoured by de Bastiani and the Verona School or by a circumferential frame described by Ilizarov and Montecelli. The latter is more cumbersome but uses finer pins and at present is undoubtedly better for intraosseous bone lengthening. Both methods allow the patient to be ambulant on crutches while the lengthening is taking place.

Lengthening may be performed by distracting the epiphysis; this is termed chondrodiastasis. The problem with this method is that once the epiphysis has been distracted, no further growth occurs at this site. In addition it appears that the bone which forms at the site of the lengthening takes longer to consolidate and, since the lengthening takes place close to joints, joint stiffness can be a problem.

Another method of lengthening is callus distraction or callotasi where the bone is carefully divided after application of the lengthening device. Callus is then allowed to form before distraction starts. This takes about 7–10 days. The callus is then slowly distracted at approximately 1 mm per day. During the process of distraction the patient is mobile on crutches and can be managed from home as an outpatient. Careful supervision of the distraction is always necessary, particularly care of the pin tracks and soft tissues. The joints must be watched for stiffness and more serious complications such as subluxation or even dislocation of adjacent joints. Neurovascular complications and failure of the bone to form satisfactorily are more major complications.

## Complications of intravenous administration of drugs

Modern chemotherapy frequently requires long-term intravenous administration of drugs by central or peripheral lines. From the orthopaedic surgeon's point of view, there are serious complications to this treatment. Intravenous lines, particularly in children whose immune status is often suppressed by the drug treatment they are receiving, are very prone to infection. The infection can involve bones and joints by either local or systemic spread, leading to severe and permanent damage in the growing child. Diagnosis of these infections is always difficult because of the overall state of the child and the suppression of the normal signs and symptoms of infection. Extravasation from the intravenous line can also cause very serious problems. Both superficial skin loss and severe compartment syndromes leading to major loss of soft tissues and neurovascular damage may occur from extravasation of toxic drugs into the soft tissues while patients are under treatment with chemotherapy. This type of injury produces long-term orthopaedic problems often with irreversible damage to muscles, tendons, neurovascular structures, bones and joints. It is most important that those involved in caring for children on intravenous infusions are aware of the signs and symptoms of early compartment syndromes from extravasation so that appropriate action can be taken to avoid such complications. As far as compartment syndromes are concerned, an important development has been that of simple compartmental pressure measuring devices which should be readily available to measure compartment pressures if the syndrome is suspected. The classical early signs and symptoms in a compartment syndrome are pain which may be severe and numbness from ischaemia of nerves within the affected compartment. The periphery of the limb may develop pallor and poor capillary return. Peripheral pulses may or may not be absent.

Early treatment by fascial decompression may reverse the ischaemic changes [18]. If the diagnosis is delayed there may be irreversible changes to muscles and nerves resulting in permanent contractures and sensory loss (Volkmann's ischaemic contracture).

# Radiation osteonecrosis

The first description of radiation necrosis is attributed to Regaud [19] in 1922 and subsequently James Ewing [20] from the United States in 1926. With modern methods of radiotherapy the complication is relatively uncommon, but when it occurs it can result in serious problems to the patient in regard to morbidity. While bone is relatively resistant to the destructive effects of irradiation, it absorbs more energy per unit volume than soft tissues because of its increased density.

The effect of radiation on bone appears to be related to the dosage. Radiation in the order of 3500–4500 cGy will impair the capacity of bone to repair. Above 5000–8000 cGy adult bone may be severely damaged [21,22].

Both animal and human studies have demonstrated the pathogenesis of the disease. Roher *et al.* [23] studied the effects of cobalt-60 irradiation on the mandible of monkeys. Blood vessels in the periosteum, bone lamellae and the medullary cavity were decreased in number. In many cases this was related to a radiation vasculitis, with obstruction to blood flow. With greater dosage of radiation there was necrosis of the osteoblasts and osteocytes in the Haversian systems within the radiation fields. This resulted in decreased bone turnover and osteoclastic resorption of dead bone lamellae and a reduced capacity for repair.

Matsubayashi *et al.* [24] examined *post mortem* specimens of patients who had been treated with radiotherapy and showed that degeneration and necrosis of tumour cells was followed by replacement with fibrous tissue. The fibrous tissue became replaced with woven bone and finally lamellar bone, providing the capacity for repair existed. The extent and rate of repair depended on the degree of radiation and volume of necrotic bone to be replaced. In a series of patients who underwent head and neck irradiation, the latent period between irradiation and the development of osteonecrosis was from 4 months to 13 years, with just over half developing the complication within the first 6 months [25].

The radiological differentiation between radiation-induced osteonecrosis and tumour recurrence may be very difficult. In both there will be areas of rarefaction and increased bone density due to islands of non-viable bone (sequestra). There may be periosteal elevation and areas of new bone formation in both disorders [26]. There is usually no significant calcified soft tissue mass in osteonecrosis

similar to that occurring in radiation-induced sarcoma. Where differentiation is not possible a bone biopsy, preferably a percutaneous needle biopsy, and histological examination will determine the underlying bone abnormality and guide future management.

With the development of radiation osteonecrosis, the bone is weakened and is unable to withstand load. This is especially the case in long bones. Some degree of protection is required to allow the bone to heal and return to its former strength. In mild cases conservative management including decreased weight-bearing will be satisfactory in most instances; in others the bone may be weakened to the extent that a pathological fracture may occur (Figure 10.4a and b). This will result in further pain and swelling together with restriction of activity. Internal fixation of the fracture may be required to support the bone and allow the patient a degree of independence. Fractures around the pelvis, acetabulum and proximal femur may result in marked restriction of activity and pain around the hip joint. This may require joint replacement in order to relieve symptoms [22].

Internal fixation is not without its complications, since successful fracture management depends on the ability of the fracture to heal. Delay or failure to obtain bone healing may result in the fixation device cutting out from the abnormal bone or the device breaking from fatigue.

Radiation-induced osteonecrosis of the femoral head is a significant complication in a small number of patients who have had radiation to the area of the groin or lower abdomen. The pathological effect on the cells is similar to that described previously with cell necrosis and vasculitis. There is bone necrosis and segmental collapse of areas of the femoral head. The articular cartilage may be preserved but subsequently becomes functionless when the head collapses and the cartilage remains loose and free from its subchondral attachments within the joint. The patient will complain of aching pain with some degree of stiffness in the early stages, even before there are radiological changes in the affected hip joint. Magnetic resonance imaging (MRI) is reported to be the most accurate method of identifying avascular necrosis before it presents on routine radiographs (see below). A technetium-99m bone scan may show a cold spot in the femoral head, but the investigation is associated with false negatives and does not appear as accurate as MRI in the early stages. In time the femoral head begins to collapse and the joint will show loss of normal architecture. In the later stages secondary changes of osteoarthritis may be present on routine radiographs.

Various methods of treatment of early avascular necrosis have been suggested including drilling of the femoral neck and head to induce vascular inflow and healing [27]. More recently, Urbaniak [28] has

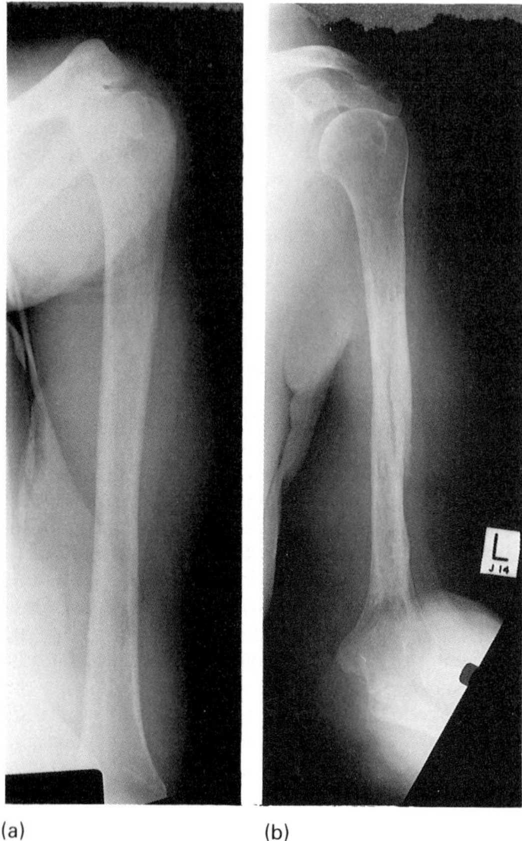

(a)                              (b)

**Figure 10.4 a** Normal humerus in patient requiring radiotherapy for a liposarcoma; **b** post-irradiation osteonecrosis with a pathological fracture

described the use of a free vascularized fibular graft placed into the neck and head of the femur to stimulate bone healing. Both these techniques require normal hip anatomy to provide a chance of success. All too often the head is beginning to flatten by the time symptoms become significant, and at this stage only a total hip replacement will offer a pain-free, mobile hip joint.

## Avascular necrosis of bone related to steroid therapy

Avascular necrosis of bone (osteonecrosis) is a well-recognized complication of steroid therapy and may occur in the treatment of several tumours including Hodgkin's disease. It usually affects the femoral head, although the distal femoral condyles, humeral head and talus may be affected. The complication occurs bilaterally in approximately 50–80% of patients.

The relationship between steroid dose and incidence of avascular necrosis has been investigated, with either a weak association or none. Felson and Anderson [29], however, showed a strong correlation between daily total dose and rate of avascular necrosis. Confirmation of these findings is awaited from other workers.

The development of avascular necrosis is associated with pain, decreased range of movement and a limp. The symptoms may develop insidiously or in a more dramatic fashion. Once avascular necrosis develops in the femoral heads, collapse of the femoral heads usually proceeds relentlessly.

While routine radiographs may show no abnormality in the early stages, MRI appears to be most useful in identifying early changes in the femoral head. Genez *et al.* [30] compared the results of MRI, radiography, proximal intramedullary pressures and biopsy specimens in seven patients with 11 painful hips with high risk of osteonecrosis. All 11 hips showed evidence of osteonecrosis on histological study but only five showed changes compatible with osteonecrosis on MRI (46% sensitivity). A routine bone scan was available in nine hips but positive in only one hip (11% sensitivity). Radiographs were sensitive in only 18% of the cases. Beltran *et al.* [31] compared MRI with radio-isotope bone scanning in a retrospective study of 49 patients (85 hips) with a clinical suspicion of avascular necrosis confirmed by biopsy or evidence on radiographs, and demonstrated a sensitivity of 89% in MRI compared with 78% in bone scans.

The importance of early diagnosis before radiological changes become significant is that early treatment may arrest the disease. Once radiological changes are present, collapse and deterioration of the joint is almost inevitable.

In the early stages, several procedures have been advocated. Core decompression has been recommended for early changes with Ficat and Arlet [32] reporting 92% good or very good results over an 8-year follow-up. The aim of core decompression is to reduce the intramedullary pressure and arrest or reverse the process of avascular necrosis before it becomes evident radiographically. Wang *et al.* [27] have produced results from experimental decompression on rabbits to confirm the normalization of femoral head blood flow following decompression. Urbaniak [28] has presented preliminary results of insertion of a free vascularized fibular graft placed into the femoral head and neck to attempt to stimulate revascularization. Longer term results are awaited before the technique can be properly evaluated.

Unfortunately the majority of patients who develop avascular necrosis of the femoral heads are detected at the late stage where the techniques described above are inapplicable and where collapse of the head becomes inevitable. In these patients a

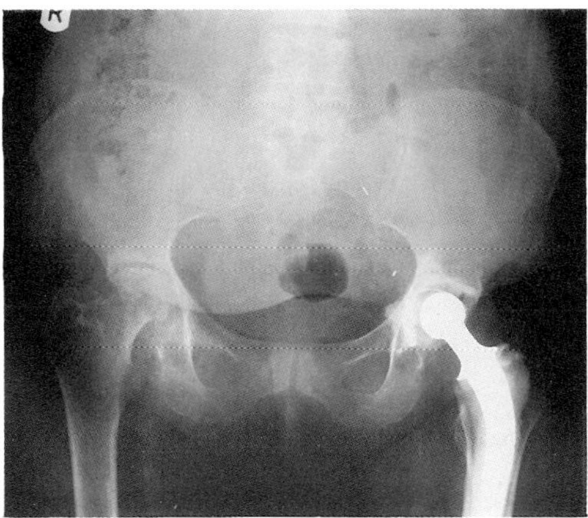

**Figure 10.5** Hip X-ray of a patient receiving high-dose steroid therapy. She developed bilateral avascular necrosis, requiring a total hip replacement on her left hip and will require a replacement on her right

total hip replacement offers a satisfactory method of pain relief and increased mobility [33] (Figure 10.5).

# Radiation-induced sarcomas

With the successes of treatment of malignant disease over the past few decades and the possibility of patients surviving 10–20 years from the time of treatment, the number of patients developing post-radiation sarcomas is likely to increase. One of the earliest descriptions of this complication was published in 1929 by Martland and Humphries [34] who described the development of osteogenic sarcomas in normal individuals who painted radium onto clock or watch dials. While radiation-induced sarcomas may arise in areas of normal bone underlying the radiation field outlined for a soft tissue tumour such as breast carcinoma, it may also develop in bone in which a benign tumour or tumour-like condition has been treated by irradiation. These disorders include giant cell tumours and aneurysmal bone cysts.

The sarcoma most frequently occurs in the sixth decade of life and often presents with sudden swelling and pain in an area of bone which was previously quiescent. An alternative presentation is through a pathological fracture.

The latent period between radiation therapy and the development of the sarcoma varies widely. A range of 3–33 years with a mean of 10.5 years was reported from the Sloan-Kettering Cancer Centre, New York [35].

It would appear that there is no direct correlation between the dose of irradiation and the subsequent development of a sarcoma, but as a rule sarcomas usually develop when at least 3000 cGy have been given over a 4-week period. However, cases of radiation-induced sarcomas have been reported after exposure to as little as 800 cGy. Presumably the radium dial workers were subjected to a chronic low dose of alpha particles of radium-226 over a long period.

Radiation-induced sarcomas may develop in almost any part of the body but commonly occur in the long bones and pelvic and shoulder girdle. Soft tissue sarcomas may occur and totalled 11% of a series of 66 patients who developed post-irradiation sarcomas reviewed by Huvos *et al.* [35]. He also gave radiation osteogenic sarcomas an incidence of 5.5% of all osteogenic sarcomas presenting to his clinic. The complication is therefore uncommon.

Histological examination most frequently demonstrates a fibrohistiocytic osteoblastic or chondrosarcomatous osteogenic sarcoma with mixed patterns being less common. There are no specific radiological or histological features which differentiate post-irradiation sarcomas from the 'idiopathic' types of osteosarcoma that may develop. The diagnosis is made on the history of previous radiotherapy.

Radiological examination will demonstrate the typical features of areas of bone destruction and repair often with dense bone, with periosteal elevation being uncommon [36]. The bone changes may be associated with a variable sized soft tissue mass (Figure 10.6a and b). It may be difficult occasionally to differentiate these features from the changes in post-irradiation bone necrosis, but in the latter soft tissue tumours are not present. Biopsy should resolve the matter.

The prognosis despite treatment is poor in patients who develop post-irradiation sarcoma. Sim *et al.* [37] from the Mayo Clinic reported a mean survival time of just over 12 months, with only two long-term survivors out of 150 cases. Huvos *et al.* [35] described a cumulative disease-free survival rate at 5 years of 17%, with a median survival of 12 months.

The various treatment modalities of chemotherapy and surgery should be considered in regard to treatment, bearing in mind the poor prognosis. Since the death rate from osteogenic sarcoma is approximately 0.5 per 100 000 of the population, the complication of post-irradiation sarcoma is extremely rare and should not be a contraindication to treatment by radiotherapy in malignant disease. However, since the disease may develop after radiotherapy to benign conditions, then surgical excision should be strongly considered as an alternative in non-malignant conditions wherever possible.

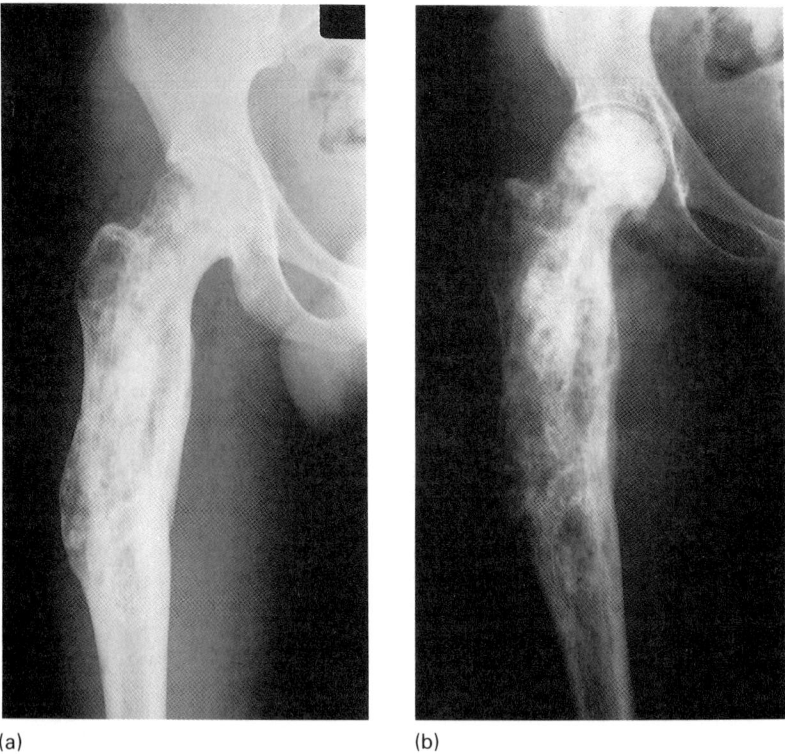



**Figure 10.6 a** Ewing's sarcoma of the proximal femur treated by radiotherapy at the age of 13 years. The tumour appears quiescent and the patient was asymptomatic; **b** at 19 years of age the patient developed pain and a limp. X-rays show activity within the bone and a large soft tissue mass. Biopsy revealed an osteosarcoma

## Metastatic bone disease

With the advances in cancer therapy in recent years, the survival time of many patients with cancer has been increased significantly. As a result the incidence of skeletal metastases has increased, and with it the frequency of pathological fractures. For example, approximately 63% of patients with breast cancer survived 5 years in 1960, whereas 15 years later the 5-year survival was 81% [38]. While skeletal metastases are not a direct complication of cancer therapy, their incidence appears to be related to successful therapy and increased survival of the patients. It is also a significant complication of malignant disease and requires comment in relation to modern orthopaedic management in which there have been significant improvements.

While almost any malignancy can spread to bone, by far the commonest primary site is breast with an incidence of approximately 50% in several series. Other primary tumours frequently spreading to bone are lung, prostate, thyroid and kidney with ovarian, colonic and oesophageal tumours metastasizing to bone infrequently [39].

While the majority of skeletal metastases are lytic, sclerotic secondaries may develop from prostatic, mammary, gastrointestinal and bladder carcinomas. Mixed lesions with areas of bone sclerosis and lysis may also occur, most commonly in mammary cancer.

With regard to the site of skeletal involvement, metastases affect the axial skeleton more frequently than the appendicular skeleton, but any bone may be involved. Most metastases originate within the red marrow and then infiltrate the cortex of the bone. The distribution of skeletal metastases has been shown to vary depending on the primary tumour, but no convincing explanation for the differences in the site of metastases has been proposed. The increased use of scintigraphy has enabled the site of metastases to be defined for individual tumours and is a most useful investigative technique [40].

Bone secondaries 10 mm in diameter may be identified on routine bone scanning, and using emission isotopic tomographic scintigraphy lesions of 2 mm in diameter have been detected [41].

The diagnosis of skeletal metastases may be

obvious from a history of pain, swelling or pathological fracture. However, in some patients these features may not be present and the skeletal metastases may not be obvious clinically. A review by Galasko [42] showed that, of 86 patients with advanced mammary carcinoma with radiological evidence of skeletal metastases only 65% complained of pain, and pathological fracture may be the first indication of skeletal involvement. Since skeletal metastases are usually multifocal, scintigraphy using technetium-99m is the most useful investigation for whole body assessment [43], although the technique is not specific and not quantitative.

In a study of women with disseminated breast cancer, 50% of women had radiographic evidence of bone secondaries, a figure which increased to 84% when they were investigated by bone scanning techniques [44]. Local specific lesions may be visualized by routine X-ray, tomograms or CT scans to provide a more accurate assessment of the size and degree of infiltration of specific secondary deposits, but whole body radiography is impractical. Edelstyn *et al.* [45] demonstrated that as much as 50% of medullary bone had to be destroyed before the lesion became apparent on routine X-rays, although a lytic area in the cortex can be detected with much less bone loss. Best *et al.* [46] reported comparative studies between X-rays, bone scans and CT scans in 30 patients. They demonstrated that a CT scan could differentiate between degenerative joint disease and metastases, both of which may produce a hot spot on a technetium-99m bone scan and which might not be visualized on routine X-rays.

Metabolic investigation is of little value in assessing secondary deposits. While alkaline phosphatase estimations were raised in 66% of 86 patients with advanced mammary cancer and skeletal metastases, the level did not relate to the extent of the bone disease and there were false positive results [42]. Cowan and Young [47] demonstrated that only 30% of patients with a positive bone scan for secondary deposits had a raised alkaline phosphatase estimation.

One of the more depressing effects of secondary deposits in bone is unremitting pain, usually made worse by weight-bearing. Fortunately most patients treated by radiotherapy to the painful secondary will be relieved of pain [48]. Occasionally pain may persist, presumably due to the osteoporosis caused by the radiotherapy together with continued microfractures in the weakened and softened bone. It may also indicate that the tumour is radio-resistant.

Following radiotherapy to a lytic metastatic lesion, there is a variable response of the bone to reossification. In clinical practice the rate of reossification of metastases treated by radiotherapy varies between 35% and approximately 60–80% [48,49]. Matsubayashi *et al.* [24] has described the sequence of events taking place in bone following radiotherapy in a series of autopsy specimens and includes necrosis of tumour cells followed by proliferation of fibrous tissue. This calcifies into woven bone which then matures into lamellar bone. Presumably in those areas not developing lamellar bone, the process is arrested at the time of tumour necrosis or the fibrous tissue is not transformed into bone.

In some patients the bone pain will be followed by a pathological fracture and one of the decisions to be made on identifying a significant lytic secondary in bone is whether prophylactic internal fixation is necessary to prevent this distressing complication. With regard to orthopaedic management of skeletal metastases in long bones, several features have been identified which, when present, make prophylactic fixation advisable. Fidler [50] has shown that the rate of pathological fracture increased with the degree of cortical destruction. If there was greater than 50% of cortical destruction in a long bone, there was a sudden increase in the frequency of pathological fracture. Another indication for fixation is the presence of continued pain in a long bone despite radiotherapy which is made worse by weight-bearing. The cumulative effect of multiple microfractures will almost inevitably result in pathological fracture. Fractures around the proximal femur are common and are related to the amount of load taken by this area on walking. A lesion 2.5 cm in diameter in the proximal femur or a pathological avulsion of the lesser trochanter are both indications that the femur is markedly weakened and that a pathological fracture is likely to develop [51]. They require internal fixation to support the bone and prevent further morbidity. Postoperative radiotherapy to the secondary is essential to prevent further bone destruction.

While prophylactic fixation of specific skeletal metastases in appropriate patients is palliative rather than curative, the quality of life for the patient will be significantly improved and the risk of pathological fracture will be decreased. With modern methods of fixation, morbidity from the procedure is low and an early return to reasonable mobility, free from pain, is to be expected.

## Pathological fractures

Pathological fractures either in the spine or long bones increase the morbidity of disseminated malignancy producing pain and loss of function. They may occur spontaneously through a previously unrecognized bony secondary deposit or through the site of a biopsy. Occasionally they may occur during or following a course of radiotherapy which may cause a temporary increased degree of osteoporosis from hyperaemia sufficient to weaken the bone at a metastasis to breaking point. The incidence of pathological fracture directly related to radiotherapy is difficult to define with certainty since the fracture may be coincidental, but is of the order of less than 2% of all pathological fractures from skeletal metastases [48]. The degree of osteoporosis following radiotherapy can, in some cases, be pronounced and may predispose the bone to fracture.

The aim of treatment in pathological fractures is to stabilize the fragments to provide sufficient strength to allow the patient to mobilize, preferably unsupported, without pain and to return function to the limb as soon as possible.

When planning fixation of a long-bone fracture, it is essential to view the whole of the bone since other deposits may be present which also require support.

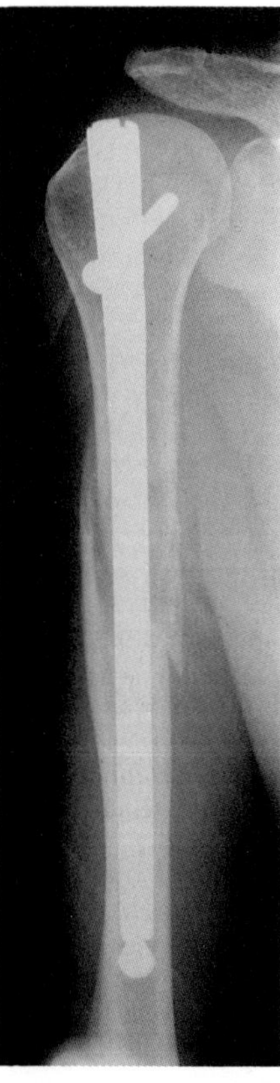

**Figure 10.7** A Seidle intramedullary locking nail used to treat an oblique pathological fracture of the midshaft of the humerus. The distal locking device is a small olive which is screwed tight into the metal rod to grip the cortex of the humerus. A proximal screw through the cortices of the humerus and the rod lock the proximal fragment

Fixation of a further fracture through an unrecognized metastasis distal to plate fixation, for example, is technically very difficult and is avoided by X-ray of the whole limb. Fractures in the proximal femur should be considered for joint replacement, whereas shaft fractures should ideally be treated by intramedullary nailing, using an interlocking nail where indicated. The advantage of a nail over a plate is that the shaft is supported along its whole length rather than within the confines of the bone beneath the plate. A nail can be inserted using a 'closed' technique, decreasing the potential morbidity of an open operation requiring a large muscle splitting incision (Figure 10.7). Even in closed nailing, if a biopsy is required from the fracture site, a curette or similar instrument can be passed down the shaft of the long bone under control of an image intensifier to retrieve tissue for histology. There is no evidence that fixation by intramedullary nailing results in spread of the tumour providing the secondary is irradiated [52,53].

In some fractures the lytic metastases may be so large that simple fixation will leave a large defect which is only supported by the fixation device. If survival is prolonged after the operation, the risk of a fatigue fracture through the fixation device will increase until the inevitable breakage through metal occurs. To prevent this complication methyl methacrylate cement has been used to fill the defect and provide support around the fixation device [54]. In its soft state after mixing, the cement can be pushed firmly into the defect and the fixation device can then be fixed either through the soft cement in the case of an intramedullary nail, or screwed into the hardened cement in the case of a plate (Figure 10.8a and b). The cement, when plastic, can be moulded into the irregular defect to fit firmly and accurately. Once the material has 'set' and the fracture fixed the patient can be mobilized immediately.

By filling the defect the cement will resist compressive forces liable to produce telescoping of the fragments and will remove some of the load from the fixation device. The fixation between cement and bone will be weakened by interposed tumour and fibrous tissue which must be carefully removed before inserting the cement.

By using cement to augment fixation of pathological fractures, Harrington *et al.* [54] reported only four failures of fixation in 323 patients with 312 pathological fractures and 63 impending fractures. The only major contraindication to surgery was a life expectancy of less than 3 months. Only six patients had a functionally poor result from pain or poor stabilization resulting in insufficient mobility. Comparing these figures with a review 25 years ago [55], the improvement in treatment of pathological fractures is dramatically demonstrated. In the latter paper only 27% of 16 patients undergoing surgery regained even partial ambulation. Thirteen patients

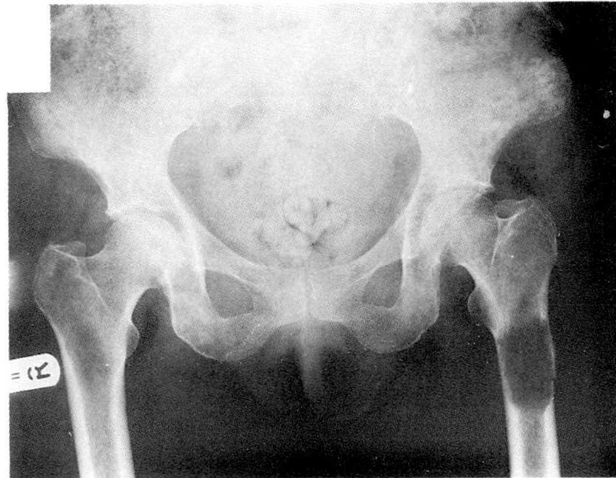

(a)

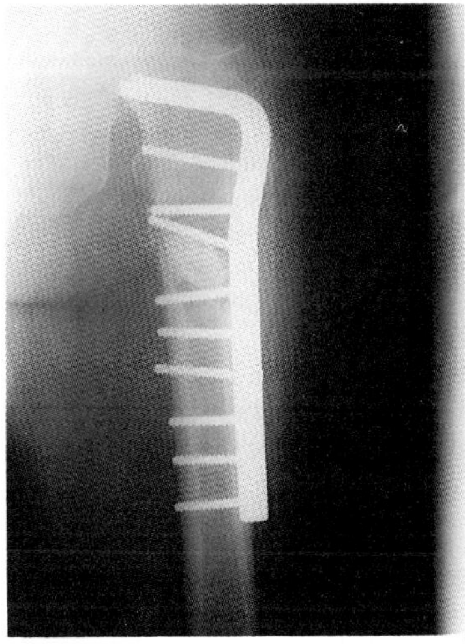

(b)

**Figure 10.8 a** A large lytic defect in the subtrochanteric area of the left hip from carcinoma of the breast; **b** cement has been used to fill the defect and a long blade-plate has been applied to the femur to support the bone

had fractures judged to be non-operable and remained immobile and in pain.

In Harrington's series 20 patients died within 4 weeks of surgery, but the mean survival time was 15.4 months. The mean survival time of patients with breast carcinoma was 19.8 months. Ten patients had survived 3 years at the time of publication. There was no difference in the results of patients allowed full weight-bearing and those allowed only partial weight-bearing following operation. Gainor and Buchert [56] showed that none of their patients with a pathological fracture from a bronchial primary survived more than 6 months.

It should be emphasized that postoperative radiotherapy is essential to prevent continued bone destruction. This is usually arranged at about 2 weeks from operation, once the wound has healed.

# References


1. Rosen, G., Marcove, R.C., Caparros, B. *et al.* Primary osteogenic sarcoma. *Cancer*, **43**, 2163–2177 (1979)
2. Rosen, G., Caparros, B., Nirenberg, A. *et al.* Ewing's sarcoma: ten year experience with adjuvant chemotherapy. *Cancer*, **47**, 2204–2213 (1981)
3. Mankin, H.J. Allograft transplantation in the management of bone tumours. In *Current Concepts of Diagnosis and Treatment of Bone and Soft Tissue Tumours* (ed. H.K. Uhthoff), Springer, Berlin, pp. 147–162 (1984)
4. Strong, L.C., Herson, J., Osborne, B.M. and Sutow, W.W. Risk of radiation. Related subsequent malignant tumours in survivors of Ewing's sarcoma. *Journal of the National Cancer Institute*, **62**, 1401 (1979)
5. Pritchard, D.J. Indications for surgical treatment of localised Ewing's sarcoma of bone. *Clinical Orthopaedics and Related Research*, **153**, 39–43 (1980)
6. Simon, M.A. Biopsy of musculo-skeletal tumours. Current concept reviews. *Journal of Bone and Joint Surgery*, **64A**, 1253–1257 (1982)
7. Serafin, J. A new operation for congenital absence of the fibula. Preliminary report. *Journal of Bone and Joint Surgery*, **49B**, 59–65 (1967)
8. Burrows, H.J. Major prosthetic replacement of bone, lessons learnt in 17 years. *Journal of Bone and Joint Surgery*, **50B**, 225–226 (1968)
9. Bradish, C.F., Kemp, H.B.S., Scales, J.T. and Wilson, J.N. Distal femoral replacement by custom made prosthesis. *Journal of Bone and Joint Surgery*, **69B**, 276–284 (1987)
10. Scales, J.C. and Sneath, R.S. The extending prosthesis. In *Bone Tumour Management* (eds R. Coombs and G. Friedlander), Butterworths, London, pp. 168–177 (1987)
11. Jofe, M.H., Gebhardt, M.C., Tomford, W.W. and Mankin, H.J. Reconstruction for defects of the proximal part of the femur using allograft arthroplasty. *Journal of Bone and Joint Surgery*, **70A**, 507–516 (1988)
12. Kotz, R. and Salzer, M. Rotation plasty for childhood osteosarcoma of the distal part of the femur. *Journal of Bone and Joint Surgery*, **64A**, 959–969 (1982)
13. Van Nes, C.P. Rotation plasty for congenital defects of the femur making use of the ankle of the shortened limb to control the knee joint of a prosthesis. *Journal of Bone and Joint Surgery*, **32B**, 12–16 (1950)
14. Enneking, W.F. and Dunham, W.K. Resection and construction for primary neoplasms involving the innominate bone. *Journal of Bone and Joint Surgery*, **60A**, 731–746 (1978)
15. Thomas, I.H., Cole, W.G., Walkers, K.D and Menelaus, M.B. Function after partial pelvic resection for Ewing's sarcoma. *Journal of Bone and Joint Surgery*, **69B**, 271–275 (1987)
16. Linberg, D.E. Interscapulo-thoracic resection for

malignant tumours of the shoulder joint region. *Journal of Bone and Joint Surgery*, **10**, 344–349 (1928)

17. Paley, D. Current techniques of limb lengthening. *Journal of Pediatric Orthopedics*, **8**, 73–92 (1988)

18. Murbarak, S.J. Principles of treating compartment syndromes. In *Compartment Syndromes and Volkmann's Contracture* (eds S.J. Murbarak and A.R. Hargens), W.B. Saunders, Philadelphia, pp. 123–132 (1981)

19. Regaud, C. Sur la necrose des os attients par un processus cancereux et traiters par les radiations. *Comptes Rendus de la Société Biologie*, **87**, 427–429 (1922)

20. Ewing, J. Radiation osteitis. *Acta Radiologica*, **6**, 399–412 (1926)

21. Woodard, H.Q. and Coley, B.C. The correlation of tissue dose and clinical response in irradiation of bone tumours and of normal bone. *American Journal of Roentgenology*, **40**, 524–534 (1938)

22. Csuka, M., Bruce, B.J., Lynch, K.L. and McCarthy, D.J. Osteonecrosis, fractures and protusio acetabulae secondary to X-irradiation therapy for prostatic carcinoma. *Journal of Rheumatology*, **14**, 165–170 (1987)

23. Roher, M.D., Kim, Y. and Fayos, J.V. The effect of cobalt-60 irradiation on monkey mandibles. *Oral Surgery*, **48**, 424 (1979)

24. Matsubayashi, T., Koga, H., Nishiyama, Y. *et al*. The reparative process of metastatic bone lesions after radiotherapy. *Japanese Journal of Clinical Oncology*, **11**(Suppl.), 253–264 (1981)

25. Epstein, J.B., Wong, F.L.W. and Stevenson-Moore, P. Osteoradionecrosis: clinical experience and a proposal for classification. *Journal of Oral and Maxillofacial Surgery*, **45**, 104–110 (1987)

26. Bragg, D.G., Shidnia, H. and Chu, F.C.U. The clinical and radiographic aspects of radiation osteitis. *Radiology*, **97**, 103–111 (1970)

27. Wang, G.J., Dughman, S.S., Reger, S.I. and Stamp, W.G. The effect of core decompression on femoral head blood flow in steroid-induced avascular necrosis of the femoral head. *Journal of Bone and Joint Surgery*, **67A**, 121–124 (1985)

28. Urbaniak, J. Treatment of avascular necrosis of the femoral head with a vascularised bone graft. *Journal of Bone and Joint Surgery*, **68B**, 677 (1986)

29. Felson, D.T. and Anderson, J.J. Across-study evaluation of association between steroid dose and bolus steroids and avascular necrosis of bone. *Lancet*, **i**, 902–906 (1987)

30. Genez, B.M., Wilson, M.R., Houk, R.W. *et al*. Early osteonecrosis of the femoral head: detection in high-risk patients with MR imaging. *Radiology*, **168**, 521–524 (1988)

31. Beltran, J., Herman, L.J., Burk, J.M. *et al*. Femoral head avascular necrosis: MR imaging with clinical, pathologic and radionuclide correlation. *Radiology*, **166**, 215–220 (1988)

32. Ficat, R.P. and Arlet, J. Ischaemia and necrosis of bone. In *Ischaemia and Necrosis of Bone* (ed. D.S. Hungerford), Williams and Wilkins, Baltimore, pp. 171–182 (1980)

33. Isono, S.S., Woolson, S.T. and Schurman, D.J. Total joint arthroplasty for steroid-induced osteonecrosis in cardiac transplant patients. *Clinical Orthopaedics and Related Research*, **217**, 201–208 (1987)

34. Martland, H.S. and Humphries, R.E. Osteogenic sarcoma in dial painters using luminous paint. *Archives of Pathology*, **7**, 406–417 (1929)

35. Huvos, A.G., Woodard, H.Q., Cahan, W.G. *et al*. Post-irradiation osteogenic sarcoma of bone and soft tissues. *Cancer*, **55**, 1244–1255 (1985)

36. Smith, J. Radiation-induced sarcoma of bone: clinical and radiographic findings in 43 patients irradiated for soft tissue neoplasms. *Acta Radiologica*, **33**, 205–221 (1982)

37. Sim, F.H., Cupps, R.E., Dahlin, D.C. and Ivins, J.C. Post-radiation sarcoma of bone. *Journal of Bone and Joint Surgery*, **54A**, 1479–1489 (1972)

38. Silverberg, E. Cancer statistics. *CA*, **35**, 19 (1985)

39. Scharberg, J. and Gainor, B.J. A profile of metastatic carcinoma of the spine. *Spine*, **10**, 19–20 (1985)

40. Tofe, A.J., Francis, M.D. and Harvey, W.J. Correlations of neoplasms with incidence and localisation of skeletal metastases. An analysis of 1355 diphosphonate bone scans. *Journal of Nuclear Medicine*, **16**, 986–989 (1975)

41. Ell, P.J., Dixon, J.H. and Abdullah, A.Z. Unusual spread of juxtacortical osteosarcoma. *Journal of Nuclear Medicine*, **21**, 190–191 (1980)

42. Galasko, C.S.B. Skeletal metastases and mammary cancer. *Annals of the Royal College of Surgeons of England*, **50**, 3–28 (1972)

43. Galasko, C.S.B. and Doyle, F.H. The detection of skeletal metastases from mammary cancer: a regional comparison between radiology and scintigraphy. *Clinical Radiology*, **23**, 295–297 (1972)

44. Galasko, C.S.B. The detection of skeletal metastases from mammary cancer by gamma camera scintigraphy. *British Journal of Surgery*, **56**, 757–764 (1969)

45. Edelstyn, G.A., Gillespie, P.J. and Grebbel, F.S. The radiological demonstration of osseous metastases: experimental observations. *Clinical Radiology*, **18**, 158–162 (1967)

46. Best, J.J.K., Forbes, W.St.C., Adam, N.M. and Isherwood, I. Computed tomographic scanning and radioisotope bone scanning: a comparison. In *Total Body Computed Tomography* (eds P. Gerhardt and G. Van Kaick), George Thieme, Stuttgart, pp. 216–220 (1979)

47. Cowan, R.J. and Young, K.A. Evaluation of serum alkaline phosphatase determination in patients with positive bone scans. *Cancer*, **32**, 887–889 (1973)

48. Cheng, D.S., Seitz, C.B. and Eyre, H.J. Non-operative management of femoral, humeral and acetabular metastases in patients with breast carcinoma. *Cancer*, **45**, 1533–1537 (1980)

49. Parrish, F.F. and Murray, J.A. Surgical treatment for secondary neoplastic fractures. A retrospective study

of 96 patients. *Journal of Bone and Joint Surgery*, **52A**, 665–686 (1970)

50. Fidler, M. Incidence of fracture through metastases in long bones. *Acta Orthopaedica Scandinavica*, **52**, 623–627 (1981)
51. Snell, W.E. and Beals, R.K. Femoral metastases and fractures from breast cancer. *Surgery, Gynecology and Obstetrics*, **119**, 22–24 (1964)
52. Fidler, M. Prophylactic internal fixation of secondary neoplastic deposits in long bones. *British Medical Journal*, **i**, 341–343 (1973)
53. Bouma, W.H., Mulder, J.H. and Hop, W.C.J. The influence of intramedullary nailing upon the development of metastases in the treatment of impending pathological fractures; an experimental study. *Clinical and Experimental Metastasis*, **1**, 205–212 (1983)
54. Harrington, K.D., Sim, F., Enis, J.E. *et al.* Methyl methacrylate as an adjunct in internal fixation of pathological fractures. *Journal of Bone and Joint Surgery*, **58A**, 1047–1055 (1976)
55. Takita, H. and Watne, A.L. Operative treatment of pathological fractures. *Surgery, Gynecology and Obstetrics*, **116**, 683–692 (1963)
56. Gainor, B. and Buchert, P. Fracture healing in metastatic bone disease. *Clinical Orthopaedics and Related Research*, **178**, 297–302 (1983)

# 11

# Sequelae of total body irradiation and bone marrow transplantation

J.E. Sanders

Prior to 1969, only a few patients who received bone marrow transplants survived. Advances in immunobiology, histocompatibility testing, immunosuppressive preparative regimens and supportive care yielded improved results. This has led to the incorporation of this therapeutic technique into the overall management of an ever increasing number of patients [1]. Thus, there is also an ever increasing number of long-term survivors.

Marrow transplant preparative regimens are designed to suppress the patient's immune system to ensure engraftment and eradicate the underlying hematological disorder or malignancy. The most frequently used regimen includes high-dose chemotherapy, usually cyclophosphamide, given with total body irradiation (TBI). Since all patients receive an infusion of bone marrow, the agents may be given in doses not limited by marrow toxicity. However, the transplant preparative regimens are associated with other toxicities, some of which occur early and others occur months to years later.

This chapter will review some of the early and late sequelae observed after marrow transplantation. These effects are categorized into those related to the transplant procedure, those related to the preparative regimen and those arising from the original disease.

## Effects related to the transplant procedure

### Engraftment

Following preparative regimens of cyclophosphamide and TBI for hematological malignancies, graft rejection usually does not occur when non-manipulated marrow from HLA matched sibling donors has been used [2]. However, when donors were non-HLA identical family members, 12% rejected the graft and factors associated with graft rejection were increasing degree of donor HLA disparity and prior allo-immunization [3]. Graft rejection has also been a relatively frequent occurrence when T cell depletion of donor marrow has been used to prevent acute graft-versus-host disease (GVHD) [4–9]. Causes of graft failure in this setting have not been clearly identified, but several investigators have suggested that more intensive preparative regimens may decrease the incidence of graft rejection after T cell-depleted marrow [7,10,11]. In both situations, detection of host lymphocytes in the majority of patients who reject their grafts suggests that residual host immunity may be the mechanism for graft rejection.

The majority of long-term survivors have stable engraftment with all hematopoietic cell lines of donor origin. Reappearance of host cells or mixed chimerism is unstable and usually followed by graft rejection or relapse of the original disease. Only rarely has mixed chimerism been followed by recovery of autologous marrow function. A study of 96 patients transplanted for aplastic anemia from HLA identical sex-mismatched donors demonstrated that 30% of the patients with mixed chimerism ultimately rejected their graft compared with 5% who were full chimeras [12]. Similarly, following transplantation for leukemia with regimens utilizing TBI, only five patients have been reported to have stable mixed chimerism for more than 6 years [13,14].

Patients given ABO-incompatible marrow grafts may produce isohemagglutinins of host origin against the ABO group of the donor up to 1 year after transplant [15]. Continuous low-grade hemolysis may result. The increased transfusion requirements may be reduced by using O packed red cell transfusions [16,17]. The marrow may show an absence of mature red cell precursors and reticulocytopenia may be present in the peripheral blood, but other cell lines are usually not affected.

## Acute graft-versus-host disease (GVHD)

Acute GVHD is usually only initiated when mature donor T lymphocytes are infused with the marrow. Murine studies [18] determined that the severity of GVHD was related to the number of mature T lymphocytes infused and degree of donor–host HLA disparity, and depletion of T lymphocytes from the donor marrow could eliminate GVHD. Human transplant studies of haplo-identical family member donors have demonstrated that the severity of acute GVHD was related to the number of disparate HLA antigens on the non-identical chromosome [19]. Patients given marrow from phenotypically matched family members have an acute GVHD incidence similar to that observed when HLA matched siblings were used. However, when donors were disparate for 2–3 antigens on the non-identical chromosome acute GVHD was significantly increased. Use of T-depleted donor marrow in man also eliminated acute GVHD [4–9].

All recipients of non-T depleted allogeneic marrow are at risk of developing acute GVHD during the first month after marrow infusion. The severity of involvement of the major target organs – skin, liver and/or gastrointestinal tract – determines the clinical grade of acute GVHD [?] Grade I is limited to less than 50% involvement of the skin only. Grade II involves the skin and also mild abnormalities of liver or gastrointestinal tract. Grades III and IV include significant involvement of the skin and liver and/or gastrointestinal systems plus a progressive decrease in clinical performance of the patient. Grade IV acute GVHD is often fatal. Attempts to prevent or modify acute GVHD have included prophylactic use of methotrexate, cyclosporine, combination of methotrexate plus cyclosporine, or antithymocyte globulin, corticosteroids, and methotrexate, and administration of anti-T cell monoclonal antibodies [20–25]. Treatment of established acute GVHD has included the use of high-dose corticosteroids, antithymocyte globulin, cyclosporine and infusion of anti-T monoclonal antibodies [26–28].

## Infections

During the initial granulocytopenic period of 20–30 days after marrow infusion, transplant patients are at highest risk for developing bacterial and/or fungal infections [29]. Nearly all patients develop fever which often indicates infection and requires systemic antibiotic treatment. Prospective studies evaluating methods of infection prevention demonstrated that prophylactic systemic antibiotics and sterile laminar air flow isolation were both effective in decreasing the septicemia rate [30]. Fungal infections are common after transplantation. A series of retrospective and prospective studies have shown a high incidence had invasive fungal infections at autopsy, a direct association between duration of severe granulocytopenia with invasive fungal infection, and an increased incidence when two or more surveillance cultures are positive for fungus [29]. Thus, when a febrile granulocytopenic patient has not responded to antibiotic therapy and has surveillance sites positive for fungus, empirical antifungal treatment should be started and continued until the patient becomes afebrile and recovers at least 500 neutrophils/mm$^3$.

Between engraftment and day 100 all patients are at risk for viral or protozoan infections. Non-bacterial or interstitial pneumonia is the most notorious and overwhelming of these [29]. Establishment of a diagnosis by bronchoalveolar lavage or open lung biopsy is important to direct therapy. Cytomegalovirus (CMV) associated pneumonia is the most common form of interstitial pneumonia. Treatment with vidarabine, acyclovir and/or alpha-interferons did not decrease the 80% mortality rate [31–33]. Although ganciclovir alone also did not decrease the mortality rate, when combined with high-titer immunoglobulin the mortality rate decreased to 20–30%. *Pneumocystis carinii* pneumonia, the most common protozoan infection, is usually not seen in patients given prophylactic trimethoprim-sulfamethoxazole (Bactrim) after engraftment. Herpes simplex and adenovirus have been isolated from a small number of patients and only rarely has a bacterial or fungal process been identified.

Any factor that increases the incidence of CMV infection also increases the risk of CMV pneumonia [34]. Cytomegalovirus infection is more common among patients who are seropositive for antibody before transplant. Among seronegative patients the infection incidence is increased if the marrow donors are seropositive. Passive immunoprophylaxis with high-titer plasma or immunoglobulins may be effective in preventing either CMV infection or CMV disease [35,36]. CMV seronegative blood products have been highly effective in preventing primary CMV infection in seronegative patients given marrow from seronegative donors [37]. Studies evaluating methods of preventing primary CMV infection for the seronegative patient who receives marrow from a seropositive donor are in progress.

Infections after 100 days are determined by the residual immune deficiency shared by all patients and by the presence of chronic GVHD. More than 40% of all transplant patients developed varicella zoster virus (VZV) infection at a median of 5 months after transplant [38,39]. Most cases occurred within the first year. One-third of patients with untreated herpes zoster developed cutaneous dissemination. Most developed herpes zoster but some had varicella-like infection. The case fatality rate ranged from 30% to 35% for untreated herpes zoster and varicella respectively. All deaths occurred during the first 9 months after transplant. Because of the high mortality rate all patients developing VZV during the first 9 months should be treated with acyclovir. Patients who develop VZV infection more than 9 months after transplant may be treated at the first sign of cutaneous dissemination if they have herpes zoster or at the first sign of visceral spread if they have varicella. The role of oral acyclovir has not yet been determined.

Severe immunodeficiency with T and B cell abnormalities have been observed in patients with chronic GVHD [40–42]. They generate non-specific suppressor T lymphocytes and have impaired humoral recovery, reconstitution of cellular immunity, opsonization and granulocyte chemotaxis. Chronic GVHD patients have an infection risk which is twice that of non-chronic GVHD patients. Sinusitis, bronchitis, otitis media, bacterial pneumonia, bacteremia and interstitial pneumonia have all been observed after day 100. Encapsulated organisms such as *S. pneumoniae* and *H. influenzae* are common while fungal infections are relatively infrequent.

Prevention of infection during chronic GVHD has focused on methods of accelerating immune reconstitution, antibiotic or intravenous immune globulin prophylaxis and immunosuppressive treatment regimens to control GVHD-induced immune dysregulation [43–45]. Daily administration of cotrimoxazole has decreased the incidence of interstitial pneumonia from 28% to 8% and has decreased pneumococcal bacteremia [46]. Long-term prophylaxis with immunoglobulin may be of benefit in patients with chronic GVHD, but this is as yet unknown.

## Chronic graft-versus-host disease

Chronic GVHD occurs in 25–50% of patients surviving 100–400 days after allogeneic marrow transplantation [47]. Most patients have had preceding acute GVHD, but 20–30% have *de novo* onset without acute GVHD. For the remainder of patients, chronic GVHD presents after a quiescent period following acute GVHD or has a progressive onset as a direct extension of acute GVHD. Factors associated with the probability of developing chronic GVHD include increasing grade of acute

GVHD, increasing patient age, and administration of viable donor buffy coat cells [48]. One report also suggests a higher risk in recipients of marrow from older donors [49]. Chronic GVHD resembles clinical, pathological and laboratory features of several naturally occurring autoimmune diseases with the exception that chronic GVHD patients do not develop CNS or renal abnormalities. Both experimental and clinical studies demonstrate the central role of donor-derived T cells in the pathogenesis of acute GVHD, but the pathogenesis of chronic GVHD is less clear [50].

The skin is nearly always involved with erythema, dyspigmentation, poikiloderma, and/or lichenoid lesions. Without therapy it will become progressively indurated and sclerotic which will lead to joint contractures and disability. The hepatocellular dysfunction is predominantly cholestatic, but the abnormalities may make it difficult to distinguish from viral hepatitis. Isolated hepatic abnormalities without other target organ involvement have not been observed. Oral lesions include erythema, atrophy and lichen planus-like findings [51]. Buccal lesions range in appearance from white reticular striae to large plaques. Mucosal atrophy, reduced keratinization and xerostomia may be present. Increased salivary sodium and decreased or absent secretory IgA may contribute to increased dental caries. Ocular abnormalities with keratoconjunctivitis sicca, conjunctivitis and uveitis also occur frequently [52]. Less frequent manifestations are desquamative esophagitis, polyserositis, vaginal stenosis and myasthenia gravis [53].

An evaluation between 80 and 100 days after transplant is most useful in diagnosing early chronic GVHD. Clinical examination of the skin with biopsies of both sun and non-sun exposed areas is important. Dermatopathology of early skin involvement reveals eosinophilic bodies, liquefactive degeneration and basal layer lichenoid reaction along the basal layer. Later dermal fibrosis and epidermal atrophy are seen. Oral examination with an oral mucosal biopsy is needed [54]. The oral biopsy findings include squamous cell necrosis and abnormalities similar to Sjogren's syndrome [54]. Liver function tests and a Schirmer's test to evaluate tear formation are also needed. Patients with limited chronic GVHD have isolated skin involvement with or without liver abnormalities [53]. Subclinical chronic GVHD patients have characteristic pathology findings on both the blind oral and skin biopsies in the absence of clinical signs or symptoms. The diagnosis of clinical chronic GVHD is made if the patient has multi-organ clinical manifestations and positive skin and oral biopsies.

Without treatment 20% of patients with clinical chronic GVHD survive with Karnofsky scores ≥70% [55]. Immunosuppressive therapy with anti-thymocyte globulin and/or corticosteroids late in the course of the disease has not altered the disease course. Treatment with thymosine, transfer factor, penicillamine, hydroxychloroquine, and electron beam irradiation have also been unsuccessful. A prospective randomized trial of early treatment with azathioprine and prednisone compared with prednisone alone demonstrated that non-relapse mortality and infections were significantly increased in patients randomized to receive combination therapy compared with those receiving prednisone alone [56]. Actuarial survival with Karnofsky scores ≥70% was significantly better (61%) for the group receiving prednisone alone compared with that achieved with dual agent therapy (47%). Patients with thrombocytopenia received prednisone alone but had a 5-year survival of only 25%. Treatment of this group of chronic GVHD patients with combination prednisone and cyclosporine increased survival to over 50% [57]. Cyclosporine as a single agent appears to have promise with three of four patients with progressive chronic GVHD responding [58]. Investigators from Baltimore have reported success with thalidomide treatment in a rat model [59].

## Immunological recovery

Repopulation of the immune and hemopoietic systems depends upon appropriate proliferation, maturation and differentiation of cells of donor origin [60–63]. Time after transplant is the most important factor. Regardless of the type of graft (autologous, allogeneic, syngeneic), underlying disease, conditioning regimen, postgrafting immunosuppression or presence of acute GVHD, all marrow graft recipients have profound impairment of most immune functions during the first 6 months after transplant. The immunological parameters of non-chronic GVHD patients return to normal about 1 year after grafting and the majority are healthy with very few infections. Patients with chronic GVHD have delayed immune reconstitution and 34% develop serious and potentially fatal infections.

Humoral immunity returns to normal 3–4 months after transplant with normal serum levels of IgG and IgM [62,64]. Levels of total hemolytic complement, the third and fourth components of complement are normal 3 months after transplant. Cellular responses and humoral responses to recall and neo-antigens recover to normal levels by 1 year in healthy recipients, but the responses remain impaired or absent among those with chronic GVHD. These patients demonstrated diminished levels of antibody response to injections of pneumococcal antigen, as well as to neo-antigens bacteriophage OX174 and keyhole limpet hemocyanin. They also fail to switch from IgM to IgG production in secondary responses.

Although the absolute numbers of T and B cells are restored to normal early, subsets of T lymphocytes repopulate at different rates [65,66]. Healthy long-term survivors have specific suppressor cells which suppress donor response to host histocompatibility antigens, but which do not interfere with immune responses to pathogens [67]. Chronic GVHD patients have non-specific suppressor cells which alter immunological responses and increase their susceptibility to pathogens. They have elevated levels of CD8 suppressor lymphocytes in peripheral blood and decreased levels of CD4 helper lymphocytes. *In vitro* studies show that T lymphocytes exert suppressor function. Additionally, B lymphocytes from chronic GVHD patients fail to proliferate or differentiate into immunoglobulin secreting cells after co-culture with putative growth factor lymphokines from supernatants of co-cultures of normal allogeneic peripheral blood mononuclear cells [63,68]. These *in vivo* and *in vitro* abnormalities are present in patients with chronic GVHD regardless of treatment. In patients with chronic GVHD, interleukin 2 production by T cells is depressed following grafting and serum thymic factor is lower.

Transfer of immunity from donor to recipient has been demonstrated and may be protective for a period of time after grafting [69]. Immune memory to diphtheria and tetanus antigens has been transferred with similar frequency into HLA-identical sibling recipients using untreated or T-depleted marrow. The percentage of patients with normal serum antibody levels to tetanus and diphtheria is the same for recipients of HLA identical or HLA nonidentical marrow. This suggests that identity at HLA is not required for response to these recall antigens. These antibody levels have been detected in patients for more than 4–5 years after transplant, but the median antibody level declines with increasing time after transplant. Thus, periodic booster immunization to tetanus will be needed for patients with low levels of serum antibody to this antigen. There is too little experience in marrow transplant recipients with the use of live virus vaccines for polio, mumps, measles or rubella to know whether they are safe to administer. If protection against polio is necessary, the inactivated vaccines may be used.

# Effects related to the preparative regimen

## Cardiac abnormalities

The most striking and devastating cardiac complication is early fatal cardiomyopathy. Cardiac toxicity of cyclophosphamide manifests as a cardiomyopathy secondary to hemorrhagic myocarditis which may occur when doses of cyclophosphamide exceed 180 mg/kg [70]. The effects occur within the first 3 weeks after therapy and late reactions are not seen. The cardiac complications of irradiation may be immediate (within days to weeks) or late (years) after exposure. One study evaluating cardiac function in 28 young adults before and after administration of cytarabine (5 mg/kg), cyclophosphamide (90 mg/kg) and TBI (900 cGy) demonstrated no significant change in cardiac function as measured by weekly echocardiography for 10 weeks post-transplant [71]. Fatal cardiac toxicity has been observed in otherwise non high-risk patients who received a combination of cytarabine (cytosine arabinoside), cyclophosphamide and TBI [72].

## Gastrointestinal abnormalities

Liver disease after marrow transplantation is complex. The common diseases, venocclusive disease (VOD) and GVHD are relatively easy to distinguish, but confusion occurs when these disease processes overlap and other factors may be contributing to abnormal liver function [73,74]. In the first few weeks after transplant, 20–40% of patients develop VOD due to the chemoradiotherapy [75]. This problem is most frequently observed in older patients with a history of hepatitis, but is also seen in any age patient receiving second transplant or intensive multi-agent conditioning regimens. It is a clinical syndrome characterized by weight gain, jaundice by day 10, liver pain and ascites. Management is supportive and nearly half of the patients will recover. From day 25–100 acute GVHD and infections occur, and after day 100 chronic GVHD and chronic viral hepatitis are usual etiologies of abnormal liver function. Throughout the post-transplant period, drug-induced injury due to cyclosporine, parenteral hyperalimentation and antibiotics may occur [76]. When possible a liver biopsy is the most accurate way of discerning which diseases are present.

Nausea, vomiting and anorexia due to chemoradiotherapy, drug toxicities, acute GVHD and/or infections occur in nearly all patients for the first 15–25 days after transplant [74,77]. Gastrointestinal bleeding occurs in about 15% of patients due to infectious or non-infectious ulcers or acute GVHD. Other than acute GVHD, diarrhea is usually related to chemoradiotherapy toxicity and/or intestinal infections. Radiographic contrast studies and/or endoscopy with biopsies and cultures are useful to establish a diagnosis. Treatment is related to the underlying cause.

## Renal abnormalities

Early post-transplant renal problems are usually related to the administration of cyclosporine and nephrotoxic antibiotic therapy [78,79]. Patients with

VOD of the liver may develop hepatorenal syndrome which results in transient renal failure and the need for dialysis. Prolonged administration of cyclosporine contributes to mild renal function abnormalities, magnesium wasting [80] and hypertension [81]. The renal function abnormalities are reversible once the nephrotoxic agents are removed.

## Pulmonary abnormalities

Pulmonary complications early after transplantation are associated with upper airway obstruction, pulmonary edema syndromes and non-bacterial pneumonias [82]. Prophylactic antibiotic administration has decreased the incidence of late interstitial pneumonia observed in patients with chronic GVHD [83]. Long-term patients who do not have chronic GVHD usually do not have compromised pulmonary function. However, those with chronic GVHD have a 20% incidence of chronic obstructive airway disease which usually becomes apparent clinically after 6 months [84]. Examination of lung tissue has shown pathological findings of bronchiolitis obliterans.

## Neuroendocrine function

Thyroid function has been studied in long-term survivors with determinations of thyroid stimulating hormone (TSH) and thyroxine ($T_4$). After a preparative regimen of high dose cyclophosphamide alone, only one of 50 children had thyroid function abnormalities [85]. Among 316 children evaluated after TBI regimens, thyroid dysfunction has been observed in 12–56% [86–89]. Patients who received 10.0 Gy single exposure TBI had 28–56% with compensated hypothyroidism and 13% had overt hypothyroidism, but patients who received fractionated TBI had 12–21% with compensated hypothyroidism and 3% with overt hypothyroidism. These apparent differences in incidences most probably reflect the shorter observation time (median of 4–5 years) after fractionated TBI schedules compared with the longer observation time (median of 8–9 years) after single exposure TBI.

Plasma 11-desoxycortisol (compound S) levels after metyrapone stimulation have been used to screen adrenocortical function [85,87]. Only one of 24 patients evaluated after cyclophosphamide only developed low compound S levels, but after TBI regimens 11% had low stimulated compound S levels. Normal ACTH and cortisol responses have been observed after insulin stimulation [90].

After marrow transplant regimens of cyclophosphamide only, longitudinal and growth velocity rates have been normal [85]. Decreased growth rates have been observed in nearly all children who received TBI regimens, and 55% have subnormal growth hormone (GH) levels determined following stimulation with insulin, arginine or L-dopa [85,87,90–92]. Growth hormone deficiency was present in 87% of patients who received previous cranial irradiation and in 42% who had not. During the first 2 years after TBI, patients with chronic GVHD grew less well than those without chronic GVHD. After the first 2 years, growth rates were similar between patients with or without chronic GVHD, but catch-up growth was not observed. Failure to achieve catch-up growth when chronic GVHD treatment was stopped suggests that irradiation effects on long bones may also contribute to decreased growth rates. Therapy with GH has resulted in some improvement in height, but usually less than observed in non-irradiated GH-deficient children.

Among patients who received a preparative regimen of cyclophosphamide only, nearly all have had normal onset and development of secondary sexual characteristics [85]. However, most patients who received preparative regimens of cyclophosphamide plus TBI had delayed puberty and elevated gonadotropin levels [85,87]. All boys who received additional testicular irradiation had very low testosterone levels. Of interest are the 30–40% of children who have normal pubertal development and normal gonadotropin levels following TBI regimens.

All women who were past puberty at time of transplant developed amenorrhea for varying lengths of time after transplant [93–95]. When a preparative regimen of cyclophosphamide only was given to women, all who were less than 26 years of age recovered ovarian function between 3 and 42 months, but among those more than 26 years of age 33% recovered ovarian function and 66% developed primary ovarian failure. Women who recover are fertile. Nine of these women have had 12 pregnancies which resulted in eight live births of normal children. Similarly, approximately 65% of men recover normal testicular function after preparative regimens of cyclophosphamide only with normal gonadotropins, testosterone and spermatogenesis. This recovery in men does not appear to be related to patient age [93,96]. Men who recover testicular function also are fertile and ten men have fathered 11 normal children.

After single exposure of 10.0 Gy TBI or fractionated exposures of 12.0–15.75 Gy TBI, all women studied have developed primary ovarian failure [93–95]. The majority have permanent ovarian failure and most have symptoms of menopause which respond to cyclic hormone therapy. Only a rare patient (five of 139) recovers ovarian function between 3 and 7 years after TBI exposure. Women who recover ovarian function after TBI may also be fertile and four have become pregnant. Only one has delivered a normal child. Most men have preservation of Leydig cell function with normal testosterone and normal luteinizing hormone levels after TBI preparative regimens. Sertoli cell function is usually abnormal and spermatogenesis is absent. A rare patient has recovered sperm production more than 6 years after irradiation and one man has fathered three children.

## Ophthalmological abnormalities

Cataracts are a well known complication of exposure to long-term steroid therapy as well as to ionizing irradiation. After TBI posterior subcapsular cataracts have occurred in 80% of patients given single exposure of 10.0 Gy TBI by 6 years and nearly all required cataract repair. Among patients given fractionated exposure TBI of 12.0–15.75 Gy, 20% developed cataracts by 5 years and 20% have required cataract repair [97].

Dry eye syndrome is another ocular complication [98]. Patients with this problem have abnormal Schirmer's testing with decreased tear formation and mild to severe corneal stippling on slit lamp examination. While the majority of these patients also have chronic GVHD, some do not. Treatment with artificial tears or other ocular lubricants is necessary to prevent corneal ulcerations.

## Dental abnormalities

Irradiation to bone produces epiphyseal, metaphyseal and diaphyseal injury which affects subsequent bone growth [99]. The effect is related to patient age at time of irradiation as well as site, dose schedule and total dose of irradiation given. Irradiation to the head and neck of the young growing child, especially those less than 6 years of age, results in altered growth of the facial skeleton and soft tissue [100,101]. Development of secondary teeth is affected with delayed or arrested tooth formation, shortening and blunting of tooth roots, incomplete calcification, premature closure of apices and dental caries.

## Central nervous system (CNS) abnormalities

Multifocal leukoencephalopathy after marrow transplant is usually due to factors which influence its development in non-transplant treatment settings [102]. Transplant patients have often received pre-transplant CNS therapy with intrathecal medications and/or cranial irradiation. Following TBI and peri-transplant intrathecal medications, one study reported a 7% incidence of leukoencephalopathy among 415 patients transplanted for acute leukemia [102]. The major risk factor was receipt of pre-transplant CNS treatment and post-transplant intrathecal therapy.

Few studies have been done on the psychological aspects of marrow transplantation. Retrospective studies in adults suggest that patients often feel anxiety, uncertainty, depression and defenceless-ness [103,104]. Most patients felt they were adequately informed about the transplant, but felt that information could be improved by discussions about the emotional and sexual problems which they would have to face. Studies among non-transplant children indicate that cognitive function abnormalities and learning disabilities are seen after cranial irradiation [105,106]. It may be anticipated that marrow transplant children who receive TBI are at risk for development of these problems.

## Secondary malignancies

Multiple factors probably contribute to the development of secondary malignancies after marrow transplantation. Studies in irradiated and non-irradiated mice given hemopoietic grafts suggested that GVHD and virus infections were major factors in the development of secondary lymphoid malignancies [107,108]. Studies in dogs and monkeys demonstrated that the relative risk of developing a malignancy was five times higher in irradiated recipients than in non-irradiated controls [109,110]. Secondary malignancies in man have been observed after marrow transplantation [111–122]. An analysis of more than 2000 marrow transplant recipients revealed that 35 patients developed secondary malignancies between 1.5 months and 13.9 years [122]. Sixteen had non-Hodgkin's lymphomas which were associated with Epstein–Barr virus in 11. Nineteen had non-lymphoid malignancies which included six leukemias of different morphological type from the original leukemia or leukemia in donor cells, three glioblastomas, three squamous cell carcinomas, three malignant melanomas, one basal cell carcinoma and three adenocarcinomas. Thirty of these 33 died of their secondary tumors. Factors associated with the development of any secondary malignancy were related to treatment of acute GVHD with antithymocyte globulin or anti-CD3 monoclonal antibody and TBI. Overall the incidence of secondary malignancies in this population was 6.8 times that observed for the incidence of primary malignancy in the state of Washington and significant elevations were seen for non-Hodgkin's lymphomas, leukemia, glioblastoma and melanoma.

## Effects related to the original disease

### Recurrence of the original disease

Relapse of leukemia continues to be a major problem. The probability of relapse varies with the stage of the patient's disease at the time of transplant with lowest relapse rates among patients transplanted while in remission (20–40%) and highest relapse rates among those transplanted while in relapse (40–70%) [123]. Once relapse occurs, the management depends on the type of recurrence. A small number of patients with Ph1 positive chronic myelogenous leukemia will have the recurrence of the Ph1 chromosome as the only sign of disease. These patients need careful follow-up since some will have spontaneous disappearance of the Ph1 chromosome whereas others will progress on to development of frank leukemia [124]. Another special small group are boys with acute lymphoblastic leukemia who develop an isolated testicular recurrence [125]. Treatment with orchiectomy and local irradiation therapy may be sufficient, but some have also received systemic chemotherapy. Approximately half of these boys have not developed any further evidence of leukemia. The majority of relapses are medullary, and treatment with chemotherapy may result in remissions of varying duration [126]. It is unlikely that these patients will be able to be cured with only chemotherapy and, thus, second marrow transplants have been considered. Successful second transplants have been reported after intensive chemotherapy preparative regimens among patients who had an initial transplant containing TBI [127–130]. These regimens have included busulfan plus cyclophosphamide (54 patients), cyclophosphamide plus melphalan (nine patients), busulphan plus etoposide (four patients) and busulphan, cyclophosphamide and etoposide (two patients). From this group of 69 patients, 21% survived in remission from 1–55 months after second transplant. Death from toxicity of the regimen and recurrent leukemia were the major causes of failure. Although these results are encouraging, improved regimens which will decrease post-transplant toxicity and relapse rate are needed.

## Graft versus leukemia effect

Barnes *et al.* observed in 1956 that transplanted marrow could destroy residual leukemia cells in lethally irradiated mice [131]. This adoptive immunotherapy suggests that there is immunological recognition by donor cells of histocompatibility or tumor-associated antigens on the malignant cells. Patients who develop acute or chronic GVHD have a higher probability of remaining in remission than patients who do not develop GVHD [132,133]. It is not known whether the apparent graft versus leukemia effect is a primary immunological event in association with GVHD or whether the lack of GVHD is simply a marker of persistent donor–host chimerism. The future challenge in transplantation biology is to determine if GVHD can be manipulated to augment the graft versus leukemia effect safely in patients at high risk for recurrent leukemia.

## Summary

Marrow transplantation has become a life-saving procedure for increasing numbers of patients during the last 15 years. Major problems are related to GVHD, infections and recurrences of the original disease. In addition, delayed effects related to the conditioning regimens are now becoming more apparent. Research efforts are being directed toward the development of more effective but less toxic transplant conditioning regimens, the elimination and/or better control of acute and chronic GVHD and improved prophylaxis and treatment of infections. As progress is made in each of these areas, greater numbers of patients will become long-term survivors who will continue to need to be carefully followed for determination and treatment of late complications. While an awareness of the acute sequelae of marrow transplantation is necessary for physicians to counsel patients prior to transplantation, an awareness of the delayed effects is especially important for all who care for survivors of marrow transplantation. These physicians are faced with diagnosing and treating late complications in this unique patient group.

## Acknowledgements

This investigation was supported by PHS Grant Numbers HL 36444 awarded by the National Heart, Lung and Blood Institute, CA 18029, CA 15704, and CA 18221 awarded by the National Cancer Institute, DHHS.

## References

1. Bortin, M.M. and Rimm, A.A. Increasing utilization of bone marrow transplantation. *Transplantation*, **42**, 229–234 (1986)
2. Thomas, E.D., Storb, R., Clift, R.A. *et al.* Bone-marrow transplantation. *New England Journal of Medicine*, **292**, 832–843, 895–902 (1975)
3. Anasetti, C., Amos, D., Beatty, P.G. *et al.* Risk factors for graft rejection of partially HLA matched haploidentical marrow transplants. In *Immunobiology of HLA* (ed. B. Dupont), Springer-Verlag, New York, pp. 516–517 (1989)
4. Mitsuyasu, R.T., Champlin, R.E., Gale, R.P. *et al.* Treatment of donor bone marrow with monoclonal anti-T-cell antibody and complement for the prevention of graft-versus-host disease. *Annals of Internal Medicine*, **105**, 20–26 (1986)
5. O'Reilly, R.J., Collins, N.H., Kernan, N. *et al.* Transplantation of marrow-depleted T cells by soybean lectin agglutination and E-rosette depletion: major histocompatibility complex-related graft resistance in leukemic transplant recipients. *Transplantation Proceedings*, **17**, 455–459 (1985)
6. Slavin, S., Waldmann, H., Or, R. *et al.* Prevention of graft-versus-host disease in allogeneic bone marrow transplantation for leukemia by T cell depletion *in vitro* prior to transplantation. *Transplantation Proceedings*, **17**, 465–467 (1985)
7. Patterson, J., Prentice, H.G., Brenner, M.K. *et al.* Graft rejection following HLA-matched T-lymphocyte depleted bone marrow transplantation. *British Journal of Haematology*, **63**, 221–230 (1986)
8. Filipovich, A.H., Vallera, D.A., Youle, R.J. *et al.* Graft-versus-host disease prevention in allogeneic bone marrow transplantation from histocompatible siblings. *Transplantation*, **44**, 62–69 (1987)
9. Martin, P.J., Hansen, J.A., Torok-Storb, B. *et al.* Graft failure in patients receiving T cell-depleted HLA-identical allogeneic marrow transplants. *Bone Marrow Transplantation*, **3**, 445–456 (1988)
10. Bozdech, M.J., Sondel, P.M., Trigg, M.E. *et al.* Transplantation of HLA-haploidentical T-cell-depleted marrow for leukemia: addition of cytosine arabinoside to the pretransplant conditioning prevents rejection. *Experimental Hematology*, **13**, 1201–1210 (1985)
11. Guyotat, D., Dutou, L., Ehrsam, A. *et al.* Graft rejection after T cell-depleted marrow transplantation: role of fractionated irradiation. *British Journal of Haematology*, **65**, 499–507 (1987)
12. Hill, R.S., Petersen, F.B., Storb, R. *et al.* Mixed hematologic chimerism after allogeneic marrow transplantation for severe aplastic anemia is associated with a higher risk of graft rejection and a lessened incidence of acute graft-versus-host disease. *Blood*, **67**, 811–816 (1986)
13. Branch, D.R., Gallagher, M.T., Forman, S.J. *et al.* Endogenous stem cell repopulation resulting in mixed hematopoietic chimerism following total body irradiation and marrow transplantation for acute leukemia. *Transplantation*, **34**, 226–228 (1982)
14. Singer, J.W., Keating, A., Ramberg, R. *et al.* Long-term stable hematopoietic chimerism following marrow transplantation for acute lymphoblastic leukemia: a case report with *in vitro* marrow culture studies. *Blood*, **62**, 869–872 (1983)
15. Witherspoon, R.P., Storb, R., Ochs, H.D. *et al.* Recovery of antibody production in human allogeneic marrow graft recipients: influence of time posttransplantation, the presence or absence of chronic graft-versus-host disease, and antithymocyte globulin treatment. *Blood*, **58**, 360–368 (1981)
16. Bensinger, W.I., Buckner, C.D., Thomas, E.D. and Clift, R.A. ABO-incompatible marrow transplants. *Transplantation*, **33**, 427–429 (1982)
17. Hows, J., Beddow, K., Easton, K. *et al.* Positive

direct antiglobulin tests in BMT recipients. *British Journal of Haematology*, **58**, 181–182 (1984)

18. Korngold, R. and Sprent, J. Lethal graft-versus-host disease after bone marrow transplantation across minor histocompatibility barriers in mice. Prevention by removing mature T cells from marrow. *Journal of Experimental Medicine*, **148**, 1687 (1978)

19. Beatty, P.G., Clift, R.A., Mickelson, E.M. *et al.* Marrow transplantation from related donors other than HLA-identical siblings. *New England Journal of Medicine*, **313**, 765–771 (1985)

20. Storb, R., Epstein, R.B., Graham, T.C. and Thomas, E.D. Methotrexate regimens for control of graft-versus-host disease in dogs with allogeneic marrow grafts. *Transplantation*, **9**, 240–246 (1970)

21. Weiden, P.L., Doney, K., Storb, R. and Thomas, E.D. Anti-human thymocyte globulin (ATG) for prophylaxis and treatment of graft-versus-host disease in recipients of allogeneic marrow grafts. *Transplantation Proceedings*, **10**, 213–216 (1978)

22. Ramsay, N.K.C., Kersey, J.H., Robison, L.L. *et al.* A randomized study of the prevention of acute graft-versus-host disease. *New England Journal of Medicine*, **306**, 392–397 (1982)

23. Deeg, H.J., Storb, R., Thomas, E.D. *et al.* Cyclosporine as prophylaxis for graft-versus-host disease: a randomized study in patients undergoing marrow transplantation for acute nonlymphoblastic leukemia. *Blood*, **65**, 1325–1334 (1985)

24. Filipovich, A.H., Krawczak, C.L., Kersey, J.H. *et al.* Graft-versus-host disease prophylaxis with anti-T-cell monoclonal antibody OKT3, prednisone and methotrexate in allogeneic bone-marrow transplantation. *British Journal of Haematology*, **60**, 143–152 (1985)

25. Storb, R., Deeg, H.J., Thomas, E.D. *et al.* Marrow transplantation for chronic myelocytic leukemia: a controlled trial of cyclosporine versus methotrexate for prophylaxis of graft-versus-host disease. *Blood*, **66**, 698–702 (1985)

26. Doney, K.C., Weiden, P.L., Storb, R. and Thomas, E.D. Treatment of graft-versus-host disease in human allogeneic marrow graft recipients: a randomized trial comparing antithymocyte globulin and corticosteroids. *American Journal of Hematology*, **11**, 1–8 (1981)

27. Remlinger, K., Martin, P.J., Hansen, J.A. *et al.* Murine monoclonal anti-T cell antibodies for treatment of steroid-resistant acute graft-versus-host disease. *Human Immunology*, **9**, 21–35 (1984)

28. Deeg, H.J., Loughran, T.P. Jr., Storb, R. *et al.* Treatment of human acute graft-versus-host disease with antithymocyte globulin and cyclosporine with or without methylprednisolone. *Transplantation*, **40**, 162–166 (1985)

29. Meyers, J.D. and Thomas, E.D. Infection complicating bone marrow transplantation. In *Clinical Approach to Infection in the Immunocompromised Host* (eds R.H. Rubin and L.S. Young), Plenum Press, New York, pp. 525–556 (1988)

30. Petersen, F.B., Buckner, C.D., Clift, R.A. *et al.* Infectious complications in patients undergoing marrow transplantation: a prospective randomized study of the additional effect of decontamination and laminar air flow isolation among patients receiving prophylactic systemic antibiotics. *Scandinavian Journal of Infectious Diseases*, **19**, 559–567 (1987)

31. Meyers, J.D., Wade, J.C., McGuffin, R.W. *et al.* The use of acyclovir for cytomegalovirus infections in the immunocompromised host. *Journal of Antimicrobial Chemotherapy*, **12**, 181–193 (1983)

32. Meyers, J.D., McGuffin, R.W., Bryson, Y.J. *et al.* Treatment of cytomegalovirus pneumonia after marrow transplant with combined vidarabine and human leukocyte interferon. *Journal of Infectious Diseases*, **146**, 80–84 (1982)

33. Meyers, J.D., Flournoy, N., Sanders, J.E. *et al.* Prophylactic use of human leukocyte interferon after allogeneic marrow transplantation. *Annals of Internal Medicine*, **107**, 809–816 (1987)

34. Meyers, J.D., Flournoy, N. and Thomas, E.D. Risk factors for cytomegalovirus infection after human marrow transplantation. *Journal of Infectious Diseases*, **153**, 478–488 (1986)

35. Winston, D.J., Pollard, R.B., Ho, W.G. *et al.* Cytomegalovirus immune plasma in bone marrow transplant recipients. *Annals of Internal Medicine*, **97**, 11–18 (1982)

36. Meyers, J.D., Leszczynski, J., Zaia, J.A. *et al.* Prevention of cytomegalovirus infection by cytomegalovirus immune globulin after marrow transplantation. *Annals of Internal Medicine*, **98**, 442–446 (1983)

37. Bowden, R.A., Sayers, M., Flournoy, N. *et al.* Cytomegalovirus immune globulin and seronegative blood products to prevent primary cytomegalovirus infection after marrow transplantation. *New England Journal of Medicine*, **314**, 1006–1010 (1986)

38. Meyers, J.D., Flournoy, N. and Thomas, E.D. Cell-mediated immunity to varicella-zoster virus after allogeneic marrow transplant. *Journal of Infectious Diseases*, **141**, 479–487 (1980)

39. Atkinson, K., Meyers, J.D., Storb, R. *et al.* Varicella-zoster virus infection after marrow transplantation for aplastic anemia or leukemia. *Transplantation*, **29**, 47–50 (1980)

40. Lapp, W.S., Ghayur, T., Mendes, M. *et al.* The functional and histological basis for graft-versus-host-induced immunosuppression. *Immunological Reviews*, **88**, 107–133 (1985)

41. Witherspoon, R.P., Lum, L.G., Storb, R. and Thomas, E.D. *In vitro* regulation of immunoglobulin synthesis after human marrow transplantation. II. Deficient T and non-T lymphocyte function within 3–4 months of allogeneic, syngeneic or autologous marrow grafting for hematologic malignancy. *Blood*, **59**, 844–850 (1982)

42. Lum, L.G. A review: the kinetics of immunologic recovery after human marrow transplantation. *Blood*, **69**, 369–380 (1987)

43. Atkinson, K., Storb, R., Ochs, H.D. *et al*. Thymus transplantation after allogeneic bone marrow graft to prevent chronic graft-versus-host disease in humans. *Transplantation*, **33**, 168–173 (1982)

44. Witherspoon, R.P., Navari, R., Storb, R. *et al*. Treatment of marrow graft recipients with thymopentin. *Bone Marrow Transplantation*, **1**, 365–371 (1987)

45. Witherspoon, R.P., Hersman, J., Storb, R. *et al*. Thymosin fraction 5 does not accelerate reconstitution of immunologic reactivity after human marrow grafting. *British Journal of Haematology*, **55**, 595–608 (1983)

46. Sullivan, K.M., Meyers, J.D., Flournoy, N. *et al*. Early and late interstitial pneumonia following human bone marrow transplantation. *International Journal of Cell Cloning*, **4**, 107–121 (1986)

47. Sullivan, K.M., Deeg, H.J., Sanders, J.E. *et al*. Late complications after marrow transplantation. *Seminars in Hematology*, **21**, 53–63 (1984)

48. Storb, R., Prentice, R.L., Sullivan, K.M. *et al*. Predictive factors in chronic graft-versus-host disease in patients with aplastic anemia treated by marrow transplantation from HLA-identical siblings. *Annals of Internal Medicine*, **98**, 461–466 (1983)

49. Lonnqvist, B., Ringden, O., Wahren, B. *et al*. Cytomegalovirus infection associated with and preceding chronic graft-versus-host disease. *Transplantation*, **38**, 465–468 (1984)

50. Tutschka, P.J. Mechanisms of chronic GVHD. In *Progress in Bone Marrow Transplantation*, (eds R.P. Gale and R. Champlin), A.R. Liss Inc, New York, pp. 457–472 (1987)

51. Schubert, M.M., Sullivan, K.M., Morton, T.H. *et al*. Oral manifestations of chronic graft-versus-host disease. *Archives of Internal Medicine*, **144**, 1591–1595 (1984)

52. Jack, M.K., Jack, G.M., Sale, G.E. *et al*. Ocular manifestations of graft-versus-host disease. *Archives of Ophthalmology*, **101**, 1080–1084 (1983)

53. Sullivan, K.M., Witherspoon, R., Storb, R. *et al*. Chronic graft-versus-host disease: pathogenesis, diagnosis, treatment and prognostic factors. In *Recent Advances and Future Directions in Bone Marrow Transplantation, (Experimental Hematology Today – 1987)* (eds S.J. Baum, G.W. Santos and F. Takaku), Springer Verlag, New York, pp. 150–157 (1988)

54. Sale, G.E., Shulman, H.M., Schubert, M.M. *et al*. Oral and ophthalmic pathology of graft versus host disease in man: predictive value of the lip biopsy. *Human Pathology*, **12**, 1022–1030 (1981)

55. Sullivan, K.M., Shulman, H.M., Storb, R. *et al*. Chronic graft-v-host disease in 52 patients: adverse natural course and successful treatment with combination immunosuppression. *Blood*, **57**, 267–276 (1981)

56. Sullivan, K.M., Witherspoon, R.P., Storb, R. *et al*. Prednisone and azathioprine compared with prednisone and placebo for treatment of chronic graft-v-host disease: prognostic influence of prolonged thrombocytopenia after allogeneic marrow transplantation. *Blood*, **72**, 546–554 (1988)

57. Sullivan, K.M., Witherspoon, R.P., Storb, R. *et al*. Alternating-day cyclosporine and prednisone for treatment of high-risk chronic graft-v-host disease. *Blood*, **72**, 555–561 (1988)

58. Bunjes, D., Heit, W., Arnold, R. *et al*. Cyclosporine as an alternative to cyclophosphamide in the treatment of chronic graft-versus-host disease. *Transplantation*, **41**, 170–172 (1986)

59. Vogelsang, G.B., Taylor, S., Gordon, G. and Hess, A.D. Thalidomide, a potent agent for the treatment of graft-versus-host disease. *Transplantation Proceedings*, **18**, 904–906 (1986)

60. Fass, L., Ochs, H.D., Thomas, E.D. *et al*. Studies of immunological reactivity following syngeneic or allogeneic marrow grafts in man. *Transplantation*, **16**, 630–640 (1973)

61. Elfenbein, G.J., Anderson, P.N. and Humphrey, R.L. Immune system reconstitution following allogeneic bone-marrow transplantation in man: a multiparameter analysis. *Transplantation Proceedings*, **8**, 641–646 (1976)

62. Witherspoon, R.P., Storb, R., Ochs, H.D. *et al*. Recovery of antibody production in human allogeneic marrow graft recipients: influence of time posttransplantation, the presence or absence of chronic graft-versus-host disease, and antithymocyte globulin treatment. *Blood*, **58**, 360–368 (1981)

63. Witherspoon, R.P., Deeg, H.J., Lum, L.G. *et al*. Immunologic recovery in human marrow graft recipients given cyclosporine or methotrexate for the prevention of graft-versus-host disease. *Transplantation*, **37**, 456–461 (1984)

64. Noel, D.R., Witherspoon, R.P., Storb, R. *et al*. Does graft-versus-host disease influence the tempo of immunologic recovery after allogeneic human marrow transplantation? An observation on 56 long-term survivors. *Blood*, **51**, 1087–1105 (1978)

65. Atkinson, K., Hansen, J.A., Storb, R. *et al*. T-cell subpopulations identified by monoclonal antibodies after human marrow transplantation. I. Helper-inducer and cytotoxic-suppressor subsets. *Blood*, **59**, 1292–1298 (1982)

66. Friedrich, W., O'Reilly, R.J. and Koziner, B. T-lymphocyte reconstitution in recipients of bone marrow transplants with and without GVHD: Imbalance of T-cell subpopulations having unique regulatory and cognitive functions. *Blood*, **59**, 696–701 (1982)

67. Lum, L.G., Seigneuret, M.C., Storb, R. *et al*. T and B cell deficiencies in patients with chronic graft-versus-host disease after HLA-identical marrow transplantation. *Transplantation Proceedings*, **13**, 1231–1232 (1981)

68. Lum, L.G., Orcutt-Thordarson, N., Seigneuret, M.C. and Storb, R. The regulation of Ig synthesis after marrow transplantation: IV. T4 and T8 subset function in patients with chronic graft-versus-host

disease. *Journal of Immunology*, **129**, 113–119 (1982)

69. Lum, L.G., Noges, J.E., Beatty, P. *et al.* Transfer of specific immunity in marrow recipients given HLA-mismatched, T cell-depleted, or HLA-identical marrow grafts. *Bone Marrow Transplantation*, **3**, 399–406 (1988)

70. Buja, M., Ferrans, V.J. and Graw, R.G. Jr. Cardiac pathologic findings in patients treated with bone marrow transplantation. *Human Pathology*, **7**, 17–45 (1976)

71. Baello, E.B., Ensberg, M.E., Ferguson, D.W. *et al.* Effect of high-dose cyclophosphamide and total-body irradiation on left ventricular function in adult patients with leukemia undergoing allogeneic bone marrow transplantation. *Cancer Treatment Reports*, **70**, 1187–1193 (1986)

72. Trigg, M.E., Finlay, J.L., Bozdech, M. and Gilbert, E. Fatal cardiac toxicity in bone marrow transplant patients receiving cytosine arabinoside, cyclophosphamide, and total body irradiation. *Cancer*, **59**, 38–42 (1987)

73. McDonald, G.B., Shulman, H.M., Wolford, J.L. and Spencer, G.D. Liver disease after human marrow transplantation. *Seminars in Liver Disease*, **7**, 210–220 (1987)

74. Wolford, J.L. and McDonald, G.B. A problem-oriented approach to intestinal and liver disease after marrow transplantation. *Journal of Clinical Gastroenterology*, **10**, 419–433 (1988)

75. McDonald, G.B., Sharma, P., Matthews, D.E. *et al.* Venocclusive disease of the liver after bone marrow transplantation: diagnosis, incidence, and predisposing factors. *Hepatology*, **4**, 116–122 (1984)

76. Yee, G.C., Kennedy, M.S., Storb, R. and Thomas, E.D. Effect of hepatic dysfunction on oral cyclosporine pharmacokinetics in marrow transplant patients. *Blood*, **64**, 1277–1279 (1984)

77. Spencer, G.D., Shulman, H.M., Myerson, D. *et al.* Diffuse intestinal ulceration after marrow transplantation: a clinico-pathological study of 13 patients. *Human Pathology*, **17**, 621–633 (1986)

78. Yee, G.C., Kennedy, M.S., Deeg, H.J. *et al.* Cyclosporine-associated renal dysfunction in marrow transplant recipients. *Transplantation Proceedings*, **17**, 196–201 (1985)

79. Zager, R.A., O'Quigley, J., Zager, B.K. *et al.* Acute renal failure following bone marrow transplantation: a retrospective study of 272 patients. *American Journal of Kidney Diseases*, **13**, 210–216 (1989)

80. June, C.H., Thompson, C.B., Kennedy, M.S. *et al.* Profound hypomagnesemia and renal magnesium wasting associated with the use of cyclosporine for marrow transplantation. *Transplantation*, **39**, 620–624 (1985)

81. Bennett, W.M. and Porter, G.A. Cyclosporine-associated hypertension. *American Journal of Medicine*, **85**, 131–133 (1988)

82. Springmeyer, S.C., Flournoy, N., Sullivan, K.M. *et al.* Pulmonary function changes in long-term survivors of allogeneic marrow transplantation. In *Recent Advances in Bone Marrow Transplantation* (ed. R.P. Gale), Alan R. Liss Inc., New York, pp. 343–353 (1983)

83. Sullivan, K.M., Meyers, J.D., Flournoy, N. *et al.* Early and late interstitial pneumonia following human bone marrow transplantation. *International Journal of Cell Cloning*, **4**, 107–121 (1986)

84. Clark, J.G., Schwartz, D.A., Flournoy, N. *et al.* Risk factors for airflow obstruction in recipients of bone marrow transplants. *Annals of Internal Medicine*, **107**, 648–656 (1987)

85. Sanders, J.E., Buckner, C.D., Sullivan, K. *et al.* Growth and development after bone marrow transplantation. In *Thalassemia: Recent Advances in Therapy – Bone Marrow Transplantation* (eds C.D. Buckner, R.P. Gale and G. Lucarelli), Alan R. Liss Inc., New York, pp. 375–382 (1989)

86. Sklar, C.A., Kim, T.H. and Ramsay, N.K.C. Thyroid dysfunction among long-term survivors of bone marrow transplantation. *American Journal of Medicine*, **73**, 688–694 (1982)

87. Sanders, J.E., Pritchard, S., Mahoney, P. *et al.* Growth and development following marrow transplantation for leukemia. *Blood*, **68**, 1129–1135 (1986)

88. Frölich, M., de Planque, M.M., Goslings, B.M. and Meinders, A.E. Thyroid function in leukaemia patients after allogeneic bone marrow transplantation. *Clinica Chimica Acta*, **165**, 127–132 (1987)

89. Bolme, P., Borgström, K. and Carlström, K. Endocrine changes in children after allogeneic bone marrow transplantation (abstract). In *Proceedings of the 27th Annual Meeting of the European Society for Paediatric Endocrinology* (1988)

90. Redman, J.R., Bajorunas, D.R., Shank, B. and O'Reilly, R.J. Endocrine dysfunction following successful bone marrow transplantation (BMT). *Blood*, **66**(Suppl. 1), 261a (1985)

91. Borgström, B. and Bolme, P. Growth and growth hormone in children after allogeneic bone marrow transplantation (abstract). In *Proceedings of the 27th Annual Meeting European Society for Paediatric Endocrinology*, 5 (1988)

92. Ranke, M.B., Blum, W.F., Dopfer, R. and Niethammer, D. Growth-related hormonal changes after allogeneic bone marrow transplantation (BMT) in children and adolescents (abstract). In *Proceedings of the 27th Annual Meeting European Society for Paediatric Endocrinology*, 59 (1988)

93. Sanders, J.E., Buckner, C.D., Leonard, J.M. *et al.* Late effects on gonadal function of cyclophosphamide, total-body irradiation, and marrow transplantation. *Transplantation*, **36**, 252–255 (1983)

94. Sklar, C.A., Kim, T.H., Williamson, J.F. and Ramsay, N.K.C. Ovarian function after successful bone marrow transplantation in postmenarcheal females. *Medical and Pediatric Oncology*, **11**, 361–364 (1983)

95. Sanders, J.E., Buckner, C.D., Amos, D. *et al.*

Ovarian function following marrow transplantation for aplastic anemia or leukemia. *Journal of Clinical Oncology*, **6**, 813–818 (1988)

96. Sklar, C.A., Kim, T.H. and Ramsay, N.K.C. Testicular function following bone marrow transplantation performed during or after puberty. *Cancer*, **53**, 1498–1501 (1984)

97. Deeg, H.J., Flournoy, N., Sullivan, K.M. *et al.* Cataracts after total body irradiation and marrow transplantation: a sparing effect of dose fractionation. *International Journal of Radiation Oncology, Biology, Physics*, **10**, 957–964 (1984)

98. Jack, M.J. and Hicks, J.D. Ocular complications in high-dose chemoradiotherapy and marrow transplantation. *Annals of Ophthalmology*, **13**, 709–711 (1981)

99. Probert, J.C. and Parker, B.R. The effects of radiation therapy on bone growth. *Radiology*, **114**, 155–162 (1975)

100. Jaffe, N., Toth, B.B., Hoar, R.E. *et al.* Dental and maxillofacial abnormalities in long-term survivors of childhood cancer: effects of treatment with chemotherapy and radiation to the head and neck. *Pediatrics*, **73**, 816–823 (1984)

101. Dahllöf, G., Barr, M., Bolme, P. *et al.* Disturbances in dental development after total body irradiation in bone marrow transplant recipients. *Oral Surgery, Oral Medicine, Oral Pathology*, **65**, 41–44 (1988)

102. Thompson, C.B., Sanders, J.E., Flournoy, N. *et al.* The risks of central nervous system relapse and leukoencephalopathy in patients receiving marrow transplants for acute leukemia. *Blood*, **67**, 195–199 (1986)

103. Gardner, G.G., August, C.S. and Githens, J. Psychological issues in bone marrow transplantation. *Pediatrics*, **60**, 625–630 (1977)

104. Hengeveld, M.W., Houtman, R.B. and Zwaan, F.E. Psychological aspects of bone marrow transplantation: a retrospective study of 17 long-term survivors. *Bone Marrow Transplantation*, **3**, 69–75 (1988)

105. Meadows, A.T., Massari, D., Fergusson, J. *et al.* Declines in IQ scores and cognitive dysfunction in children with acute lymphocytic leukemia treated with cranial irradiation. *Lancet*, i, 1015–1018 (1981)

106. Rowland, J.H., Glidewell, O.J., Sibley, R.F. *et al.* Effects of different forms of central nervous system prophylaxis on neuropsychologic function in childhood leukemia. *Journal of Clinical Oncology*, **2**, 1327–1335 (1984)

107. Cole, L.J. and Nowell, P.C. Parental-F₁ hybrid bone marrow chimeras: high incidence of donor-type lymphomas. *Proceedings of Society for Experimental Biology and Medicine*, **134**, 653–657 (1970)

108. Gleichmann, E., Gleichmann, H. and Schwartz, R.S. Immunologic induction of malignant lymphoma. Identification of donor and host tumors in the graft-versus-host model. *Journal of the National Cancer Institute*, **54**, 107–116 (1975)

109. Deeg, H.J., Prentice, R., Fritz, T.E. *et al.* Increased incidence of malignant tumors in dogs after total body irradiation and marrow transplantation. *International Journal of Radiation Oncology, Biology, Physics*, **9**, 1505–1511 (1983)

110. Broerse, J.J., Hollander, C.R. and Van Zwieten, M.J. Tumor induction in rhesus monkeys after total body irradiation with X-rays and fission neutrons. *International Journal of Radiation Biology*, **40**, 671–676 (1981)

111. Fialkow, P.J., Thomas, E.D., Bryant, J.I. and Neiman, P.E. Leukaemic transformation of engrafted human marrow cells *in vivo*. *Lancet*, i, 251–255 (1971)

112. Thomas, E.D., Bryant, J.I., Buckner, C.D. *et al.* Leukaemic transformation of engrafted human marrow cells *in vivo*. *Lancet*, i, 1310–1313 (1972)

113. Goh, K. and Klemperer, M.R. *In vivo* leukemic transformation: cytogenetic evidence of *in vivo* leukemic transformation of engrafted marrow cells. *American Journal of Hematology*, **2**, 283–290 (1977)

114. Elfenbein, G.J., Brogaonkar, D.S. and Bias, W.B. Cytogenetic evidence for recurrence of acute myelogenous leukemia after allogeneic bone marrow transplantation in donor hematopoietic cells. *Blood*, **52**, 627–636 (1978)

115. Newburger, P.E., Latt, S.A. and Pesando, J.M. Leukemia relapse in donor cells after allogeneic bone-marrow transplantation. *New England Journal of Medicine*, **304**, 712–714 (1981)

116. Schubach, W.H., Hackman, R., Neiman, P.E. *et al.* A monoclonal immunoblastic sarcoma in donor cells bearing Epstein–Barr virus genomes following allogeneic marrow grafting for acute lymphoblastic leukemia. *Blood*, **60**, 180–187 (1982)

117. Sanders, J., Sale, G.E., Ramberg, R. *et al.* Glioblastoma multiforme in a patient with acute lymphoblastic leukemia who received a marrow transplant. *Transplantation Proceedings*, **14**, 770–774 (1982)

118. Deeg, H.J., Sanders, J., Martin, P. *et al.* Secondary malignancies after marrow transplantation. *Experimental Hematology*, **12**, 660–666 (1984)

119. Witherspoon, R.P., Schubach, W., Neiman, P. *et al.* Donor cell leukemia developing six years after marrow grafting for acute leukemia. *Blood*, **65**, 1172–1174 (1985)

120. Klingemann, H-G., Storb, R., Sanders, J. *et al.* Acute lymphoblastic leukaemia after bone marrow transplantation for aplastic anaemia. *British Journal of Haematology*, **63**, 47–50 (1986)

121. Zutter, M.M., Martin, P.J. Sale, G.E. *et al.* Epstein–Barr virus lymphoproliferation after bone marrow transplantation. *Blood*, **72**, 520–529 (1988)

122. Witherspoon, R.P., Fisher, L., Martin, P. *et al.* Secondary malignancies following bone marrow transplantation for aplastic anemia or hematologic malignancy (abstract). *Blood*, **72**(Suppl. 1), 1562 (1988)

123. Thomas, E.D. Marrow transplantation for malignant disease. *American Journal of the Medical Sciences*, **30**, 75–79 (1987)

# 12

# Cardiovascular system morbidity of radiotherapy

Klaus-Rüdiger Trott

The vascular system plays a dominant role in the pathogenesis of acute and chronic side effects of radiotherapy. Although most acute side effects of radiotherapy are caused primarily by radiation effects on the parenchymal cells in the various tissues, e.g. in the basal cells of the epidermis, the mucosal epithelia or the haemopoietic cells of the bone marrow, substances like histamine are released during the expression of this parenchymal radiation injury which lead to a secondary inflammatory response of the vascular system with vascular dilatation, increased capillary permeability and interstitial oedema. These secondary reactions of the vascular system may sometimes be more conspicuous even than the primary injury to the parenchyma, e.g. in skin where erythema is the main manifestation of acute radiation response.

Quite apart from these acute secondary responses of the vascular system to acute parenchymal tissue injury, direct radiation effects on the vascular system mainly on the capillary bed and the arterioles take a long time to become manifest and are usually progressive. Gradually they lead to reduced capillary density in the irradiated tissues and a decrease in blood perfusion resulting in secondary parenchymal atrophy. A typical morphological sign of these degenerative changes in the capillary system is the gradual appearance of telangiectasis, i.e. greatly enlarged but functionally deficient dilated capillaries which may be found after long latency periods in most heavily irradiated tissues but which are most readily seen in skin.

These vascular changes are ubiquitous and are common to all organs in the body after irradiation. Their clinical significance may vary as may their contribution to the pathogenesis of gross clinical side effects. Since they play such an integral role in the side effects of all organs after radiotherapy they will not be analysed in more detail here. This chapter therefore will concentrate on the side effects of radiotherapy in the heart and the major blood vessels.

## Radiation effects in the heart

### Clinical presentation of radiation-induced heart disease

For a long time the heart was classified as a radio-resistant organ. This was due to the fact that until recently long-term survival of those patients who received high radiation doses homogenously to the mediastinum, including more than 50% of the heart, was uncommon. However, as early as 1924, Schweizer [1] described the typical features of radiation-induced heart disease in a patient who had received two courses of mediastinal radiotherapy for recurrent Hodgkin's disease.

The full extent of potential radiation injury to the heart was only recently revealed in numerous clinical reports which followed the first extensive study on a number of Hodgkin's patients from Stanford published by Cohn et al. [2]. The clinical features and the incidence of cardiac side effects of radiotherapy to the mediastinum and the chest wall is thus now well documented. In mediastinal radiotherapy usually more than 50% of the heart is included in the 90% isodose, whereas in postoperative radiotherapy of the chest wall for breast cancer it is only about 20%. These differences in the topographical distribution of radiation dose are reflected in differences in clinical presentation and incidence of cardiac side effects.

Cardiac side effects may arise primarily in the pericardium, the myocardium, or in the coronary

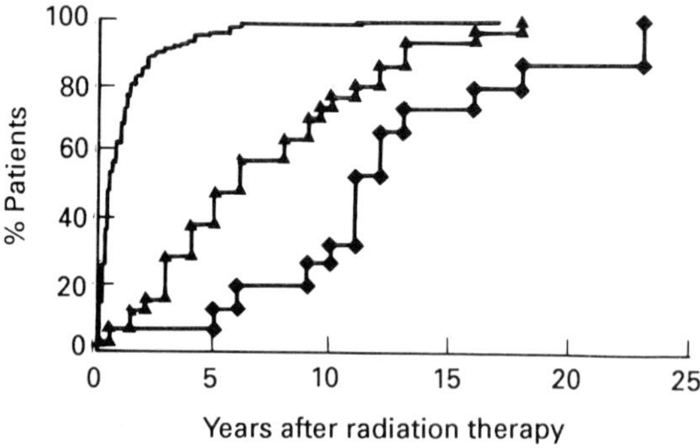


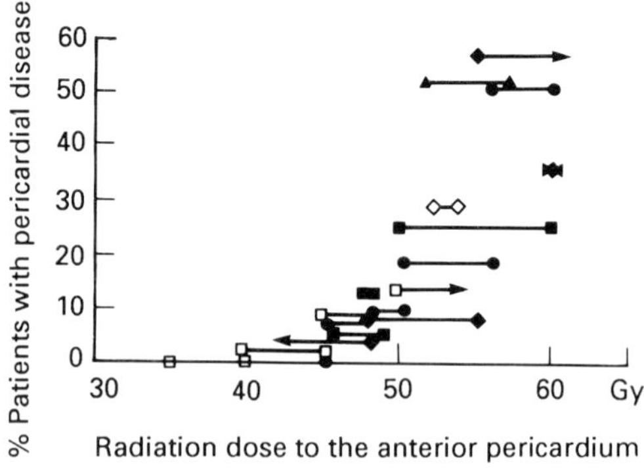


**Figure 12.1** Cumulative latency times until onset of symptoms of radiation-induced pericarditis (—), coronary heart disease (▲—▲) or conduction defects (◆—◆) with post-irradiation time. Compiled by Lauk [3]

**Figure 12.2** Incidence of pericarditis as a function of total dose to the anterior pericardium. Compiled by Lauk [3]

arteries. Besides their clinical presentation, these side effects differ in their latency. In an extensive compilation of the published literature, Lauk [3] estimated a median latency in 196 cases of radiation-induced pericarditis of about 1 year (Figure 12.1). Of the 32 reported cases of radiation-induced coronary artery disease 50% occurred within 5 years whereas severe conduction defects as signs of severe myocardial injury occurred even later.

## Radiation pericarditis

Transient, asymptomatic pericardial effusions diagnosed on routine chest X-rays or at echocardiography are the most common form of cardiac side effects of mediastinal radiotherapy. One-third of these asymptomatic pericardial effusions clear completely within 2–5 months [4]. However, persistent effusions may require surgical intervention before constrictive pericarditis occurs which has been described in about one-third of all cases of radiation-induced pericarditis. Overall lethality of radiation-induced pericarditis is 6% (11/196).

The incidence of pericarditis increases with radiation dose in a steep dose-response curve. Lauk [3] estimated the radiation dose to the anterior pericardium from nine reports on cardiac side effects of mediastinal radiotherapy of Hodgkin's disease and plotted this against the reported incidence of pericarditis. Despite the great dosimetric uncertainties it appears that the risk is low at doses below 40 Gy and rises to about 10% at 50 Gy and further to about 50% at 60 Gy (Figure 12.2). It may be of interest to note that all patients in this study were planned to receive tumour doses to their mediastinum of only about 40 Gy and the large differences in pericardial doses arose entirely from differences in radiation

energy, in source skin distance and in weighting of anterior and posterior fields.

The recorded incidence of pericarditis is also influenced by the sensitivity of the diagnostic procedure. Whereas in a chest X-ray significant enlargement of the heart can be discovered only when at least 250–500 ml have accumulated, echocardiography permits the detection of only 10% of this volume. Thus, by echocardiography small, asymptomatic pericardial effusions may be detected in one-third of breast cancer patients 6 months after postoperative radiotherapy to the chest wall [5]; however, their clinical relevance is uncertain.

## Radiation-induced myocardial changes

The most common clinical presentation of early but asymptomatic myocardial radiation injury consists of flattening or inversion of the T wave in the ECG [6]. It may become apparent by 4 months after radiotherapy and usually resolves after 1 year.

Severe conduction defects have been reported to develop after 6–23 years (Figure 12.1), the most common being a right bundle branch block. In the only study where patients were systematically investigated later than 10 years after radiotherapy for Hodgkin's disease four out of 28 patients (14%) had severe conduction defects [7].

Studies of heart function by radionuclide angiography or heart catheterization 5–15 years after radiotherapy have demonstrated a reduced ventricular function at even lower doses than pericardial reactions. With 30–36 Gy mean heart dose, the incidence was about 10–20% [8,9], whereas mean organ doses of 50 Gy led to decreased ventricular ejection fraction 5–15 years after radiotherapy in about one-third of the patients [10].

## Radiation-induced coronary artery disease

There are 32 case reports summarized by Lauk [3] describing young patients under 42 years with myocardial infarction that appeared to be due to previous heart irradiation because few or no other risk factors for coronary artery disease were found. Radiation doses to the mediastinum were typically between 30 and 50 Gy. Although the clinical presentation of radiation-induced coronary artery disease is not much different from that associated with other risk factors, Lauk concluded that heart irradiation appeared to be a risk factor in its own right for coronary artery disease at 5 years or more after treatment. In young irradiated patients there is more often only one artery narrowed than in non-irradiated patients. Yet since coronary artery disease following irradiation does not have any specific clinical characteristics, it is not possible clinically to attribute disease in an individual patient to previous heart irradiation.

## Histopathology

The most consistent finding at autopsy of patients after high dose mediastinal radiotherapy is thickening of the pericardium and endocardium [11]. Collagen replaces adipose tissue and in most cases fibrinous exudate, a large number of fibroblasts and fibrous adhesions are seen. In addition to the pericardial changes, Fajardo, Stewart and Cohn [11] observed areas of diffuse interstitial fibrosis in the myocardium where individual myocardial fibres were separated from each other by thick bands of collagen. The severity as well as the extent and location of fibrosis varied widely. In the vessels, endothelial cell proliferation was a common finding. Brosius, Waller and Roberts [12] looked specifically at the coronary arteries and found that of a total of 64 coronary arteries from 16 autopsies of patients on average 55 months after radiotherapy 16 were narrowed by more than 75%, mostly caused by intimal fibrosis. The most specific change in irradiated patients was the loss of medial smooth muscle cells which is only rarely observed in atherosclerosis patients.

Similar histopathological findings of the epicardium were also found in some experimental animals such as rabbits [13], rats [14] and dogs [15], often accompanied by pericardial effusions. Yet diffuse interstitial fibrosis which is the most characteristic histopathological picture in humans after heart irradiation is not commonly observed in experimental animals after local heart irradiation except for rabbits [13]. In rats, however, focal myocardial degeneration and myocardial cell necrosis is very prominent with only a small amount of replacement fibrosis. Vascular damage in rat hearts was only found within areas of degeneration.

## Pathogenesis and pathophysiology

Recent experimental studies in rabbits and, above all, in rats after local heart irradiation have elucidated the major steps in the pathogenesis of radiation-induced heart disease.

Radiation pericarditis appears to develop independently from myocardial radiation injury after a well defined latency period which, in the Wistar Nhg rat is 16 weeks and, as in patients, may clear spontaneously if it does not aggravate cardiac insufficiency from myocardial damage which develops later [14]. The experimental observations are consistent with an inflammatory response of the subepicardial tissue to mesothelial denudation and subsequent fibrous organization of the fibrinous exudate, very similar to the radiation response of other surface epithelia but very much delayed due to the slow turnover of the pericardial mesothelium.

Myocardial injury after irradiation is secondary to radiation damage to the capillary bed in rabbits [16] and in rats [14]. Capillary density in rat hearts starts to decrease already about 1 month after a single dose of 20 Gy whereas myocardial damage is not observed before 70 days when capillary density is well below 50% of normal. Thus, severe reduction of the capillary network is present before any other morphological or functional signs of radiation damage to the myocardium are observed [17]. Even before the capillary density is significantly decreased a proliferative response in capillary endothelial cells is elicited about 20 days after irradiation [18] which may actually precipitate loss of endothelial cells and disappearance of capillaries. In rats the change in microvascular anatomy is accompanied by loss of alkaline phosphatase activity from surviving capillary endothelial cells [17]. Enzyme loss occurred simultaneously with disappearance of capillaries in defined, randomly distributed areas of the myocardium; when myocardial degeneration occurred it was always within areas of enzyme loss. The sequence of these events after a single dose of 20 Gy to the heart of Wistar Nhg rats is summarized in Figure 12.3. Similar changes have been observed in other rat strains [19,20]. After sublethal radiation doses there was complete structural and functional recovery of the capillary network after the initial damage which was complete after about 1 year; at higher doses decrease in capillary density was continuously progressive. However, the rate of capillary damage was clearly dose-dependent as was also the latency to a level when gross myocardial injury became apparent. In rats the mean latency to congestive heart failure appears to be the best clinical end point of myocardial radiation injury (Figure 12.4) which, however, at high radiation doses reaches a plateau which is consistent with the latency period for radiation-induced pericarditis.

Whereas the primary effect of radiation to the

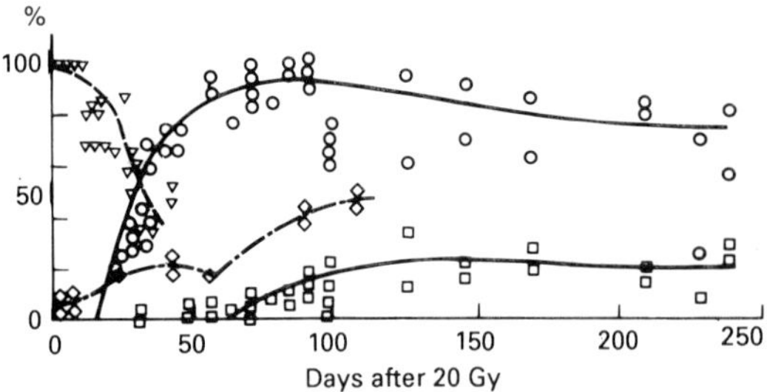

Figure 12.3 Time course of morphological changes following irradiation with 20 Gy to the heart of Wistar Nhg rats: ○, percentage section area where alkaline phosphatase activity was lost; □, percentage section area of myocardial degeneration and necrosis; ▽, volume density of capillaries (percentage of normals); ◇, labelling index of capillary endothelial cells

## Fractionation response of radiation-induced heart disease

Lauk [3] analysed published reports with regard to the dependence of pericarditis incidence on dose per fraction (Figure 12.5). For similar total doses to the anterior pericardium, the incidence of pericarditis appeared to increase sharply as the dose per fraction

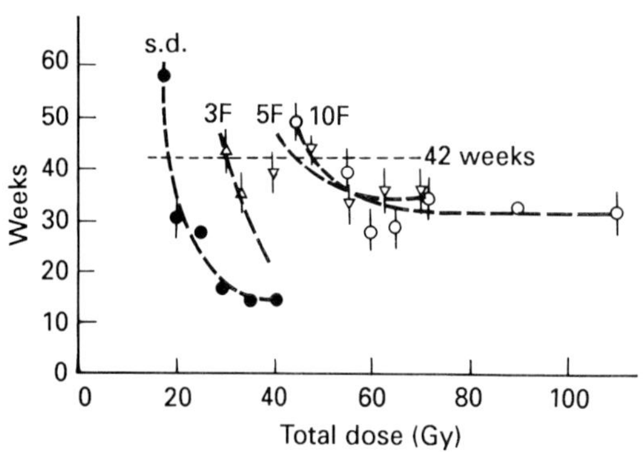

Figure 12.4 Mean survival times and standard errors after single dose and fractionated irradiation in Wistar Nhg rats [23]

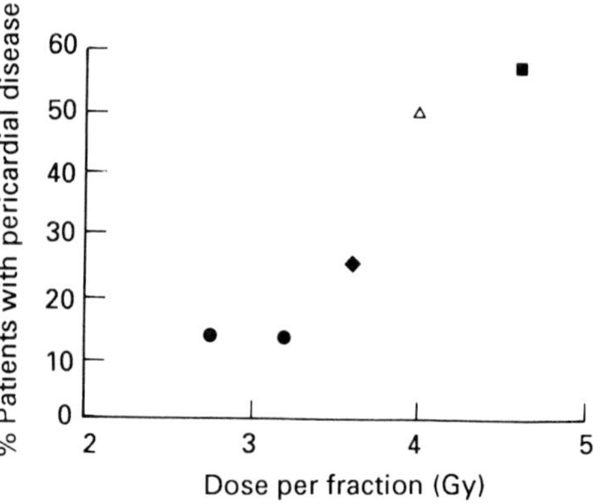

Figure 12.5 Variation of incidence of pericarditis with dose per fraction to the anterior heart surface through the anterior treatment port. Total doses at 2 cm depth were 50–60 Gy [3]

heart in all experimental models was capillary loss, the morphological and functional consequences to the myocardium may be different in different animals. Thus the development of interstitial fibrosis in humans and in rabbits appears to be secondary to myocardial atrophy and degeneration. Whereas cardiac output was found to decrease in dogs [15] and in Sprague-Dawley rats, it was increased in Wistar rats [20] which appears to be a compensatory reaction to improve the impaired ventricular blood flow, possibly mediated by an increase in alpha- and beta-adrenergic receptors [3]. Non-invasive examination of cardiac function in awake animals showed a reduced functional reserve capacity in the myocardium long before gross clinical signs of congestive heart failure became apparent [21].

exceeded 3 Gy. In a more complex analysis of all published data Lauk [3] concluded that for pericarditis an $\alpha/\beta$ value of about 2 Gy is most consistent with the clinical experience. A similar value was estimated from experimental studies in dogs [22] and in rats [23] (Figure 12.4).

## Interaction of heart irradiation and doxorubicin chemotherapy

The most severe side effect of chemotherapy with doxorubicin (Adriamycin) is heart damage. The incidence shows a gradual increase with increasing total dose [24], but a total dose of 450 mg/m$^2$ is generally recommended as the maximal cumulative dose which is consistent with a 3–5% incidence of doxorubicin cardiopathy.

In contrast to radiation-induced heart disease, doxorubicin cardiopathy is due to direct myocardial injury; however, the exact mechanism is not known. It has a higher lethality (about 50%) than radiation-induced heart disease, and it appears earlier after treatment with a median of about 4 weeks.

Some clinical reports suggest an increased cardiotoxicity of the combination of radiotherapy and doxorubicin chemotherapy. Gilladoga *et al.* [25] reported that four of 42 children who received more than 500 mg/m$^2$ doxorubicin alone developed serious cardiomyopathy while four of eight did so after the same dose of doxorubicin in combination with mediastinal radiotherapy.

In two series of Hodgkin's patients, no increased incidence of cardiac side effects was detected if the mediastinal radiation dose was kept below 40 Gy and the doxorubicin dose below 250 mg/m$^2$ [26,27].

Le Chevalier *et al.* [28] found pericardial effusions in 50% of patients after treatment for small cell lung cancer with 45 Gy to the thorax and chemotherapy including a total of 240–320 mg/m$^2$ doxorubicin which suggests a marked increase in the risk of radiation-induced pericarditis.

The only quantitative analysis of combined mediastinal radiotherapy and doxorubicin chemotherapy is the study by Billingham [29]. In 84 patients percutaneous endomyocardial biopsies were performed 3 weeks to 4 years after doxorubicin treatment with doses of 90–610 mg/m$^2$; 15 patients had been irradiated 11 years to 6 months before doxorubicin chemotherapy with doses between 25 and 60 Gy. A semiquantitative histological score increased with doxorubicin dose but in each dose group pre-irradiated patients had a higher score (Figure 12.6). Irradiated patients who had 200–300 mg/m$^2$ doxorubicin showed a similar score to non-irradiated patients at 400–500 mg/m$^2$. No other quantitative data on the interaction of doxorubicin and mediastinal radiation in patients have been published. Information from experimental studies is also scarce but pilot experiments in rabbits [30] and in rats [31] suggest a markedly increased cardiotoxicity even if both treatments are separated by a long gap. There is definitely a need for more experimental data on the problem of reduced tolerance of the heart to doxorubicin or radiotherapy in patients previously treated with the other modality, and the relationship of this with dose and time.

## Radiation effects in the major blood vessels

Radiation injury of the major blood vessels has not been well documented and the available clinical reports show that the injuries are often complicated by tumour invasion or infection. Fajardo [32] analysed 90 reported cases of 'spontaneous' rupture of irradiated large arteries, especially carotid artery, aorta and femoral arteries, but found that most of these vascular perforations were associated with local surgical complications such as fistulas, abscesses, etc. In only five of them did direct radiation injury appear to be the cause of vessel rupture.

The main manifestation of damage in the major vessels is haemorrhage which occurred 1–7 years after doses of 40–70 Gy in the three cases described by Fajardo and Lee [33]. However, Drescher, Basche and Schumann [34] described a thrombosis of the iliac artery 7 years after a dose of 50 Gy to the para-aortic lymph nodes for metastatic seminoma. The histopathological features of radiation-induced damage to the major vessels are not much different from those of atheromatosis and are somewhat non-specific.

However, in intraoperative radiotherapy, radiation injury to the major vessels may become a major limitation. Gilette *et al.* [35] reported that intraoperative radiation doses to the aorta of dogs of 25 Gy or more led to a high incidence of dissecting aneurysms and thrombosis as late as 5 years after irradiation. At 5 years, a 50% incidence of thrombosis or disruption of branch arteries was observed

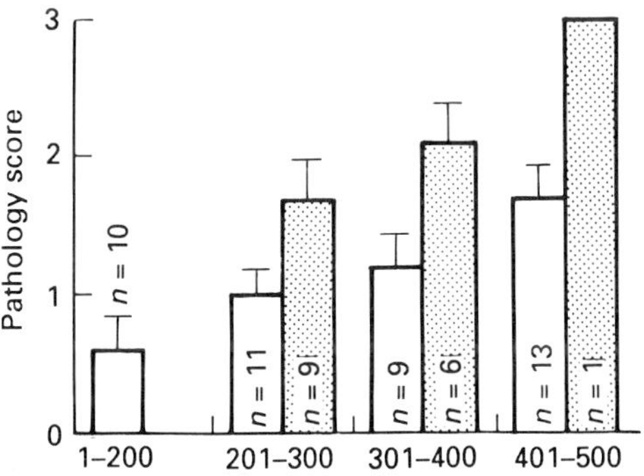


**Figure 12.6** Comparison of histopathology scores in myocardial biopsies from unirradiated (□) and irradiated (□) patients for different ranges of cumulative doxorubicin doses [29]

after about 25 Gy intraoperative irradiation alone or after about 20 Gy if this followed 30–50 Gy fractionated external beam radiotherapy.

## References


1. Schweizer, E. Ueber spezifische Roentgenschaedigungen des Herzmuskels. *Strahlentherapie*, **18**, 812–828 (1924)

2. Cohn, K.E., Stewart, J.R., Fajardo, L.F. and Hancock, E.W. Heart disease following radiation. *Medicine*, **46**, 281–298 (1967)

3. Lauk, S. Radiation injury to the heart. In *Radiation Pathology of Organs and Tissues*, (eds E. Scherer, C. Streffer and K.R. Trott), Springer, Heidelberg (1990)

4. Pierce, R.H., Haferman, M.D. and Kagan, A.R. Changes in the transverse cardiac diameter following irradiation for Hodgkin's disease. *Radiology*, **93**, 619–624 (1960)

5. Ikaheimo, S.M., Niemela, M/.M., Linnaluoto, M.M. *et al*. Early cardiac changes related to radiation therapy. *American Journal of Cardiology*, **56**, 943–946 (1985)

6. Catterall, M. and Evans, W. Myocardial injury from therapeutic irradiation. *British Heart Journal*, **22**, 168–174 (1960)

7. Pohjola-Sintonen, S., Tottermann, K.J., Salmo, M. and Siltanen, P. Late cardiac effects of mediastinal radiotherapy in patients with Hodgkin's disease. *Cancer*, **60**, 31–37 (1987)

8. Gomez, G.A., Park, J.J., Panahon, A.M. *et al*. Heart size and function after radiation therapy to the mediastinum in patients with Hodgkin's disease. *Cancer Treatment Reports*, **67**, 1099–1103 (1983)

9. Morgan, G.W., Freeman, A.P., McLean, R.G. *et al*. Late cardiac thyroid and pulmonary sequelae of mantle radiotherapy for Hodgkin's disease. *International Journal of Radiation Oncology, Biology, Physics*, **11**, 1925–1931 (1985)

10. Gottdiener, J.S., Katin, M.J., Borer, J.S. *et al*. Late cardiac effects of therapeutic mediastinal irradiation. Assessment by echocardiography and radionuclide angiography. *New England Journal of Medicine*, **308**, 569–588 (1983)

11. Fajardo, L.F., Stewart, J.R. and Cohn, K.E. Morphology of radiation-induced heart disease. *Archives of Pathology*, **86**, 512–519 (1968)

12. Brosius, F.C., Waller, B.F. and Roberts, W.L. Analysis of 16 young (aged 15–33 years) necropsy patients who received over 3500 rads to the heart. *American Journal of Medicine*, **70**, 519–530 (1981)

13. Fajardo, L.F. and Stewart, J.R. Experimental radiation-induced heart disease. *American Journal of Pathology*, **59**, 299–316 (1970)

14. Lauk, S., Kiszel, Z. and Trott, K.R. Radiation-induced heart disease in rats. *International Journal of Radiation Oncology, Biology, Physics*, **11**, 801–808 (1985)

15. McChesney, S.L., Gillette, E.L. and Powers, B.E. Radiation-induced cardiomyopathy in the dog. *Radiation Research*, **113**, 120–132 (1988)

16. Fajardo, L.F. and Stewart, J.R. Capillary injury preceding radiation-induced myocardial fibrosis. *Radiology*, **101**, 429–433 (1971)

17. Lauk, S. Endothelial alkaline phosphatase activity loss as an early stage in the development of radiation-induced heart disease in rats. *Radiation Research*, **110**, 118–128 (1987)

18. Fajardo, L.F. and Stewart, J.R. Pathogenesis of radiation-induced myocardial fibrosis. *Laboratory Investigation*, **29**, 244–257 (1973)

19. Lauk, S. Strain differences in the radiation response of the rat heart. *Radiotherapy and Oncology*, **5**, 333–335 (1986)

20. Yeung, T.K., Lauk, S., Simmonds, R.H. *et al*. Morphological and functional changes in the rat heart after X-irradiation: strain differences. *Radiation Research*, **119**, 489–499 (1989)

21. Geist, B.J., Lauk, S., Bornhausen, M. and Trott, K.R. Physiological consequences of local heart irradiation in rats. *International Journal of Radiation Oncology, Biology, Physics*, **18**, 1107–1113 (1990)

22. Gillette, E.L., McChesney, S.L. and Hoopes, P.J. Isoeffect curves for radiation-induced cardiomyopathy in the dog. *International Journal of Radiation Oncology, Biology, Physics*, **11**, 2091–2097 (1985)

23. Lauk, S., Rueth, S. and Trott, K.R. The effects of dose fractionation on radiation-induced heart disease in rats. *Radiotherapy and Oncology*, **8**, 363–367 (1987)

24. Von Hoff, D.D., Layard, M.W., Basa, P. *et al*. Risk factors for doxorubicin-induced congestive heart failure. *Annals of Internal Medicine*, **91**, 710–717

25. Gilladoga, A.C., Corazon, M., Tan, C.C. *et al*. Cardiotoxicity of adriamycin in children. *Cancer Chemotherapy Reports*, Part 3, Vol. 6, 209–215 (1975)

26. LaMonte, C.S., Yeh, S.D.J. and Straus, D.J. Long-term follow-up of cardiac function in patients with Hodgkin's disease treated with mediastinal irradiation and combination chemotherapy including doxorubicin. *Cancer Treatment Reports*, **70**, 439–444 (1986)

27. Santoro, A., Bonnadonna, G., Valagussa, P. *et al*. Long-term results of combined chemotherapy–radiotherapy approach in Hodgkin's disease: superiority of ABVD plus radiotherapy versus MOPP plus radiotherapy. *Journal of Clinical Oncology*, **5**, 27–37 (1987)

28. LeChevalier, T., Arriagada, R., deThe, H. *et al*. Combination of chemotherapy and radiotherapy in limited small cell lung carcinoma: results of alternating schedule in 109 patients. *NCI Monograph*, **6**, 335–338 (1988)

29. Billingham, M.E. Endomyocardial changes in anthracycline-treated patients with and without irradiation. *Frontiers of Radiation Therapy and Oncology*, **13**, 67–81 (1979)

30. Eltringham, J.R., Fajardo, L.F. and Stewart, J.R. Adriamycin cardiomyopathy: enhanced cardiac dam-

age in rabbits with combined drug and cardiac irradiation. *Radiology*, **115**, 471–472 (1975)

31. Trott, K.R. Radiation–chemotherapy interactions. *International Journal of Radiation Oncology, Biology, Physics*, **12**, 1409–1413 (1986)

32. Fajardo, L.F. *Pathology of Radiation Injury*, Masson, New York (1982)

33. Fajardo, L.F. and Lee, H.A. Rupture of major vessels after radiation. *Cancer*, **36**, 904–913 (1975)

34. Drescher, W., Basche, S. and Schumann, E. Arterielle Spaetkomplikationen nach Strahlentherapie. *Strahlentherapie*, **160**, 505–507 (1984)

35. Gillette, E.L., Powers, B.E., McChesney, S.L., Park, R.D. and Withrow, S.J. Response of aorta and branch arteries to experimental intraoperative irradiation. *International Journal of Radiation Oncology, Biology, Physics*, **17**, 1247–1255 (1989)

# 13

# Cardiac morbidity of chemotherapy

T.J. McElwain

## Introduction

Compared with some organs and tissues such as the bone marrow and gastrointestinal endothelium, the heart is injured by a relatively small number of cytotoxic drugs. However, this number is growing, particularly with the introduction of new anthracyclines. Furthermore, as more cancer patients are considered eligible for treatment with chemotherapy, particularly in the adjuvant setting, the immediate and long-term morbidity of cardiotoxic drugs becomes increasingly important. As older patients with established cardiac disease are recipients of cancer chemotherapy, great vigilance on the part of oncologists will be required if unacceptable cardiotoxic effects are to be avoided, and, where a relatively small proportion of a group of patients may be expected to benefit from cardiotoxic chemotherapy, as for example in the adjuvant therapy of post-surgical breast cancer, consideration of risk of iatrogenic morbidity compared with possible benefit from treatment becomes paramount.

A further important consideration is what exactly is meant by cardiotoxicity since this can range from temporary reversible ECG changes to fully established irreversible cardiac failure. Here the notion of what is meant by a 'safe' dose of a particular treatment requires careful definition; clearly to regard such a dose as that which brings the patient to the edge of clinical cardiac failure is of questionable value, although it may permit crude comparison between drugs of a particular class such as anthracyclines when the choice of drug for use in a particular clinical setting is being made.

Finally, the therapist must constantly be aware of the causes, often far more common than cytotoxic drugs, of cardiac complications in cancer patients. These include not only established ischaemic heart disease but also anaemia, septicaemia, nutritional disorders and previous radiation damage to the pericardium and myocardium. This chapter will focus on those cytotoxic drugs which directly damage the heart.

## Anthracyclines

These include doxorubicin (Adriamycin), daunorubicin, epirubicin and idarubicin. Doxorubicin and daunorubicin are the most long established drugs in clinical practice. Their major cardiac effects can be divided into various non-specific electrocardiographic changes and arrhythmias related to acute drug administration and the development of a cardiomyopathy related to the cumulative dose of drug administered. The latter is largely irreversible and manifests in its late stage as congestive cardiac failure.

### Doxorubicin

Doxorubicin is widely used in the treatment of acute leukaemia, lymphomas including Hodgkin's disease, many tumours of childhood and adolescence including Wilms' tumour, rhabdomyosarcoma, Ewing's sarcoma, osteosarcoma, germ cell tumours and neuroblastoma. Breast cancer, some lung cancers, myeloma and soft tissue sarcomas are also responsive. Indeed, there are probably no human tumours in which the use of this drug has not been investigated.

## Electrocardiographic (ECG) changes

ECG changes are observed during and after drug administration. Commonly these include low voltage QRS complexes, non-specific ST and T wave changes, sinus tachycardia, prolongation of the QT interval, premature atrial and ventricular beats and supraventricular arrhythmias. These and many other abnormalities have been observed: the frequency of their observation broadly increases with the level of monitoring, being less frequently seen when the period of monitoring is short, and more frequently noted in patients in whom continuous monitoring is performed over a long time period. The frequency of ECG abnormalities probably also increases in the presence of pre-existing ischaemic and other heart disease. Sudden death associated with doxorubicin administration has rarely been reported.

The ECG changes most commonly occur during or within a few days of drug administration and reverse spontaneously. However, in some patients abnormalities may persist for longer and, particularly in the case of patients with heart disease predating the administration of doxorubicin, may represent an indication for discontinuing the drug.

In the review by Minow, Benjamin and Gottlieb [1], changes in the ECG were noted in 160 of 1051 patients (15.2%) receiving doxorubicin. The changes were all non-specific and were seen at all dose levels, irrespective of schedule and, apart from the low QRS voltage, resolved within 2 months of discontinuing the drug. There was no relationship between ECG changes and the subsequent development of congestive cardiac failure.

Other workers have noted the absence of a relationship between the development of ECG changes and the development of doxorubicin-induced cardiomyopathy apart from an association between low voltage QRS complexes and the subsequent development of cardiomyopathy. From the point of view of the management and cardiac monitoring of patients receiving doxorubicin the very important conclusion is that, by themselves, serial electrocardiograms are a totally inadequate way of diagnosing and thus preventing the early development of myopathic changes in the heart.

## Doxorubicin-induced cardiomyopathy

In patients dying from doxorubicin cardiomyopathy the heart is enlarged, pale and flabby [1]. The ventricles are dilated and may be mildly hypertrophied. There is no doxorubicin-related coronary artery or valvular damage. In 46 patients who had received various doses of doxorubicin but who had not died from cardiomyopathy, Cortes *et al.* [2] found that 26% of patients showed pathological evidence of cardiotoxicity. The changes were less severe than those seen in patients who had died with congestive cardiac failure.

Billingham and co-workers [3] first described the myocardial changes associated with doxorubicin toxicity by means of light and electron microscopical analysis of endomyocardial biopsies obtained from patients undergoing treatment. These are non-specific and may be seen in other cardiomyopathies. The changes are dose-related and can be seen in nearly all patients who have received a total dose of doxorubicin in excess of $240\,mg/m^2$. The pathological process is characterized by myocyte degeneration and oedema which is accompanied by partial or total myofibrillar loss.

Sarcotubular dilatation with vacuole formation is also seen and may occur with or without myofibrillary changes. Early on mitochondria may remain relatively intact but later there is mitochondrial degeneration, crystolysis and appearance of myelin bodies. Myocyte death ultimately leads to interstitial fibrosis. Billingham [3] has proposed a pathological grading system which is shown in Table 13.1 and this can be used in conjunction with information obtained from cardiac catheterization and phonocardiography [4] to assess the risk of congestive cardiac failure in patients. Bristow and co-workers [4] studied 33 patients and found that doxorubicin administration was associated with a dose-related increase in the degree of myocyte damage. In 27 of 28 patients receiving cumulative doxorubicin doses greater than $240\,mg/m^2$, degenerative changes were identified on right ventricular endomyocardial biopsy. The pre-ejection period to left ventricular ejection time ratio (PEP/LVET) did not begin to increase until a threshold of $400\,mg/m^2$ had been reached. Seven patients with catheterization-proven cardiac failure had a significantly greater amount of myocyte damage on biopsy than dose-matched control subjects. Mediastinal irradiation and age greater than 70 years were risk factors for heart failure.

The mechanisms of doxorubicin and other anthracycline-induced myocardial damage is still not clear but there is increasing evidence that it is associated with the production of free radicals such as superoxide and hydroxyl radicals. *In vitro*, cytochrome P450 in the nuclear membrane and microsomes reduces anthracyclines to form a semiquinone intermediate radical which then uses oxygen to form the superoxide and hydroxyl radicals. Furthermore, anthracyclines can chelate iron transferred from ferritin to form a complex which causes oxygen radical formation and lipid peroxidation; damage to nucleic acids, endoplasmic reticulum and mitochondria results and may lead to myocyte damage, although this is not established *in vivo* [5–10].

## The influence of dose on cardiac failure

In 1979 Von Hoff and his colleagues reported 3941 patients who had received doxorubicin of whom 88 had developed congestive cardiac failure (CCF) [11]. In this landmark paper they examined the relationship between the cumulative probability of developing CCF and the total cumulative dose of doxorubicin. They have reviewed these data and those of other workers [12] and state that the overall reported frequency of doxorubicin cardiomyopathy ranges from 0.4 to 9% for patients receiving the drug on a variety of dosages and schedules. Total dose, schedule, age, pre-existing heart disease, prior mediastinal radiotherapy and possibly treatment with other cytotoxic drugs are risk factors for cardiomyopathy. For patients receiving a cumulative dose of doxorubicin of less than $550\,mg/m^2$ the incidence of congestive cardiac failure ranged from 0.1 to 1.2%. About 30% of patients who received more than $550\,mg/m^2$ (range $560–1155\,mg/m^2$) developed CCF. From their own study [11] it was clear that, although this was true, there was a continuum of increasing risk of CCF with increasing dose of doxorubicin, but there was no absolute cut-off point that should not be exceeded in any circumstances within this dose range. This has led them to suggest that in circumstances where there is a therapeutic indication to exceed a total dose of $550\,mg/m^2$, cardiac investigations may assist the physician in deciding whether to continue with administration of the drug.

## Assessment of cardiomyopathy

Right ventricular endomyocardial biopsy has already been described. The criteria of Billingham *et al.* [3] may be applied to assign patients to risk categories. If a further $100\,mg/m^2$ of doxorubicin above the dose of $550\,mg/m^2$ is administered, the risk of CCF is 3.2%, 12.5% and 45% respectively in risk categories 1, 2 and 3 (see Table 13.1).

**Table 13.1 Pathologic grades of myocardial toxicity due to anthracyclines**

| Grade | Features |
|---|---|
| 0 | Normal |
| 1 | Scanty early myofibrillar loss and/or distended sarcoplasmic reticulum |
| 2 | Groups of cells with marked myofibrillar loss and/or cytoplasmic vacuolization |
| 3 | Diffuse cell damage with total loss of contractile elements, loss of organelles, mitochondrial and nuclear degeneration |

Adapted from Billingham *et al.* [3]

However, this approach is not widely applicable and suffers from the disadvantage that it may miss severe myocardial damage in those patients in whom it develops at cumulative dosages well below $550\,mg/m^2$.

Serial chest X-rays, cardiac enzymes and electrocardiograms are all unreliable ways of predicting the development of CCF and are only likely to become consistently abnormal when the patient is in established heart failure [12]. For this reason they cannot be recommended.

Radionuclide angiography (MUGA scanning) is generally agreed to be the most sensitive way of detecting subclinical cardiac failure. The method is widely available and can be used serially to monitor patients receiving repeated courses of doxorubicin. Schwartz and co-workers [14] have reported guidelines for monitoring which are summarized in Table 13.2. McKillop *et al.* [15] from Stanford University have published a more complex monitoring scheme which employs radionuclide scanning, exercise testing and cardiac catheterization.

The work of both Schwartz and McKillop clearly demonstrates that to minimize the risk of doxorubicin-related CCF, cardiac function must be monitored; the use of empirical 'safe' dose limits is dangerous and inappropriate. Even when functional monitoring is employed a few patients will develop

**Table 13.2 Guidelines for monitoring patients receiving doxorubicin, using radionuclide angiography (MUGA scanning)**

| Findings | Action |
|---|---|
| Normal baseline LVEF (50% or greater) No risk factors | Determine second LVEF after $250–300\,mg/m^2$ and again at $450\,mg/m^2$. Sequential studies then done before each subsequent dose |
| Normal baseline LVEF Risk factors – heart disease, abnormal ECG, radiation, cyclophosphamide | Determine second LVEF after $250–300\,mg/m^2$ and again at $400\,mg/m^2$. Sequential studies then done before each subsequent dose |

Discontinue treatment if there is an absolute decrease in LVEF of 10% or more, or a decline to 50% or less.

| | |
|---|---|
| Abnormal baseline LVEF | Sequential studies before each dose |

Discontinue treatment if there is an absolute decrease of LVEF of 10% or more and/or a final LVEF of 30% or less.

From Schwartz *et al.* [14]

CCF and the risk of this is far greater if rule-of-thumb only dosage schemes are employed. Furthermore, some patients who would benefit from further therapy will be underdosed.

## Daunorubicin

Daunorubicin is used almost exclusively in the treatment of the acute leukaemias. From the standpoint of cardiac toxicity it can be regarded as virtually identical with doxorubicin although there have been relatively fewer patients subjected to extensive pathological and physiological studies than those receiving doxorubicin [12]. Of interest are the observations that elderly patients [16,17] and young children [18] may be more likely to develop daunorubicin-induced CCF and the suggestion that patients receiving high doses over short time periods are more likely to develop CCF than those receiving the drug at slower dose rates [19]. Daunorubicin has also been implicated in the development of pericarditis with acute myocarditis in young patients at low cumulative doses in the range of $60$–$180\,mg/m^2$, leading to CCF and death [20,21]. For what it is worth the cumulative 'safe dose' of daunorubicin has been stated to be $600\,mg/m^2$.

## Idarubicin

Idarubicin is 4-demethoxydaunorubicin. It can be given orally or intravenously and has been mostly investigated in the treatment of acute leukaemia. In mice it has been shown to be less cardiotoxic than other anthracyclines and in phase II trials, summarized by Weiss and others [22], it has exhibited a marked absence of cardiotoxicity although occasional CCF and reduction in LVEF have been observed in patients previously treated with other anthracyclines. It is most commonly used at a dose of $45\,mg/m^2$ over 3 days every 3 weeks. Few patients have received a total dose of more than $200\,mg/m^2$. At present there is not enough clinical data on previously untreated patients to conclude that idarubicin is less cardiotoxic than daunorubicin or doxorubicin given in equivalently tumouricidal doses.

## Epirubicin

Epirubicin is 4'-epidoxorubicin, differing from doxorubicin in the epimerization of the hydroxyl group in the 4' position of the aminosugar daunosamine. Its mechanism of action is similar to that of doxorubin but it has been shown to be less cardiotoxic dose for dose than doxorubicin in experimental animals [23,24]. In clinical studies, predominantly in patients with advanced breast cancer, it has been shown to produce life-threatening cardiac toxicity at

doses around $1000\,mg/m^2$ compared with $550\,mg/m^2$ for doxorubicin [16,25].

In the study by Jain *et al.* [25], 54 patients with advanced breast cancer who had failed prior non-anthracycline containing treatment were randomized to receive either epirubicin $85\,mg/m^2$ or doxorubicin $60\,mg/m^2$ intravenously every 3 weeks. The antitumour response rate was the same (25%) in each patient group. Cardiotoxicity was monitored by radionuclide scanning. The median doses to the development of cardiac toxicity, defined as a decrease in resting left ventricular ejection fraction of more than 10% from baseline value or 5% or more with exercise, were $935\,mg/m^2$ for epirubicin and $468\,mg/m^2$ for doxorubicin. Four patients treated with epirubicin and five treated with doxorubicin developed CCF. The mean cumulative doses at which CCF developed were $1134\,mg/m^2$ for epirubicin and $492\,mg/m^2$ for doxorubicin. This study suggests that although the equitherapeutic dose of epirubicin is 40% greater than that of doxorubicin, the equitoxic dose is approximately 100% greater, which leaves a therapeutic 'window' of safety for epirubicin.

A later study by the Italian Multicentre Breast Study [26] compared epirubicin $50\,mg/m^2$ or doxorubicin $50\,mg/m^2$ in combination with fluorouracil and cyclophosphamide for the treatment of breast cancer. There was no difference in response rate or survival in the two arms but there was one case of CCF in the epirubicin-containing arm compared with four in patients receiving doxorubicin. This again suggests that, at least in breast cancer, epirubicin is as effective as doxorubicin while less cardiotoxic.

What is not clear is whether epirubicin is superior to doxorubicin in the treatment of other tumours such as lymphomas, lung cancer, leukaemia, ovarian cancer and soft tissue sarcomas since, although it has been used in these settings, the equitherapeutic doses for these tumours are not established. Endomyocardial biopsy has been used to assess the relative toxicity of doxorubicin and epirubicin by Torti *et al.* [27]. They showed that milligram for milligram epirubicin caused less endomyocardial injury than doxorubicin, although the pattern of endomyocardial damage caused by both drugs was the same. On the basis of the available evidence epirubicin is less toxic than doxorubicin at equal doses. What is still not clear is the therapeutic efficacy of the former drug or its optimal combination and scheduling, so that whether it can replace doxorubicin in all therapeutic settings is still to be determined.

## Mitoxantrone

Mitoxantrone is an anthraquinone which binds to DNA and RNA by intercalation like doxorubicin

[28,29]. It is structurally related to doxorubicin but lacks an aminosugar moiety [30,31]. It causes DNA breakage by stabilizing a complex formed between DNA and topoisomerase II [32,33]. In the clinic it is active against leukaemia, breast cancer, lymphomas and possibly myeloma. Since mitoxantrone is structurally similar to doxorubicin it might be expected to possess myocardial toxicity and this has proved to be the case, although there is an impression, which needs to be further investigated, that it is less clinically cardiotoxic than doxorubicin in the doses that are currently employed.

In beagle dogs treated with mitoxantrone or doxorubicin the doxorubicin-treated group showed low voltage QRS abnormalities on ECG and the animals died of CCF whereas the mitoxantrone-treated group showed no evidence of this [34]. Similarly, a beagle study in which endomyocardial biopsies were examined showed the typical changes due to doxorubicin whereas mitoxantrone led to dilatation of the sarcoplasmic reticulum without other ultrastructural changes [35]. Other animal studies have demonstrated cardiac damage due to mitoxantrone [36].

In an interesting study by Gray and Novak [37] mitoxantrone was shown to inhibit the rate of doxorubicin-stimulated oxygen consumption while the same group have shown that it is a potent antioxidant that inhibits both basal and drug-induced peroxidation of lipids [38]. These observations would lead to the prediction that mitoxantrone should produce less cardiac damage than doxorubicin if free radical formation and lipid peroxidation are important in the production of cardiotoxicity [7].

In the clinic mitoxantrone has shown evidence of cardiotoxicity although this has only been seen in a relatively small proportion of patients. Previous exposure to doxorubicin increases the risk of cardiac complications as does prior mediastinal irradiation or prior cardiovascular disease. For a full review of the therapeutic usefulness of mitoxantrone and its cardiac and other side effects the reader is referred to the paper by Shenkenberg and Von Hoff [39].

## Prevention of anthracycline-related cardiotoxicity

Dose limitation as a means of preventing cardiotoxicity has already been dealt with. Notions of 'safe dose' are inherently unsatisfactory since they lead to the overdosing of patients who are particularly susceptible such as the very young, the old, the previously irradiated and those with underlying heart disease, while those patients who could benefit from higher doses without sustaining unacceptable cardiac damage may be underdosed. Empirical dosing must, therefore, be combined with monitor-

ing of the type advocated by Schwartz and listed in Table 13.2.

Scheduling of anthracyclines may reduce cardiotoxicity. Thus Legha *et al.* [40] have shown that prolonged continuous intravenous infusion of doxorubicin reduced cardiotoxicity while Torti *et al.* [41] have demonstrated that weekly compared with 3-weekly scheduling allowed greater doses of doxorubicin to be given.

This is an area of cancer therapeutics which will repay further investigation and which needs to be done for the newer anthracyclines as well as the original ones.

## Cardioprotection

Attempts to protect the heart against the toxic effects of anthracyclines have been made with many compounds. These include prednisone [42] and digoxin [42,43], coenzyme Q10, an enzyme required for oxidative metabolism [44], vitamin E (free radical scavenger) [45], *N*-acetyl cysteine (glutathione-like free radical protector), liposome encapsulation of the drug [46] and calcium channel blockade (to block intracellular transport). None of these approaches has shown convincing cardioprotection in well-designed clinical trials.

The most promising cardioprotective compound is ICRF 187. This is a bispiperazinedione which is hydrolysed intracellularly to form a bidentate chelator resembling EDTA. It was shown to protect against daunorubicin- and doxorubicin-induced cardiomyopathy in laboratory animals when the drugs were given within a short time of one another and in a clinical study by Speyer *et al.* [47] it has been tested in a randomized trial in 92 women with advanced breast cancer.

Patients were randomized to receive either fluorouracil, doxorubicin and cyclophosphamide or this combination preceded 30 min before by the administration of ICRF 187, 1000 mg/m$^2$ intravenously over 15 min. Treatments were repeated at 3-weekly intervals. There was no difference in anti-tumour effect or survival between the two arms of the study, but in the group receiving ICRF 187 there was a reduction in the number of patients who developed CCF (2 versus 11). The mean decrease in left ventricular ejection fraction was reduced when the cumulative dose of doxorubicin was 250–399 mg/m$^2$ (1% versus 7%, $P=0.02$), 400–499 mg/m$^2$ (1% versus 16%, $P=0.001$) and 500–599 mg/m$^2$ (3% versus 16%, $P=0.003$). The Billingham biopsy score was two or more in five of 13 patients not receiving ICRF 187 ($P=0.03$).

This study provides highly suggestive, albeit not conclusive, evidence that ICRF 187 is cardioprotective against doxorubicin without protecting the breast cancer. Further studies on larger numbers of patients and those with other tumours are clearly indicated.

## Management of anthracycline-related cardiomyopathy

There is no specific treatment for anthracycline-related cardiomyopathy. Conventional treatment with digoxin, diuretics and vasodilators may lead to improvement of cardiac function and should be pursued vigorously. Stabilization of cardiac function can occur [4,48,49]; younger patients with intractable heart failure have successfully received cardiac transplants.

## Anthracycline-induced pericarditis

A rare complication of the use of daunorubicin and doxorubicin in young adults is the pericarditis-myocarditis syndrome [41]. It occurs at low cumulative doses in the range 60–180 mg/m$^2$ and is seen within 3 weeks of the administration of the drug. The patients have no previous history of heart disease and the onset is sudden being characterized by arrhythmias associated with severe congestive cardiac failure often leading to death. Autopsy reveals acute inflammatory changes in the epimyocardium and pericardium [50]. The mechanism of the development of this syndrome is unknown.

## Alkylating agents

The alkylating agents include cyclophosphamide, ifosfamide, nitrogen mustard, melphalan, chlorambucil, busulphan, thiotepa and mitomycin C. Most are not associated with significant cardiac toxicity although there are case reports of endomyocardial fibrosis in a patient treated with busulphan [51], radiation-like injury in patients treated with mitomycin C [52] and arrhythmias due to nitrogen mustard in high dose [53]. The use of chlorambucil, thiotepa and melphalan, even in very high doses (when given alone), has not been linked to cardiac toxicity.

## Cyclophosphamide

Until the use of very high-dose chemotherapy, often associated with the concomitant use of other drugs in high dose or irradiation with or without autologous or allogeneic bone marrow transplantation, cyclophosphamide was not associated with cardiac injury. Since its use in this setting a characteristic syndrome has been observed in a small proportion of patients [54–57]. This is characterized by the development of acute congestive cardiac failure with a pericardial effusion, occurring within 2 weeks of the administration of doses of 90–270 mg/kg of cyclophosphamide. The clinical picture is one of an acute cardiomyopathy although cardiac tamponade may also be a feature. With energetic treatment, including pericardial drainage, the condition may resolve completely leaving no sign of residual cardiac damage but in most patients the heart failure is intractable and leads to death.

The risk of developing the syndrome is increased by irradiation and other drugs, particularly carmustine (BCNU), given concomitantly and possibly by prior exposure to anthracyclines.

At autopsy the findings are an acute haemorrhagic myocarditis with necrosis associated with pericarditis and bloodstained pericardial effusion [54–58]. It is thought that cyclophosphamide exerts its toxic effect upon the vascular endothelium of the myocardium leading to massive endomyocardial haemorrhage.

It is of interest that this toxic effect has not been seen clinically with the closely related drug ifosfamide.

## Other drugs

The vinca alkaloids vincristine, vinblastine and vindesine have very rarely been associated with the development of ischaemic changes and myocardial infarction [59–62]. A drug more commonly implicated in the genesis of angina pectoris and myocardial infarction is 5-fluorouracil (5-FU) [63, 64, 65]. As with the vinca alkaloids there is sometimes a history of previous heart disease or cardiac irradiation, but in some patients there is no previous history of any cardiac abnormality. The symptoms of angina usually develop some hours after administration of the drug but the time course may be very variable ranging from minutes to days later. The administration of coronary artery vasodilators has sometimes relieved the angina. In view of the frequency of myocardial infarction in patients who develop 5-FU-associated angina (approximately 20%) the drug should be discontinued if this symptom develops.

Etoposide [66] has been reported to be associated with a myocardial infarction in a 27-year-old woman with Hodgkin's disease who had received previous mediastinal radiotherapy and MOPP (mechlorethamine, vincristine (Oncovin), procarbazine and prednisone), so it is impossible to judge whether the drug was responsible.

Finally, *m*-AMSA (amsacrine) [67] has been shown in children to be associated with fatal congestive cardiac failure in four out of 25 patients who had previously received anthracycline therapy, and with echocardiographic evidence of diminished left ventricular function in a much higher proportion

(64%). Since *m*-AMSA has a mode of action similar to anthracyclines, it is clearly very important to monitor its cardiac effects with the greatest care in patients who have received previous anthracycline therapy. The incidence of CCF in previously untreated patients is stated by Torti and Lum [68] to be none out of 683 compared with 0.2% in patients previously treated with other drugs, mostly anthracyclines.

## Conclusions

Cardiac toxicity from cytotoxic drugs is a serious problem mainly for those patients receiving anthracyclines and high-dose cyclophosphamide. Cardiac monitoring is essential in these patients and there is a pressing need to reduce anthracycline-related cardiotoxicity either through the development of less cardiotoxic analogues or more effective cardioprotective agents. There is early evidence that this goal is beginning to be achieved but there is still a long way to go before toxicity to the heart ceases to be a problem in cancer chemotherapy.

## References


1. Minow, R.A., Benjamin, R.S. and Gottlieb, J.A. Adriamycin (NSC-123127) cardiomyopathy. An overview with determination of risk factors. *Cancer Chemotherapy Reports*, **6**, 195–201 (1975)
2. Cortes, E.P., Lutman, G., Wanka, J. *et al.* Adriamycin (NSC-123127) cardiotoxicity: a clinicopathologic correlation. *Cancer Chemotherapy Reports*, **6**, 215–225 (1975)
3. Billingham, M.E., Mason, J.W., Bristow, M.R. and Daniels, M.R. Anthracycline cardiomyopathy monitored by morphologic changes. *Cancer Treatment Reports*, **62**, 865–872 (1978)
4. Bristow, M.R., Mason, J.W., Billingham, M.E. and Daniels, J.R. Doxorubicin cardiomyopathy: evaluation by phonocardiography, endomyocardial biopsy and cardiac catheterisation. *Annals of Internal Medicine*, **88**, 168–175 (1978)
5. Bachur, N.R., Gordon, S.L. and Gee, M.V. Anthracycline antibiotic augmentation of microsomal electron transport and free radical formation. *Molecular Pharmacology*, **13**, 901–910 (1977)
6. Sato, S., Iwaizumi, M., Handa, K. *et al.* Electron spin resonance study on the mode of generation of free-radicals of daunomycin, Adriamycin and carboquone in NAD(P)H-microsome systems. *Gann*, **68**, 603–608 (1977)
7 Meyers, C.E., Liss, R.H., Ifrim, J. *et al.* The role of lipid peroxidation on cardiac toxicity and tumour response. *Science*, **197**, 165–167 (1977)
8. Thomas, C.E. and Aust, S.D. Release of iron from ferritin by cardiotoxic anthracycline antibiotics. *Archives of Biochemistry and Biophysics*, **246**, 684–689 (1986)
9. Gutteridge, J.M.C. Lipid peroxidation and possible hydroxyl radical formation stimulated by self-reduction of a doxorubicin–iron(III) complex. *Biochemical Pharmacology*, **33**, 1725–1728 (1984)
10. Bachur, N.R., Gordon, S.L. and Gee, M.V. A general mechanism for microsomal activation of quinone anticancer agents to free radicals. *Cancer Research*, **38**, 1745–1750 (1978)
11. Von Hoff, D.D., Layard, M.W., Basa, P. *et al.* Risk factors for doxorubicin-induced congestive heart failure. *Annals of Internal Medicine*, **91**, 710–717 (1979)
12. Tokaz, L.K. and Von Hoff, D.D. The cardiotoxicity of anticancer agents. In *Toxicity of Chemotherapy* (eds M.C. Perry and J.W. Yarbro), Grune and Stratton, Orlando, pp. 199–226 (1984)
13. Bristow, M.R., Lopez, M.B., Mason, J.W. *et al.* Efficacy and cost of cardiac monitoring in patients receiving doxorubicin. *Cancer*, **50**, 32–41 (1982)
14. Schwartz, R.G., McKenzie, W.B., Alexander, J. *et al.* Congestive heart failure and left ventricular dysfunction complicating doxorubicin therapy. Seven-year experience using radionuclide angiography. *American Journal of Medicine*, **82**, 1109–1118 (1987)
15. McKillop, J.H., Bristow, M.R., Goris, M.L. *et al.* Sensitivity and specificity of radionuclide ejection fractions in doxorubicin cardiotoxicity. *American Heart Journal*, **106**, 1048–1056 (1983)
16. Bonadonna, G. and Monfardini, S. Cardiac toxicity of daunorubicin. *Lancet*, **i**, 837 (1969)
17. Malpas, J.S. and Scott, R.B. Daunorubicin in acute myelocytic leukaemia. *Lancet*, **i**, 469–470 (1969)
18. Von Hoff, D.D., Rozencweig, M., Layard, M. *et al.* Daunomycin-induced cardiotoxicity in children and adults: a review of 110 cases. *American Journal of Medicine*, **62**, 200–208 (1977)
19. Wiernik, P.H., Schimpff, S.C., Schiffer, C.A. *et al.* Randomised clinical comparison of daunorubicin (NSC 82151) alone with a combination of daunorubicin, cytosine arabinoside, 6-thioguanine and 6-pyrimethamine for the treatment of acute non-lymphocytic leukaemia. *Cancer Treatment Reports*, **60**, 41–53 (1976)
20. Harrison, D.T. and Sanders, L.A. Pericarditis in a case of early daunorubicin cardiomyopathy. *Annals of Internal Medicine*, **85**, 339–340 (1976)
21. Bristow, M.R., Billingham, M.R., Mason, J.W. *et al.* Clinical spectrum of anthracycline cardiotoxicity. *Cancer Treatment Reports*, **62**, 873–879 (1978)
22. Weiss, G.R., Arteaga, C.L., Bailes, J.S. *et al.* New anticancer agents. In *Cancer Chemotherapy and Biological Response Modifiers Annual 10* (eds H.M. Pinedo, D.L. Longo and B.A. Chabner), Elsevier, Amsterdam, p. 93, (1988)
23. Casazza, A.M. Experimental evaluation of anthra-

cycline analogs. *Cancer Treatment Reports,* **63**, 835–844 (1979)

24. Casazza, A.M., Di Marco, A., Bonadonna, G. *et al.* Effect of modifications in position 4 of the chromophore or position 4′ of the aminosugar, on the antitumour activity and toxicity of daunorubicin and doxorubicin. In *Anthracyclines: Current Status and New Development* (eds S.T. Crooke and S.D. Reich), Academic, San Diego, pp. 403–430 (1980)

25. Jain, K.K., Casper, E.S., Geller, N.L. *et al.* A prospective randomised comparison of epirubicin and doxorubicin in patients with advanced breast cancer. *Journal of Clinical Oncology,* **3**, 818–826 (1985)

26. Italian Multicentre Breast Study with Epirubicin. Phase III randomised study of fluorouracil, epirubicin and cyclophosphamide v. fluorouracil, doxorubicin and cyclophosphamide in advanced breast cancer: an Italian multicentre trial. *Journal of Clinical Oncology,* **6**, 976–982 (1988)

27. Torti, F., Bristow, M.M., Lum, B.L. *et al.* Cardiotoxicity of epirubicin and doxorubicin: assessment by endomyocardial biopsy. *Cancer Research,* **46**, 3722–3727 (1986)

28. Traganos, F., Evenson, D.P., Staiano-Coico, L. *et al.* Action of dihydroxyanthraquinone on cell cycle progression and survival of a variety of cultured mammalian cells. *Cancer Research,* **40**, 671–680 (1980)

29. Lown, J.W., Hanstock, C.C., Bradley, R.D. and Scraba, D.G. Interactions of the antitumour agents mitoxantrone and bisantrene with deoxyribonucleic acids studied by electron microscopy. *Molecular Pharmacology,* **25**, 178–184 (1984)

30. Johnson, R.K., Zee-Cheng, R.K-Y., Lee, W.W. *et al.* Experimental antitumour activity of amino anthraquinones. *Cancer Treatment Reports,* **63**, 425–439 (1979)

31. Trissel, I.L.A., Davignon, J.P., Kleinman, L.M. *et al. NCI Investigational Drugs – Pharmaceutical Data 1985.* NIH Publication No. 82-2141, US Department of Health and Human Services, Bethesda, Maryland, pp. 165–166 (1985)

32. Nelson, E.M., Tewey, K.M. and Liu, L.F. Mechanism of antitumour drug action: poisoning of mammalian DNA topoisomerase II on DNA by 4′-(9-acridinylamino)-methansulfon-*m*-anisidide. *Proceedings of the National Academy of Sciences of USA,* **81**, 1361–1365 (1984)

33. Tewey, K.M., Rowe, T.C., Yang, L. *et al.* Adriamycin-induced DNA damage is mediated by mammalian DNA topoisomerase II. *Science,* **226**, 466–468 (1984)

34. Henderson, B.M., Dougherty, W.J., James, V.C. *et al.* Safety assessment of a new anticancer compound, mitoxantrone, in beagle dogs: comparison with doxorubicin. I. Clinical observations. *Cancer Treatment Reports,* **66**, 1139–1143 (1982)

35. Sparano, B.M., Gordon, G., Hall, C. *et al.* Safety assessment of a new anticancer compound, mitoxantrone, in beagle dogs. Comparison with doxorubicin. II. Histologic and ultrastructural pathology. *Cancer Treatment Reports,* **66**, 1145–1148 (1982)

36. Perkins, W.E., Schroeder, R.L., Carrano, R.A. and Imondi, A.R. Myocardial effects of mitoxantrone and doxorubicin in the mouse and guinea pig. *Cancer Treatment Reports,* **68**, 841 (1984)

37. Gray, M.A. and Novak, R.F. Comparative studies of the antioxidant properties of mitoxantrone, ametantrone and bisantrene (abstract). *Proceedings of the American Association of Cancer Research,* **26**, 223 (1985)

38. Novak, R.F. and Kharasch, E.D. Mitoxantrone: propensity for free radical formation and lipid peroxidation – implications for cardiotoxicity. *Investigational New Drugs,* **3**, 95–99 (1985)

39. Shenkenberg, T.D. and Von Hoff, D.D. Mitoxantrone: a new anticancer agent with significant clinical activity. *Annals of Internal Medicine,* **105**, 67–81 (1986)

40. Legha, S., Benjamin, R., MacKay, B. *et al.* Reduction of doxorubicin cardiotoxicity by prolonged continuous intravenous injection. *Annals of Internal Medicine,* **96**, 113–119 (1982)

41. Torti, F.M., Bristow, M.R., Howes, A.E. *et al.* Reduced cardiotoxicity of doxorubicin delivered on a weekly schedule: assessment by endomyocardial biopsy. *Annals of Internal Medicine,* **99**, 745–749 (1983)

42. Gupta, M., Cortes, E.P. and Mundia, A. Systolic time interval (STI) in adriamycin (ADM) treated patients on digoxin or prednisone cardioprophylaxis (abstract). *Proceedings of the American Society for Cancer Research and ASCO,* **17**, 269 (1976)

43. Williams, C.J. Doxorubicin cardiotoxicity: role of digoxin in prevention (letter). *British Medical Journal,* **i**, 176 (1978)

44. Cortes, E.P., Gupta, M., Chou, C. *et al.* Adriamycin cardiotoxicity: early detection by systolic time interval and possible prevention by coenzyme Q10. *Cancer Treatment Reports,* **62**, 887–891 (1978)

45. Legha, S., Benjamin, R., Wang, Ȳ. *et al.* Evaluation of 2-tocopherol against Adriamycin cardiotoxicity in humans (abstract). *Proceedings of the American Association for Cancer Research,* **21**, 176 (1981)

46. Olson, F., Mayhew, E., Maslow, D. *et al.* Characterisation, toxicity and therapeutic efficacy of Adriamycin encapsulated in liposomes. *European Journal of Cancer and Clinical Oncology,* **18**, 167–176 (1982)

47. Speyer, J.L., Green, M.D., Kramer, E. *et al.* Protective effect of the bispiperazinedione ICRF-187 against doxorubicin-induced cardiac toxicity in women with advanced breast cancer. *New England Journal of Medicine,* **319**, 745–752 (1988)

48. Gottdeiner, J.S., Mathisen, D.J., Borer, J.S. *et al.* Doxorubicin cardiotoxicity: assessment of late left ventricular dysfunction by radionuclide cineangiography. *Annals of Internal Medicine,* **94**, 430–435 (1981)

49. Friedman, J.J., Ewy, G.A., Jones, S.E. *et al.* 1-year

follow up of cardiac status after adriamycin therapy. *Cancer Treatment Reports,* **63**, 1809–1816 (1979)

50. Bristow, M.R., Billingham, M.E., Mason, J.W. *et al.* Clinical spectrum of anthracycline antibiotic cardiotoxicity. *Cancer Treatment Reports,* **62**, 873–879 (1978)

51. Weinberger, A., Pinkhas, J., Sandbank, V. *et al.* Endocardial fibrosis following busulfan treatment (abstract). *Journal of the American Medical Association,* **231**, 495 (1975)

52. Ravry, M.J.R. Cardiotoxicity of mitomycin C in man and animals (letter). *Cancer Treatment Reports,* **63**, 555 (1979)

53. Hartmann, D.W., Robinson, W.A., Mangauk, A. *et al.* Unanticipated side effects from treatment with high dose mechlorethamine in patients with malignant melanoma. *Cancer Treatment Reports,* **65**, 327–328 (1981)

54. Applebaum, F.R., Strauchen, J.A., Graw, R.G. *et al.* Acute lethal carditis caused by high dose combination chemotherapy: a unique clinical and pathological entity. *Lancet,* **i**, 58–67 (1967)

55. Goldberg, M.A., Antin, J.H., Guinan, E.C. and Rappeport, J.M. Cyclophosphamide cardiotoxicity: an analysis of dose as a risk factor. *Blood,* **68**, 1114–1118 (1986)

56. Gottdiener, J.S., Applebaum, F.R., Ferrens, V.J. *et al.* Cardiotoxicity associated with high dose cyclophosphamide therapy. *Archives of Internal Medicine,* **141**, 758–763 (1981)

57. Trigg, M.E., Finlay, J.L., Bozdech, M. *et al.* Fatal cardiac toxicity in bone marrow transplant patients receiving cytosine arabinoside, cyclophosphamide and total body irradiation. *Cancer,* **59**, 38–42 (1987)

58. Steinherz, I.J., Steinherz, P.G., Margia-Casale, D. *et al.* Cardiac changes with cyclophosphamide. *Medical and Pediatric Oncology,* **9**, 417–422 (1981)

59. Harris, A.L. and Wong, C. Myocardial ischaemia, radiotherapy and vinblastine. *Lancet,* **i**, 787 (1981)

60. Mandel, E.M., Lewinski, U. and Djaletti, M. Vincristine-induced myocardial infarction. *Cancer,* **36**, 1979–1982 (1975)

61. Somers, G., Abramow, M., Wittek, M. *et al.* Myocardial infarction: a complication of vincristine treatment? *Lancet,* **ii**, 690 (1976)

62. Yancey, R.S. and Talpaz, M. Vindesine-associated angina and ECG changes. *Cancer Treatment Reports,* **66**, 587–589 (1982)

63. Dent, R.G. and McColl, I. 5-fluorouracil and angina. *Lancet,* **i**, 347–348 (1975)

64. Labianca, R., Beretta, G., Clerici, M. *et al.* Cardiac toxicity of 5-fluorouracil: a study on 1083 patients. *Tumori,* **68**, 505–510 (1982)

65. Burger, A.J. and Mannino, S. 5-fluorouracil-induced coronary vasospasm. *American Heart Journal,* **114**, 433–436 (1987)

66. Schechter, J.P. and Jones, S.E. Myocardial infarction in a 27-year-old woman: possible complication of treatment with VP16-213, mediastinal irradiation, or both. *Cancer Chemotherapy Reports,* **59**, 887–888 (1975)

67. Steinherz, L.J., Steinherz, P.G., Mangiacasale, D. *et al.* Cardiac abnormalities after AMSA administration. *Cancer Treatment Reports,* **66**, 483–488 (1982)

68. Torti, F.L. and Lum, B.L. Cardiac toxicity. In *Cancer: Principles and Practice of Oncology* (eds V.T. De Vita, S. Hellman and S.A. Rosenberg), J.B. Lippincott, Philadelphia, pp. 2153–2162 (1969)

# 14

# Renal and genitourinary system morbidity of radiotherapy

**M.E.C. Robbins and J.W. Hopewell**

## Introduction

It is now well recognized that radiotherapy for abdominal tumours is frequently limited by the adverse reactions of the normal tissues included within the treatment volume. This fact was not readily appreciated in early studies. Although experimental evidence as to the deleterious effects of radiation on the kidney was reported as early as 1904 [1], such data were largely ignored. Indeed, statements such as that by McQuarrie and Whipple [2]: 'We feel confident that the clinician may use the X-rays over the kidney areas with confidence that renal tissue is resistant to the hard Roentgen rays' implied no clinical problems associated with renal irradiation. There was however, some disagreement. It was inferred, from experimental results [3], that patients who either had some impairment of renal function, or whose kidneys were 'under special strain' should not be treated with radiation or should be followed-up closely after X-ray exposure. Not until the excellent experimental studies by Hartman, Bolliger and Doub [4,5] was it appreciated that renal tissue was indeed radiosensitive. This was confirmed in their later clinical report [6].

Any radiotherapeutic procedure in which renal tissue is included within the treatment volume carries with it the potential risk of radiation-induced damage to the kidney. In children the most common tumours are Wilms' tumour or nephroblastoma; this may require irradiation of the total renal mass. Paediatric patients with neuroblastoma, or peritoneal involvement with rhabdomyosarcoma, may also require abdominal irradiation. The treatment of Hodgkin's lymphoma in adults may require abdominal, stomach or spleen irradiation, where one or both kidneys could be in the treatment volume. The irradiation of both kidneys may also occur in the treatment of ovarian carcinoma or seminoma. Radiation therapy for the treatment of pancreatic cancer requires the inclusion of a portion of one or both kidneys in the treatment volume. More recently, the development of total body irradiation (TBI) for bone marrow ablation, as a prerequisite to bone marrow transplantation (BMT) for treatment of leukaemias has produced another radiotherapeutic procedure in which radiation-induced damage to the kidney may produce adverse, potentially dose-limiting reactions.

As with the kidney, there are a number of clinical situations in which radiotherapy may result in radiation damage to the urinary tract. Treatment of advanced carcinoma of the cervix with intracavitary irradiation will result in irradiation of the base of the bladder. Similarly, radiotherapeutic treatment of anorectal carcinoma may well include the bladder in the treatment volume during at least part of the irradiation. Radical external irradiation will inevitably result in a high dose to the bladder base. Although endometrial carcinoma is usually treated surgically, advanced cases may be treated by external radiotherapy together with intracavitary caesium, with a resultant high dose to part of the bladder. In all these situations the urinary tract damage induced by radiotherapy will limit the total dose that can be safely applied.

## The kidney

### Clinical pattern of radiation-induced damage to the kidney

Probably the first report of radiation-induced renal damage in a patient appeared in 1927. Domagk [7] described a 9-year-old girl who received abdominal irradiation for tuberculous mesenteric lymph nodes; she died 6 months later with symptoms of renal

reviewed previously [8,9]. Radiation-induced alterations in the vasculature, tubules and glomeruli have all been highlighted. The degeneration and sclerosis of small arteries and arterioles with secondary tubular degeneration were observed in the rat [50,51]. In contrast Warren [52] stated that the tubules were preferentially damaged by radiation. This statement was supported by Davey, Hamilton and Steele [53] who suggested that the proximal and distal convoluted tubules were more sensitive to radiation than the glomeruli. A number of experimental observations support this suggestion [54–56].

Zuelzer, Palmer and Newton [14] described different stages of both glomerular and tubular damage in children who had died 3–7 months after radiotherapy. These ranged from complete scarring and glomerular obliteration to early degenerative changes and acute tubular necrosis, indicative of recurrent renal injury. The glomerular lesions consisted of endothelial cell damage, basement membrane thickening, obstruction of capillary loops by eosinophilic material, and focal necrosis. Glomerular changes have consistently been reported in more recent clinical cases [57–61]. These have shown an increase in the mesangial cells and matrix, and thickening and splitting of the glomerular capillary walls leading eventually to necrosis. EM studies have revealed a marked widening of the subendothelial space as a result of the deposition of amorphous fluffy material. This material may be produced by the damaged endothelial cells [58], or could represent aggregated blood proteins that had accumulated under the damaged endothelial cells [61]. Similar glomerular changes have been observed in experimental studies [62,63]. Thus these findings would appear to suggest that the glomerulus, and particularly the endothelial cell, is the primary site of radiation damage.

The results of an extensive series of studies in the rat by Madrazo *et al.* [62–64] have suggested that both glomerular endothelial cells and tubular epithelial cells were equally radiosensitive. Glomerular endothelial cells exhibited cytoplasmic degeneration, detachment from the basement membrane with collapse of the capillary lumina, and a marked tortuosity of the basement membrane. Epithelial tubular cells showed degenerative changes, with atrophic collapsed tubules and areas of necrosis. In contrast to earlier studies these findings indicated a lack of vascular damage in the initial stages; vascular damage was a late effect.

In view of these differing histological observations it is not surprising that the question of the mechanisms responsible for the development of radiation nephropathy remains unanswered. Rubin and Casarett [51] proposed that the principal lesion in radiation nephropathy was arteriolonephrosclerosis, with the vascular damage leading to vessel occlusion, ischaemia and *secondary* tubular degeneration.

It has been shown, however, that such arteriolar changes are an uncommon feature, arteriolar lesions being either less severe when compared with the tubular or the glomerular lesions [44], or even absent. It is unlikely that the tubular degeneration evident in radiation nephropathy is due primarily to ischaemia resulting from occlusion of large blood vessels. However, focal vascular effects could bring about a more generalized tubular lesion.

This apparent lack of a role for vascular injury in the pathogenesis of radiation nephropathy was cited by Withers, Mason and Thames [65]. They proposed that radiation nephropathy resulted from tubular cell depletion alone. This hypothesis was based on the assumption that since acute radiation effects resulted from the sterilization of rapidly dividing parenchymal cells, then the development of radiation nephropathy with its long latent period represented a similar but slower loss of parenchymal cells, i.e. the tubular epithelium. The cells of the proximal convoluted tubule do appear to be the most radioresponsive, with cell loss being evident within several weeks of irradiation [66,67]. An *in vivo* assay was developed which, it was claimed, measured the clonogenic cell survival of the tubule epithelial cells. The $D_0$ for these clonogens was estimated to be 1.5 Gy, a value similar to that found for other mammalian cells *in vivo* and *in vitro*. There are a number of points which militate against this proposal. It still remains to be proven that the tubules counted in this assay are truly regenerated tubules; they may simply represent persisting tubules. Moreover this proposal ignores the wealth of clinical and experimental reports showing glomerular damage either before or concomitant with the development of tubular damage. Thus, in addition to the tubular epithelium, the role of the glomerular endothelial cell should be considered.

The mechanism(s) by which damage to this cell results in subsequent radiation nephropathy remains ill-defined. It has been suggested that radiation causes endothelial cell swelling, resulting in capillary occlusion [68]. Keane *et al.* [59] were impressed by the similarity between the subendothelial accumulation of amorphous material found in radiation nephropathy and that reported in thrombocytopenic purpura and hameolytic uraemic syndrome, where intravascular coagulation may be important. They speculated that radiation-induced endothelial cell damage caused local activation of the coagulation system with subsequent thrombosis in the renal microvasculature. Later findings have supported this hypothesis [30,69]. More recently radiation-induced changes in eicosanoid metabolism have been noted. It has been shown that irradiation decreased endothelial epoprostenol (prostacyclin) production [70]: the resultant decrease in levels of epoprostenol, a potent vasodilator, may result in vasoconstriction. Thus radiation-induced endothelial cell damage may cause potential changes in capillary thrombosis and vasoconstriction, both leading to capillary occlusion. These occlusive changes will result in ischaemia and the secondary loss of tubular epithelial cells.

It is thus likely that radiation damages both tubular epithelial and glomerular endothelial cells. The resulting lesions will interact and further exacerbate the overall pathology. Associated with these changes will be the added complication of late vascular damage, resulting in a secondary ischaemic insult and the possible development of hypertension. Moreover, the progressive reduction in renal function, which is likely to be reflected in the progressive loss of nephrons, may lead to compensatory hyperfiltration by the remaining nephrons [71]. This itself causes glomerular damage due to increased capillary pressure and flow. Thus the kidney becomes locked in a pathogenic circle of increasing nephron loss and damage. The final result is the destruction of the renal parenchyma, glomerulosclerosis and fibrosis.

## Influence of dose fractionation on the radiation tolerance of the kidney

Clinically the kidney is regarded as a radiosensitive organ, a total dose of 20 Gy being considered the upper limit of radiation 'tolerance' [72]. This dose would appear to have been adopted somewhat arbitrarily, it being applied over a broad range of dose fractionation schedules. Experimental studies [73–80] have indicated that the kidney has an extensive capacity for repair of sublethal radiation damage. The size of the dose per fraction markedly influences the total tolerance dose. There is a marked increase in the tolerance dose with decreasing size of the dose per fraction.

In an attempt to predetermine the tolerance dose for normal tissues for differing fractionation regimens Ellis [81] proposed the Nominal Standard Dose (NSD) concept:

$$\text{Total dose} = \text{NSD } N^{0.24}\, T^{0.11}$$

where $N$ = fraction number and $T$ = overall treatment time. It has been shown experimentally [82] that the NSD formula does not accurately predict the variation in total radiation dose with dose fraction. With treatment times of approximately 6 weeks, $N$ exponents of 0.4–0.5 have been obtained [73,76–80] (Figure 14.1). Shorter overall treatment times gave lower values of 0.2–0.3 [75,78,82] (Figure 14.1). Stewart *et al.* [80] showed that the size of the $N$ exponent declined as the fraction number increased. This, they stated, is what would be expected if the underlying cell survival curves for the target cell responsible for the development of renal damage were fitted by a linear

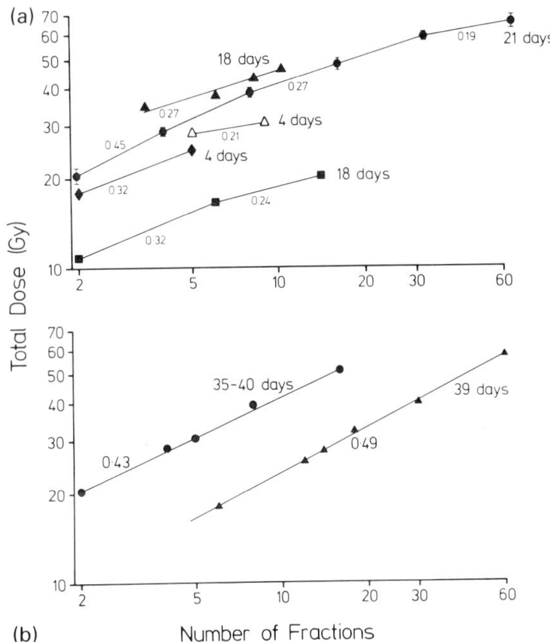


**Figure 14.1** Isoeffect plots for renal irradiation damage as a function of fraction number. The treatment time is given with the associated slope (fraction exponent): **a** the changes in isoeffect dose with fraction number for treatments given in 4–21 days (■—■ [76]; △8△, ▲—▲ [75]; ●—● [79]; ◆—◆ [78]); **b** the change in isoeffect dose with fraction number for treatments given in 35–40 days (●—● [78]; ◆—◆ [76] plus some previously unpublished data)

quadratic (LQ) model of cell survival. Thus renal fractionation data can be analysed using the LQ formula where the effect ($E$) produced by a dose per fraction ($d$) is such that $E = \alpha d + \beta d^2$ [83,84]. This equation allows determination of the $\alpha/\beta$ ratio, a direct measure of the extent of curvature on the underlying cell survival curve. Generally experimental renal fractionation data have been well described by the LQ model; the $\alpha/\beta$ ratio is 2–3 Gy [78–80,85].

At doses of <1–2 Gy per fraction, major deviations from the values predicted by the LQ model were observed in the derived isoeffect doses [80]. This may in part reflect incomplete repair of sublethal damage between fractions, since short interfraction intervals of 5 h were used. However, a reduction in repair capacity after multiple irradiations or the presence of a small population of radiosensitive cells cannot be excluded.

It should be noted that the LQ analysis ignores the time factor associated with the differing fractionation regimens. The influence of overall treatment time on renal tolerance is much less important

## The potential for the treatment of radiation nephropathy

Radiation nephropathy can obviously be reduced or prevented by limiting the volume of renal tissue irradiated and the total dose administered. When clinical radiation nephropathy occurs, however, there are several procedures available to minimize the magnitude of the effect. In general, the clinical management consists of a treatment that will theoretically carry the patient through an acute phase, with the view that some of the functional impairment is reversible. Placing the patient on a low protein diet may be helpful [51,126]. However, this suggestion is still unsubstantiated. The experimental findings outlined previously indicate that radiation nephropathy is a chronic, progressive and possibly irreversible lesion [66,95]. However, a scientific rationale for the clinical use of low protein diets to reduce the functional load on the kidney has come from studies on the pathogenic consequences of renal hyperfiltration [71]. A reduced nephron number, as found in a number of nephropathies, results in a deleterious compensatory hyperfiltration in the remaining nephrons. This itself leads to progressive glomerulosclerosis. Low protein diets, which prevent hyperfiltration, have proved to be successful experimentally in preventing a progressive loss of renal function [127]. A similar manoeuvre has been useful in the prevention of experimental radiation nephropathy [128]. The clinical use of this approach should be encouraged. It is worth noting, however, that as yet there is little evidence to suggest that such treatment would result in regeneration and/or repair of the radiation-induced damage; it may simply prevent its expression and progression, and therefore the kidneys in such patients may well remain permanently compromised.

The successful protection of the irradiated kidney with renal arterial adrenaline infusion has been reported [129]. Again this does not appear to have been widely used. Steroids have been reported to provide some symptomatic help [130] but did not modify the progressive renal insufficiency. More importantly, experimental evidence has indicated that such a treatment potentiates radiation effects on the renal vasculature [131,132]. Attempts at treatment with tri-iodothyronine [133] have similarly caused the potentiation of radiation effects in the kidney.

In chronic radiation nephropathy, hypertension should be treated aggressively (see p. 195) since the presence of hypertension suggests a poor prognosis. Low protein diets should be used to prevent hyperfiltration and severe anaemia may require transfusion. Renal dialysis or transplantation may be practical in a patient with severe bilateral involvement.

In general, the irradiated kidney should be managed by a reduction in its functional load. It may well be that the function in all irradiated kidneys is compromised to varying degrees. Exposure of the irradiated kidney to any additional nephrotoxins should be viewed with extreme caution.

## The bladder

### Clinical pattern of radiation-induced damage to the bladder

Three types of radiation-induced reaction were initially observed in the bladder after the completion of radiotherapy [134,135]; these were defined as acute, subacute and chronic damage. More recently this classification has been simplified [126]; acute effects were said to be seen up to 4 months after the start of radiotherapy and late, chronic effects, were most commonly seen 1–4 years after the completion of radiotherapy. In general the term subacute could be used to cover the interim period between the expression of the early acute and the late chronic effects.

The acute changes are often referred to as 'radiation cystitis'. This term covers a variety of lesions and symptoms. Radiation cystitis is observed 4–6 weeks after radiotherapy, but may present earlier if high doses of radiation are employed. The symptoms are those of acute cystitis with dysuria, frequency and nocturia; the capacity of the bladder may be reduced. The reaction is generally mild, and may even pass unnoticed by the patient. However, with increasing dose the severity of radiation cystitis increases. Severe cystitis may present due to the presence of secondary bacterial infection, and can then progress to hydronephrosis, pyelonephritis, uraemia and death if not successfully treated. The most common causative bacterial organisms have been reported to be *E. coli*, *S. faecalis*, *Ps. pyocyaneus* and *B. proteus mirabilis* [136]. In addition to infection, factors such as an extensive ulcerated tumour, previous surgery with radiotherapy treatment, and urinary tract obstruction can exacerbate acute radiation cystitis [137].

If perforation of the bladder or a vesicovaginal fistula develops during the course of radiotherapy, this reflects an invasive tumour with resultant damage to the bladder wall or vesicovaginal septum. It can usually be identified in patients who present with a sudden cessation in frequency and nocturia.

Subacute clinical changes, in the form of trigonal ulceration, are seen between approximately 6 months and 2 years after therapy. The main symptom is a painless haematuria due to the rupture of telangiectatic vessels in the ulcer. Ulceration of the trigone may develop as a result of vascular ischaemia due to the obliteration of the smaller arterioles. Damage to larger vessels leads to necrosis of the bladder wall and the septum leading to the development of a fistula. Secondary infection may be associated with the area of ulceration. Oedema may result in ureteral occlusion and hydronephrosis. This is reversible when the infection has been controlled.

During this subacute period cystoscopy frequently reveals dilated and tortuous blood vessels, with the presence of a thin atrophic epithelium. Radiation-induced ulcers have been described as having sharply demarcated walls; in contrast, in recurrent cancer the mucosa appears to be heaped or rolled up [138].

The late phase of bladder damage is generally seen 1–10 years after radiotherapy [50]. It is characterized by a contracted bladder with a reduced capacity. This results from a combination of infection and fibrosis of the submucosal and muscle layers. Telangiectasia of the bladder mucosa, often at the site of the tumour, has also been reported [136].

Radiation damage to the bladder has been reported in several animal models. In the mouse a dose-dependent increase in urination frequency has been described [139]. This occurred at least 5 months after irradiation, with maximum damage being found by 12 months. A reduction in bladder capacity was noted 18 months after irradiation. Recently, an *in vivo* cystometric technique has been used to demonstrate an acute, reversible reduction in the bladder volume of the mouse within 6–14 days of irradiation after single doses of 15–30 Gy [140]. This was followed by a later, irreversible reduction in bladder volume 2–3 months following irradiation. In the pig an acute reduction in the inflatability of the bladder was seen by 1 month after irradiation (Hopewell, unpublished data). A decreased bladder distensibility was noted in dogs up to 6 months after doses of 11–36 Gy intraoperative irradiation (IOR) followed by 50 Gy in 5 weeks [141]. However, later studies with IOR alone using single doses of up to 40 Gy failed to identify any reduction in the contractility or volume of the canine bladder up to 4 years after IOR [142].

Intracavitary therapy for cervical cancer may also result in bladder damage. This is particularly true in cases where there has been some asymmetry in the insertion with a resultant high dose to a relatively small volume [143]. More accurate localization of the various structures would result in a more accurate placing of sources and planning of tumour masses. Techniques such as computed tomography and ultrasound scanning [144,145] should improve tumour cure and reduce late normal tissue injury.

The similarities in the anatomy of the urogenital tract tissues within the pelvis between pig and man suggested that this species might be useful for evaluating bladder damage following intracavitary irradiation [146]. However, pigs failed to develop severe bladder damage although ureteral strictures were seen. This reflects the problem of postural differences between the two species which caused the ureters to receive a higher dose than the bladder. These findings highlight the difficulties associated with extrapolating animal findings to man.

## Incidence of radiation-induced bladder lesions

A number of clinical studies have reported on the incidence of late radiation-induced bladder damage such as vesicovaginal fistulation, haemorrhagic cystitis and bladder contraction [136,147–150]. In general, the incidence of these complications increases both with the volume of bladder irradiated and the total dose used, particularly to the anterior wall [151]. The incidence of late effects appears to be in the order of 1.5–7% [147,149]. However, increased doses to the bladder will increase the incidence of complications, e.g. Koeck and Hillsinger [152] reported a 3% complication rate in patients who received 50–60 Gy to the bladder given in daily fractions over a 7 week period; increasing the total dose to 60–70 Gy given over 8 weeks increased the complication rate to 11%. Complication rates of between 6 and 30% have been noted in dose-seeking studies using total doses of from 50 Gy for a 10 cm field to 57.5 Gy for 8 cm field given in 20 fractions over 4 weeks [153]. The incidence of late effects after 57.5 Gy was considered unacceptable and the dose was reduced to 54 Gy.

Based on the findings of a postal questionnaire Parkin, Davis and Symonds [154] reported that 26% of all patients treated for cervical carcinoma complained of severe symptoms of bladder dysfunction. They also suggested that many earlier retrospective analyses of case records may have underestimated the extent of this problem. Bladder dysfunction appeared to reflect detrusor instability rather than a contracted bladder. Thus radiotherapy which includes the bladder in the treatment volume can cause severe morbidity, particularly when combined with surgery [137]. This can be reduced by limiting the dose and the volume of bladder irradiated.

## Histological changes and pathogenesis

Gowing [155] described the major pathological changes seen in the bladder of patients following irradiation. A total of 35 cystectomy specimens, taken between 5 months and 9 years after therapy from cases of proven bladder carcinoma, were evaluated. Macroscopically all showed bladder contraction and a reduction in the luminal capacity with fibrosis and thickening of the bladder wall. Mucosal oedema and hyperaemia were evident, the latter characterized by prominent telangiectatic vessels. The surface epithelium showed focal areas of atrophy alternating with areas of thickening and hypertrophy. The subepithelial tissues were oedematous with dilated capillaries. There were increased amounts of fibrous tissue which occasionally contained cells with enlarged nuclei, described as 'radiation fibroblasts'. The muscle layers showed areas of necrosis, hyalinization and replacement by fibrous tissue; vascular changes consisted of hyperaemia and telangiectasia. Small arteries often exhibited fibrous thickening of the intima with luminal narrowing.

These clinical observations are of limited value in defining the pathogenesis of radiation-induced bladder injury since the time sequence of these changes was ill-defined. Such detailed information necessitates the use of experimental studies (Table 14.1) [139,156,157]. In the mouse the initial lesion, seen in the bladder 5–10 months after irradiation, was epithelial desquamation with the cells lining the bladder lumen being lost. This coincided with a reduction in bladder function, as seen in terms of an increase in urination frequency [139]. After 9–12 months there was a burst of epithelial proliferation which produced a hyperplastic epithelium. This was associated with a recovery in function. However, 18 months after irradiation the bladder was fibrotic and exhibited a reduced capacity. These findings have been confirmed in an extensive study in rats [155]. In this species the epithelial damage was accompanied by ongoing damage to the vasculature, the smooth muscle and nerves, causing fibrosis and increased bladder rigidity. Although a much earlier development of epithelial changes had been reported in the rat bladder after irradiation [158], these bladders were infected with a parasitic roundworm which possibly aggravated and precipitated the radiation response.

Stewart, Michael and Denekamp [139] noted a correlation between epithelial desquamation and the time of onset of functional damage 5–6 months after irradiation and inferred a causal relationship. Thus the observed latent period of several months before functional damage was evident reflected the

**Table 14.1 Time-related changes in the morphology and function of the irradiated rodent bladder**

| Species (reference) | Radiation dose (Gy) | Time after irradiation | Histological and functional changes in the irradiated bladder |
|---|---|---|---|
| Mouse [139] | 15–40 | 5–10 months | Epithelial desquamation and loss of specialized surface cells. Increased urination frequency |
| | 15–40 | 9–12 months | Epithelium hyperplastic |
| | 15–40 | 18 months | Bladder wall fibrosis; reduced bladder capacity |
| Rat [157] | 20 | 1 week–1 month | Necrosis of some epithelial cells. Occasional binucleate basal cells evident |
| | 20 | 3 months | Subcellular damage involving intermediate and basal epithelial cells. Blood vessels contain oedematous endothelial cells. Focal destruction of bladder wall smooth muscle cells. Collagen deposition within and around nerve fibre bundles |
| | 20 | 6 months | Focal epithelial hyperplasia. Multilayering of basal luminae around capillaries. More extensive destruction of bladder wall smooth muscle cells with marked collagen deposition |
| | 20 | 12 months | Subepithelial capillary endothelial cells hyperplastic; prominent vascular fibrosis. Continued degeneration of muscle coat and replacement by fibrous tissue. Binucleated fibroblasts evident |
| | 20 | 20 months | Blood vessels have thickened walls consistent with previous occlusion and recanalization. Marked degeneration of muscle layers and fibrosis. Fibroblasts prominent in bladder wall |

slow turnover of the bladder epithelial cells [159]. However, the administration of cyclophosphamide 1 week after irradiation, which itself induces an immediate wave of epithelial cell death and proliferation, failed to precipitate functional radiation damage [160]. This would suggest that epithelial cell depletion was not the primary event leading to late bladder damage. An alternative suggestion is that late bladder damage reflects damaged vasculature and a disruption of the histohaematic barrier due to the development of perivascular fibrosis and a multilayering of the basal lamina [157].

It is possible that acute or subacute radiation damage results from the loss of epithelial cells, exacerbated by the presence of infection. This is followed by a chronic period characterized by a slowly progressive deterioration of the fine vasculature as a result of endarteritis with fibrosis and sclerosis of vessels. This leads to occlusive changes and an increase in the histohaematic connective tissue barrier, which causes ischaemia, progressive epithelial atrophy and necrosis with ulceration and, in some cases, fistula formation. The fibrosis and induration of the bladder wall leads to contraction and a reduction in bladder capacity.

## Influence of dose fractionation on the radiation tolerance of the bladder

There has been only one major experimental study on the response of the bladder to fractionated radiation [161,162]. Mouse bladders were irradiated with electrons given in 1–20 fractions in an overall treatment time of 1–2 weeks (Figure 14.3). These studies showed that the bladder has an extensive

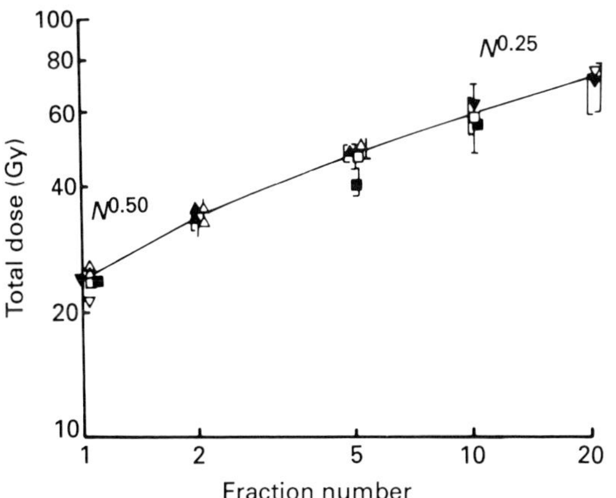


**Figure 14.3** Isoeffective doses assessed from urination frequency (ope symbols) or bladder volume (closed symbols) as a function of fraction number ($\triangle$. $\blacktriangle$ [161], $\square$, $\blacksquare$, $\triangledown$. $\blacktriangledown$ [162]). Drawn from ref. [162]

capacity for the repair of sublethal radiation damage. Thus the number of dose fractions would appear to be more important than the overall treatment time in determining the tolerance of the bladder to fractionated radiotherapy. Analysis of the data using the LQ model produced an $\alpha/\beta$ ratio of between 5 and 10 Gy, higher than that generally reported for late responding normal tissues. This confirms the view that a therapeutic benefit might be expected in treatments that involve irradiating the bladder with a large number of small dose fractions [84].

In a recent clinical study [163], patients with T2–T4 bladder carcinoma received either $3 \times 1\,\mathrm{Gy}$ fractions per day or a more conventional $2\,\mathrm{Gy}$ fraction daily treatment schedule. Survival was improved significantly in patients with T3 tumours receiving the hyperfractionation regimen compared with those treated conventionally. The normal tissue reactions were similar. Thus hyperfractionation in radiotherapy may hold the promise of an increased therapeutic gain in the treatment of bladder carcinoma.

## Effects of high LET radiation

The results of a number of clinical studies involving irradiation with fast neutrons for the treatment of bladder cancer have been reported [164–167]. Although Griffin *et al.* [166] found some therapeutic advantage from the use of neutron therapy in a group of 26 patients with bladder carcinoma, a randomized comparison was not made. Other studies have shown no therapeutic advantage when using neutrons. Indeed, in some of these studies severe late bladder damage, e.g. contracture and fistulization have been reported [165,167]. This may be due to the use of an inappropriate RBE value for the calculation of safe tolerance doses, these being based on the acute effects of normal tissues rather than late responses. The RBE for late morbidity may be significantly higher in some normal tissues [165].

Experimental studies have shown that the RBE value ($4\,\mathrm{MeV}_{d\to\mathrm{Be}}$ *versus* $4\,\mathrm{MeV}$ electrons) varies from 3.2 to 5.4 for electron doses of between 24 and 5 Gy per fraction [168]. Theoretical predictions based on the LQ model suggest a maximum RBE value of ~8 at clinically relevant doses per fraction for these relatively low energy neutrons [168].

## Influence of radiosensitizers and radioprotectors

In the MRC trial of hyperbaric oxygen and irradiation in the treatment of carcinoma of the cervix [169] it was found that treatment in hyperbaric oxygen, as opposed to air, was associated with an improvement in local control and survival of patients. However, there was an increase in morbidity due to radiation-induced bladder damage. This increase might have resulted from an increase in bladder radiosensitivity due to an increase in the tissue $PO_2$ concentration. Experimental studies in the mouse have also shown that the radiosensitivity of the bladder can be modified by varying the inspired oxygen concentration [170]. Mice were irradiated whilst breathing nitrogen, air, or 7–95% oxygen; as the oxygen concentration was increased the radiosensitivity of the bladder was also increased. An oxygen enhancement ratio of ~2.6 was obtained by irradiation in the presence of the sensitizer misonidazole, or was reduced by the radioprotector WR2721 [170]. The mouse bladder does appear, to some extent at least, to be radiobiologically hypoxic under normal conditions.

## Chemotherapeutic drug interactions

Examples of specific drug cytotoxicity in the bladder are rare. However, cyclophosphamide does cause bladder damage in a number of species, including man [171,172]. This is due to the direct contact of cyclophosphamide metabolites with the bladder epithelium during their excretion [173]. Bladder damage, characterized by ulceration, epithelial desquamation and haemorrhage, presents within several days of cyclophosphamide administration. Several authors contend that the bladder epithelium shows complete recovery within 2 weeks [173,174]; others suggest that increased proliferative activity is still present 2–3 months after drug administration [175].

Cyclophosphamide is used clinically, in combination with pelvic irradiation, for the treatment of ovarian cancer [176]. In such a situation there is the possibility of increased bladder damage [177,178]. Experimental studies have shown that a fixed dose of cyclophosphamide, given up to 9 months before or after bladder irradiation, caused an early X-ray dose-related expression of damage due to precipitation of latent radiation injury [179]. There was also increased late bladder damage seen 9–12 months after treatment. The results suggested a dose-enhancement factor of ~1.3. This increased late damage was thought to represent additive drug and radiation toxicities. These studies suggest that the use of cyclophosphamide should be avoided in clinical situations where the bladder has been irradiated.

## The ureter

### Clinical pattern of radiation-induced damage to the ureter

The close proximity of the lower urinary tract to the distal vagina and the cervix results in the potential for development of damage after radiotherapeutic treatment for cervical cancer. Radiation-induced bladder injuries such as radiation cystitis, ulceration and fistulization are well recognized and have been discussed previously. However ureteral changes, as studied by intravenous or retrograde pyelography, have proved vital in the pre- and post-treatment evaluation of patients presenting with cervical carcinoma. Despite this the post-therapeutic alterations in ureteral structure and function have received scant attention, except in an attempt to diagnose tumour recurrences. Thus the significance of radiation-induced obstruction has been largely neglected, despite its clinical importance. The most common cause of death in progressive cervical carcinoma is uraemia following ureteral obstruction [180,181]. Alfert and Gillenwater [180] reported that ureteral obstruction occurred in ~70% of patients with cervical carcinoma, ~75% of whom died of renal complications. Although oncologists have generally felt that radiation is rarely the underlying reason for this obstructive nephropathy, scarring and stenosis as a direct effect of radiation is a potential cause.

The first case of ureteral stricture, secondary to radiation-induced fibrosis, was reported by Schmitz in 1930 [182]. Since then several investigators have reported that the incidence of radiation-induced ureteral fibrosis is approximately 1% [147,180,183,184]. When surgery was combined with radiotherapy the incidence of ureteral stricture increased to ~6% [185]. The ureteral epithelium, which like the bladder is transitional stratified epithelium, appeared to be less radiosensitive than that of the bladder [51], possibly due to its relatively poor vascular supply rendering it radiobiologically hypoxic.

Experimental data on the effects of localized radiation on the ureter are somewhat limited. Early studies in the rat [186,187] were complicated by the use of invasive surgical techniques during irradiation. However, ureteral irradiation did produce hydronephrosis due to ureteral occlusion. Albers *et al.* [188] failed to observe any marked ureteral changes in dogs after fractionated irradiation with $^{60}$Co gamma rays, although they did report a marked deleterious effect on the subsequent tolerance of the ureter following surgical intervention. More recently IOR has been used to study radiation-induced ureteral injury in the dog [141,189,190]. The ureter, along with the kidney, appeared to be the most radiosensitive of the retroperitoneal structures. The relatively high radiosensitivity of the ureter has also been confirmed recently in the rat [191–193]. A dose of only 10 Gy to a 1.5 cm length of ureter caused a high incidence of hydronephrosis. It would appear that the rat ureter is more radiosensitive than that of either the dog [141,188] or man [194].

## Histological changes and pathogenesis

The histological changes observed following irradiation to the ureter were described by Cosbie [195]. Three phases in the development of radiation ureteritis were reported. Acute ureteritis was seen both during and up to several weeks after irradiation. All layers of the ureteral wall exhibited an acute, reversible oedema and hyperaemia. Degeneration of epithelial cells as well as damage to the fine vasculature were noted. Endothelial cells showed evidence of degeneration, necrosis and proliferation which caused vascular occlusion. There was also subendothelial and medial vascular occlusion. Fibrous tissue extended into the muscularis and replaced ureteral muscle tissue which had degenerated, a process believed to be mediated via vascular insufficiency. The oedema and hyperaemia may cause a transient obstruction of the ureter with the development of hydronephrosis in some 50–60% of patients. This appears to resolve with time. This acute phase was followed by a subacute phase, during which time there was continued epithelial degeneration and progressive vascular changes; infiltration with inflammatory cells may also occur. In the late stage chronic obstruction develops, seen approximately 1–4 years after irradiation [183,196]. The underlying pathogenesis of this late stage is again believed to be the obliteration of the vasculature by a radiation-induced endarteritis. This decreases the blood supply to the distal ureter; the subsequent atrophy of ureteral muscle and epithelium with tissue fibrosis results in ureteral stricture.

Histological changes in the rat ureter following irradiation have also been reported [192]. The lesion consisted of the following features to a varying degree; urothelial hyperplasia, fibrosis of the ureteral wall and vascular damage. The urothelial hyperplasia ranged from a mild, fairly uniform thickening to an extensive lesion with large polypoid outgrowths or multiple tubule formations. Urothelial cells sometimes extended deep into the lamina propria and muscle layer. This possibly represents a healing or healed ulcerated area. The associated fibrosis and muscle damage support this hypothesis. Two types of fibrosis were noted. Most commonly the ureteral wall was greatly thickened by fibrous tissue external to the muscle layer. However, on occasions an extremely dense collagenous scar tissue was seen. This was usually directly below the urothelium, in the lamina propria, but also extending peripherally through the muscle layer. The vascular damage was mainly arterial, and included vessel wall thickening, peri-arterial and fibrinoid necrosis, with the complete occlusion of vessels in some instances.

Studies of IOR in the dog [141] have demonstrated a variety of ureteral changes including stenosis, obstruction, thickening, dilatation, atrophy and shortening. Decreased lumen size and/or an increase in the diameter of the ureter results from oedema, inflammation and most commonly fibrosis. The loss of small arterioles in the adventitia resulted in medial necrosis and intimal proliferation [190].

## Factors modifying the development of ureteral stricture

Radiation-induced ureteral damage has most commonly been seen in patients treated for cervical carcinoma, particularly in those who receive interstitial irradiation [197]. The packing of the vagina may distort the local anatomy; the displacement of a radiation source so that it is 1 cm closer to the ureter can increase the dose received by 65% [196]. This increased irradiation dose to the ureter will be associated with an increased risk of damage. The anatomy of individual patients will also influence the radiation dose received by organs during intracavitary irradiation [198]. Several reports suggest that patients presenting with pelvic disease or urinary tract complications prior to irradiation are more likely to develop radiation-induced ureteral damage [181,199]. Infection is a potent predisposing factor to ureteral damage [199]. Quiescent salpingitis may be exacerbated by radiotherapy and patients in whom this occurs have a poor prognosis, i.e. a 22% 5-year survival rate compared with a 62% survival rate in patients without such an infection. A recrudescence of pelvic inflammation or upper urinary tract infection during radiotherapy may also predispose to ureteral damage [181]. Surgical intervention, whether before [200], during [201], or after [188] radiotherapy dramatically increases the incidence of ureteral damage.

## Management and treatment

The development of post-irradiation ureteral obstruction, along with its underlying cause, should be evaluated as soon as possible and be treated appropriately. A poor outcome will result if treatment is inadequate or delayed [202,203]. Several authors have stressed the value of regular IVP follow-up after irradiation [196,203]; serum creatinine is not useful for assessing renal function in hydronephrosis [187]. The IVP should be performed annually in asymptomatic patients, and earlier in patients with flank and lower abdominal pain [196]. The development of gamma camera renography techniques may also be useful in the clinical detection of hydronephrosis. Recent studies in the rat [204] have indicated that early changes in renal transit time indices, assessed by gamma camera renography, were excellent predictors of later chronic hydronephrosis. Since it is highly important to treat ureteral obstruction as soon as possible, the application of such techniques to patients following radiotherapy involving the urinary tract may prove beneficial. Once obstruction has been diagnosed and the presence of recurrent malignancy excluded, then surgical intervention is required. If the obstruction is partial or near the ureterovesical junction, cystoscopic ureteral dilation may be sufficient [183,196], although permanent correction often requires more extensive measures. If the obstruction results in a hydronephrotic kidney found to be non-functioning then UN is appropriate; if the kidney is still functioning reimplantation of the ureter into the bladder is possible. Failure of this procedure is likely to be due to radiation injury of the ureter [205]. Ileal conduit and cutaneous ureterostomy offer all the disadvantages of an external urinary diversion; ureteroileoneocystostomy has given good results with no apparent deleterious renal effects [181].

## References


1. Baerman, G. and Linser, P. Beitrage zur chirurgischen Behandlung und histologie der roentgenulzera. *Munchen Medizin Wochnschr.*, **51**, 918–920 (1904)
2. McQuarrie, I. and Whipple, G.H. Study of renal function of roentgen ray intoxication; resistance of renal epithelium to direct radiation. *Journal of Experimental Medicine*, **35**, 225–242 (1922)
3. Edsall, D.L. The attitude of the clinician in regard to exposing patients to the X-ray. *Journal of the American Medical Association*, **47**, 1425–1429 (1906)
4. Hartman, F.W., Bolliger, A. and Doub, H.P. Experimental nephritis produced by irradiation. *American Journal of Medical Science*, **172**, 487–500 (1926)
5. Hartman, F.W., Bolliger, A. and Doub, H.P. Functional studies throughout course of roentgen-ray nephritis in dogs. *Journal of the American Medical Association*, **88**, 139–145 (1927)
6. Doub, H.P., Hartman, F.W. and Bolliger, A. Relative radiosensitivity of kidney to irradiation. *Radiology*, **8**, 142–148 (1927)
7. Domagk, G. Roentgenstrahlenschadigurgen der Niere beim Menschen. *Medical Klinics*, **23**, 345–347 (1927)
8. Grossman, B.J. Radiation nephritis. *Journal of Pediatrics*, **47**, 424–433 (1955)
9. Redd, B.L. Jr. Radiation nephritis. Review, case report and animal study. *American Journal of Roentgenology*, **83**, 88–106 (1960)
10. Kunkler, P.B., Farr, R.F. and Luxton, R.W. The limit of renal tolerance to X-rays. *British Journal of Radiology*, **25**, 190–201 (1952)
11. Luxton, R.W. Radiation nephritis. *Quarterly Journal of Medicine*, **22**, 215–242 (1953)
12. Luxton, R.W. Radiation nephritis. A long-term study of 54 patients. *Lancet*, **ii**, 1221–1224 (1953)
13. Luxton, R.W., Effects of irradiation on the kidney. In *Diseases of the Kidney* (eds M.B. Strauss and L.G. Welt), Little Brown, Boston, pp. 1049–1070 (1973)
14. Zuelzer, W.W., Palmer, H.D. and Newton, W.A., Jr. Unusual glomerulonephritis in young children, probably radiation nephritis; report of three cases. *American Journal of Pathology*, **26**, 1019–1039 (1950)
15. Zeigerman, J.H., Tulsky, E.G. and Makler, P. Post-irradiation nephritic syndrome. *Obstetrics and Gynecology*, **9**, 542–548 (1957)
16. Glatstein, E., Fajardo, L.F. and Brown, J.M. Radiation injury in the mouse kidney I. Sequential light microscopic injury. *International Journal of Radiation Oncology, Biology, Physics*, **2**, 933–943 (1977)
17. Avioli, L.V., Lazor, M.Z., Cotlove, E. *et al.* Early effects of radiation on renal function in man. *American Journal of Medicine*, **34**, 329–337 (1963)
18. Le Bourgeois, J.P., Meignan, M., Parmentier, C. and Tubiana, M. Renal consequences of irradiation of the spleen in lymphoma patients. *British Journal of Radiology*, **52**, 56–60 (1979)
19. Quinn, J.L., Meschan, I., Blake, D.D. and Witcovski, R.L. The usefulness of the radioisotopic renogram in radiation therapy. *Radiology*, **78**, 266–268 (1962)
20. Kim, T.H., Freeman, C.R. and Webster, J.H. The significance of unilateral radiation nephropathy. *International Journal of Radiation Oncology, Biology, Physics*, **6**, 1567–1571 (1980)
21. Kim, T.H., Somerville, P.J. and Freeman, C.R. Unilateral radiation nephropathy – the long-term significance. *International Journal of Radiation Oncology, Biology, Physics*, **10**, 2053–2059 (1984)
22. Raulston, G.L., Gray, K.N., Gleiser, C.A. *et al.* A comparison of the effects of $50\,MeV_{d\rightarrow Be}$ neutron and cobalt-60 irradiation on the kidneys of rhesus monkeys. *Radiology*, **128**, 245–249 (1978)
23. Mendelsohn, M.L. and Caceres, E. Effect of X-ray to the kidney on renal function of the dog. *American Journal of Physiology*, **173**, 351–354 (1953)
24. Robbins, M.E.C., Hopewell, J.W. and Gunn, Y. Effects of single doses of X-rays on renal function in unilaterally irradiated kidneys. *Radiotherapy and Oncology*, **4**, 143–151 (1985)
25. Ewen, C. and Hendry, J.H. Functional assessment of long-term tubule and vascular injury in the irradiated kidney. *International Journal of Radiation Biology*, **53**, 1005 (1988)
26. Robbins, M.E.C., Campling, D., Rezvani, M. *et al.* Nephropathy in the mature pig following the irradiation of a single kidney. *International Journal of Radiation Oncology, Biology, Physics*, **16**, 1519–1528 (1989)
27. Coburn, J.W., Rubini, M.E. and Kleeman, C.R. Renal concentrating defect in canine radiation nephritis. *Journal of Laboratory and Clinical Medicine*, **67**, 209–223 (1966)
28. Jongejan, H.T.M., van der Kogel, A., Provoost, A.P. and Molenaar, J.C. Radiation nephropathy in

young and adult rats. *International Journal of Radiation Oncology, Biology, Physics*, **13**, 225–232 (1987)

29. Cullen, B.M., Burgin, J., Reeves, B. and Michalowski, A. Functional assessments of radiation nephropathy. *British Journal of Cancer*, **53**, Supplement VII, 292–294 (1986)

30. Steele, B.T. and Lirenman, D.S. Acute radiation nephritis and the haemolytic syndrome. *Clinical Nephrology*, **11**, 272–274 (1979)

31. Tarbell, N.J., Guinan, E.C., Niemeyer, C. *et al.* Late onset of renal dysfunction in survivors of bone marrow transplantation. *International Journal of Radiation Oncology, Biology, Physics*, **15**, 99–104 (1988)

32. Osnes, S. Experimental study of an erythropoietic principle produced in the kidney. *British Medical Journal*, **i**, 650–658 (1959)

33. Fisher, J.W., Roh, B. and Sherap, K. Influence of X-irradiation of the dog kidney on erythropoietin production. *Sangre*, **9**, 112–117 (1964)

34. Alpen, E.L. and Stewart, F.A. Radiation nephritis and anaemia: a functional assay for renal damage after irradiation. *British Journal of Radiology*, **57**, 185–187 (1984)

35. Koury, S.T., Bondurant, M.C. and Koury, M.J. Localisation of erythropoietin synthesising cells in murine kidneys by *in situ* hybridisation. *Blood*, **71**, 524–527 (1988)

36. Lacombe, C., DaSilva, J.L., Bruneval, P. *et al.* Peritubular cells are the site of erythropoietin synthesis in the murine hypoxic kidney. *Journal of Clinical Investigation*, **81**, 620–623 (1988)

37. Thompson, P.L., Mackay, I.R., Robson, G.S.M. and Wall, A.J. Late radiation nephritis after gastric X-irradiation for peptic ulcer. *Quarterly Journal of Medicine*, **XL**, 145–157 (1971)

38. Dean, A.L. and Abels, J.C. Study by newer renal function tests of unusual case of hypertension following irradiation of one kidney and relief by nephrectomy. *Journal of Urology*, **52**, 497–501 (1944)

39. Crummy, A.B. Jr., Hellman, S., Stazel, H.C. and Hukill, H.B. Renal hypertension secondary to unilateral radiation damage relieved by nephrectomy. *Radiology*, **84**, 108–111 (1965)

40. Shapiro, A.P., Cavallo, T., Cooper, W. *et al.* Hypertension in radiation nephritis. *Archives of Internal Medicine*, **137**, 848–851 (1977)

41. Wacholz, B.W. and Casarett, G. Radiation hypertension and nephrosclerosis. *Radiation Research*, **41**, 39–56 (1970)

42. Asscher, A.W., Wilson, C. and Anson, S.G. Sensitization of blood vessels to hypertensive damage by X-irradiation. *Lancet*, **i**, 580–583 (1961)

43. Robbins, M.E.C., Campling, D., Rezvani, M. *et al.* Radiation nephropathy in mature pigs following the irradiation of both kidneys. *International Journal of Radiation Biology*, **56**, 83–98 (1989)

44. Wilson, C., Ledingham, J.H. and Cohen, M. Hypertension following X-irradiation of the kidneys. *Lancet*, **i**, 9–16 (1958)

45. Fisher, E.R. and Hellstrom, H.R. Pathogenesis of hypertension and pathological changes in experimental renal irradiation. *Laboratory Investigation*, **19**, 530–538 (1968)

46. Ljungqvist, A., Unge, G., Lagergren, C. and Nolter, G. The intrarenal vascular alteration in radiation nephritis and their relationship to the development of hypertension. *Acta Pathologica Microbiologica Scandinavica*, **79**, 629–638 (1971)

47. Scanlon, G.T. Vascular alteration in the irradiated rabbit kidney: a microangiographic study. *Radiology*, **94**, 401–406 (1970)

48. Tobian, L., Thompson, J., Twedt, R. and Janeck, J. The granulation of juxtaglomerular cells in renal hypertension. *Journal of Clinical Investigation*, **37**, 660–671 (1958)

49. Minton, J., McIvor, J., Capuccio, F.P. *et al.* Case report: renovascular hypertension following radiotherapy and chemotherapy treated by transluminal angioplasty. *Clinical Radiology*, **37**, 399–401 (1986)

50. Casarett, G.W. Histopathology of alpha radiation from internally administered polonium. US Atomic Energy Commission Document UR 201 (1950)

51. Rubin, P. and Casarett, G.W. *Urinary Tract: The Kidney, Clinical Radiation Pathology*, Vol. 1, W.B. Saunders, Philadelphia, pp. 293–333 (1968)

52. Warren, S. Effects of radiation on normal tissues. VII. Effects of radiation on the urinary system. *Archives of Pathology*, **34**, 1079–1084 (1942)

53. Davey, P.W., Hamilton, J.D. and Steele, H.D. Radiation injury of the kidney. *Canadian Medical Association Journal*, **67** 648–650 (1952)

54. Philips, T.L. and Ross, G. A quantitative technique for measuring renal damage after irradiation. *Radiology*, **109**, 457–462 (1973)

55. Jordan, S.W., Key, C.R., Gomez, L.S. *et al.* Late effects of radiation on the mouse kidney. *Experimental and Molecular Pathology*, **29**, 115–129 (1978)

56. Michalowski, A., Cullen, B.M., Burgin, J. and Rogers, M.A. Development of structural renal damage and its quantification. *British Journal of Cancer*, **53**, Supplement VII, 295–297 (1986)

57. Rubenstone, A.I. and Fitch, L.B. Radiation nephritis. A clinicopathologic study. *American Journal of Medicine*, **33**, 545–554 (1962)

58. Rosen, S., Swerdlow, M.A., Muehrcke, R.C. and Piriani, C.L. Radiation nephritis: light and electron microscopic observations. *American Journal of Clinical Pathology*, **41**, 487–502 (1964)

59. Keane, W.F., Crosion, J.T., Staley, W.A. *et al.* Radiation-induced renal disease: a clinicopathologic study. *American Journal of Medicine*, **60**, 127–137 (1976)

60. Kapur, S., Chandra, R. and Antonvych, T. Acute radiation nephritis: light and electron microscopic observations. *Archives of Pathology and Laboratory Medicine*, **101**, 469–473 (1977)

61. Bergstein, J., Andreoli, S.P., Provisor, A.J. and Yum, M. Radiation nephritis following total-body

irradiation and cyclophosphamide in preparation for bone marrow transplantation. *Transplantation*, **41**, 63–66 (1986)

62. Madrazo, A.A. and Churg, J. Radiation nephritis. Chronic changes following moderate doses of radiation. *Laboratory Investigation*, **34**, 283–290 (1976)

63. Madrazo, A.A., Susuki, Y. and Churg, J. Radiation nephritis: acute changes following high dose of radiation. *American Journal of Pathology*, **54**, 507–527 (1969)

64. Madrazo, A.A., Susuki, Y. and Churg, J. Radiation nephritis II: chronic changes after high doses of radiation. *American Journal of Pathology*, **61**, 37–56 (1970)

65. Withers, H.R., Mason, K.A. and Thames, H.D. Jr. Late radiation response of kidney assayed by tubule-cell survival. *British Journal of Radiology*, **59**, 587–595 (1986)

66. Michalowski, A. The pathogenesis of the late side-effects of radiotherapy. *Clinical Radiology*, **37**, 203–207 (1986)

67. Hoopes, P.J. Gillette, E.L. and Benjamin, S.A. The pathogenesis of radiation nephropathy in the dog. *Radiation Research*, **104**, 404–419 (1985)

68. Fajardo, L.F. and Stewart, J.R. Capillary injury preceding radiation-induced myocardial fibrosis. *Radiology*, **101**, 429–433 (1971)

69. Fajardo, L.F., Brown, M.J. and Glatstein, E. Glomerular and juxtaglomerular lesions in radiation nephropathy. *Radiation Research*, **68**, 177–183 (1976)

70. Allen, J.B., Sagermann, R.H. and Stuart, M.J. Irradiation decreases vascular prostacyclin formation with no concomitant effect on platelet thromboxane production. *Lancet*, **ii**, 1193–1196 (1981)

71. Brenner, B.M., Meyer, T.W. and Hostetter, T.H. Dietary protein intake and the progressive nature of kidney disease. *New England Journal of Medicine*, **307**, 652–659 (1982)

72. Greenberger, J.S., Weichselbaum, R.R. and Cassady, J.R. Radiation nephropathy. In *Cancer and the Kidney* (eds R.E. Reiselbach and M.B. Garnich), Lea Febiger, Philadelphia, pp. 814–823 (1982)

73. Caldwell, W.L. Time-dose factors in fatal post-irradiation nephritis. In *Cell Survival after Low Doses of Radiation. Theoretical and Clinical Complications* (ed. T. Alper), John Wiley, New York, pp. 328–334 (1975)

74. Hopewell, J.W. and Berry, R.J. Radiation tolerance of the pig kidney: a model for determining overall time and fraction factors for preserving overall renal function. *International Journal of Radiation Oncology, Biology, Physics*, **1**, 61–68 (1975)

75. Glatstein, E., Brown, R.C., Zanelli, G.D. and Fowler, J.F. The uptake of rubidium-86 in mouse kidneys irradiated with fractionated doses of X-rays. *Radiation Research*, **61**, 417–426 (1975)

76. Hopewell, J.W. and Wiernik, G. Tolerance of the pig kidney to fractionated X-irradiation. In *Radiobiological Research and Radiotherapy*, IAEA, Vienna, pp. 65–73 (1977)

77. Williams, M.V. and Denekamp, J. Radiation-induced renal damage in mice: influence of overall treatment time. *Radiotherapy and Oncology*, **1**, 355–367 (1984)

78. Williams, M.V. and Denekamp, J. Radiation-induced renal damage in mice: influence of fraction size. *International Journal of Radiation Oncology, Biology, Physics*, **10**, 885–893 (1984)

79. Stewart, F.A., Soranson, J.A., Alpen, E.L. *et al.* Radiation-induced renal damage. The effects of hyperfractionation. *Radiation Research*, **98**, 407–420 (1984)

80. Stewart, F.A., Oussoren, Y., Luts, A. *et al.* Repair of sublethal radiation injury after multiple small doses in mouse kidney: an estimate of flexure dose. *International Journal of Radiation Oncology, Biology, Physics*, **13**, 765–772 (1987)

81. Ellis, F. Dose, time and fractionation: a clinical hypothesis. *Clinical Radiology*, **20**, 1–7 (1969)

82. Hopewell, J.W. and Berry, R.J. The predictive value of the NSD system for renal tolerance to fractionated X-irradiation in the pig. *British Journal of Radiology*, **47**, 679–690 (1974)

83. Douglas, B.G. and Fowler, J.F. The effect of multiple small doses of X-rays on skin reactions in the mouse and a basic interpretation. *Radiation Research*, **66**, 401–426 (1976)

84. Fowler, J.F. What next in fractionated radiotherapy? *British Journal of Cancer*, **49**, Supplement VI, 285–300 (1984)

85. Jordan, S.W., Anderson, R.E., Lane, R.G. and Brayer, J.M. Fraction size, dose and time dependence of X-ray induced late renal injury. *International Journal of Radiation Oncology, Biology, Physics*, **11**, 1095–1101 (1985)

86. Moulder, J.E. Response of rat kidney to fractionated radiation: lack of evidence for a time factor or for slow repair. *Radiation Research*, **91**, 370 (1982)

87. Williams, M.V., Stewart, F.A., Soranson, J.A. and Denekamp, J. The influence of overall treatment time on renal injury after multifraction irradiation. *Radiotherapy and Oncology*, **4**, 87–96 (1985)

88. Hopewell, J.W. and Robbins, M.E.C. The time factor in the radiation response of the kidney. *Radiotherapy and Oncology*, **5**, 75–78 (1986)

89. Geraci, J.P., Thrower, P.D. and Mariano, M. Cyclotron fast neutron RBE for late kidney damage. *Radiology*, **126**, 519–520 (1978)

90. Stewart, F.A., Soranson, J., Maughan, R. *et al.* The RBE for renal damage after irradiation with 3 MeV neutrons. *British Journal of Radiology*, **57**, 1009–1021 (1984)

91. Hopewell, J.W., Barnes, D.W.H., Goodhead, D.T. *et al.* The relative biological effectiveness of fast neutrons ($42\,\text{MeV}_{d\to Be}$) for early and late normal tissue injury in the pig. *International Journal of Radiation Oncology, Biology, Physics*, **8**, 2077–2081 (1982)

92. Joiner, M.C. and Johns, H. Renal damage in the mouse: the effect of $d(4)$-Be neutrons. *Radiation Research*, **109**, 456–468 (1987)

93. Robbins, M.E.C., Hopewell, J.W., Barnes, D.W.H. *et al*. The relative biological effectiveness of fractionated doses of fast neutrons ($42\,\mathrm{MeV}_{d\to\mathrm{Be}}$) for normal tissues in the pig. III. Effects on the kidney. *British Journal of Radiology*, in press

94. Moulder, J.E. Kidney tolerance in split-course radiation schedules. *International Journal of Radiation Oncology, Biology, Physics*, **9**, Supplement 1, 107–108 (1983)

95. Stewart, F.A., Lebesque, L.V. and Hart, A.A.M. Progressive development of radiation damage in mouse kidneys and the consequences for reirradiation tolerance. *International Journal of Radiation Biology*, **53**, 405–415 (1988)

96. Soranson, J.A. and Denekamp, J. Precipitation of latent renal radiation injury by unilateral nephrectomy. *British Journal of Cancer*, **53**, Supplement VII, 268–272 (1986)

97. Phemister, R.D., Thomassen, R.W., Nordin, R.W. and Jaenke, R.S. Renal failure in perinatally irradiated beagles. *Radiation Research*, **55**, 399–410 (1973)

98. Donaldson, S.S., Moskowitz, P.S., Canty, E.L. and Efron, B. Radiation-induced inhibition of compensatory renal growth in the weanling mouse kidney. *Radiology*, **128**, 491–495 (1978)

99. Wachtel, L.W., Cole, L.J. and Rosen, V.J. X-ray induced glomerulosclerosis in rats: modification of lesion by food restriction, uninephrectomy and age. *Journal of Gerontology*, **21**, 442–448 (1966)

100. Eisenbrandt, D.L. and Phemister, R.D. Radiation injury in the neonatal canine kidney. *Laboratory Investigation*, **37**, 437–446 (1977)

101. Rubin, P., van Houtte, P. and Constine, L. Radiation sensitivity and organ tolerance in pediatric oncology: a new hypothesis. *Frontiers of Radiation Therapy and Oncology*, **16**, 62–82 (1982)

102. Asscher, A.W. The delayed effects of renal irradiation. *Clinical Radiology*, **15**, 320–325 (1964)

103. Bolliger, A. and Laidley, J.W.S. Experimental renal disease produced by X-rays. Histologic changes in the kidney exposed to a measured amount of unfiltered rays of medium wavelength. *Medical Journal of Australia*, **1**, 136–147 (1930)

104. Robbins, M.E.C. and Hopewell, J.W. Effects of single doses of X-rays on renal function in the pig after the irradiation of both kidneys. *Radiotherapy and Oncology*, **11** 253–262 (1988)

105. Dicker, S.E. and Shirley, D.G. Compensatory renal growth after unilateral nephrectomy in the new-born rat. *Journal of Physiology*, **228**, 193–202 (1973)

106. Rubin, P. Late effects of chemotherapy and radiation therapy: a new hypothesis. *International Journal of Radiation Oncology, Biology, Physics*, **10**, 5–34 (1984)

107. Arneil, G.C., Emmanuel, I.G., Flatman, G.E. *et al*. Nephritis in two children after irradiation and chemotherapy for nephroblastoma. *Lancet*, **i**, 960–963 (1974)

108. Moskowitz, P.S., Donaldson, S.S. and Canty, E. Chemotherapy-induced inhibition of compensatory renal growth in the immature mouse. *American Journal of Roentgenology*, **134**, 491–496 (1980)

109. Einhorn, L.H. and Donohue, J. *Cis*-diamminodichloroplatinum, vinblastine and bleomycin combination chemotherapy in disseminated testicular cancer. *Annals of Internal Medicine*, **87**, 293–298 (1977)

110. Wiltshaw, E. and Kroner, T. Phase II study of *cis*-dichlorodiammineplatinum (II) (NSC-119875) in advanced carcinoma of the ovary. *Cancer Treatment Reports*, **60**, 55–60 (1976)

111. Gonzalez-Vitale, J.C., Hayes, D.M., Cvitkovic, E. and Sternberg, S. The renal pathology in clinical trials of *cis*-platinum (II) diamminedichloride. *Cancer*, **39**, 1362–1371 (1977)

112. Hayes, D.M., Cvitkovic, E., Golbey, R.B. *et al*. High dose *cis*-platinum diamminedichloride. *Cancer*, **39**, 1372–1381 (1977)

113. Groth, S., Neilsen, H., Sorensen, J.B. *et al*. Acute and long-term nephrotoxicity of *cis*-platinum in man. *Cancer Chemotherapy and Pharmacology*, **17**, 191–196 (1986)

114. Daugaard, G., Rossing, N. and Rorth, M. Effects of cisplatin on special measures of glomerular function in the human kidney with special emphasis on high-dose. *Cancer Chemotherapy and Pharmacology*, **21**, 163–167 (1988)

115. Robbins, M.E.C., Campling, D., Hopewell, J.W. and Michalowski, A. Cisplatin-induced reductions in porcine renal reserve following unilateral nephrectomy. *Cancer Chemotherapy and Pharmacology*, in press

116. Read, G. Reduction in renal radiation tolerance by combination chemotherapy including *cis*-platinum. *British Journal of Cancer*, **45**, 634 (1982)

117. Robbins, M.E.C., Robinson, M., Rezvani, M. *et al*. The response of the pig kidney to the combined effects of cisplatin and unilateral renal irradiation. *Radiotherapy and Oncology*, **11**, 271–278 (1988)

118. Stewart, F.A., Luts, A., Oussoren, Y. *et al*. Renal damage in mice after treatment with cisplatin and X-rays: comparison of fractionated and single-dose studies. *NCI Monographs*, **6**, 23–27 (1988)

119. van Rongen, E., Kuijpers, W.C. and van der Kogel, A.J. Interaction of cisplatin and X-rays in rat kidney. *NCI Monographs*, **6**, 19–22 (1988)

120. Moulder, J.E. and Fish, B.L. Effect of sequencing on combined toxicity of renal irradiation and cisplatin. *NCI Monographs*, **6**, 35–41 (1988)

121. Landuyt, W., van der Kogel, A.J., De Roo, H. *et al*. Unilateral kidney irradiation and late retreatments with *cis*-dichloro-diammineplatinum (II): functional measurements with 99m-technetium-dimercaptosuccinic acid. *International Journal of Radiation Oncology, Biology, Physics,* **14**, 95–101 (1988)

122. Stewart, F.A., Luts, A. and Begg, A.C. Tolerance of previously irradiated mouse kidneys to cisplatinum. *Cancer Research*, **47**, 1016–1021 (1987)

123. Mihatsch, M.J., Thiel, G. and Ryffel, B. Brief review of the morphology of cyclosporin nephropathy. *Contributions to Nephrology*, **51**, 156–161 (1986)

124. Schulman, H., Striker, G., Deeg, H.J. *et al.* Nephrotoxicity of cyclosporin A after allogeneic marrow transplantation. *New England Journal of Medicine*, **305**, 1392–1395 (1981)

125. Atkinson, K., Biggs, J.C., Hayes, J. *et al.* Cyclosporin A associated nephrotoxicity in the first 100 days after allogeneic bone marrow transplantation: three distinct syndromes. *British Journal of Haematology*, **54**, 59–67 (1983)

126. Maier, J.G. Effects of radiation on kidneys, bladder and prostate. *Frontiers of Radiation Therapy and Oncology*, **6**, 196–227 (1972)

127. Anderson, S., Meyer, T.W. and Brenner, B.M. The role of haemodynamic factors in the initiation and progression of renal disease. *Journal of Urology*, **133**, 363–368 (1985)

128. Mahler, P.A., Rasey, J.S. and Yatvin, M.B. Influence of protein nutrition on dose-survival relationship following rat kidney irradiation. *Radiation Research*, **109**, 238–244 (1987)

129. Steckel, R.J., Collins, J.D., Snow, H.D. *et al.* Radiation protection of the normal kidney by selective arterial infusion. *Cancer*, **34**, 1046–1058 (1974)

130. Schreiner, B.F. and Greendyke, R.M. Radiation nephritis: report of a fatal case. *American Journal of Medicine*, **26**, 146–151 (1959)

131. Berdjis, C.C. Cortisone and radiation. III. Histopathology of the effect of cortisone on the irradiated rat kidney. *Archives of Pathology*, **69**, 431–439 (1960)

132. Caldwell, W.L. The effect of prednisolone on fatal post-irradiation nephritis in rabbits. *Radiology*, **98**, 431–433 (1971)

133. Caldwell, W.L., Thomassen, R.W. and Bosch, A. Effects of triiodothyronine in altering the response of kidneys to cobalt-60 radiation. *Radiology*, **81**, 657–663 (1963)

134. Dean, A.L. Ulceration of the urinary bladder as a late effect of radium applications to uterus. *Journal of the American Medical Association*, **89**, 1121–1124 (1927)

135. Dean, A.L. Injury of the urinary bladder following irradiation of the uterus. *Journal of Urology*, **29**, 559–575 (1933)

136. Morrison, R. and Deeley, T.J. The treatment of carcinoma of the bladder by supervoltage X-rays. *British Journal of Radiology*, **38**, 449–458 (1965)

137. Bloedorn, F.G., Young, J.D., Cuccia, C.A. *et al.* Radiotherapy in carcinoma of the bladder: possible complications and their prevention. *Radiology*, **79**, 576–581 (1962)

138. Mallik, M.K. Study of radiation necrosis of the urinary bladder following treatment of carcinoma of the cervix. *American Journal of Obstetrics and Gynecology*, **83**, 393–400 (1962)

139. Stewart, F.A., Michael, B.D. and Denekamp, J. Late radiation damage in the mouse bladder as measured by increased urination frequency. *Radiation Research*, **75**, 649–659 (1978)

140. Lundbeck, F., Ulso, N., Overgaard, J. and Djurhuus, J.C. Cystometry in mice: an *in vivo* model for evaluating early and late radiation damage to the urinary bladder. In *Proceedings of the 8th International Congress of Radiation Research*, Vol. 1 (eds E.M. Fielden *et al.*), Taylor Francis, London, p. 253 (1987)

141. Gillette, E.L., Hoopes, P.J., Withrow, S.J. and Park, R.D. Comparison of response of canine ureter and bladder to intraoperative and fractionated radiation. *International Journal of Radiation Oncology, Biology, Physics*, **10**, (Supplement 2), 103 (1984)

142. Kinsella, T.J., Sindelar, W.F., DeLuca, A.M. *et al.* Tolerance of the canine bladder to intraoperative radiation therapy: an experimental study. *International Journal of Radiation Oncology, Biology, Physics*, **14**, 939–946 (1988)

143. Unal, A., Hamberger, A.D., Seski, J.C. and Fletcher, G.H. An analysis of the severe complications of irradiation of carcinoma of the uterine cervix: treatment with intracavitary radium and parametrial irradiation. *International Journal of Radiation Oncology, Biology, Physics*, **7**, 999–1004 (1981)

144. Rothwell, R.I., Ash, D.V. and Thorogood, J. An analysis of the contribution of computed tomography to the treatment outcome in bladder cancer. *Clinical Radiology*, **36**, 369–372 (1985)

145. Mak, A.C.A., van t'Reit, A., Ypma, A.F.G.V.M. *et al.* Dose determination in bladder and rectum during intracavitary irradiation of cervix carcinoma. *Radiotherapy and Oncology*, **10**, 97–100 (1987)

146. Sullivan, M.F., Beamer, J.L., Cross, F.T. *et al.* Pathologic effects of intracavitary irradiation with californium-252. *International Journal of Radiation Oncology, Biology, Physics*, **6**, 1613–1627 (1980)

147. Kottmeir, H.L. Complications following radiation therapy in carcinoma of the cervix and their treatment. *American Journal of Obstetrics and Gynecology*, **88**, 854–864 (1964)

148. Villasanta, U. Complications of radiotherapy for carcinoma of the uterine cervix. *American Journal of Obstetrics and Gynecology*, **114**, 717–726 (1972)

149. Jones, C.R., Woodhouse, C.R.J. and Hendry, W.F. Urological problems following treatment of carcinoma of the cervix. *British Journal of Urology*, **56**, 609–613 (1984)

150. Horiot, J.C., Pigneux, J., Pourquier, H. *et al.* Radiotherapy alone in carcinoma of the intact uterine cervix according to G.H. Fletcher guidelines: a French cooperative study of 1313 cases. *International Journal of Radiation Oncology, Biology, Physics*, **14**, 605–611 (1988)

151. Dewit, L., Ang, K.K. and van der Schueren, E. Acute side effects and late complications after radiotherapy of localised carcinoma of the prostate. *Cancer Treatment Reviews*, **10**, 79–89 (1983)

152. Koeck, G.P. and Hillsinger, W.R. Dosage tolerance of pelvic structures with cobalt-60 rotation radiation

therapy. *American Journal of Roentgenology*, **111**, 260–268 (1971)

153. Quilty, P.M., Duncan, W. and Kerr, G.R. Results of a randomised study to evaluate influence of dose on morbidity in radiotherapy for bladder cancer. *Clinical Radiology*, **36**, 615–618 (1985)

154. Parkin, D.E., Davis, J.A. and Symonds, R.P. Long-term bladder symptomatology following radiotherapy for cervical carcinoma. *Radiotherapy and Oncology*, **9**, 195–199 (1987)

155. Gowing, N.F.C. Treatment of carcinoma of the bladder. III. Pathological changes in the bladder following irradiation. *British Journal of Radiology*, **33**, 484–487 (1960)

156. Heuper, W.C., Fisher, C.V., de Carvajel-Ferero, J. and Thompson, J.R. The pathology of experimental roentgencystitis in dogs. *Journal of Urology*, **47**, 156–167 (1942)

157. Antonakopoulos, G.N., Hicks, R.M., Hamilton, E. and Berry, R.J. Early and late morphological changes (including carcinoma of the urothelium) induced by irradiation of the rat urinary bladder. *British Journal of Cancer*, **46**, 403–416 (1984)

158. Zhuravlev, A.V. Changes in transitional epithelium subject to ionizing radiation. *Arkhiv Anatomii Gistologii i Embriologi*, **45**, 59–66 (1963)

159. Stewart, F.A., Denekamp, J. and Hirst, D.G. Proliferation kinetics of the mouse bladder after irradiation. *Cell and Tissue Kinetics*, **13**, 75–89 (1980)

160. Stewart, F.A. The proliferative and functional response of mouse bladder to treatment with radiation and cyclophosphamide. *Radiotherapy and Oncology*, **4**, 353–362 (1985)

161. Stewart, F.A., Randhawa, V.S., Michael, B.D. and Denekamp, J. Repair during fractionated irradiation ot the mouse bladder. *British Journal of Radiology*, **54**, 799–804 (1981)

162. Stewart, F.A., Randhawa, V.S. and Michael, B.D. Multifraction irradiation of mouse bladders. *Radiotherapy and Oncology*, **2**, 131–140 (1984)

163. Edsmyr, F., Andersson, L., Esposti, P.L. *et al.* Irradiation therapy with multiple small fractions per day in urinary bladder cancer. *Radiotherapy and Oncology*, **4**, 197–203 (1985)

164. Batterman, J.J., Results of d + t fast neutron irradiation on advanced tumours of bladder and rectum. *International Journal of Radiation Oncology, Biology, Physics*, **8**, 2159–2164 (1982)

165. Duncan, W., Arnot, S.J., Orr, J.A. and Kerr, G.R. The Edinburgh experience of fast neutron therapy. *International Journal of Radiation Oncology, Biology, Physics*, **8**, 2155–2158 (1982)

166. Griffin, T.W., Laromore, G.E., Hussey, D.H. *et al.* Fast neutron beam radiation therapy in the United States. *International Journal of Radiation Oncology, Biology, Physics*, **8**, 2165–2168 (1982)

167. Pointon, R.S., Read, G. and Greene, D. A randomised comparison of photons and 15 MeV neutrons for the treatment of carcinoma of the bladder. *British Journal of Radiology*, **58**, 219–224 (1985)

168. Stewart, F.A., Randhawa, V.S. and Maughan, R. The RBE for mouse bladders after irradiation with 1–8 fractions of 3 MeV neutrons. *British Journal of Radiology*, **59**, 61–68 (1986)

169. Watson, E.R., Halnan, K.E., Dische, S. *et al.* Hyperbaric oxygen and radiotherapy: a Medical Research Council trial in carcinoma of the cervix. *British Journal of Radiology*, **51**, 879–887 (1978)

170. Stewart, F.A. Mechanism of bladder damage and repair after treatment with radiation and cytostatic drugs. *British Journal of Cancer*, **53**, Supplement VII, 280–291 (1986)

171. Forni, A.M., Koss, L.G. and Geller, W. Cytological study of the effect of cyclophosphamide on the epithelium of the urinary bladder in man. *Cancer*, **17**, 1348–1355 (1964)

172. Farsund, T. Cell kinetics of mouse urinary bladder epithelium II. *Virchows Archives B. Cell Pathology*, **21**, 279–298 (1976)

173. Philips, F.S., Sternberg, S.S., Cronin, A.P. and Vidal, P.M. Cyclophosphamide and urinary bladder toxicity. *Cancer Research*, **21**, 1577–1589 (1961)

174. Koss, L.G. and Lavin, P. Effect of a single dose of cyclophosphamide on various organs in the rat II. Response of urinary bladder epithelium according to strain and sex. *Journal of the National Cancer Institute*, **44**, 1195–1200 (1970)

175. Stewart, F.A. The proliferative and functional response of mouse bladder to treatment with radiation and cyclophosphamide. *Radiation and Oncology*, **4**, 353–362 (1985)

176. Rizal, S., Biran, S., Antely, S. *et al.* Combined modality treatment for stage III ovarian carcinoma. *Radiotherapy and Oncology*, **3**, 237–244 (1985)

177. Hustu, H.O., Pinkel, D. and Pratt, C.B. Treatment ot clinically localised Ewing's sarcoma with radiation and combination chemotherapy. *Cancer*, **30**, 1522–1527 (1972)

178. Jayalakshmamma, B. and Pinkel, D. Urinary bladder toxicity following pelvic irradiation and simultaneous cyclophosphamide therapy. *Cancer*, **38**, 701–707 (1976)

179. Edrees, G., Luts, A. and Stewart, F.A. Bladder damage in mice after combined treatment with cyclophosphamide and X-rays. The influence of timing and sequence. *Radiotherapy and Oncology*, **11**, 349–360 (1988)

180. Alfert, H.J. and Gillenwater, J.Y. The consequences of ureteral irradiation with special reference to subsequent ureteral injury. *Journal of Urology*, **107**, 369–371 (1972)

181. Perry, P., Massey, F.M., Moore, T.N. and Eriksson, C.A. Treatment of irradiation injury to the ureter by ileal substitution. *Obstetrics and Gynecology*, **46**, 517–522 (1975)

182. Schmitz, H. Complications in the urinary tract due to carcinoma of the uterine cervix or radiation treatment. *American Journal of Roentgenology*, **24**, 47–53 (1930)

183. Shingleton, H.M., Fowler, W.C., Pepper, F.D. and

adriamycin and cyclophosphamide in previously untreated patients and as a single agent in previously treated patients. *Cancer Treatment Reports*, **63**, 1745–1753 (1979)

48. Stewart, A.F., Keating, T. and Schwartz, P.E. Magnesium homeostasis following chemotherapy with cisplatin: a prospective study. *American Journal of Obstetrics and Gynecology*, **153**, 660–665 (1985)

49. Ozols, R.F., Cordon, B.J., Jacobs, J. *et al*. High-dose cisplatin in hypertonic saline. *Annals of Internal Medicine*, **100**, 19–24 (1984)

50. Blumenreich, M.S., Woodcock, T.M., Jones, M. *et al*. High-dose cisplatin in patients with advanced malignancies. *Cancer*, **55**, 1118–1122 (1985)

51. Vannetzel, J.M., Baillent, F., Misset, J.L. *et al*. Toxicity of high-dose *cis*-DDP administered in hypertonic saline. *Proceedings of the American Society of Clinical Oncology*, **2**, 270 (1983)

52. Daugaard, G., Strandgaard, S., Holstein-Rathlou, N.H. *et al*. The renal handling of sodium and water is not affected by the standard-dose cisplatin treatment for testicular cancer. *Scandinavian Journal of Clinical and Laboratory Investigation*, **47**, 455–459 (1987)

53. Daugaard, G., Abildgaard, U., Holstein-Rathlou, N.H. *et al*. Renal tubular functions in patients treated with high-dose cisplatin. *Clinical Pharmacology and Therapeutics*, **44**, 164–172 (1988)

54. Sørensen, P.G., Nissen, M.H., Groth, S. and Rørth, M. Beta-2-microglobulin excretion: an indicator of long term nephrotoxicity during *cis*-platinum treatment? *Cancer Chemotherapy and Pharmacology*, **14**, 247–249 (1985)

55. Goren, M.P., Forastiere, A.A., Wright, R.K. *et al*. Carboplatin, iproplatin, and high-dose cisplatin in hypertonic saline evaluated for tubular nephrotoxicity. *Cancer Chemotherapy and Pharmacology*, **19**, 57–60 (1987)

56. Hacke, M., Schmoll, H.J., Alt, J.M. *et al*. Nephrotoxicity of *cis*-diamminedichloroplatinum with or without ifosfamide in cancer treatment. *Clinical Physiology and Biochemistry*, **1**, 17–26 (1983)

57. Cohen, A.I., Harberg, J. and Citrin, D.L. Measurement of urinary $\beta_2$-microglobulin in the detection of cisplatin nephrotoxicity. *Cancer Treatment Reports*, **65**, 1083–1085 (1981)

58. Dentino, M., Luft, F.C., Yum, M.N. *et al*. Long-term effect of *cis*-diamminedichloride platinum (CDDP) on renal function and structure in man. *Cancer*, **41**, 1274–1281 (1978)

59. Goren, M.P., Wright, R.K. and Horowitz, M.E. Cumulative renal damage associated with cisplatin nephrotoxicity. *Cancer Chemotherapy and Pharmacology*, **18**, 69–73 (1986)

60. Schilsky, R.L., Barlock, A. and Ozols, R.F. Persistent hypomagnesemia following cisplatin chemotherapy for testicular cancer. *Cancer Treatment Reports*, **66**, 1767–1769 (1980)

61. Schilsky, R.L. and Anderson, T. Hypomagnesemia and renal magnesium wasting in patients receiving *cis*-diamminedichloroplatinum(II). *Annals of Internal Medicine*, **90**, 929–931 (1979)

62. Mavichak, V., Wong, N.L.M., Quamme, G.A. *et al*. Studies on the pathogenesis of cisplatin-induced hypomagnesemia in rats. *Kidney International*, **28**, 914–921 (1985)

63. Massry, S.G., Coburn, J.W., Chapman, L.W. and Kleeman, C.R. Effect of NaCl infusion on urinary calcium and magnesium during reduction in their filtered loads. *American Journal of Physiology*, **213**, 1218–1244 (1967)

64. Wong, N.L.M., Quamme, G.A., Sutton, R.A.L. and Dirks, J.H. Effect of mannitol on water and electrolyte transport in the dog kidney. *Journal of Laboratory and Clinical Medicine*, **94**, 563–692 (1979)

65. Bar, R.S., Wilson, H.E. and Mazzaferri, E.I. Hypomagnesemic hypocalcemia, secondary to renal magnesium wasting: a possible consequence of high dose gentamycin therapy. *Annals of Internal Medicine*, **82**, 646–649 (1975)

66. Ward, J.N. and Fauvie, K.A. The nephrotoxic effect of *cis*-diamminedichloroplatinum(II) (NSC-119875) in male F344 rats. *Toxicology and Applied Pharmacology*, **38**, 535–547 (1976)

67. Dobyan, D.C., Levi, J., Jacobs, C. *et al*. Mechanism of *cis*-platinum nephrotoxicity: II Morphologic observations. *Journal of Pharmacology and Experimental Therapeutics*, **7**, 551–556 (1980)

68. Gonzales-Vitale, J.C., Hayes, D.M., Cvitkovic, E. and Sternberg, S.S. The renal pathology in clinical trial of *cis*-platinum (II) diamminedichloride. *Cancer*, **39**, 1362–1371 (1977)

69. Daugaard, G., Abildgaard, U., Holstein-Rathlou, N.H. *et al*. Acute effect of cisplatin on renal hemodynamics and tubular function in dog kidneys. *Renal Physiology*, **9**, 303–316 (1986)

70. Daugaard, G., Holstein-Rathlou, N.H. and Leyssac, P.P. Effects of cisplatin on proximal convoluted and straight segments of the rat kidney. *Journal of Pharmacology and Experimental Therapeutics*, **244**, 1081–1085 (1988)

71. Daugaard, G., Abildgaard, U., Larsen, S. *et al*. Functional and histopathological changes in dog kidneys after administration of cisplatin. *Renal Physiology*, **10**, 54–64 (1987)

72. Chopra, S., Kaufman, J.S., Jones, T.W. *et al*. Cis-diamminedichloroplatinum-induced acute renal failure in the rat. *Kidney International*, **21**, 54–64 (1982)

73. Safirstein, R., Miller, P., Dikman, S. *et al*. Cisplatin nephrotoxicity in rats: defect in papillary hypertonicity. *American Journal of Physiology*, **241**, F175–F185 (1982)

74. Phelps, J.S., Gandolfi, A.J., Brendel, K. and Dorr, R.I. Cisplatin nephrotoxicity: *in vitro* studies with precision-cut rabbit renal cortical slices. *Toxicology and Applied Pharmacology*, **90**, 501–512 (1987)

75. Gordon, J.A. and Gattone, V.H. Mitochondrial alterations in cisplatin-induced acute renal failure.

*American Journal of Physiology*, **250**, F991–F998 (1986)

76. Safirstein, R., Winston, J., Moel, D. *et al.* Cisplatin nephrotoxicity: insights into mechanism. *International Journal of Andrology*, **10**, 325–346 (1987)

77. Uozumi, J. and Litterst, C.L. The effect of cisplatin on renal ATPase activity *in vivo* and *in vitro*. *Cancer Chemotherapy and Pharmacology*, **15**, 93–96 (1985)

78. Hanneman, J. and Baumann, K. Cisplatin-induced lipid peroxidation and decrease of gluconeogenesis in rat kidney cortex: different effects of antioxidants and radical scavengers. *Toxicology*, **51**, 119–132 (1988)

79. Stark, J.J. and Howell, S.B. Nephrotoxicity of *cis*-platinum(II)-dichlorodiammine. *Clinical Pharmacology and Therapeutics*, **23**, 461–466 (1978)

80. Goldstein, R.S. and Mayor, G.H. Minireview: the nephrotoxicity of cisplatin. *Life Sciences*, **32**, 685–690 (1982)

81. Pera, M.F. and Harder, H.C. Effects of furosemide and mannitol-induced diuresis on the nephrotoxicity and physiologic disposition of *cis*-dichlorodiammineplatinum in rats. *Proceedings of the American Association of Cancer Research*, **19**, 100 (1978)

82. Cvitkovic, K., Spaulding, J., Bethume, V. *et al.* Improvement of *cis*-dichlorodiammineplatinum (NSC 119875): therapeutic index in an animal model. *Cancer*, **39**, 1357–1361 (1977)

83. Pera, M.F., Zook, B.C. and Harder, H.C. Effects of mannitol or furosemide diuresis on the nephrotoxicity and physiological disposition of *cis*-diammine platinum(II) in rats. *Cancer Research*, **29**, 1269–1278 (1979)

84. Hayes, D.M., Cvitkovic, E., Golbey, R.B. *et al.* High-dose *cis*-platinum diammine dichloride: amelioration of renal toxicity by mannitol diuresis. *Cancer*, **39**, 1372–1381 (1977)

85. Al-Sarraf, M., Fletcher, W., Oishi, N. *et al.* Cisplatin hydration with and without mannitol diuresis in refractory disseminated malignant melanoma: a Southwest Oncology Group Study. *Cancer Treatment Reports*, **66**, 31–35 (1982)

86. Lehane, D., Winston, A., Gray, R. and Daskal, V. The effect of diuretic pre-treatment on clinical, morphological and ultrastructural *cis*-platinum-induced nephrotoxicity. *International Journal of Radiation Oncology, Biology, Physics*, **5**, 1393–1399 (1979)

87. Ward, J.M., Grabin, M.E., LeRoy, A.F. and Young, D.M. Modification of the renal toxicity of *cis*-dichlorodiammineplatinum(II) with furosemide in male F344 rats. *Cancer Treatment Reports*, **61**, 375–379 (1977)

88. McMurty, R.J. and Mitchell, J.R. Renal and hepatic necrosis after metabolic activation of 2-substituted furans and thiophenes including furosemide and cephaloridine. *Toxicology and Applied Pharmacology*, **42**, 285–300 (1977)

89. Heidemann, H.Th., Gerkens, J.F., Jackson, E.K. and Branch, R.A. Attenuation of cisplatinum-induced nephrotoxicity in the rat by high salt diet, furosemide and acetazolamide. *Archives of Pharmacology*, **329**, 201–205 (1985)

90. Daley-Yates, P.T. and McBrian, D.C.H. A study of the protective effect of chloride salts on cisplatin nephrotoxicity. *Biochemical Pharmacology*, **34**, 2363–2369 (1985)

91. Earhart, R.H., Martin, P.A., Tutsch, K.D. *et al.* Improvement in the therapeutic index of cisplatin (NSC 119875) by pharmacologically induced chloruresis in the rat. *Cancer Research*, **43**, 1187–1194 (1983)

92. Litterst, C.L. Alterations in the toxicity of *cis*-dichlorodiammineplatinum(II) and in tissue localization of platinum as a function of NaCl concentration in the vehicle of administration. *Toxicology and Applied Pharmacology*, **61**, 99–108 (1981)

93. Safirstein, R. Correspondence re R.H. Earhart *et al.* Improvement in the therapeutic index of cisplatin (NSC 119875) by pharmacologically induced chloruresis in the rat. *Cancer Research*, **44**, 5455–5456 (1984)

94. Gonzales-Vitale, J.C., Hayes, D.M., Cvitcovic, E. and Sternberg, S.S. Acute renal failure after *cis*-dichlorodiammineplatinum(II) and gentamicin-cephalothin therapies. *Cancer Treatment Reports* **62**, 693–698 (1978)

95. Salem, P.A., Jaboury, K.W. and Khalil, M.F. Severe nephrotoxicity: A probable complication of *cis*-dichlorodiammineplatinum(II) and cephalothin-gentamicin therapy. *Oncology*, **39**, 31–32 (1982)

96. Haas, A., Anderson, L. and Lad, T. The influence of aminoglycosides on the nephrotoxicity of *cis*-diamminedichloroplatinum in cancer patients. *Journal of Infectious Diseases*, **147**, 363 (1983)

97. Engineer, M.S., Bodey, G.P., Newman, R.A. and Ho, D.W. Effects of cisplatin-induced nephrotoxicity on gentamicin pharmacokinetics in rats. *Drug Metabolism and Disposition*, **15**, 329–334 (1987)

98. Kawamura, J., Soeda, A. and Yoshida, O. Nephrotoxicity of *cis*-diamminedichloroplatinum(II) (*cis*-platinum) and the additive effect of antibiotics: morphological and functional observation in rats. *Toxicology and Applied Pharmacology*, **58**, 475–482 (1981)

99. Jongejan, H.T.M. Provoost, A.P. and Molenaar, J.C. Potentiation of *cis*-diamminedichloroplatinum nephrotoxicity by amikacin in rats. *Cancer Chemotherapy and Pharmacology*, **22**, 178–180 (1988)

100. Dorr, R.T. and Soble, M.J. Cimetidine enhances cisplatin toxicity in mice. *Journal of Cancer Research and Clinical Oncology*, **114**, 1–2 (1988)

101. Mulder, P.O.M., Sleijfer, D.T., de Vries, E.G.E. *et al.* Renal dysfunction following high-dose carboplatin treatment. *Journal of Cancer Research and Clinical Oncology*, **114**, 212–214 (1988)

102. Lelieveld, P., van der Vijgh, W.J.F., Veldhuizen, R.W. *et al.* Preclinical studies on toxicity, antitumour

activity and pharmacokinetics of cisplatin and three recently developed derivatives. *European Journal of Cancer and Clinical Oncology*, **20**, 1087–1104 (1984)

103. Creaven, P.J., Madajewicz, S., Pendyala, L. *et al.* Phase I clinical trial of *cis*-dichloro-trans-dihydroxy-bis-isopropylamine platinum IV (CHIP). *Cancer Treatment Reports*, **67**, 794–796 (1983)

104. Pendyala, L., Madajewicz, S., Shashikant, B. *et al.* Evaluation of the nephrotoxicity of iproplatin (CHIP) in comparison to cisplatin by the measurement of urinary enzymes. *Cancer Chemotherapy and Pharmacology*, **15**, 203–207 (1985)

105. Rozencweig, M., Nicaise, C., Beer, M. *et al.* Phase I study of carboplatin given on a five-day intravenous schedule. *Journal of Clinical Oncology*, **1**, 621–626 (1983)

106. Gore, M.E., Calvert, A.H. and Smith, I.E. High dose carboplatin in the treatment of lung cancer and mesothelioma: a phase I dose escalation study. *European Journal of Cancer and Clinical Oncology*, **23**, 1391–1397 (1987)

107. Trump, D.L., Grem, J.L., Tutsch, K.D. *et al.* Platinum analogue combination chemotherapy: cisplatin and carboplatin – a phase I trial with pharmacokinetic assessment of the effect of cisplatin administration on carboplatin excretion. *Journal of Clinical Oncology*, **5**, 1281–1289 (1987)

108. Evans, B.D., Rajn, K.S., Calvert, A.H. *et al.* Phase II study of JM-8, a new platinum analog, in advanced ovarian carcinoma. *Cancer Treatment Reports*, **67**, 997–1000 (1983)

109. Liegler, D.G., Henderson, E.S., Halan, M.A. and Oliverio, V.T. The effect of organic acids on renal clearance of methotrexate in man. *Clinical Pharmacology and Therapeutics*, **10**, 849–857 (1969)

110. Bleyer, W.A. The clinical pharmacology of methotrexate: new application of an old drug. *Cancer*, **41**, 36–51 (1978)

111. Pratt, C.B., Roberts, D., Shanks, E.C. and Warmath, F.L. Clinical trials and pharmacokinetics of intermittent high-dose methotrexate – 'leucoverin rescue' for children with malignant tumors. *Cancer Research*, **34**, 3326–3331 (1974)

112. Condit, P.T., Chanes, R.E. and Joel, W. Renal toxicity of methotrexate. *Cancer*, **23**, 127–131 (1969)

113. Howell, S.B. and Carmody, J. Changes in glomerular filtration rate associated with high-dose methotrexate therapy in adults. *Cancer Treatment Reports*, **61**, 1389–1391 (1977)

114. Weinblatt, M.E. Toxicity of low dose methotrexate in rheumatoid arthritis. *Journal of Rheumatology (Suppl.)*, **12**, 35–39 (1985)

115. Von Hoff, D.D., Penta, J.S., Helman, L.J. and Slavik, M. Incidence of drug related death secondary to high-dose methotrexate and citrovorum factor administration. *Cancer Treatment Reports*, **61**, 745–748 (1977)

116. Jacobs, S.A., Stoller, R.G., Chabner, P.A. and Johns, D.G. 7-hydroxymethotrexate as a urinary metabolite in human subjects and rhesus monkeys receiving high-dose methotrexate. *Journal of Clinical Investigation*, **57**, 734–738 (1976)

117. Huang, K.C., Wenczak, B.A. and Liu, Y.K. Renal tubular transport of methotrexate in the rhesus monkey and dog. *Cancer Research*, **39**, 4843–4848 (1979)

118. Abelson, H.T. and Garnick, M.B. Renal failure induced by cancer chemotherapy. In *Cancer and the Kidney* (eds R.E. Rieselbach and M.B. Garnick), Lea and Febiger, Philadelphia, pp. 769–813 (1982)

119. McKenzie, A.W. and Aitken, C.V.E. Psoriasis and folic acid antagonists. *British Journal of Dermatology*, **79**, 122–123 (1967)

120. Ryan, T.J. and Vickers, H.R. Psoriasis and folic acid antagonists. *British Journal of Dermatology*, **78**, 612–613 (1966)

121. Pitman, S.W., Parker, L.M., Tattersall, M.H.N. *et al.* Clinical trial of high-dose methotrexate (NSC-740) with citrovorum factor (NSC-3590) – toxicologic and therapeutic observations. *Cancer Chemotherapy Reports*, **6**, 43–49 (1975)

122. Pitman, S.W. and Frei, E. Weekly methotrexate-calcium leucovorin rescue: effect of alkalinization of nephrotoxicity; pharmacokinetics in the CNS; and use in CNS non-Hodgkin's lymphoma. *Cancer Treatment Reports*, **61**, 695–701 (1977)

123. Goren, M.P., Wright, R.K., Horowitz, M.E. and Meyer, W.H. Enhancement of methotrexate nephrotoxicity after cisplatin therapy. *Cancer*, **58**, 2617–2621 (1986)

124. Wang, Y., Sutow, W.W., Romsdahl, M.M. and Perez, C. Age-related pharmacokinetics of high-dose methotrexate in patients with osteosarcoma. *Cancer Treatment Reports*, **63**, 405–410 (1979)

125. Frei, E. Methotrexate revisited. *Medical and Pediatric Oncology*, **2**, 227–241 (1976)

126. Gibson, T.P., Reich, S.D., Krumolovsky, F.A. and Ivanovich, P. Hemoperfusion for methotrexate removal. *Clinical Pharmacology and Therapeutics*, **23**, 351–355 (1978)

127. Hande, K.R., Balow, J.E., Drake, J.C. *et al.* Methotrexate and hemodialysis. *Annals of Internal Medicine*, **87**, 495–496 (1977)

128. Ahmad, S., Shen, F. and Bleuer, W.A. Methotrexate-induced renal failure and ineffectiveness of peritoneal dialysis. *Archives of International Medicine*, **138**, 1146–1147 (1978)

129. Mandel, M.A. The synergistic effect of salicylates on methotrexate toxicity. *Plastic and Reconstructive Surgery*, **57**, 733–737 (1976)

130. Bourke, R.S., Cheda, G., Bremer, A. *et al.* Inhibition of renal tubular transport of methotrexate by probenecid. *Cancer Research*, **35**, 110–116 (1975)

131. Preiss, R., Brovtsyn, V.K., Perevodchikova, N.I. *et al.* Effects of methotrexate on the pharmacokinetics and renal excretion of cisplatin. *European Journal of Clinical Pharmacology*, **34**, 139–144 (1988)

132. Crom, W.R., Pratt, C.B., Green, A.A. *et al.* The

effect of prior cisplatin therapy on the pharmacokinetics of high-dose methotrexate. *Journal of Clinical Oncology*, **2**, 655–661 (1984)

133. Allen, L.M. and Creaven, P.J. Effect of microsomal activation on interaction between iphosphamide and DNA. *Journal of Pharmaceutical Sciences*, **61**, 2009–2011 (1972)

134. Cox, P.J. Cyclophosphamide cystitis: identification of acrolein as the causative agent. *Biochemical Pharmacology*, **28**, 2045–2049 (1979)

135. Scheef, W., Klein, H.O., Brock, N. *et al.* Controlled clinical studies with an antidote against the urotoxicity of oxazaphosphorines: preliminary results. *Cancer Treatment Reports*, **63**, 501–503 (1979)

136. Bryant, B.M., Jarman, M., Ford, H.T. and Smith, I.E. Prevention of ifosfamide-induced urothelial toxicity with 2-mercaptoethane sulphonate sodium (mesnum) in patients with advanced carcinoma. *Lancet*, **ii**, 657–659 (1980)

137. Barnett, D. Preclinical toxicology of ifosfamide. *Seminars in Oncology*, **9**, 8–13 (1982)

138. Stuart-Harris, R.C., Harper, P.G., Parsons, C.A. *et al.* High-dose alkylation therapy using ifosfamide infusion with mesna in the treatment of adult advanced soft-tissue sarcoma. *Cancer Chemotherapy and Pharmacology*, **11**, 69–72 (1983)

139. Cohen, M.H., Creaven, P.J., Tejada, F. *et al.* Phase I clinical trial of ifosfamide (NSC-109724). *Cancer Treatment Reports*, **59**, 751–755 (1975)

140. Fosså, S.D. and Talle, K. Treatment of metastatic renal cancer with ifosfamide and mesnum with and without irradiation. *Cancer Treatment Reports*, **64**, 1103–1108 (1980)

141. Goren, M.P., Wright, R.K., Horowitz, M.E. and Pratt, C.B. Ifosfamide-induced subclinical tubular nephrotoxicity despite mesna. *Cancer Treatment Reports*, **71**, 127–130 (1987)

142. Bremner, D.N., McCormick, J.S. and Thomson, J.W.W. Clinical trial of ifosfamide (NSC-109724) – results and side effects. *Cancer Chemotherapy Reports*, **58**, 889–893 (1974)

143. DeFonzo, R.A., Abeloff, M., Braine, H. *et al.* Renal dysfunction after treatment with isophosphamide (NSC-109724). *Cancer Chemotherapy Reports*, **58**, 375–382 (1974)

144. Sangster, G., Kaye, S.B., Calman, K.C. and Dalton, J.F. Failure of 2-mercaptoethane sulphonate sodium (mesna) to protect against ifosfamide nephrotoxicity. *European Journal of Cancer and Clinical Oncology*, **20**, 435–436 (1984)

145. Loehrer, P.J., Williams, S.D., Einhorn, L.H. and Ansari, R. Ifosfamide: an active drug in the treatment of adenocarcinoma of the pancreas. *Journal of Clinical Oncology*, **3**, 367–372 (1985)

146. van Dyk, J.J., Falkson, H.C., van der Merwe, A.M. and Falkson, G. Unexpected toxicity in patients treated with ifosfamide. *Cancer Research*, **32**, 921–924 (1972)

147. Niederle, N., Scheulen, M.E., Cremer, M. *et al.* Ifosfamide in combination chemotherapy for sarcomas and testicular carcinomas. *Cancer Treatment Reviews*, **10**, 129–135 (1983)

148. Wheeler, B.M., Loehrer, P.J., Williams, S.D. and Einhorn, L.H. Ifosfamide in refractory male germ cell tumors. *Journal of Clinical Oncology*, **4**, 28–34 (1986)

149. Hacke, M., Schmoll, H.J., Alt, J.M. *et al.* Nephrotoxicity of cis-diamminedichloroplatinum with or without ifosfamide in cancer treatment. *Clinical Physiology and Biochemistry*, **1**, 17–26 (1983)

150. Goren, M., Wright, R.K., Pratt, C.B. *et al.* Potentiation of ifosfamide neurotoxicity, hematotoxicity, and tubular nephrotoxicity by prior cis-diamminedichloroplatinum(II) therapy. *Cancer Research*, **47**, 1457–1460 (1987)

151. Philips, F.S., Sternberg, S.S., Cronin, A.P. and Vidal, P.M. Cyclophosphamide and urinary bladder toxicity. *Cancer Research*, **21**, 1577–1589 (1961)

152. Stillwell, T.J. and Benson, R.C. Cyclophosphamide-induced hemorrhagic cystitis. *Cancer*, **61**, 451–457 (1988)

153. DeFonzo, R.A., Colvin, O.M., Braine, H. *et al.* Cyclophosphamide and the kidney. *Cancer*, **33**, 483–491 (1974)

154. Bode, U., Seif, S.M. and Levine, A.S. Studies on the antidiuretic effect of cyclophosphamide: vasopressin release and sodium excretion. *Medical and Pediatric Oncology*, **8**, 295–303 (1980)

155. Murray-Lyon, I.M., Eddleston, A.L.W.F., Williams, R. *et al.* Treatment of multiple-hormone-producing malignant islet-cell tumor with streptozotocin. *Lancet*, **ii**, 26, 895–898 (1968)

156. Adolphe, A.B., Glasofer, E.D., Troetel, W.M. *et al.* Fate of streptozotocin in patients with advanced cancer. *Cancer Chemotherapy Reports*, **59**, 547–556 (1975)

157. Bhuyan, B.K., Kuentzel, S.L., Gray, L.G. *et al.* Tissue distribution of streptozotocin. *Cancer Chemotherapy Reports*, **58**, 157–165 (1974)

158. Karunanayake, E.H., Hearse, D.J. and Mellows, G. The metabolic fate and elimination of streptozotocin. *Biochemical Society Transactions*, **3**, 410–414 (1975)

159. Sadoff, L. Nephrotoxicity of streptozotocin. *Cancer Chemotherapy Reports*, **54**, 457–459 (1970)

160. Carter, S.K., Broder, L. and Friedman, M. Streptozotocin and metastatic insulinoma. *Annals of Internal Medicine*, **74**, 445–446 (1971)

161. Stolinsky, D.C., Sadoff, L., Braunwald, J. *et al.* Streptozotocin in the treatment of cancer. *Cancer*, **30**, 61–67 (1972)

162. Broder, L.E. and Carter, S.K. Pancreatic islet cell carcinoma. *Annals of Internal Medicine*, **79**, 108–118 (1973)

163. Hall-Craggs, M., Brenner, D., Vigortia, R. *et al.* Renal ultrastructure following streptozotocin nephrotoxicity. *Proceedings of the American Association of Cancer Research*, **22**, 201 (1981)

164. Fennell, J.S. and Falls, W.F. Streptozotocin nephrotoxicity. *Clinical Nephrology*, **15**, 97–101 (1981)

165. Moertel, C.G., Reitemeier, R.J., Schutt, A.J. *et al.* Phase II study of streptozotocin in the treatment of advanced gastrointestinal cancer. *Cancer Chemotherapy Reports*, **55**, 303–307 (1971)

166. DuPriest, R.W., Huntington, M.C., Massey, W.H. *et al.* Streptozotocin therapy in 22 cancer patients. *Cancer*, **35**, 358–367 (1975)

167. Myerowitz, R.L., Sartiano, G.P. and Cavallo, T. Nephrotoxic and cytoproliferative effects of streptozotocin. *Cancer*, **38**, 1550–1555 (1976)

168. Loftus, L., Cupagge, F.E. and Hoogstraten, B. Clinical and pathological effects of streptozotocin. *Journal of Laboratory and Clinical Medicine*, **84**, 407–413 (1974)

169. Denine, E.P., Harrison, S.D. and Peckham, J.C. Qualitative and quantitative toxicity of sublethal doses of methyl-CCNU in BDF1 mice. *Cancer Treatment Reports*, **61**, 409–417 (1977)

170. Schaeppi, U., Fleichman, R.W. and Phelan, R.S. *et al.* CCNU (NSC-79037): preclinical toxicologic evaluation of a single intravenous infusion in dogs and monkeys. *Cancer Chemotherapy Reports*, **5**, 53–64 (1974)

171. Weiss, R.B., Posada, J.G., Kramer, R.A. and Boyd, M.R. Nephrotoxicity of semustine. *Cancer Treatment Reports*, **67**, 1105–1112 (1983)

172. Nichols, W.C. and Moertel, C.C. Nephrotoxicity of methyl-CCNU. *New England Journal of Medicine*, **301**, 1181 (1979)

173. Silver, H.K.B. and Morton, D.L. CCNU nephrotoxicity following sustained remission in oat cell carcinoma. *Cancer Treatment Reports*, **63**, 226–227 (1978)

174. Micetich, K.C., Jensen-Akula, M., Mandard, J.C. and Fischer, R.I. Nephrotoxicity of semustine (MeCCNU) in patients with malignant melanoma receiving adjuvant chemotherapy. *American Journal of Medicine*, **71**, 967–972 (1981)

175. Schacht, R.G., Feiner, H.D., Gallo, G.R. *et al.* Nephrotoxicity of nitrosourea. *Cancer*, **48**, 1328–1334 (1981)

176. Harmon, W.E., Cohen, H.J., Schneeberger, E.E. and Grupe, W.E. Chronic renal failure in children treated with methyl CCNU. *New England Journal of Medicine*, **300**, 1200–1203 (1979)

177. Berglund, J. Progredierande njurinsufficiens efter CCNU-behandling. *Läkartidningen*, **77**, 1760 (1980)

178. Ellis, M.E., Weiss, R.B. and Kuperminc, M. Nephrotoxicity of lomustine. *Cancer Chemotherapy and Pharmacology*, **15**, 174–175 (1985)

179. Crooke, S.T. and Bradner, W.T. Mitomycin C: a review. *Cancer Treatment Reviews*, **3**, 121–139 (1976)

180. Philips, F.S., Schwartz, H.S. and Sternberg, S.S. Pharmacology of mitomycin C: I. Toxicity and pathologic effects. *Cancer Research*, **20**, 1354–1361 (1960)

181. Matsuyama, M., Suzumori, K. and Nakamura, T. Induction of hydronephrosis by prolonged intraperitoneal injections of subtoxic dose of mitomycin C in mice. *Nature*, **202**, 99–100 (1964)

182. Hanna, W.T., Krauss, S., Regester, R.F. and Murphy, W.M. Renal disease after mitomycin C therapy. *Cancer*, **48**, 2583–2588 (1981)

183. Cantrell, J.E., Philips, T.M. and Schein, P.S. Carcinoma-associated hemolytic-uremic syndrome: a complication of mitomycin C chemotherapy. *Journal of Clinical Oncology*, **3**, 723–734 (1985)

184. Lempert, K.D. Haemolysis and renal impairment syndrome in patients on 5-fluorouracil and mitomycin-C. *Lancet*, **ii**, 369–370 (1980)

185. Rumpf, K.W., Rieger, J., Lankisch, P.G. *et al.* Mitomycin-induced haemolysis and renal failure. *Lancet*, **ii**, 1037–1038 (1980)

186. Hamner, R.W., Verani, R. and Weinman, E.J. Mitomycin-associated renal failure. *Archives of Internal Medicine*, **143**, 803–807 (1983)

187. Verwey, J., De Vries, J. and Pinedo, H.M. Mitomycin C-induced renal toxicity, a dose-dependent side effect? *European Journal of Cancer and Clinical Oncology*, **23**, 195–199 (1987)

188. D'Elia, J.A., Aslani, M., Schermer, S. *et al.* Hemolytic-uremic syndrome and acute renal failure in metastatic adenocarcinoma treated with mitomycin: a case report and literature review. *Renal Failure*, **10**, 107–113 (1987)

189. Valavaara, R. and Nordman, E. Renal complications of mitomycin C treatment with special reference to the total dose. *Cancer*, **55**, 47–50 (1985)

190. Proia, A.D., Harden, E.A. and Silberman, H.R. Mitomycin-induced hemolytic-uremic syndrome. *Archives of Pathology and Laboratory Medicine*, **108**, 959–962 (1984)

191. Catell, V. Mitomycin-induced hemolytic uremic kidney. *American Journal of Pathology*, **121**, 88–95 (1985)

192. Webster, J., Rees, A.J., Lewis, P.J. and Hensby, C.N. Prostacyclin deficiency in hemolytic uremic syndrome. *British Medical Journal*, **ii**, 271 (1980)

193. Kennedy, B.J. Metabolic and toxic effects of mithramycin during tumor therapy. *American Journal of Medicine*, **49**, 494–503 (1970)

194. Fillastre, J.P., Maitrot, J., Cannone, M.A. *et al.* Renal function and alterations in plasma electrolyte levels in normocalcaemic and hypercalcaemic patients with malignant diseases, given an intravenous infusion of mithramycin. *Chemotherapy*, **20**, 280–295 (1974)

195. Sternberg, S.S. Cross-striated fibrils and other ultrastructural alterations in glomeruli of rats with daunomycin nephrosis. *Laboratory Investigation*, **23**, 39–51 (1970)

196. Buss, H. and Lamberts, B. The kidney glomerulus of the rat during experimental daunomycin nephrosis. A comparative transmission scanning electron microscopic study. *Beitrage zur Pathologie*, **148**, 360–387 (1973)

197. Serpick, A.A. and Henderson, E.S. Observations on toxicity and clinical trials with daunomycin. *Pathologie Biologie*, **15**, 909–912 (1967)

198. Fajardo, L.F., Eltringham, J.R., Stewart, J.R. and Klauber, M.R. Adriamycin nephrotoxicity. *Laboratory Investigation*, **43**, 242–253 (1980)

199. Bernard, J., Boeron, P.R., Jacgiullat, C. and Maral, R. Rubidomycin. A new agent against cancer. *Recent Results in Cancer Research*, **20**, 101–113 (1969)

200. Von Hoff, D.D., Rozencweig, M. and Slavik, M. Daunomycin, an anthracycline antibiotic effective in acute leukemia. *Advances in Pharmacology and Chemotherapy*, **15**, 1–50 (1978)

201. Burke, J.F., Laucius, J.F., Brodovsky, H.S. and Soriano, R.Z. Doxorubicin hydrochloride-associated renal failure. *Archives of Internal Medicine*, **137**, 385–388 (1977)

202. Ho, M., Bear, R.A. and Garvey, M.B. Symptomatic hypophosphatemia secondary to 5-azacytidine therapy of acute nonlymphocytic leukemia. *Cancer Treatment Reports*, **60**, 1400–1402 (1976)

203. Peterson, B.A., Collins, A.J., Vogelzang, N.J. and Bloomfield, C.D. 5-Azacytidine and renal tubular dysfunction. *Blood*, **57**, 182–185 (1981)

# 16

# Lung morbidity of radiotherapy

E.L. Travis

The treatment with radiation of a large number of different malignant diseases encompasses some portion of the lung in the treatment portal. In addition to the treatment of lung cancer, in which the tumor arises from the critical normal tissue, the treatment of other diseases with radiation, e.g. breast cancer or Hodgkin's disease, delivers radiation to the lung incidentally, i.e. the tumor is located elsewhere, but the lung is by necessity included in the treatment field. This situation also pertains to head and neck patients most of whom have the apices of both lungs irradiated in the supraclavicular fields. The entire lung also is treated frequently as part of the management of Wilms' tumor or Ewing's sarcoma in children. More recently, the use of total body irradiation in the management of both hematopoietic and non-hematopoietic malignancies has increased the number of patients who receive radiation to the entire lung as part of their treatment regimen.

In all of these situations concerns about lung toxicity influence radiation therapy technique, thus imposing limits on the amount of radiation that can be delivered to the tumor. Despite the large numbers of treatments that involve irradiating either a part of the lung (the most common situation) or the whole lung (a less frequent scenario), clinical expression of lung damage is infrequent and few patients exhibit severe life-threatening complications. However, radiation pneumonitis and fibrosis can be fatal. For example, in a series of 72 patients who received more than 40 Gy preoperative radiotherapy for lung carcinoma, acute radiation pneumonitis was the cause of death or a major contributor to it in 8% of the patients [1]. In another study involving single doses of irradiation to the whole lung, 17.9% of the patients (44/245) developed the clinical syndrome of radiation pneumonitis that was fatal in 84% of cases [2].

Lung irradiation damage is related to the total dose, fractionation regimen, volume of tissue irradiated, and previous radiation therapy or chemotherapy. Accurate clinical data on the influence of each of these parameters on morbidity are required if the radiotherapist is to either reduce the morbidity of current treatment techniques or develop new regimens that improve tumor control while affording the same morbidity as current ones. Because the lung does not manifest radiation damage until a relatively long time after the completion of radiotherapy, no compensation can be made during treatment for severe reactions. The challenge to the radiotherapist then is to cure the malignant disease in the chest without causing severe, life-threatening sequelae to the patient.

## Lung architecture and morbidity

In clinical circumstances the radiotherapist accepts some lung damage, either pneumonitis or fibrosis, because of the large functional reserve of this organ. The whole organ does not fail if part of it is destroyed, thus damage and morbidity may not be closely related. This is in contrast to other tissues, such as the spinal cord, in which partial destruction results in complete functional failure. Although failure in all tissues ultimately results from killing and depletion of groups of sensitive cells critical to tissue survival, the clinical morbidity of a given treatment depends not only on the survival of a sufficient number of cells to maintain tissue function but the proper organization of these cells into subunits that perform the function of the tissue. The spatial arrangement of these functional subunits differs between tissues and is critical to the relationship between the damage produced and the resultant morbidity of the treatment [3–5].

Functional subunits in tissues can be arranged either in a series or in parallel. Like Christmas tree lights, if one light in a series arrangement burns out, the whole strand fails. However, if one light in a parallel strand burns out, it goes unnoticed. An example of a tissue in which the functional subunits are arranged in series is the spinal cord. In this and other tissues similarly organized, the functional integrity of the tissue is dependent on the integrity of each subunit and the destruction of only one subunit will result in complete failure of the organ. In those tissues in which the functional subunits are arranged in series, estimates of damage will be closely correlated with morbidity.

The lung, however, consists of structurally well-defined subunits arranged in parallel. Architecturally, the lung is a system of branching ducts and accompanying blood vessels that ultimately terminate in the alveolus (Figure 16.1) [6]. The functional

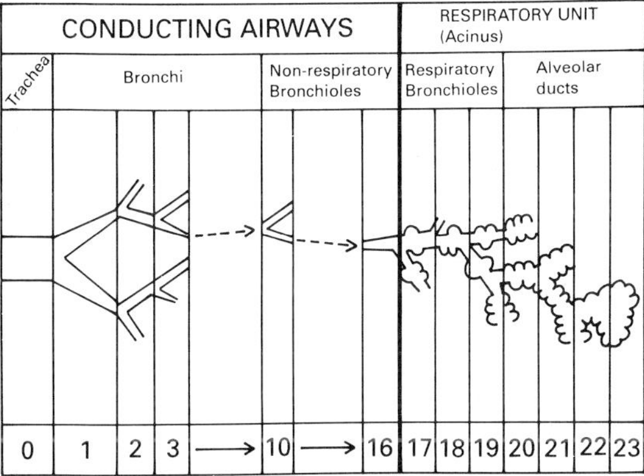



**Figure 16.1** Schematic of the organization of the lung from the trachea to the alveoli. Numbers at the bottom indicate the approximate number of generations from trachea to alveoli. The respiratory unit consisting of respiratory bronchioles and alveolar ducts is most likely the functional subunit of the lung. Alveoli appear in progressively larger numbers beginning from the 17th branching of airways; thus gas exchange occurs along the whole length of the respiratory bronchioles and alveolar ducts. Reproduced with permission from ref. [6]

subunit of the lung is most likely the acinus, which is structurally well-defined, beginning at the ramification of the terminal bronchiole to the respiratory bronchioles and terminating in the alveolar sacs, each bearing numerous alveoli. Alveoli appear in increasing numbers along the acinus; gas exchange thereby occurs along its entire length. It has been estimated that the human lung contains approximately 300 million alveoli. Each acinus is a self-contained entity independent of its neighbor, and

although the survival of each acinus is dependent on the survival of a critical number of target cells in the structure, obliteration of one acinus will have no measurable effect on lung function. The integrity of the lung as a whole is not dependent on maintaining the integrity of each subunit. This alone accounts for the large functional reserve of the lung and the fact that destruction of a part of the lung does not cause significant damage to the lung as a whole. In tissues like the lung in which the functional subunits are arranged in parallel, estimates of damage may not always agree well with clinically expressed morbidity.

## What is morbidity?

Morbidity is a clinical term that describes how an individual patient feels and/or how well a specific organ functions. Clinical morbidity of a treatment is determined by three factors:

1. The effect of the treatment on the tissue, i.e. the damage incurred.
2. The impact of this damage on organ function.
3. The impact of both of the above on the patient's well-being and life style.

Clearly, life-threatening morbidity is related to observable changes in the lung, but estimates of morbidity will vary dependent on the criteria used to assess the damage. For example, damage does occur in the lungs of practically all patients treated with radiation for lung, breast or esophageal tumor. Thus, quantitating the number of patients who exhibit histological or radiographic evidence of lung damage after thoracic irradiation is one way to assess damage. Yet, what is critical to the individual is how such damage affects the ability of the lung to exchange oxygen and carbon dioxide. Sophisticated pulmonary function tests may demonstrate only minimal dysfunction. But a true measure of morbidity must reflect the impact of these deficits on the patient's health and lifestyle. Small changes in pulmonary function that pose little problem for most people may seriously compromise the lifestyles of more active individuals, e.g. construction workers, long distance runners, or of individuals with diminished reserve due to pre-existing damage.

Morbidity, then, is a subjective end point; however, both the damage produced by irradiation and the resulting functional deficits can be assessed by objective criteria. A goal of this chapter is to relate the objective criteria for assessing the effects of radiation on the human lung – the damage – to the more subjective criteria of clinical morbidity. All clinical studies suffer from the disadvantages of restricted numbers of patients, confounding clinical and treatment variables, type of tumor, smoking history, underlying lung disease, and inconsistencies in treatment technique and time and dose fractionation parameters. In addition, most studies rely on sophisticated pulmonary function tests but fail to correlate such tests with radiographic or histological evidence of lung damage or with subjective functional assessments. Nonetheless, there are sufficient reports in the literature that some estimate of lung damage and the resultant morbidity incurred by the patient after thoracic radiotherapy can be made.

# Lung damage after irradiation

## Histology

Irradiation of the lung produces two separate and distinct histological phases of damage [7–13]. The first, radiation pneumonitis, appears within 6 months after irradiation and for this reason is referred to as the 'acute phase' of the response. Histologically radiation pneumonitis has been well characterized in both experimental animals and man. The acute phase is characterized by edema, the deposition of fibrin-like material in the alveolar spaces forming hyaline membranes, and swelling and degeneration of the epithelial cells lining the alveolar walls, specifically the type 2 cells. Hyaline membranes are commonly found in humans after lung irradiation; this change is less frequently observed in those animals commonly used in studies of lung response after irradiation. In both man and animals the histological changes are not accompanied by an inflammatory cell infiltrate, which makes them somewhat unique and differentiates them from the usual inflammatory condition in the lung.

The predominant lesion of the chronic phase in humans appears to be a progressive diffuse fibrosis of the septa, causing a progressive widening of the alveolar walls which, if severe, leads to a complete obliteration of the air spaces. If the total dose has been high or multiple courses of radiation have been given, then the predominant pathology is an organizing lesion that leads to eventual replacement of the lung parenchyma with scar tissue. Clearly, changes in the pulmonary vascular bed such as thromboses or vascular sclerosis occur concomitantly, but neither the parenchymal nor the vascular changes are indicative of the underlying pathogenesis [7–12].

Although there is a clear consensus on the pathology of the later fibrotic stage in man, no clear consensus exists concerning this later stage of damage in mouse lungs [13–16]. In an elegant and detailed study of histological changes after irradiation of the lungs of nine different strains of mice, Sharplin and Franko [16] found that not all late damage in mice was characterized by fibrosis.

Fundamental differences existed in the amount of fibrosis and scarring between the mouse strains studied, ranging from extensive fibrosis and contracted scarring to few late fibrotic scars. In the latter situation, the major, albeit infrequently observed pathology was multifocal clusters of tightly packed 'foamy cells' and small accumulations of lymphocytes. A third subset showed a combination of both pathologies, exhibiting some areas of focal fibrosis accompanied by cellular infiltrates in other areas. Regardless of the pathology, mice of all strains died during this chronic phase.

Although these data may appear to challenge the validity of the mouse as an appropriate model for studying late radiation-induced lung damage, the mouse still provides a useful if imperfect model of chronic lung damage after irradiation.

## Pathophysiology

The histological changes of radiation pneumonitis and fibrosis produce clinical symptoms. In fact, it is these clinical manifestations of the histological damage that are commonly referred to as radiation pneumonitis. Clinically, radiation pneumonitis is characterized by a deterioration in lung function, dyspnea and cough. These symptoms usually heal within 2–3 months if the dose has not been high nor the volume of lung irradiated very large. If the latter is the case, the patient becomes progressively dyspneic and cyanotic, all of which may lead to the demise of the patient. In those patients who survive this initial pneumonitis phase, a chronic progressive fibrosis may develop. This chronic phase also occurs in patients who never exhibited the acute clinical syndrome. The patients who manifested the acute phase usually exhibit a more severe form of the chronic phase.

Although the chronic phase also may be symptomatic dependent on the volume of lung involved, most often little change is found in lung function despite radiographic changes. If the fibrosis involves an extensive area of the lung, the patient will exhibit symptoms such as cough and shortness of breath. This is an extremely unusual situation, however, with few patients exhibiting disabling symptoms.

# Damage and its relationship to morbidity

The accurate assessment of damage and morbidity critically depends on techniques that clearly identify first any change from normal in the lung as due to irradiation, i.e. provide a *qualitative* assessment of the damage, and second, and more importantly, *quantify* these changes in terms of incidence, the numbers of patients who exhibit the change, and the severity of the changes. In addition, the optimum technique for assessing post-irradiation lung changes in humans must be non-invasive.

## Assessment of lung damage

The pathological changes of radiation pneumonitis and fibrosis would be expected to increase lung opacity and density; thus, plain chest radiographs should detect these abnormalities and provide an estimate of the incidence of the damage in any group of irradiated patients. Radiographic changes in the lungs may occur in any patient who receives radiation therapy to the thorax, but the radiographic appearance of these changes is not specific and must be differentiated from recurrent tumor, lymphangitic spread, and infection. In addition, these radiological changes do not necessarily agree with the incidence of the clinical syndrome of radiation pneumonitis. The radiological diagnosis of radiation-induced damage can be made with reasonable certainty only when a pretreatment radiograph was normal and the post-treatment film shows an area of increased density that corresponds to the size and shape of the treatment fields.

Although the chest X-ray is the most frequent initial form of assessment of radiation lung damage, it is a relatively insensitive indicator of radiation damage in the lung. In a recent comparison of the sensitivity of two diagnostic imaging techniques to detect post-irradiation changes in the chest, Bell *et al.* [17] found that, in 50% of the irradiated patients, chest X-rays failed to detect even the most obvious change – lung opacity – which subsequently was detected by computed tomographic examination. More importantly, in this same study the findings on chest X-rays did not correlate well with functional deficits, a better indicator of morbidity, in the same patients. Thus, although the chest X-ray is non-invasive, it is, not surprisingly, of relatively little value for assessing morbidity in patients who have received radiotherapy to the lungs.

Computed tomography (CT), on the other hand, provides data on the incidence of pneumonitis in humans as well as a quantitative estimate of the severity of this damage [18–20]. CT works for the same reason that chest radiographs do, i.e. radiation damage in the lung is expressed as an increase in the density of the lung parenchyma. However, whereas a chest film images the whole volume of the lung, CT observes only a small slice through this volume; thus, better resolution of any lung damage should be possible. In addition, this technique is well suited to the assessment of pulmonary damage in humans because of its high sensitivity to changes in attenuation and its non-invasive nature. Radiation-induced changes in the lung can be observed on CT as irregular radio-opacities in the irradiated area, which subsequently can be quantitated by assigning CT numbers to the changes in lung density. Quantitative increases in lung density have been shown to be dose-dependent in mice and in humans [18–20], making this a potentially useful tool. CT has the further advantage over chest films that it can better differentiate between post-irradiation change and tumor recurrence. In addition, in the study by Bell *et al.* [17] good agreement was found between the changes detected by CT and those demonstrated by ventilation and perfusion scans of the irradiated area.

Despite the limitations of these techniques for assessing morbidity, both chest X-rays and CT are useful. First, they can be useful in diagnosing symptomatic patients. Second, quantitative CT in particular can be used to verify radiobiological models. For example, it has been suggested that new fractionation techniques using doses per fraction of less than the conventional 2 Gy given more than once a day may increase the therapeutic ratio by sparing late-responding tissues like the lung more than the tumor. Clearly, the radiotherapist is reluctant to irradiate a large volume of lung using an unproven technique for fear of inducing clinically significant morbidity. Quantitative CT permits assessment of the damage in a small lung volume without exposing the patient to the risk of unacceptable morbidity. In addition, because drugs are frequently used with radiation to treat those malignant diseases for which the lung is dose limiting, e.g. Hodgkin's disease, dose enhancement factors can be estimated from the data obtained from these techniques.

Imaging techniques provide qualitative and quantitative assessment of lung injury after irradiation. However, these data may bear little relationship to functional deficits and/or the morbidity of the treatment because of the large functional reserve of the lung. Even severe changes as measured by CT may have little, if any, effect on lung function if they occur in only small lung volumes. A better indicator of morbidity are tests of pulmonary function.

## Assessment of pulmonary function

Pulmonary function may be the most often tested parameter of a morbidity related to radiation treatment. Pulmonary function has been assessed in every possible scenario involving radiation treatment of all or part of the lung [21–27]. In all of these studies minimal functional deficits have been reported. It is exactly for this reason that these data are critical, because they stress the importance of determining the functional impact of the damage observed in this organ. In general, the pathological changes of radiation pneumonitis and fibrosis would be expected to produce restrictive lung disease,

**Table 16.1 Some commonly used tests of pulmonary function after irradiation**

| Tests | Method |
|---|---|
| Lung volumes: | |
| Functional residual capacity | Nitrogen washing |
| | Body plethysmography |
| Vital capacity and subdivisions | Water- or dry-seal spirometer |
| | |
| Lung mechanics: | |
| Forced vital capacity | |
| Forced expired volumes | Water- or dry-seal spirometer |
| Forced expiratory flows | with graphic recorder |
| Flow-volume loops | |
| Maximal voluntary ventilation | |
| Airway resistance | Body plethysmography |
| Pulmonary compliance | Esophageal balloon/transducers |
| Closing volume | Single-breath $N_2$ elimination |
| Gas dependent flow-volume loops | Helium-oxygen spirometry |
| | |
| Gas diffusion: | |
| Diffusing capacity | CO single-breath diffusion |
| Membrane/intracapillary diffusion | |
| | |
| Gas distribution | |
| Distribution of ventilation | Multibreath nitrogen washout |
| | Radionuclide ventilation scanning* |
| | Single-breath $N_2$ elimination* |
| Distribution of perfusion | Radionuclide perfusion scanning* |
| Distribution of ventilation/ | Arterial blood gases* |
| perfusion scans | |

All tests assess total lung function except for those marked with an asterisk which provide information on regional function. Adapted from ref. [92]

abnormalities of gas transfer, and ventilation-perfusion mismatches. Yet these functional deficits are infrequent, and those that do occur are rarely disabling. It is now clear that this is largely due to the spatial organization of the functional subunits in the lung, which affords the organ a large functional redundancy. Thus, if only a part of the lung is irradiated, little change in total lung function may occur even though that one area may be obliterated. In addition, such changes would be most profound in patients who began treatment with insufficient pulmonary reserve, i.e. patients with lung cancer or those with pre-existing lung disease.

Function tests most commonly used to assess functional lung deficits after irradiation include spirometry (forced vital capacity (FVC), forced expiratory volume ($FEV_1$, $FEV_1$/FVC)), lung volumes (total lung capacity, residual volume, and functional residual capacity), and diffusing capacity for carbon monoxide ($D_LCO$) (Table 16.1). Because lung irradiation produces restrictive lung disease, few tests assess obstructive changes, although forced vital capacity can be useful in determining whether restrictive lung disease is accompanied by obstructive changes as well. Functional changes indicative of obstructive lung disease have been observed in irradiated lungs, but a reduction of air flow through the conducting airways is probably secondary to changes in the pulmonary parenchyma rather than being due to primary effects of irradiation on the large airways.

It is important to distinguish between those tests that provide an index of the overall functional status of the lung and those that delineate abnormalities in a specific area. If morbidity is an indicator of the state of wellbeing of the organ, then tests of total lung function are more appropriate indicators of clinical morbidity. For example, diffusing capacity ($D_LCO$) is determined by the number of functioning alveoli in contact with red blood cells. If the number of these units is reduced, as might be expected during pneumonitis or fibrosis, $D_LCO$ will be proportionately reduced in that area. However, when the diffusing capacity per liter volume is calculated it may be normal, indicating that the remaining alveolar units are normal. Also, in restrictive lung disorders such as pulmonary fibrosis, spirometry data such as FEV may be reduced. Yet when FEV is expressed as a percentage of forced vital capacity, normal or increased values may be found.

Tests of total lung function may give the poorest

**Table 16.2 Tests used to assess distribution and matching of ventilation and perfusion**

| *Physiological variable* | *Tests* |
| --- | --- |
| Overall distribution of ventilation | Multibreath $N_2$ washout<br>Single-breath $N_2$ test<br>Helium mixing time |
| Localized distribution of ventilation | $^{133}$Xe ventilation scan<br>Lateral position test<br>Bronchospirometry |
| Distribution of perfusion | $^{99m}$Tc-HAM perfusion scan |
| Relationship of ventilation to perfusion | $^{133}$Xe ventilation/perfusion scan<br>Physiological dead space<br>Physiological shunt<br>Single-breath $CO_2$ test |

Reproduced with permission from ref. [92]

agreement with damage assessed by chest X-rays or CT. However, as in the Christmas tree light analogy, if enough of the individual units fail, the overall effectiveness is diminished and assays of damage and total lung function then will show clearer correlation.

Data from regional lung function tests, on the other hand, will be in better agreement with those obtained from imaging techniques, but they will not necessarily be good indicators of clinical morbidity. Even severe damage in small volumes will have little effect on total pulmonary function. Perhaps this is why very few studies show profound changes in pulmonary function in patients after radiotherapy for diseases such as breast cancer, lung cancer, esophageal cancer, or mediastinal tumors – situations in which only a part of the lung is irradiated. For example, only small changes in total lung function, including decreases in static and dynamic lung volumes and diffusing capacity, have been reported in patients who received irradiation to the lung for the management of breast cancer [28]. In these same patients, however, tests of regional lung function, i.e. blood flow, ventilation/perfusion scans, showed that function was severely compromised in the irradiated region as early as 1 month after the initiation of radiotherapy. Thus, after irradiation of only part of the lung, tests of regional function will give a very different picture of functional status from those which measure total lung function. Table 16.2 lists those tests commonly used to assess regional and total gas distribution and ventilation.

Clearly, greater changes in total lung function would be expected in patients whose whole lung is irradiated, e.g. in Wilms' tumor or from the treatment of hemopoietic malignancies using total body irradiation. In these patients, tests of total lung function would be the best indicator of morbidity.

Because of careful dose selection, only minimal pulmonary dysfunction has been reported in these patients too.

It is tempting to associate the changes in lung function with the underlying pathogenesis of radiation-induced lung damage. Although the changes in lung function clearly are related to the pathological changes in the lung, they do not provide information on the pathogenesis of this damage, e.g. is it vascular or parenchymal? The pathological changes and concomitant changes in pulmonary function are related to damage in all tissue components, i.e. the vasculature, the epithelium, most likely type 2 cells, and the interstitium. Because both vascular and parenchymal injury are manifested after irradiation, it is difficult to define how much of any given change is due to vascular pathology or parenchymal pathology. In other words, these functional changes are related to the pathological changes but are not indicative of the degree of damage in the various tissue components.

# Dose-response relationships for human lung

One goal of radiotherapy treatment is to deliver as high a total dose to malignant diseases in the thoracic area as possible while maintaining the functional integrity of the lung. This can only be accomplished if the relationship between the incidence of morbidity and dose is well defined.

The relationship of lung damage to radiation dose to the whole lung is well established for a number of small animal systems using assays that assess morbidity (lethality) [29,30], lung function (breathing rate [31], CO uptake [32]), and damage (histological changes) [13,16,31]. For all species studied, the incidence of pneumonitis rises very steeply with dose after whole lung irradiation, producing steep, well-defined dose-response curves. In addition, a comparison of mouse and human data indicates that the shape of the dose-response curves for the two species is similar, but the absolute dose level for the response varies, generally in the direction of a lower isoeffect dose in humans (Figure 16.2). Thus, there is an urgent need to define the

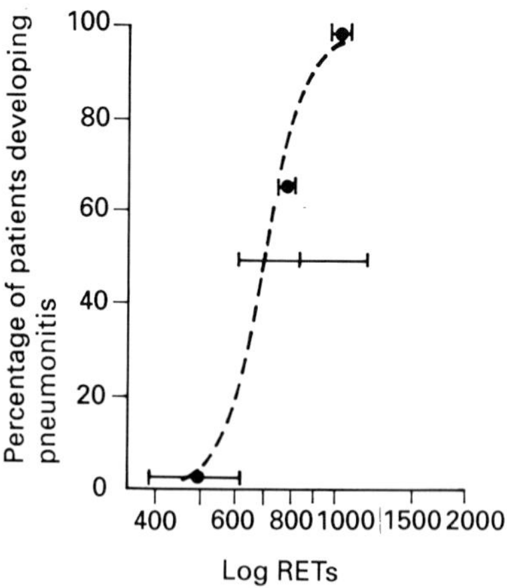


**Figure 16.3** Percentage of patients developing pneumonitis as a function of dose in Roentgen Equivalent Therapy units (RETs). Reproduced with permission from ref. [33]

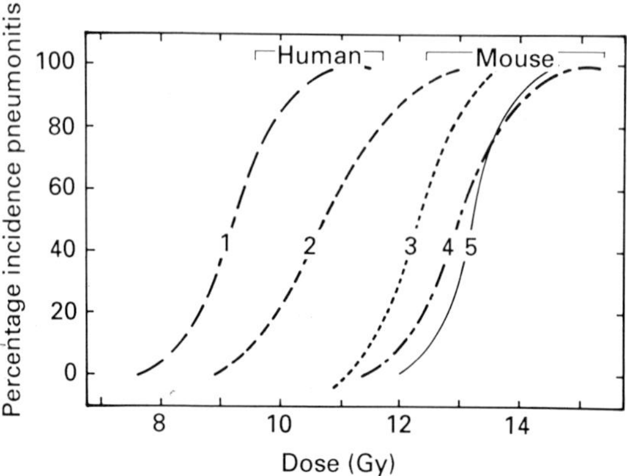


**Figure 16.2** Dose-response curves for incidence of pneumonitis in humans and from several studies in mice. 1, ref. [34]; 2, ref. [93]; 3, ref. [4]; 4, ref. [94]; 5, ref. [29]. Modified with permission from ref. [95]

dose-response relationship for radiation pneumonitis in humans accurately and concisely, particularly because of the implied steepness of the dose-response curves as derived from animal data.

The development and use of objective end points for quantitating lung damage and morbidity after irradiation in man has allowed the establishment of the dose-response relationship for pneumonitis in humans. Wara *et al.* [33] published the first dose-response curve for radiation pneumonitis in humans in 1973. Patients entered into this study were being treated for metastatic disease and had at least 75% of one whole lung irradiated. They had to exhibit both the clinical syndrome characteristic of pneumonitis – cough, fever, or dyspnea – as well as show definite changes on the chest radiograph. Treatments were given using various dose fractionation schedules, thus either the Ellis normal standard dose (NSD) or equivalent dose model was used to estimate the single dose equivalent of fractionation schedules with equivalent biological effect. This curve is shown in Figure 16.3 and, as with the mouse data, the dose-response curve for pneumonitis in humans appeared to be steep, although both the slope and placement of the curve were uncertain, as

each depended on one data point obtained from a small sample size.

Recent treatment techniques employing large single doses to the upper half body or total body have provided a larger data base to better resolve the dose-response relation for radiation pneumonitis in man [2,34–36]. Dose-response curves for the incidence of pneumonitis in humans after single doses of radiation have been well defined in a retrospective study of 150 patients treated at the Princess Margaret Hospital in Toronto with large single doses of radiation to the upper half body for widespread metastatic disease [2,34]. Patients with significant previous and subsequent lung irradiation, previous lung disease and tumor in the lung were excluded from the analysis. All doses were corrected for inhomogeneities. The actuarial incidence of radiation pneumonitis versus dose to lung was evaluated using probit analysis. A clear well-defined, dose-response relationship was demonstrated that does not differ significantly in shape from that of Wara *et al.* [33] (Figure 16.4). The curve for human lung is very steep; the dose range spanning 10–90% incidence in van Dyk's study [34] was only about 2 Gy. The incidence of pneumonitis rises from 5% to 50% with an increase in dose of about 1 Gy. Thus, small increases in dose could significantly increase morbidity if the doses given are on the steeply rising portion of the dose-incidence curve.

These data exemplify the need for an accurate description of the dose-incidence curve for pneumonitis after fractionated irradiation, the most frequent clinical situation. Because only a part of the lung is usually irradiated, morbidity as assessed by clinically expressed pneumonitis or even tests of total lung function may not be good end points. Instead, quantification of damage or changes in regional lung function are more appropriate. In addition, the fractionation regimens must encompass a range of total doses to obtain dose-response data while at the same time using similar sizes of doses per fraction

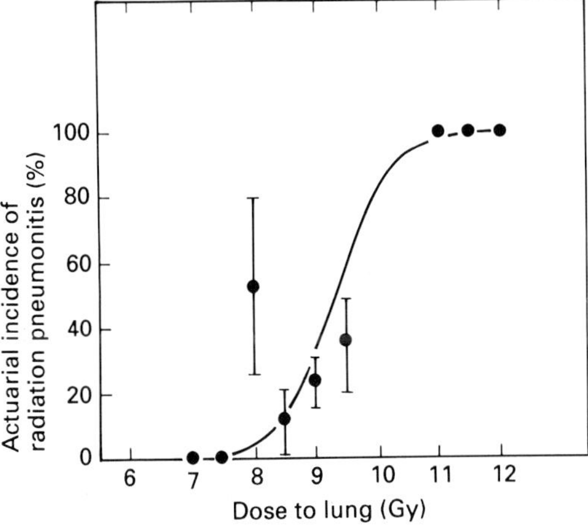

**Figure 16.4** Percentage of radiation pneumonitis as a function of single doses to the whole lung based on all patients 1960–1978, excluding those with significant additional radiation, previous lung disease or lung cancer. The curve is the best fit probit regression line to the actual data points. Reproduced with permission from ref. [34]

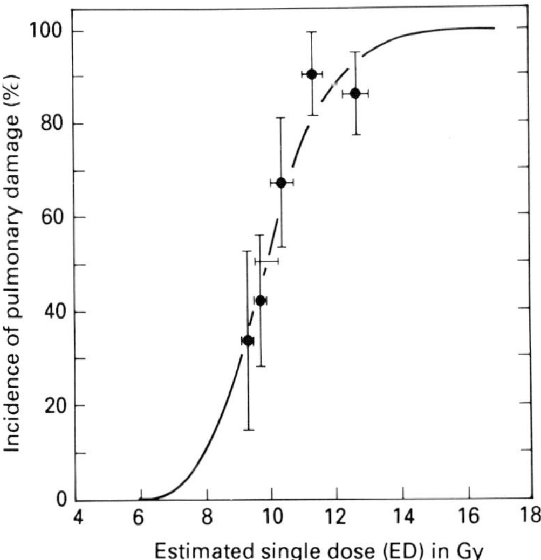

**Figure 16.5** Dose-response curve for the incidence of lung damage in humans after fractionated irradiation. The curve is the best fit to the solid data points as determined by probit regression. The $ED_{50}$ is approximately 10 Gy with a standard error of 0.40 Gy (horizontal error bar on the curve). Vertical error bars are the standard deviation of the points. Reproduced with permission from ref. [37]

to exclude the influence of the dose per fraction dependence of repair. Clinical studies by Mah *et al.* [37] and van Dyk *et al.* [38] fit these criteria and have the added advantage of being prospective. Mah *et al.* assessed lung damage in patients using CT to quantify the increase in lung density in the irradiated area. The effective single dose model was used to determine fractionation schedules with equivalent biological effects. These data, given in Figure 16.5, show that the incidence of damage increased steeply with dose: a 5% increase in lung dose produced a 12% increase in the incidence of damage. In fact, the whole range of the response from 10% to 90% occurred over a dose range of only 3 Gy. Although a direct comparison of these data with those obtained in the single upper half body irradiation study of van Dyk *et al.* [34] is difficult because of the different end points used and the retrospective nature of the van Dyk study [34], the similarities in both the slopes of the two dose-response curves and the doses that gave a 50% incidence of morbidity and damage, 9.3 Gy and 10 Gy respectively, indicate that quantifying lung damage in small volumes may be useful in predicting morbidity of a given treatment when a larger volume is irradiated.

# Modifying lung damage and morbidity

## Fractionation response of the lung

It is well established that one of the most significant factors in sparing the lung from radiation damage is the size of the dose per fraction used in radiotherapy. Based on the time at which damage is expressed, normal tissues have been divided into two categories – acutely responding and late responding – the lung being an example of the latter [39]. It is now established that these two classes of tissue exhibit differential responses to changes in dose fractionation and that tissues classified as late responding are relatively more sensitive to changing the size of the dose per fraction used in clinical radiotherapy than are acutely responding tissues [39]. Abundant clinical data show that when the dose per fraction is increased and the total dose adjusted to produce the same level of acute reactions, more damage to late responding normal tissues is observed. Conversely, decreasing the size of dose per fraction should produce less damage in late than in acutely responding tissues. This concept is illustrated in Figure 16.6 in which total dose versus dose per fraction is plotted for 50% incidence of radiation pneumonitis in mouse lung from a number of different authors. Also shown on the same plot is crypt survival in the jejunum, an acutely responding normal tissue. The curve for pneumonitis rises

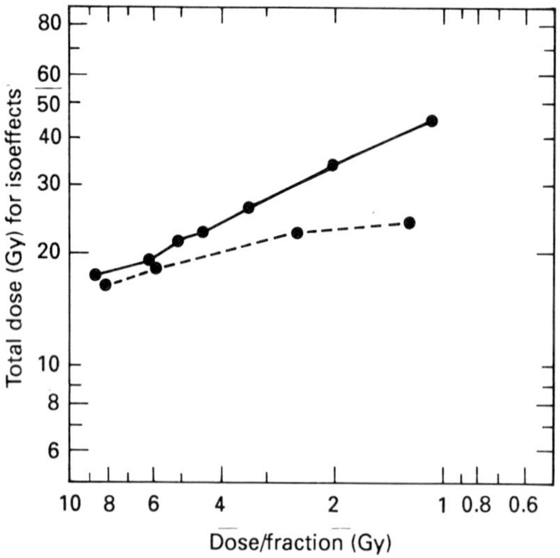

**Figure 16.6** Plot of total dose for radiation pneumonitis
and gut lethality in mice as a function of dose per fraction.
It is clear that the same change in dose per fraction has a
bigger effect on the total dose for isoeffect in the lung
(●—●) than the jejunum (●---●)

steeply as the dose per fraction increases, whereas
that for gut is more shallow. The clinical significance
of these data is that the lung behaves as a late
responding tissue and that decreasing the dose per
fraction should allow an increase in the total dose
given with little, if any, increase in morbidity.
Conversely, large reductions in total dose will be
necessary to achieve the comparable degree of
damage in the lung if the dose per fraction is
increased.

This knowledge has been the single most important factor in changing radiotherapeutic practice in
the last 5 years and has spawned the development
of new fractionation regimens using more than one
fraction per day [39–41]. Critical to the use of these
regimens in radiotherapy is the assumption that
most malignant tumors will exhibit a fractionation
response more like acutely responding tissues than
late responding tissues. Thus, decreasing the size of
dose per fraction used in radiotherapy should
improve the therapeutic ratio by decreasing reactions in late responding normal tissues while not
changing tumor cell kill and, therefore, tumor
control. The term hyperfractionation has been used
to describe schedules in which two or more fractions
per day are given with doses per fraction of less than
2 Gy in the same overall (or somewhat shorter)
treatment time. Higher total doses may be given in
expectation of decreased effect in tissues like the
lung. The use of an increased number of small
fractions should diminish the effect on the lung
without sacrificing tumor control and may in fact

increase tumor control because of the higher total
doses given.

Based on these considerations, the Radiation
Therapy Oncology Group (RTOG) initiated clinical
trials of hyperfractionation in the thoracic region,
two of which involved treatment of lung cancer [42–
44]. Although the findings are preliminary, a
number of tentative conclusions are already apparent.

1. There is no evidence of more severe reactions in
   the lung in the patients treated in the hyperfractionated protocols.
2. Tumor control in the hyperfractionation arms is
   at least as good as that in the standard fractionation arms.

Although more data are needed before definitive
statements can be made, the preliminary data
suggest that hyperfractionated radiotherapy may be
useful for treating diseases in which the lung is a
critical normal tissue. Radiobiology also indicates
that the use of large dose fractions is relatively
contraindicated when the lung is in the treatment
field, particularly in the treatment of diseases that
have a high probability of long-term cure.

## Volume

It is well known clinically that one of the single most
effective ways of changing the morbidity of lung
irradiation for a given dose is to change the volume
of tissue irradiated. Both the incidence in the
irradiated population and severity of symptomatic
pneumonitis in an individual patient will increase as
the volume increases. This volume effect, generally
considered to be 'large' for the lung, is not surprising, considering the parallel arrangement of the
functional subunits in the lung. However, few
quantitative data, either clinical or experimental,
are available that define the relationship between
volume of lung irradiated and morbidity.

In a study of breast cancer patients who had
various volumes of the lungs irradiated with equivalent doses, Rothwell *et al.* [45] have attempted to
address the issue of the relationship of volume of
lung treated to the incidence and severity of
pneumonitis. In these studies the dose given was
constant. The severity of pneumonitis was graded
subjectively, ranging from radiographic changes
only to marked symptoms requiring treatment. One
category, grade 1, included patients who exhibited
definite radiographic evidence of lung damage but
were clinically asymptomatic. The volumes of lung
irradiated were estimated from CT scans. The
incidence of all grades of pneumonitis was increased
as the volume irradiated increased, as shown in
Figure 16.7. Adjustments in dose would be necessary if morbidity was not to be exceeded as the

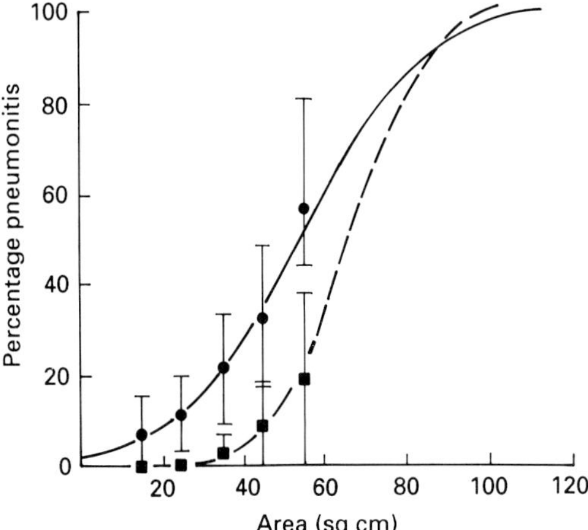

**Figure 16.7** Probit analysis curve relating area irradiated to incidence of pneumonitis for all grades (●——●) or for only grade 3 pneumonitis (●---●). Grade 3 included only those patients with marked symptoms requiring treatment (see text for further discussion). It is clear that the incidence of all grades of pneumonitis significantly increases as the volume of lung irradiated increases. Modified from ref. [45]

volume irradiated increased. Of course the radiotherapist must still rely on his clinical judgement when adjusting dose and volume.

The exact relationship between dose and volume and clinically expressed morbidity in the lung is unknown. It has been shown that a dose given to a modest volume of lung tissue will produce minimal morbidity but that this same total dose given to a large volume will result in unacceptable morbidity [46,47]. More recent clinical studies by the RTOG [42–44] supported these data and showed that when the total dose to the lung was increased from 60 Gy to 74 Gy, clinically expressed morbidity as assessed by radiation pneumonitis or fibrosis was not increased after the higher total doses, if the volume irradiated remained modest. Based on these data, it was suggested that the volume of lung irradiated is a more significant factor in clinically expressed lung damage than is total dose. This is most likely a correct assumption if the total dose given is beyond the steep portion of the dose-response curve. However, changes in volume would be expected to significantly affect morbidity if the total dose given was on the steeply rising portion of the curve.

## Specific treatment-related morbidity

### Lung cancer

Approximately 50% of patients with lung cancer receive radiation to the lung at some point in the management of their disease. Because these patients generally have had large volumes of lung treated to large total doses they are ideal candidates for morbidity assessment, and data on both the incidence and severity of radiation pneumonitis can be obtained [47–54]. However, long-term survival in this group of patients is poor; thus, few data can be derived concerning radiation fibrosis. In addition, the interpretation of radiation-induced lung damage in this patient population is plagued by numerous difficulties. First is the problem of residual disease in the lung. Second, some patients receive chemotherapy as part of the management of their disease, further confounding any attempts to determine the role of radiation alone on the incidence and severity of lung damage [55]. Lastly, the functional reserve of the lung is compromised at the outset of treatment in this population composed primarily of heavy smokers, clearly a factor in assessing treatment-related morbidity.

Despite these complicating factors, estimates of the incidence of damage and morbidity can be obtained. The incidence of damage, i.e. radiographic evidence of pneumonitis or fibrosis, is high. However, the incidence of associated functional changes is low. A study by Brady *et al.* [46] showed that total doses of 20–60 Gy given over a period of 11–40 days produced few significant changes in pulmonary mechanics, ventilation, volume and blood gases, indicating that morbidity is low even in these aggressively treated patients.

Cox [42] has clearly identified the critical problem in estimating treatment-related morbidity in malignancies with low and short post-treatment survival times, of which lung cancer is an example. The risks in such patient populations may be underestimated because the total number of patients treated with the particular regimen is often used for the denominator. In trials for cancer of the lung this may be particularly misleading because a large proportion of these patients die of their neoplasm before enough time has elapsed for lung damage to be expressed.

### Hodgkin's disease

The treatment of Hodgkin's disease with the mantle field technique frequently involves irradiating substantial volumes of lung. This patient population is relatively young, and 80–90% of these patients will be cured of their disease and will be long-term survivors placing them at risk for chronic sequelae. For this reason, morbidity of lung irradiation as measured by pulmonary function tests has most often been assessed in these patients. Both prospective and retrospective studies have shown that pulmonary sequelae after mantle field technique are minimal both in incidence and severity [21–23,56–60].

Smith *et al.* [22] prospectively studied 30 patients who were evaluated prior to irradiation and at 3, 6, and 12 months after the completion of therapy and yearly thereafter. Twenty patients were tested 4 years after treatment. This study showed that although most patients experience an early decrease (within the first 6 months to 1 year) in all lung function parameters tested, all values return to within 10% of normal values within 5 years after treatment. Based on this careful analysis, no significant changes in pulmonary function attributable to mantle irradiation were observed at long intervals after treatment.

These function tests were performed at rest and not during exercise, when one might expect the probability of the expression of lung dysfunction to be increased. Watchie *et al.* [23] have performed lung function tests retrospectively on 57 patients both at rest and during exercise who were treated with mantle field irradiation alone or combined with chemotherapy. Follow-up time in this study was at least 1 year, with a median of 5 years. A comparison of these data from patients treated with irradiation only with those receiving chemotherapy at the completion of radiotherapy showed that resting lung function values were normal in all treatment groups and that exercise values were no more than 20% below normal. Thus, even exercise tolerance was not significantly affected by irradiation.

The precise role of radiation in the lung morbidity of mantle field irradiation is confounded by many other factors including smoking history, extensive intrathoracic disease and chemotherapy. Unfortunately, there is no clear consensus on the effect of most of these factors on morbidity. For example, in one study only patients who smoked exhibited a significant progressive decrease in $FEV_1/FVC$ consistent with a progressive obstructive ventilatory defect [22]. In other studies no significant difference in pulmonary function was found in smoking versus non-smoking patients [59]. The one factor that has been found to increase morbidity in all studies is chemotherapy. In some of those studies in which patients who received combined chemotherapy plus radiation were separated from those who received radiation only, the combined therapy treatment produced significantly more morbidity than radiation alone.

It seems apparent that the incidence of pulmonary dysfunction following mantle field radiotherapy for Hodgkin's disease is small. The most significant factor in increasing the morbidity of this treatment may be concomitant chemotherapy, although smoking remains a strong candidate too. Although patients with extensive intrathoracic disease might be expected to experience increased morbidity, this appears to be true only if they received chemotherapy and radiation therapy.

The general consensus of all of these studies can be stated quite simply: extensive treatment to the mantle field results in, at most, minimal pulmonary dysfunction in less than one-third of the patients.

## Breast cancer

Pulmonary and pleural changes secondary to irradiation have been recognized since 1923 when Groover, Christie and Merritt [61] first reported such changes in breast cancer patients. The occurrence and severity of the lung damage was related to the type of irradiation given, the specific treatment technique used, the size and shape of the treatment field, the dose of radiation, and the fractionation regimen. It is in this group of patients that the largest discrepancies in estimates of morbidity can be found, depending on the criteria used. The percentage of patients who develop radiographic evidence of lung damage secondary to irradiation for breast cancer ranges from a low of 10% to a high of 90% [24–26,28,62]. The abnormalities are confined and are most common in the apical regions of the lung (due to the supraclavicular fields used) and the paramediastinal area (due to the internal mammary fields). Thus, studies using radiographic changes or tests of regional lung function will show a high incidence of damage. However, minimal, if any, pulmonary dysfunction will be observed if total lung function is assessed. Few of these patients are symptomatic and morbidity is minimal. It is particularly important that this distinction between damage and morbidity be recognized because radiation therapy is now an important form of treatment after conservative surgery for early stage breast cancer.

## Total body irradiation

High-dose chemo-radiotherapy followed by bone marrow transplantation (BMT) has become a popular treatment for many patients with hematological malignancies. One of the major life-threatening complications after BMT is interstitial pneumonitis. Although about half of the occurrences are caused by an infectious agent, no clear cause can be found in the other half and these are referred to as idiopathic pneumonitis.

It is difficult, if not impossible, to assess the role of radiation in these cases. The bone marrow transplant registry has identified six factors that influence the incidence of pneumonitis in these patients [63]. Although radiation was identified as one of those factors, at the total doses, dose rates and doses per fraction used, it was found to exert a minimal influence on this treatment complication and when it was implicated, the relationship did not depend on the radiation factors but rather on the combined effect of radiation and the drugs employed. In addition, a high incidence of interstitial pneumonia occurs in BMT patients who have not had irradiation.

It is, therefore, particularly difficult to ascertain the exact role of radiation in this multifactorial problem. Nonetheless it is important to understand the relationship of pulmonary irradiation in this clinical setting because one limit to the total dose of total body irradiation (TBI) is the lung [64,65].

It is now clear that the optimum technique for TBI is to use either fractionated irradiation or low dose rate irradiation [66–77]. The rationale for the use of fractionated or low dose rate TBI is based on the now well-known differences between the shapes of the survival curves for the target cells of hemopoietic origin and lung (Figure 16.8) [66]. The lung would thereby be spared more by either dose fractionation or low dose rate irradiation than the leukemic cells.

In clinical practice, however, a 50% incidence of pneumonitis still occurs after a total dose of only 12 Gy given at a low dose rate. This cannot be attributed to radiation alone, as the total doses given in TBI using either fractionated dose regimens or low dose rates are all significantly below those known to cause pneumonitis in humans after high dose rates. For example, the single dose for 50% incidence of pneumonitis in humans [34] is about 9.3 Gy after irradiation using high dose rates of >1 Gy/min. Assuming a dose rate effect of 1.8, the dose that would give the same incidence of pneumonitis after low dose rate irradiation would be ~17 Gy. Total doses in TBI rarely exceed 10 Gy after low dose rates. Lopez-Cardozo *et al.* [78] and others [74,75,77] have demonstrated very clearly that after irradiation with low dose rate, idiopathic pneumonitis in humans would not be expected after lung doses <14 Gy.

One possible explanation of this surprisingly high incidence of pneumonitis is that TBI is combined with chemotherapy [64]. Figure 16.9 shows the

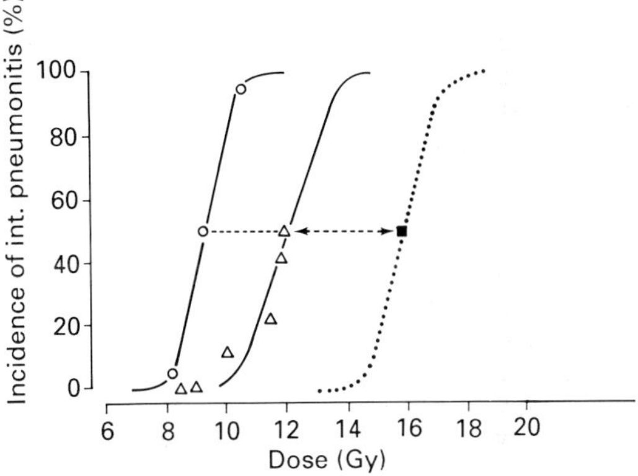



**Figure 16.9** The incidence of pneumonitis as a function of single dose irradiation at a high dose rate (○), low dose rate plus drugs (△), or low dose rate alone (■). It is clear that low dose rate irradiation significantly spares the lung. The single dose ED$_{50}$ after high dose rate is 9.3 Gy [34] whereas after low dose rate irradiation it is >15 Gy. However drugs significantly reduce the ED$_{50}$ even after low dose rate irradiation. Reproduced with permission from ref. [64]

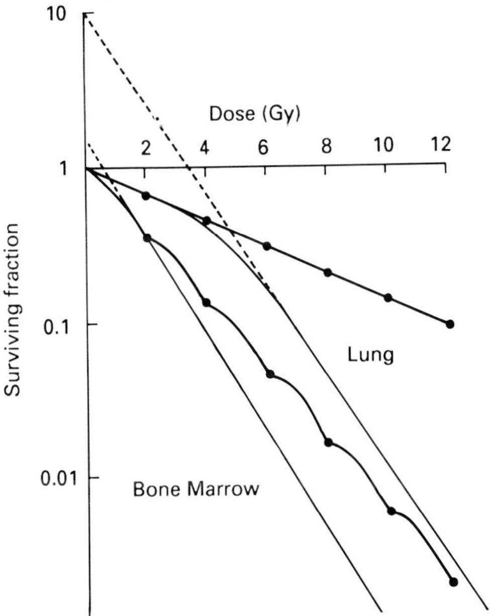



**Figure 16.8** The effect of fractionation on the lung and bone marrow. It is clear that dose fractionation spares the lung more than the bone marrow and thus will be more useful than single dose irradiation in the TBI setting. Reproduced with permission from ref. [96]

incidence of pneumonitis in BMT patients after chemotherapy and low dose rate TBI. It is clear that the chemotherapy significantly reduces the dose that can be given to the lung in this setting. These data are supported by animal studies in which it has been demonstrated that the dose to the lungs can be increased by as much as a factor of 1.8 over the clinically relevant dose rate range of 0.05–0.4 Gy/min if prior chemotherapy had not been given [79]. Cyclophosphamide, a cytotoxic agent often used in preparative regimens, is of particular interest because it is given at intervals quite close to irradiation. It is well established in animals that administration of cyclophosphamide near the time of low dose rate TBI at the least reduces, and has been shown to totally abolish, the sparing effect on the lung of low dose rate irradiation. The sparing effects of low dose rate irradiation on the incidence of radiation pneumonitis can be abrogated by the chemotherapeutic agents used in the preparative regimens.

An alternative to low dose rate irradiation in TBI regimens is to give more than one fraction a day using a smaller dose per fraction, i.e. hyperfractionation. Experimental data from studies with mice have shown that fractionated irradiation at conventional dose rates ($>1.0$ Gy/min) are as efficient at sparing the lungs as TBI given at a low dose rate of 0.25 Gy/min [67]. Clinically, the former would be preferable for reasons of both patient comfort and machine scheduling. A number of centers are now giving TBI in a hyperfractionated regimen using doses per fraction of 1.2–1.75 Gy [80,81] to a total dose of 10.5–10.8 Gy.

One pulmonary complication associated with preparative regimens for BMT that is not radiation-related occurs within days of irradiation and is characterized by severe inflammation, acute pulmonary edema and a complete white-out of the lungs on a radiograph. This form of acute respiratory distress syndrome shows no dose response over the dose range commonly used in TBI, 9–14 Gy, and thus is not radiation-related. It is most likely a result of multiple insults with high-dose chemotherapy the major causative agent with a small contribution from radiation.

## Children

Irradiation of the lungs in children represents a special situation, particularly in children under the age of 3 years [82]. The lungs of young children are in a period of rapid growth, particularly in terms of the number of alveoli. Unlike the airways, which are fully formed in gestational life and increase only in size but not number during childhood, the number of alveoli increases rapidly during the first few years of life. Radiation given during this time of rapid cellular proliferation can be expected to kill large numbers of these cells and to limit their ability to proliferate. The ultimate result of this reduction in the number of cells in the alveoli of the lung would be pulmonary hypoplasia and commensurate changes in lung function.

There are relatively few pediatric studies assessing lung function and/or morbidity at long term after irradiation. The lung may be irradiated in young children for a number of pediatric solid tumors, but most frequently lung irradiation is for pulmonary metastases from Wilms' tumour, Ewing's sarcoma and osteosarcoma [83–91]. In children, unlike

adults, in whom the common situation is irradiation of only a portion of the lung, treatment of the lung for pediatric tumors most often involves the whole lung either prophylactically or definitively.

The difficulty of assessing the effects of lung irradiation on young children is compounded by the fact that most of these children receive chemotherapy at some time in the clinical management of their disease. Because tumors in the lung are the target of this treatment, the drugs most commonly used are known pulmonary toxins in their own right or they interact with radiation, enhancing its deleterious effects.

Perhaps the largest number of pediatric patients who received lung irradiation and were followed for treatment outcome, including toxic effects, were those entered into the first and second National Wilms' Tumor Study (NWTS) Group [83–85]. The incidence of significant clinically demonstrable lung toxicity in these two studies was remarkably small. In the first NWTS study [83], of the 24 patients (total number of patients = 359) who had lung irradiation, seven had clinically manifested lung damage (29%). In the second NWTS study [84,85], 49 patients had the whole lung irradiated and four of these 49 developed clinically manifested lung toxicity; three of these four died from this complication.

Both NWTS studies concentrated on severe morbidity. Other studies have concentrated on subclinical toxic effects, e.g. changes in pulmonary function tests. The studies of Wohl *et al.* [86] and Benoist *et al.* [87] on long-term survivors of Wilms' tumor with follow-up times ranging from 2 to 17 years, showed changes in pulmonary function that were consistent with restrictive lung disease and thoracic hypoplasia. The studies of Benoist *et al.* [87] are particularly interesting as these investigators performed sequential lung function tests on the same patients for up to 4 years after treatment. Based on their data, they described three phases of lung function change (Figure 16.10). The first acute phase occurred 3–6 months after the completion of treatment and was characterized by a progressive deterioration of lung function. This was followed by a period of stability in lung function up to 2 years, after which time lung function again decreased. At this time the number of patients exhibiting changes in pulmonary function also increased. Chest radiographs in these same patients, however, revealed no lung abnormalities. Both Wohl *et al.* [86] and Benoist *et al.* [87] found functional lung changes only in those patients who received pulmonary irradiation; those patients who were managed without lung irradiation all had normal lung function at all times tested after completion of their treatment.

These findings are in contrast with those of Miller *et al.* [91] who, in a follow-up of long-term survivors of various types of pediatric tumors, including

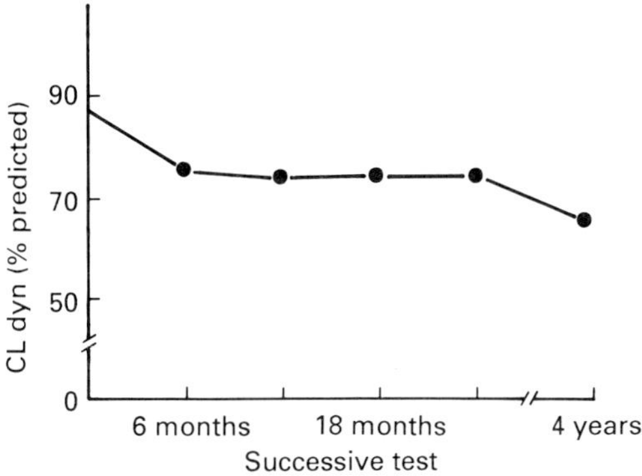

**Figure 16.10** Change in dynamic lung compliance (CL dyn) in children up to 4 years after treatment with whole lung radiation and actinomycin D for Wilms' tumor. Three phases of lung response are shown: early lung disease within the first 6 months followed by a plateau up to 2 years and a subsequent progressive decrease in lung compliance up to 4 years after treatment. Modified from ref. [87]

Wilms' tumor, neuroblastoma and leukemia, found that 48% of the 29 survivors demonstrated abnormal pulmonary function tests. Only four of 29 survivors had received thoracic irradiation without chemotherapy. However, these authors also found a 38% incidence of abnormal lung function in patients who had not received thoracic irradiation leading them to conclude that radiation is not the sole factor contributing to abnormal lung function in long-term survivors of childhood cancers.

Interpretation of the data from all of these studies is confounded by the concurrent administration of chemotherapy with radiation, a situation that appears to predispose the lung to enhanced radiation response.

Perhaps the most important lessons to be learned from the few but comprehensive studies on long-term survivors of pediatric tumors are those on the pathogenesis of damage in a developing organ. In Benoist's study [87], the progressive deterioration in lung function after 2 years was not due to fibrosis in the lung, as determined by the appropriate lung function tests (normal PSSV curves, exercise $PaO_2$ normal). Wohl *et al.* [86] also could not attribute their findings to lung fibrosis, although they could not exclude this lesion as a possible causative factor of the late function changes. Because most of these children develop skeletal abnormalities [89], it is most likely that these changes contribute to the later reduction in lung volume.

In general, the incidence of clinically manifested pulmonary morbidity after irradiation of the whole thorax in young children is low. In addition, lung function is well preserved in these children despite doses considered close to tolerance. Most importantly, any changes in lung function in these children is probably consistent with a proportionate interference with the growth of both the chest wall and the lung.

## Conclusions

Despite the fact that the clinical expression of lung radiation damage is infrequent, pulmonary complications of radiotherapy are a significant consideration in the treatment of malignant diseases in which the lung must be irradiated. Such damage can be serious and life-threatening. Thus it is important to better understand the nature of the damage in the lung and to develop both biological and physical methods of reducing lung toxicity. It is now well established that the two parameters which most critically influence toxicity are dose, particularly dose per fraction, and volume of lung irradiated. All doses to the lung should be corrected for tissue inhomogeneity since lung doses are appreciably higher than the values calculated without this correction. The extra dose may range from 40% for a large patient treated with $^{40}$Co to only a few percent for small patients treated with a 10 MV linear accelerator. Increases in dose of about 20% are common and because the dose-response curve for radiation pneumonitis is steep, failure to correct for the low density of lung tissue can make the difference between occurrence or avoidance of pulmonary toxicity.

Another primary way of reducing toxicity is to reduce the volume of lung irradiated. CT planning and custom blocks for individual patients could contribute much to tailoring the field to each patient, thus reducing the volume of tissue irradiated.

Since the lung does impose significant limitations to the dose of radiation that can be given for the treatment of malignant disease, it is important that clinical and experimental data continue to be reported. However, a clear distinction must be made between damage and morbidity, since a direct correlation between these two parameters does not necessarily exist for the lung.

## Acknowledgements

This work is supported by NIH Research Grant CA-38106 and CA-06294. I wish to thank my clinical colleagues Drs Lester Peters, Ritsuko Komaki and James Cox for helpful discussions. I owe a particular thanks to Dr Patricia Eifel whose input was invaluable to this chapter. I also wish to thank Shelia

Buckner and Lori Verhalen for their assistance in preparation of this chapter.

## References


1. Bennett, D.E., Million, R.R. and Ackerman, L.V. Bilateral radiation pneumonitis: a complication of the radiotherapy of bronchogenic carcinoma. *Cancer*, **23**, 1001–1018 (1968)

2. Fryer, C.J.H., Fitzpatrick, P.J., Rider, W.D. and Poon, P. Radiation pneumonitis: experience following a large single dose of radiation. *International Journal of Radiation Oncology, Biology, Physics*, **4**, 931–936 (1978)

3. Travis, E.L. The tissue rescuing unit. In *Proceedings of the 8th International Congress of Radiation Research*, Vol. 2 (eds E.M. Fielden, J.F. Fowler, J.H. Hendry and D. Scott), Taylor and Francis, London, pp. 795–800 (1987)

4. Travis, E.L. and Tucker, S.L. The relationship between functional assays of radiation response in the lung and target cell depletion. *British Journal of Cancer*, **53**, 304–319 (1986)

5. Withers, H.R., Taylor, J.M.G. and Maciejewski, B. Treatment volume and tissue tolerance. *International Journal of Radiation Oncology, Biology, Physics*, **14**, 751–759 (1988)

6. Weibel, E.R. *Morphometry of the Lung*, Academic Press, New York (1963)

7. Moss, W.T., Brand, W.N. and Fattifora, H. (eds) The lung and thymus. In *Radiation Oncology: Rationale, Technique, Results*, 5th edn, C.V. Mosby, St. Louis, pp. 253–288 (1979)

8. Fajardo, L.F. (ed.). Respiratory system. In *Pathology of Radiation Injury*, Masson, New York, pp. 34–46 (1982)

9. Gross, N.J. Pulmonary effects of radiation therapy. *Annals of Internal Medicine*, **86**, 81–92 (1977)

10. Cox, J.D., Byhardt, R.W., Wilson, J.F. *et al*. Complications of radiation therapy and factors in their prevention. *World Journal of Surgery*, **10**, 171–188 (1986)

11. Fennessy, J.J. Irradiation damage to the lung. *Journal of Thoracic Imaging*, **2**, 68–79 (1987)

12. Rubin, P. and Casarett, G.W. (eds). *Clinical Radiation Pathology*, Vol. 1. W.B. Saunders, Philadelphia (1968)

13. Travis, E.L. The sequence of histological changes in mouse lungs after single doses of X-rays. *International Journal of Radiation Oncology, Biology, Physics*, **6**, 345–347 (1980)

14. Travis, E.L., Meistrich, M.L., Finch-Neimeyer, M.V. *et al*. Late functional and biochemical changes in mouse lung after irradiation: Differential effects of WR-2721. *Radiation Research*, **103**, 219–231 (1985)

15. Parkins, C.S. Assessment of late lung damage. *International Journal of Radiation Oncology, Biology, Physics*, **55**, 479–481 (1989)

16. Sharplin, J. and Franko, A.J. A quantitative histology study of strain-dependent differences in the effects of irradiation on mouse lung during the intermediate and late phases. *Radiation Research*, **119**, 15–31 (1989)

17. Bell, J., McGovern, D., Bullimore, J. *et al*. Diagnostic imaging of post-irradiation changes in the chest. *Clinical Radiology*, **39**, 109–119 (1988)

18. Mah, K., Poon, P.Y., van Dyk J. *et al*. Assessment of acute radiation-induced pulmonary changes using computed tomography. *Journal of Computer Assisted Tomography*, **10**, 736–743 (1986)

19. Mah, K. and van Dyk, J. Quantitative measurement of changes in human lung density following irradiation. *Radiotherapy and Oncology*, **11**, 169–179 (1988)

20. Lehnert, S. and El-Khatib, E. The use of CT densitometry in the assessment of radiation-induced damage to the rat lung: A comparison with other endpoints. *International Journal of Radiation Oncology, Biology, Physics*, **16**, 117–124 (1989)

21. Abbatucci, J.S., Boulier, A., Fabre, J. and Lozier, J.C. Functional evaluation of pulmonary bilateral irradiation effects. *European Journal of Cancer*, **14**, 781–785 (1978)

22. Smith, L.M., Mendenhall, N.P., Cicale, M.J. *et al*. Results of a prospective study evaluating the effects of mantle irradiation on pulmonary function. *International Journal of Radiation Oncology, Biology, Physics*, **16**, 79–84 (1989)

23. Watchie, J., Coleman, N., Raffin, T.A. *et al*. Minimal long-term cardiopulmonary dysfunction following treatment for Hodgkin's disease. *International Journal of Radiation Oncology, Biology, Physics*, **13**, 517–524 (1987)

24. Rothwell, R.I., Kelley, S.A. and Joslin, C.A.F. Radiation pneumonitis in patients treated for breast cancer. *Radiotherapy and Oncology*, **4**, 9–14 (1985)

25. Kaufman, J., Gunn, W., Hartz, A.J. *et al*. The pathophysiologic and roentgenologic effects of chest irradiation in breast carcinoma. *International Journal of Radiation Oncology, Biology, Physics*, **12**, 887–893 (1986)

26. Polansky, S.M., Ravin, C.E. and Prosnitz, L.R. Pulmonary changes after primary irradiation for early breast carcinoma. *American Journal of Radiology*, **134**, 101–105 (1980)

27. Springmeyer, S.C., Flournoy, N., Sullivan, K.M. *et al*. Pulmonary function changes in long-term survivors of allogeneic marrow transplantation. In *Recent Advances in Bone Marrow Transplantation* (ed. R.P. Gale), Alan R. Liss, New York, pp. 343–353 (1983)

28. Prato, F.S., Kurdyak, R., Saibil, E.A. *et al*. Regional and total lung function in patients following pulmonary irradiation. *Investigative Radiology*, **12**, 224–237 (1977)

29. Phillips, T.L. and Margolis, L. Radiation pathology and the clinical response of lung and esophagus. In *Frontiers of Radiation Therapy and Oncology*, Vol. 6 (ed. J.M. Vaeth). S. Karger, Basel, p. 254 (1972)

30. Siemann, D.W., Hill, R.P. and Penney, D.P. Early

and late pulmonary toxicity in mice evaluated 180 and 420 days following localized lung irradiation. *Radiation Research*, **89**, 396–407 (1982)

31. Travis, E.L., Down, J.D., Holmes, S.J. and Hobson, B. Radiation pneumonitis and fibrosis in mouse lung assayed by respiratory frequency and histology. *Radiation Research*, **84**, 133–143 (1980)

32. Depledge, M.H., Collis, C.H. and Barrett, A. The technique for measuring carbon monoxide uptake in mice. *International Journal of Radiation Oncology, Biology, Physics*, **7**, 485–489 (1981)

33. Wara, W.M., Phillips, T.L., Margolis, L.W. and Smith, V. Radiation pneumonitis: a new approach to the deterioration of time-dose factors. *Cancer*, **32**, 547–552 (1973)

34. Van Dyk, J., Keane, T.J., Kan, S. *et al.* Radiation pneumonitis following large single dose irradiation: a re-evaluation based on absolute dose to lung. *International Journal of Radiation Oncology, Biology, Physics*, **7**, 461–467 (1981)

35. Prato, F.S., Kurdyak, R., Saibil, E.A. *et al.* The incidence of radiation pneumonitis as a result of single fraction upper half body irradiation. *Cancer*, **39**, 71–78 (1976)

36. Fitzpatrick, P.J. and Rider, W.D. Half body radiotherapy. *International Journal of Radiation Oncology, Biology, Physics*, **1**, 197–207 (1976)

37. Mah, K., Van Dyk, J., Keane, T. and Poon, P.Y. Acute radiation-induced pulmonary damage; a clinical study on the response to fractionated radiation therapy. *International Journal of Radiation Oncology, Biology, Physics*, **13**, 179–188 (1987)

38. Van Dyk, J., Mah, K. and Keane, T.J. Radiation-induced lung damage: dose-time-fractionation considerations. *Radiotherapy and Oncology*, **14**, 55–69 (1989)

39. Thames, H.D., Withers, H.R., Peters, L.J. and Fletcher, G.H. Changes in early and late radiation responses with altered dose fractionation: implication for dose survival relationships. *International Journal of Radiation Oncology, Biology, Physics*, **8**, 219–226 (1982)

40. Thames, H.D. Jr., Peters, L.J., Withers, H.R. and Fletcher, G.H. Accelerated fractionation vs. hyper-fractionation: rationales for several treatments per day. *International Journal of Radiation Oncology, Biology, Physics*, **9**, 127–138 (1983)

41. Withers, H.R., Peters, L.J., Thames, H.D. and Fletcher, G.H. Hyperfractionation. *International Journal of Radiation Oncology, Biology, Physics*, **8**, 1807–1809 (1982)

42. Cox, J.D. Presidential address. Fractionation: a paradigm for clinical research in radiation oncology. *International Journal of Radiation Oncology, Biology, Physics*, **13**, 1271–1281 (1987)

43. Perez, C.A., Stanley, K., Rubin, P. *et al.* A prospective randomized study of various irradiation doses and fractionation schedules in the treatment of inoperable non-oat-cell carcinoma of the lung. *Cancer*, **45**, 2744–2753 (1980)

44. Seydel, H.G., Diener-West, M., Urtasun, R. *et al.* Radiation Therapy Oncology Group (RTOG). Hyperfractionation in the radiation therapy of unresectable non-oat cell carcinoma of the lung: preliminary report of an RTOG pilot study. *International Journal of Radiation Oncology, Biology, Physics*, **11**, 1841–1847 (1985)

45. Rothwell, R.I., Kelley, S.A. and Joslin, C.A.F. Radiation pneumonitis in patients treated for breast cancer. *Radiotherapy and Oncology*, **4**, 9–14 (1985)

46. Brady, L.W., Cancer, L., Evans, G.C. and Forest, D.S. Carcinoma of the lung: results of supervoltage radiation therapy. *Archives of Surgery*, **90**, 90–94 (1965)

47. Brady, L.W., German, P.A. and Cancer, L. The effects of radiation therapy on pulmonary function in carcinoma of the lung. *Radiology*, **85**, 130–134 (1965)

48. Urtasun, R.C., Belch, A. and Bodnar, D. Hemibody radiation: an active therapeutic modality for the management of patients with small cell lung cancer. *International Journal of Radiation Oncology, Biology, Physics*, **9**, 1575–1578 (1983)

49. Salazar, O.M., Slawson, R.G., Poussin-Rosillo, H. *et al.* A prospective randomized trial comparing once-a-week versus daily radiation therapy for locally-advanced, non-metastatic, lung cancer: a preliminary report. *International Journal of Radiation Oncology, Biology, Physics*, **12**, 779–787 (1986)

50. Simpson, J.R., Bauer, M., Wasserman, T.H. *et al.* Large fraction irradiation with or without misonidazole in advanced non-oat cell carcinoma of the lung: a phase III randomized trial of the RTOG. *International Journal of Radiation Oncology, Biology, Physics*, **13**, 861–867 (1987)

51. Powell, B.L., Jackson, D.V., Scarantino, C.W. *et al.* Sequential hemibody irradiation integrated into a chemotherapy-local radiotherapy program for limited disease small cell lung cancer. *International Journal of Radiation Oncology, Biology, Physics*, **12**, 1951–1956 (1986)

52. Petrovich, Z., Mietlowski, W., Ohanian, M. and Cox, J. Clinical report on the treatment of locally advanced lung cancer. *Cancer*, **40**, 72–77 (1977)

53. Choi, N.C.H. and Doucette, J.A. Improved survival of patients with unresectable non-small-cell bronchogenic carcinoma by an innovated high-dose en-block radiotherapeutic approach. *Cancer*, **48**, 101–109 (1981)

54. Payne, D.G., Yeoh, L., Feld, R. *et al.* Upper half body irradiation (UHBI) for extensive small cell carcinoma of the lung. *International Journal of Radiation Oncology, Biology, Physics*, **9**, 1571–1574 (1983)

55. Papac, R.J., Son, Y., Bien, R. *et al.* Improved local control of thoracic disease in small cell lung cancer with higher dose thoracic irradiation and cyclic chemotherapy. *International Journal of Radiation Oncology, Biology, Physics*, **13**, 993–998 (1987)

56. Carmel, R.J. and Kaplan, H.S. Mantle irradiation in Hodgkin's disease: an analysis of technique, tumor eradication, and complications. *Cancer*, **37**, 2813–2825 (1976)

57. Host, H. and Vale, J.R. Lung function after mantle field irradiation in Hodgkin's disease. *Cancer*, **32**, 328–332 (1973)

58. do Pico, G.A., Wiley, A.L. Jr., Rao, Pradeep and Dickie, H.A. Pulmonary reaction to upper mantle radiation therapy for Hodgkin's disease. *Chest*, **75**, 688–692 (1979)

59. Morgan, G.W., Freeman, A.P., McLean, R.G. *et al.* Late cardiac, thyroid and pulmonary sequelae of mantle radiotherapy for Hodgkin's disease. *International Journal of Radiation Oncology, Biology, Physics*, **11**, 1925–1931 (1985)

60. Slanina, J., Musshoff, K., Rahner, T. and Stiasny, R. Long-term side effect in irradiated patients with Hodgkin's disease. *International Journal of Radiation Oncology, Biology, Physics*, **2**, 1–19 (1977)

61. Groover, T.A., Christie, A.C. and Merritt, E.A. Intrathoracic changes following roentgen treatment of breast carcinoma. *American Journal of Radiology*, **10**, 471–476 (1923)

62. Groth, S., Zarick, A., Sorensen, P.B. *et al.* Regional lung function impairment following post-operative radiotherapy for breast cancer using direct or tangential field techniques. *British Journal of Radiology*, **59**, 445–451 (1986)

63. Weiner, R.S., Bortin, M.M., Gale, R.P. *et al.* Interstitial pneumonitis after bone marrow transplantation. *Annals of Internal Medicine*, **104**, 168–175 (1986)

64. Molls, M., Budach, V. and Bamberg, M. Total body irradiation: the lung as critical organ. *Strahlentherapie und Onkologie*, **162**, 226–232 (1986)

65. Bortin, M. and Hartz, A.J. Influence of radiation regimens on the risk of interstitial pneumonitis in leukemia patients treated with allogeneic bone marrow transplantation. In *Innovations in Radiation Oncology*, (eds H.R. Withers and L.J. Peters). Springer-Verlag, Berlin, pp. 107–111 (1988)

66. Peters, L.H., Withers, H.R., Cundiff, J.H. and Dicke, K.A. Radiobiological considerations in the use of total-body irradiation for bone-marrow transplantation. *Radiology*, **131**, 243–247 (1979)

67. Lehnert, S. and Rybka, W.B. Dose-rate dependence of response of mouse lung to irradiation. *British Journal of Radiology*, **58**, 745–749 (1985)

68. Fang, M.Z., Travis, E.L., Peters, L.J. and Barkely, H.T. The effect of continuous vs. fractionated low dose-rate total body irradiation on bone marrow and late tissue responses. In *Abstracts of Papers for the 34th Annual Meeting of the Radiation Research Society*, p.149 (1986)

69. Depledge, M.H. and Barrett, A. Dose-rate dependence of lung damage after total body irradiation in mice. *International Journal of Radiation Biology*, **41**, 325–334 (1982)

70. Hill, R.P. Response of mouse lung to irradiation at different dose rates. *International Journal of Radiation Oncology, Biology, Physics*, **9**, 1043–1047 (1983)

71. Travis, E.L., Peters, L.J., McNeill, J. *et al.* Effect of dose rate on total body irradiation: lethality and pathologic findings. *Radiotherapy and Oncology*, **4**, 341–351 (1985)

72. Down, J.D., Easton, D.F. and Steel, G.G. Repair in the mouse lung during low dose-rate irradiation. *Radiotherapy and Oncology*, **6**, 29–42 (1986)

73. Deeg, H.J., Storb, R., Longton, G. *et al.* Single dose or fractionated total body irradiation and autologous marrow transplantation in dogs: effects of exposure rate, fraction size, and fractionation interval on acute and delayed toxicity. *International Journal of Radiation Oncology, Biology, Physics*, **15**, 647–653 (1988)

74. Kim, T.H., Rybka, W.B., Lehnert, S. *et al.* Interstitial pneumonitis following total body irradiation for bone marrow transplantation using two different dose rates. *International Journal of Radiation Oncology, Biology, Physics*, **11**, 1285–1291 (1985)

75. Barrett, A., Depledge, M.H. and Powles, R.L. Interstitial pneumonitis following bone marrow transplantation after low dose rate total body irradiation. *International Journal of Radiation Oncology, Biology, Physics*, **9**, 1029–1033 (1983)

76. Lichter, A.S., Tutschka, P.J., Wharma, M.D. *et al.* The use of fractionated radiotherapy as preparation for allogeneic bone marrow transplantation. *Transplantation Proceedings*, **11**, 1492–1494 (1979)

77. Thomas, E.D., Clift, R.A., Hersman, J. *et al.* Marrow transplantation for acute nonlymphoblastic leukemia in first remission using fractionated or single-dose irradiation. *International Journal of Radiation Oncology, Biology, Physics*, **8**, 817–821 (1982)

78. Lopez-Cardozo, B.L., Zoetelief, H., Van Bekku, D.W. *et al.* Lung damage following bone marrow transplantation: I. The contribution of irradiation. *International Journal of Radiation Oncology, Biology, Physics*, **11**, 907–914 (1985)

79. Lockhart, S.P., Down, J.D. and Steel, G.G. The effect of low dose-rate and cyclophosphamide on the radiation tolerance of the mouse lung. *International Journal of Radiation Oncology, Biology, Physics*, **12**, 1437–1440 (1986)

80. Shank, B., Chu, F.C.H., Dinmore, R. *et al.* Hyper-fractionation total body irradiation for bone marrow transplantation: results in 70 leukemia patients with allogeneic transplants. *International Journal of Radiation Oncology, Biology, Physics*, **9**, 1607–1611 (1983)

81. Shank, B., Hopfan, S., Kim, J.H. *et al.* Hyperfractionated total body irradiation for bone marrow transplantation. I. Early results in leukemia patients. *International Journal of Radiation Oncology, Biology, Physics*, **7**, 1109–1115 (1981)

82. Makipernaa, A., Heino, M., Laitinen, L.A. and Siimes, M.A. Lung function following treatment of malignant tumors with surgery, radiotherapy, or cyc-

lophosphamide in childhood: a follow-up study after 11 to 27 years. *Cancer*, **63**, 625–630 (1989)

83. Tefft, M. Radiation related toxicities in National Wilms' Tumor Study number 1. *International Journal of Radiation Oncology, Biology, Physics*, **2**, 455–463 (1977)

84. Thomas, P.R.M., Tefft, M., D'Angio, G.J. and Norkool, P. Acute toxicities associated with radiation in the Second National Wilms' Tumor Study. *Journal of Clinical Oncology*, **6**, 1694–1698 (1988)

85. Jones, B., Breslow, N.E. and Takashima, J. Toxic deaths in the Second National Wilms' Tumor Study. *Journal of Clinical Oncology*, **2**, 1028–1033 (1984)

86. Wohl, M.E.B., Griscom, T., Traggis, D.G. and Jaffe, N. Effects of therapeutic irradiation delivered in early childhood upon subsequent lung function. *Pediatrics*, **55**, 507–514 (1975)

87. Benoist, M.R., Lemerle, J., Jean, R. *et al.* Effects on pulmonary function of whole lung irradiation for Wilms' tumor in children. *Thorax*, **37**, 175–180 (1982)

88. Littman, P., Meadows, A.T., Polgar, G. *et al.* Pulmonary function in survivors of Wilms' tumor: patterns of impairment. *Cancer*, **37**, 2773–2776 (1976)

89. Breur, K., Cohen, P., Schweisguth, O. and Hart, A.M.M. Irradiation of the lungs as an adjuvant therapy in the treatment of osteosarcoma of the limbs: An EORTC randomized study. *European Journal of Cancer*, **14**, 461–471 (1978)

90. Blatt, J. and Bleyer, W.A. Late effects of childhood cancer and its treatment. In *Principles and Practice of Pediatric Oncology* (eds P.A. Pizzo and D.G. Poplack). J.B. Lippincott, Philadelphia, pp. 1003–1025 (1989)

91. Miller, R.W., Fusner, J.E., Fink, R.J. *et al.* Pulmonary function abnormalities in long-term survivors of childhood cancer. *Medical and Pediatric Oncology*, **14**, 202–207 (1986)

92. Conrad, S.A., Kinasewetz, G.T. and George, R.B. *Pulmonary Function Testing*, Churchill Livingstone, New York (1984)

93. Field, S.B. and Hornsey, S. Damage to mouse lung with neutrons and X-rays. *European Journal of Cancer*, **10**, 621–627 (1974)

94. Rubin, P., Siemann, D.W., Shapiro, D.L. *et al.* Surfactant release as a predictor and measure of radiation pneumonitic injury. *International Journal of Radiation Oncology, Biology, Physics*, **9**, 1669–1674 (1983)

95. Rubin, P. Late effect of chemotherapy and radiation therapy: a new hypothesis. *International Journal of Radiation Oncology, Biology, Physics*, **10**, 5–34 (1984)

96. Peters, L.J. The radiobiological basis of TBI. *International Journal of Radiation Oncology, Biology, Physics*, **6**, 785–787 (1980)

# 17

# Chemotherapy-related morbidity to the lungs

C.H. Collis

Lung damage was a relative newcomer amongst the toxicities of cytotoxic chemotherapy agents until the late 1960s. Though first described with busulphan in 1961 [1], the rather sporadic and infrequent occurrence meant it remained something of a medical curiosity until late in the decade. Subsequently methotrexate lung damage [2] and more importantly bleomycin lung damage [3] which was dose-limiting, were reported. Since then it has become evident that lung damage can occur with a large number of the currently available cytotoxic drugs though with most drugs it occurs infrequently and hence has taken some time to come to light (Table 17.1).

Since 1980 when it would have been reasonable to say just three agents were of practical importance – bleomycin, busulphan and methotrexate [4] – BCNU (carmustine) has also been established as a frequent cause of lung damage [5]. Pneumonitis has also become important as a cause of death following bone marrow transplantation, an increasingly frequent method of treatment. Though initially put down to irradiation and/or infection, high-dose cytotoxic drugs themselves can cause pneumonitis which is dose-limiting with BCNU [6] and with cytarabine (Ara-C) [7]. With the increasing tendency towards dose intensification and high-dose chemotherapy, lung toxicity may become a still more frequent dose-limiting side effect.

In this chapter we shall concentrate on parenchymal and reactive changes in the lung in response to chemotherapy. However cytotoxic drugs can affect the lungs in other ways. Chest infections occur indirectly as a result of drug-induced marrow suppression and immunocompetence. Metastases may cavitate [8]. Hexamethyl melamine has been reported to cause respiratory dyskinesia [9], and pneumothorax and pleurisy have been reported [10,11]. There is even the possibility that cytotoxic drugs may enhance metastases as has been shown in certain experimental animal models [12,13].

The definitive diagnosis of lung damage due to cytotoxic drugs depends on three factors: a history of drug exposure, demonstration of lung damage, and exclusion of other causes of lung damage. To fulfil these criteria it is necessary to have obtained a clear history, to have carried out a thorough search

**Table 17.1 Lung damage from cytotoxic drugs: reports in chronological order**

|  | Date of first report | Date of initial use |
|---|---|---|
| Busulphan | 1961 | 1953 |
| Cyclophosphamide | 1967 | 1958 |
| 6-Mercaptopurine | 1968 | 1953 |
| Methotrexate | 1969 | 1948 |
| Bleomycin | 1969 | 1969 |
| Thioguanosine | 1971 | 1971 |
| Procarbazine | 1972 | 1963 |
| Azathioprine | 1972 | 1961 |
| Melphalan | 1972 | 1958 |
| Chlorambucil | 1972 | 1955 |
| Carmustine (BCNU) | 1976 | 1962 |
| Vinblastine | 1976 | 1963 |
| Mitomycin C | 1978 | 1957 |
| Uracil mustard | 1978 | 1960 |
| Semustine (methyl-CCNU) | 1978 | 1971 |
| Zinostatin | 1978 | 1971 |
| VM-26 | 1979 | 1972 |
| Peplomycin | 1980 | 1980 |
| Cytarabine (Ara-C) | 1981 | 1966 |
| Chlorozotocin | 1981 | 1976 |
| Lomustine (CCNU) | 1982 | 1971 |
| Vindesine | 1985 | 1976 |

for microorganisms, and to have lung histology. The most common presenting symptoms are dyspnoea, a dry cough and fever, and there is also frequently malaise, anorexia and weight loss. At first a common chest infection may be considered, but disproportionate dyspnoea, the presence of bilateral crepitations and diffuse bilateral shadowing on the chest radiograph suggest a more generalized disorder. Abnormal lung function tests, typically a restrictive ventilatory defect and a diffusion defect, are non-specific.

The differential diagnosis usually lies between a generalized infection such as *Pneumocystis carinii* or a viral pneumonia, tumour infiltration, or interstitial pneumonitis with or without fibrosis, the most common type of pathology seen with cytotoxic drugs. Bronchial brushings and transbronchial biopsy via the fibreoptic bronchoscope will be diagnostic in the majority of cases [14]. Occasionally open lung biopsy may be necessary to obtain adequate histology.

The cytotoxic drugs reported to cause pulmonary damage can be grouped into five categories: antibiotic cytotoxics, nitrosoureas, alkylating agents, antimetabolites and others. These are shown in Table 17.2. Reported estimates of the percentage frequency are available for four drugs as shown. When the incidence is low, but a large number of case reports have been published they are shown as (++). For the rest there have only been a few sporadic cases of lung damage: these are shown as (+). The drugs reported to cause lung damage will be described individually below.

# Cytotoxic antibiotics

## Bleomycin

### Incidence

Bleomycin is the most important cytotoxic drug to cause lung damage, since lung toxicity occurs relatively frequently and is a major and often dose-limiting side effect. Reports of the incidence of pneumonitis and fibrosis vary from 3% to 40% [15,16]. Clearly the reported incidence depends on how hard damage is searched for, but in reviewing over 1700 patients throughout the world Blum, Carter and Agre [17] found the overall incidence to be 10%. More sensitive assessments with carbon monoxide diffusion capacity and computed tomography have demonstrated damage in 20–35% [18,19]. Progressive fatal pleural fibrosis occurs in about 1%.

## Clinical features, radiology and respiratory function tests

The characteristic symptoms (dyspnoea, sometimes with a dry cough and fever) usually develop over a few weeks 1–3 months after treatment. Although these features usually regress on stopping the drug they may progress or actually develop despite stopping the treatment [20,21]. Bilateral basal crepitations may be heard in the lower zone.

An early chest radiograph may show a fine reticular or reticulomicronodular pattern in the lower zones [16]. Features supporting the underlying fibrosing and restrictive pathology include elevation of the diaphragm, pleural reactions and thickening of the interlobular fissures [22]. Later the changes may become widespread, with patchy linear infiltrates indistinguishable from secondary infection, tumour spread, radiation change or heart failure. Neither pleural effusions nor hilar lymphadenopathy have been noted. Gallium-67 scintigraphy has been reported as a sensitive means of assessing lung damage but is non-specific [23].

Computed tomography (CT) has greatly improved both the sensitivity and specificity of radiological diagnosis. Changes which correlate well with the measurement of lung volumes can be picked up well before any conventional radiological changes are seen and the appearances are characteristic [24]. The changes affect mainly the posterior

**Table 17.2 Cytotoxic drugs causing lung damage**

| Group | Drug | Incidence (%) |
|---|---|---|
| Antibiotic cytotoxics | Bleomycin | 10 |
| | Peplomycin | + |
| | Liblomycin | |
| | Mitomycin C | 3 |
| | Zinostatin | + |
| Alkylating agents | Busulphan | 2.5 |
| | Cyclophosphamide | ++ |
| | Chlorambucil | ++ |
| | Melphalan | + |
| Nitrosoureas | Carmustine (BCNU) | 20 |
| | Lomustine (CCNU) | + |
| | Semustine (methyl-CCNU) | + |
| | Chlorozotocin | + |
| Antimetabolites | Methotrexate | 7 |
| | Cytarabine (Ara-C) | ++ |
| | 6-Mercaptopurine | + |
| | Azathioprine | + |
| Other drugs | Procarbazine | + |
| | Vinblastine | + |
| | Vindesine | + |
| | Uracil mustard | + |
| | Thioguanosine | + |
| | VM-26 | + |

+, Few sporadic cases of lung damage; ++, incidence low but a large number of case reports

aspects of the lungs and are predominantly subpleural [25,26]. There is often a relatively translucent zone between the pleura and the zone of maximal opacification. This opacification may be streaky or reticular [27], but may also have a nodular appearance which can be difficult to distinguish from pulmonary metastases [28,29]. CT monitoring which can be enhanced by density measurements as well as by visual assessments [30] shows complete resolution of most cases of minor or moderate damage, but in patients with severe damage, residual abnormality remains [24,26] and there may be progression of such lesions in about 20% of the cases [27].

Respiratory function tests probably remain the most sensitive method of detecting early toxicity in clinical practice. There is a restrictive ventilatory defect as shown by a reduced forced vital capacity (FVC) and a diffusion defect which can be shown by reduced carbon monoxide diffusion capacity ($D_L CO$) and there is often arterial hypoxaemia. A reduced $D_L CO$ is the most sensitive indicator of clinical toxicity but minor changes should be interpreted with caution [19]. If the respiratory function is monitored at 2–4-weekly intervals lung damage may be able to be minimized by the early withdrawal of bleomycin [31], though this is not always the case [32,33].

### Histological features

Light microscopy shows an interstitial pneumonitis with oedema of the alveolar walls and interstitial tissues, atypical proliferation of the alveolar epithelial cells, collapse of the alveoli and hyaline membrane formation within the alveoli. There is hyperplasia and migration of type II (granular) pneumocytes and macrophages into the alveolar lumen. Type I (membranous) pneumocytes are reduced. In more advanced cases there is collagen and reticulin deposition around the basement membrane. Hyperplasia of the bronchiolar muscle fibres and squamous metaplasia of the bronchiolar epithelium are also present [16,34,35]. Low grade dysplasia can be seen on sputum cytology in 37% of bleomycin-treated patients compared with 10% of the controls [36].

Electron microscopy confirms interstitial oedema, collagen deposition, accumulation of fibroblasts, lack of type I pneumocytes and proliferation of type II pneumocytes. The abnormalities of type II cells have been thought to be consistent with surfactant impairment [37]. Further nuclear, nucleolar and cytoplasmic abnormalities have been described but their significance is difficult to interpret [38].

Although interstitial pneumonitis is the usual histopathological finding described, a 'hypersensitivity' pneumonitis or eosinophilic pneumonia has been reported. A patchy eosinophilic infiltrate surrounds the small airways and distal air spaces and peripheral eosinophilia may also be a feature. This variant is particularly notable because of its favourable response to steroid therapy [39,40]. However, in one case which was antedated by eosinophilia, fulminant fatal angio-oedema unresponsive to steroids occurred [41].

### Factors predisposing to pulmonary toxicity

A number of factors influence the likelihood of pulmonary toxicity occurring following bleomycin therapy. There is a greater incidence of lung toxicity with high doses as shown in Figure 17.1 [42]. With

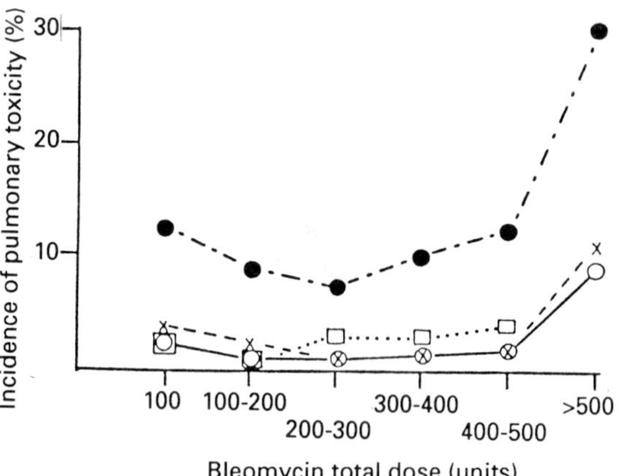


**Figure 17.1** The relationship between the total cumulative bleomycin dose and pulmonary toxicity: ●, overall; ×, definite; □, autopsy; ○, probable. Reproduced with permission from ref. [42]

cumulative doses above 500 mg Samuels *et al.* [43] reported a 20% incidence and a mortality of up to 5%. It is therefore most important to take into account any previous bleomycin therapy [44]. When the total dose of bleomycin is restricted to less than 300 mg, the incidence falls from 10% to 3–5%. In general the lower the total dose of bleomycin, the less the likelihood of lung toxicity [17,45]. Against this apparent dose relationship is the fact that occasionally, even with low total doses, symptomatic pneumonitis may occur as an idiosyncratic response. Reversible damage has been reported in a child after only 30 mg [46] and fatal pulmonary toxicity has been reported with 100–150 mg bleomycin [45,47], and when bleomycin was given with other cytotoxic drugs fatal toxicity at only 50 mg/m$^2$ has recently been reported [48].

The route of administration and schedule may affect the incidence of lung toxicity. In a study of lymphomas there was less toxicity in patients receiving intramuscular injections than intravenous and it was suggested that the likelihood of lung toxicity is related to peak blood levels [45]. Animal studies confirm that intravenous bleomycin produces more toxicity than equivalent doses given by intraperitoneal injection [49]. Animal studies have also shown that continuous infusion produces less lung damage and more inhibition of growth of the Lewis lung carcinoma than the same total dose given as an intermittent schedule [50]. Although initial studies in man of continuous intravenous infusion (CIVI) were encouraging, recent studies have shown little reduction in the incidence of lung damage [51]. In a further study, although efficacy may have been enhanced, pulmonary toxicity occurred in 39% of cases receiving bleomycin by CIVI [15]. On the other hand in a comparative study, continuous subcutaneous infusion (CSCI) has resulted in less pulmonary toxicity than CIVI, but with an equivalent antitumor effect [52].

Elderly patients, over the age of 70 are more susceptible to pulmonary toxicity [17,53]. It has also been reported that lung toxicity occurs more frequently in patients with pre-existing poor lung function [53]. However, Yagoda and Krakoff [54] found that the initial pulmonary function was unrelated to the subsequent occurrence of lung toxicity.

Pulmonary irradiation in itself insufficient to produce overt lung damage increases the incidence of bleomycin lung damage. Following early anecdotal reports, a number of studies showed a higher incidence of lung damage in those treated by chemotherapy and prior irradiation compared with chemotherapy alone [43,55,56]. On reviewing the literature for patients treated with concurrent bleomycin and irradiation, Catane *et al.* [57] found 22 (19%) of 115 patients developed pulmonary toxicity, and in 11 (10%) it was fatal. The clinical reports suggest that concurrent administration of bleomycin with pulmonary irradiation leads to the greatest enhancement and that, though prior irradiation also leads to enhancement, this is less. Animal studies have also shown increased damage from combined treatment. In our study the effect was not time-dependent [49] but Von der Maase, Overgaard and Vaeth [58] in a different strain of mice have demonstrated time dependency. These studies also show how the onset may be earlier and more abrupt than with either agent alone.

A number of reports have suggested that bleomycin lung damage is enhanced by other cytotoxic drugs [59,60] but in most cases the effect is not very great. Mitomycin C itself can cause lung damage (see below) and in combination with bleomycin the likelihood of lung damage is somewhat increased

[61,62]. Another worrying report was of fatal pneumonitis in five out of 19 (25%) cases of non-Hodgkin's lymphoma following low-dose bleomycin ($<50\,\mu g/m^2$) given as part of a regime of bleomycin, vincristine and prednisolone alternating with cyclophosphamide and mitoxantrone [48]. Carmustine (BCNU) also may be expected to increase pulmonary toxicity and a new experimental mouse model measuring lung hydroxyproline levels [63] has demonstrated an additive effect of bleomycin and carmustine. Another important interaction that has been reported has been with cisplatin [64], but this appears to be indirect, being related to impaired renal function (see below).

Over-oxygenation during or following anaesthesia may result in severe lung toxicity, frequently fatal even many months after bleomycin [65–67]. High-dose steroids can control the condition if given early [68]. Experimental studies in laboratory hamsters indicate synergism if oxygen and bleomycin are given together, but little effect if a month elapses between the two [69]. However, as stated above, in man many of the fatalities occurred many months after bleomycin.

Impaired renal function now appears to be a further factor that increases the likelihood of lung damage. Bennett, Pastore and Houghton [64] reported a fatal case of pulmonary bleomycin toxicity in a patient with unrecognized cisplatin-induced acute renal failure. Subsequently a fatality with a bleomycin dose of only 60 mg has been reported in a patient with renal insufficiency [70]. In searching for a predictive factor for lung damage in patients with testicular tumours receiving bleomycin and cisplatin, Bell, Meredith and Gill [32] found the carbon monoxide diffusing capacity disappointing, but noted the two fatal cases in their study had had reduced renal function. Van Barneveld *et al.* [18] concluded that patients with the combination of a low normal creatinine clearance and a decreased vital capacity and alveolar volume without a decrease in pulmonary capillary blood volume were at high risk.

## Management and prevention

Although there are no absolute contraindications, careful consideration should be given before treating the elderly, those with poor lung function, those receiving more than 300 mg total dose and those who have had previous lung irradiation. Particular caution should be taken in treating patients in renal failure (and in those concurrently on cisplatin). Anaesthetists should always be forewarned of the risks of over-oxygenation. Concurrent irradiation may also increase the likelihood of lung damage.

Patients at risk should be monitored every 2–4 weeks. Signs and symptoms should be sought; chest

X-rays, CT scans, lung function studies with the FVC and $D_LCO$, and renal function should be monitored. If following a non-invasive investigation a diagnosis of bleomycin-induced lung damage remains in doubt, histological confirmation, preferably via fibreoptic bronchoscopy, should be sought. In this way lung toxicity can be identified as early as possible. Bleomycin should be stopped and avoided in further therapy. Prednisone, 60–100 mg daily, reverses pulmonary damage in a number of cases [21]. There is little information on the outcome of pulmonary damage but it may be concluded from the incidence figures that about one in ten symptomatic cases may be fatal.

Much work has gone into the search for an agent to prevent lung damage. New derivatives such as peplomycin and liblomycin have been evaluated (see below). As noted above bleomycin damage is enhanced by high oxygen levels, and it is thought that lung damage may result from the production of toxic oxygen radicals during enzymic redox cycling of Fe(III)-bleomycin [71]. Desferroxamine, an iron chelating agent, has been shown to reduce the collagen content of the lung of laboratory animals following intratracheal bleomycin [72] and *N*-acetylcysteine, which maintains tissue levels of glutathione, protected mice against lung damage from the combined effects of hyperbaric oxygen and bleomycin [73]. Both agents appear promising.

Although steroids failed to prevent bleomycin lung damage in animal experiments [17], concurrent therapy with prednisone prevented side effects, including lung toxicity, in a series of 40 patients receiving a total dose of 420 mg of bleomycin [74]. At present this is probably the best 'prophylactic' agent available. Indomethacin is another agent that may be of value. It considerably reduced pulmonary fibrosis produced by endotracheal administration of bleomycin in rats but has not yet been formally tested in man. The extent of damage was assessed by measuring the vascular permeability and hydroxyproline content of lung tissue, and by counting the number of eosinophils in the peripheral blood [75].

### Pathogenesis

The development of bleomycin-induced lung toxicity has been extensively examined in animals. It was initially observed in dogs [76] but most of the subsequent work has been done on rodents. Adamson and Bowden [77] examined the lungs of mice by light and electron microscopy at weekly intervals during and following a 4-week course of twice weekly bleomycin. They found similar histological changes to those seen in man. The initial site of injury appeared to be the intima of the pulmonary arteries and veins. The endothelial cells became oedematous and were separated from the basement membrane by large blebs. Lymphocytes and plasma cells infiltrated the perivascular spaces. These changes were seen at 2 weeks. At 4 weeks similar changes were seen in the capillaries and there was multifocal necrosis of type I pneumocytes. There was diffuse interstitial oedema and the air spaces contained numerous vacuolated macrophages. From 4 weeks onwards there was hypertrophy of the type II pneumocytes and progressive intra-alveolar and septal fibrosis. Similar changes have been reported by others not only in mice [50,78,79], but also in hamsters in which the drug was given endotracheally [80,81], in baboons [82] and in pheasants [83].

These histological changes are consistent with a direct toxic effect of bleomycin on the lung, and are probably not specific for bleomycin but represent a general reaction of the lung to injury [79,83]. Indirect support for this mechanism of action is the fact that the occurrence of damage is dose-related in man and the extent of lung damage is dose-related in experimental animals [49], and also the finding of relatively high level of bleomycin in the lungs as well as in skin. The reason bleomycin accumulates in the lung is due to low levels of the bleomycin deactivating enzyme, bleomycin hydrolase, in the lung and particularly in the type II pneumocytes [84]. The mechanism of injury may be via toxic oxygen radicals [71] as discussed above, and supportive evidence is the protection from damage by desferroxamine and *N*-acetylcysteine [72,73]. Bleomycin has also been shown to increase procollagen synthesis, although decreasing cell growth of cultured fibroblasts [85].

## Peplomycin and liblomycin

These second (peplomycin) and third generation (liblomycin) analogues of bleomycin have been developed largely in the hope of reducing lung toxicity. Though peplomycin has satisfactory antitumour activity it also causes lung toxicity which is dose-limiting [86]. Liblomycin appears to cause less pulmonary toxicity and hopefully may prove therapeutically superior to bleomycin. Phase I studies are currently ongoing in Japan [87,88].

## Mitomycin C

### Incidence

Until 1978 pulmonary toxicity was not recognized as a clinical complication of mitomycin C [89], although lung damage had been recorded in two out of 40 dogs tested during early toxicity studies and also in rodents [90]. Subsequent reports [91–93] substantiated the problem, and there have been now over 40 cases reported in the literature [94–97]. In retrospectively reviewing 200 cases treated with mitomycin-containing drug regimes, Gunstream *et al.* [98] found six cases of substantiated toxicity giving an incidence of 3%. Many of these cases had been receiving concurrent 5-fluorouracil or sometimes a vinca alkaloid but in no case bleomycin, carmustine or busulphan.

### Diagnostic features and histology

The symptoms are usually dyspnoea and a dry cough sometimes associated with a chill, pleuritic chest pain or with weight loss and develop after 3–6 months of mitomycin treatment or occasionally several months after stopping mitomycin [99]. The patients are usually afebrile and bilateral basal crepitations may be heard. Chest radiographs show diffuse reticular infiltrates, sometimes with fine nodularity. Occasional pleural effusions have been described and pulmonary hilar prominence may be seen.

Histology has generally shown interstitial pneumonitis with moderate fibrosis, with a rather non-specific pattern of diffuse alveolar damage progressing along the final common path to interstitial fibrosis [92,98].

### Management course and prognosis

In some cases resolution occurs on stopping mitomycin, and about 50% will respond to steroids. However in one-third to one-half progression is relentless, unresponsive to steroids and fatal. Friedman [99] reported seven fatal cases of lung toxicity which were associated with renal failure and anaemia. Three of these developed after stopping mitomycin. In a further three cases early lung damage was followed by fatal mitomycin-induced microangiopathic haemolytic uraemic syndrome [100].

In order to minimize toxicity it is important to be aware of potential mitomycin lung damage and to stop mitomycin early should there be any suggestion of lung damage. There is some evidence that dexamethasone given prior to mitomycin reduces the incidence of clinically evident damage [101]. There is also some evidence from experimental studies that the lungs are circadian in their susceptibility to toxicity, toxicity being least in the period of 'late activity' and most in 'mid–late sleep' [102].

### Zinostatin

Zinostatin (carcinostatin), an antibiotic cytotoxic, was first investigated in the early 1980s. Encouraging initial Japanese reports of its efficacy failed to be confirmed by phase I and II studies against leukaemias and solid tumours in the USA, and it has little clinical role. However these clinical studies did reveal pulmonary toxicity similar to bleomycin lung damage in two reported cases [103,104].

# Alkylating agents

## Busulphan

### Incidence

Interstitial pulmonary fibrosis was reported in 1961 [1] which was the first time that a cytotoxic drug had been shown to cause lung damage. Many further reports of lung toxicity have followed which have been reviewed [20,42,105].

The incidence of the true 'busulphan lung syndrome', i.e. symptomatic lung damage histologically confirmed, is difficult to assess, but is probably not more than about 2.5% [106]. If only *post mortem* histology is considered, the incidence may appear as high as six out of 14 (43%) [107].

### Clinical features and investigations

The clinical features are similar to those of bleomycin pulmonary toxicity, but the development is usually more insidious. Dyspnoea, sometimes associated with a dry cough and fever, usually develops after several months 3–4 years after the onset of treatment, although it has been reported as early as 9 months and as late as 10 years [108]. Occasionally the onset may be fulminant, acute or subacute [109] but such an apparent acute onset may be due to a supervening infection [110]. Cyanosis, basal crepitations and rarely Addisonian signs may be found [111]. Chest radiographs show similar changes to those seen with bleomycin lung damage, with an early reticulonodular pattern or more often linear opacities. In addition, pleural effusions or even virtually normal radiographs have been reported [112]. Impaired respiratory function is reflected by arterial hypoxaemia and a reduced $D_LCO$. However, although Littler and Ogilvie [108] reported six out of 21 cases with a reduced $D_LCO$, only one was subsequently confirmed to have interstitial pneumonitis. Sometimes a restrictive ventilatory defect is found although this occurs less often than with bleomycin lung toxicity [20].

### Histological features

On reviewing the *post mortem* histology of 81 cases of chronic myeloid leukaemia, only half of whom had received busulphan, Kirschner and Esterly [106] found many characteristic features of interstitial pneumonitis such as fibrinous oedema, interstitial fibrosis, alveolar epithelialization and atypism of alveolar cells, occurring equally in both groups. A few features such as hyaline membrane formation and dysplasia of the bronchial epithelium were predominant in the busulphan-treated groups. Although distinctive large cells with hyperchromatic nuclei, so-called 'busulphan cells', were seen in four patients, all of whom had received busulphan, only one out of the 40 patients that had received busulphan had associated pulmonary fibrosis and respiratory distress. The explanation of the findings in the control group is not clear, but such findings emphasize the fact that many of the reported lesions may be due to other drugs or unknown factors.

## Factors predisposing to pulmonary toxicity

Few factors have been reported that influence the development of pulmonary damage. Although lung damage usually follows prolonged drug administration, no critical total dose has been cited. Added toxicity from combined treatment with other cytotoxic drugs does seem likely [113]. Fatal radiation pneumonitis has been reported in a patient following a split course of mantle irradiation, 40 Gy fractionated over 50 days [114]. The patient had been treated with a total dose of busulphan of 480 mg over the previous 6 years for polycythaemia rubra vera.

## Diagnosis, management and outcome

Diagnosis should be histologically confirmed. Sputum cytology and bronchial brushings may be useful [115] but the definitive diagnosis may require transbronchial biopsy. Following early diagnosis busulphan should be withdrawn. Despite this the lung damage frequently progresses and the patient dies [105], the median survival from onset of symptoms being 5 months [110]. Steroids are often given, but it is doubtful whether they affect the course of pulmonary disease.

## Pathogenesis

Busulphan-induced lung damage has not been reproduced in experimental animals. The theories about pathogenesis and aetiology are based only on clinical observations and the histological and the electron microscopical (EM) findings in man. Oliner *et al.* [1] likened the response to that of hexamethonium, and suggested the response was a hypersensitivity reaction to busulphan. However, following an EM study of 'busulphan lung', Littler *et al.* [116] considered it most likely to be a direct chemically-induced alveolitis. It was thought that the presence of large atypical cells which are also seen in many other organs of the busulphan-treated patient represent a non-specific response of the type II (granular) pneumocytes to injury [106,107].

# Cyclophosphamide
## Prevalence

It is now well substantiated that the commonly used alkylating agent cyclophosphamide can cause pulmonary toxicity [117], and there have been a number of case reports since it was first reported [20,117–125]. However these are rare and sporadic cases, and considering the widespread use of the drug, the likelihood of developing pulmonary toxicity is extremely low.

## Clinical features, investigations and histology

Dyspnoea often associated with dry cough and fever has developed from 3 weeks to 3 years [117] and in one case 8 years [122] after commencing cyclophosphamide treatment, and in four cases from 2 months [119] to 6 years [122] after stopping cyclophosphamide. The symptoms develop over a period of a few days to a few weeks. The time course is thus intermediate between that of busulphan and bleomycin lung damage [117]. Bilateral basal crepitations may be heard, and the radiological features are similar to those of bleomycin and busulphan. Similar histological changes, such as bronchoalveolar cell dysplasia, alveolar septal thickening with a mild mononuclear cell infiltrate and interstitial fibrosis are found.

## Factors predisposing to pulmonary toxicity

The influence of dose and schedule is not clear from the limited number of case reports. It is interesting that pulmonary toxicity had not been a major side effect of high-dose cyclophosphamide [126].

Combined treatment with other cytotoxic drugs may increase the incidence of pulmonary toxicity, since cyclophosphamide was a common drug included in many of the schedules of combination therapy described below in which pulmonary toxicity was reported and particularly when it has been used with bleomycin.

Radiation-induced lung damage in man has not yet been clearly shown to be enhanced by cyclophosphamide. However it has been included in several schedules of combination chemotherapy reported to have enhanced radiation lung damage. In some the enhancement was attributed to bleomycin [55,127], and in another actinomycin D and doxorubicin [128–130]. A number of the cases reported as cyclophosphamide-induced lung damage had, in fact, received previous mantle irradiation [118,121,122] but many of the cases had not received irradiation. Very high-dose cyclophosphamide has been reported to enhance radiation-induced lung fibrosis in treatment of small cell carcinoma of the lung [131]. The potential enhancement of radiation lung damage by cyclophosphamide is particularly important in view of the frequent use of high-dose cyclophosphamide prior to total body irradiation. Pneumonitis is the major cause of death from such programmes, but in fact there is little evidence that the cyclophosphamide increases the risk of lung damage over and above the effects of radiation alone, despite the results of the experimental studies which will be described below.

## Management and outcome

On stopping cyclophosphamide pulmonary damage resolved in about half the cases, although in one this took several months [20,117,120,123]. Concurrent steroids may aid recovery [20,117]. In the other half of the cases, some of whom have been children [119,122,125], the pulmonary damage progressed relentlessly.

## Pathogenesis and experimental animal studies

Cyclophosphamide-induced lung damage has been extensively studied in experimental animals, in which lung damage can be readily produced. In this respect it differs markedly from the lung damage seen in man. It was first reported in dogs who died of pulmonary oedema within 4–6 h from administration [132]. However this may have been due to myocardial toxicity which was also seen. Pulmonary oedema occurred in mice treated with high-dose cyclophosphamide and this effect was greatly enhanced by potassium iodide, resulting in death within a few hours of drug administration [133]. However the pathogenesis of the pulmonary oedema was not elucidated.

Gould and Miller [134] discovered that sclerosing alveolitis occurred in rats treated with cyclophosphamide. Perivascular oedema, septal thickening and minute haemorrhages were evident as early as 48 h after drug administration. By 4–7 days after treatment many of the alveoli contained debris and macrophages. Focal hyaline membrane formation was seen and there was alveolar cell hyperplasia with increased septal cellularity and increased interstitial material. Subsequently these changes persisted and septal fibrosis progressed. The histological changes seen in experimental laboratory mice are very similar and the extent of damage can be quantified either histologically or more easily by

measurement of a crude respiratory function test ventilation rate.

A large number of studies have been carried out searching for manoeuvres or agents that might modify or reduce lung damage. The extent of lung damage has been shown to be schedule-dependent. By 'priming', i.e. giving a small dose 12 h prior to the main dose, some degree of protection can be obtained in CBA mice [135]. Bone marrow recovery could also be enhanced by this 'priming' manoeuvre but unfortunately does not help clinically. In C3H mice, sodium thiosulphate, mesna and epsilon-aminocaproic acid have been evaluated and have little effect, but mice given WR2721, a radio-protector, before cyclophosphamide were protected [136].

In male CBA mice cyclophosphamide has been shown to enhance radiation lung damage. The extent of lung damage varied considerably with the timing of administration of cyclophosphamide in relation to irradiation: greatest enhancement occurred when cyclophosphamide was given 12 h before irradiation [137]. Von der Maase, Overgaard and Vaeth [58] have also reported enhanced lung damage with concurrent irradiation in $C_3D_2F_1$/BOM mice, but little enhancement when the gap between irradiation and drug was more than 6 h. In the male CBA mice the enhancing effect of cyclophosphamide appears to be dose rate-dependent, reducing the relative sparing effect of low dose rate irradiation compared with high dose rate irradiation [138]. A similar effect was reported in laboratory rats when cyclophosphamide was given 24 h before radiotherapy [139]. These investigations demonstrate the great complexity of the interaction of cytotoxic drugs with irradiation but unfortunately cannot be directly translated to the human situation.

## Chlorambucil

Pulmonary fibrosis following chlorambucil similar to that seen with other alkylating agents was first briefly reported in four cases by Rubio [140]. Subsequently more than ten further cases have been reported [141–149] which have been reviewed by Carr [150]. Most cases have occurred in patients with chronic lymphatic leukaemia on oral chlorambucil, having received a total dose of 540–4300 mg given for 5–56 months.

Dyspnoea, fatigue, weakness, anorexia and weight loss usually develop subacutely over a period of 2–3 weeks. Fever may be present and the signs, radiographic findings and lung function defects are similar to those seen with the other alkylating agents. Light and electron microscopy also show similar changes to those seen with busulphan and cyclophosphamide [145]. In one case lung damage had followed high-dose chlorambucil [146]. In another the onset of symptoms did not occur until several months after stopping chlorambucil [150].

Although the prognosis has been poor (over 50% of the patients died), recovery may occur on stopping the drug and instigating high-dose steroids [145,148,150]. Therefore, although the condition is rare, it is important to obtain a diagnosis made by lung biopsy.

## Melphalan

There have been some seven cases of melphalan-induced lung damage reported [151–155]. However the occurrence of some degree of damage may be higher: Taetle, Dickman and Feldman [152] reported atypical epithelial proliferation in six out of 11 cases of myeloma treated with melphalan, but in none of a matched control group of myeloma patients, and Giles *et al.* [156] have shown reduced respiratory function in seven out of ten non-smoking myeloma patients recently studied.

The symptoms develop over 2–10 days, following 2–36 months of oral melphalan. Despite withdrawal of oral melphalan and treatment with steroids, most of the patients deteriorated and died within a few weeks of the onset of symptoms. One patient improved a little and stabilized following steroids [154], and one, who had had only two cycles of melphalan, appeared to recover completely [153].

## Nitrosoureas

### Carmustine (BCNU; 1,3-bis(2-chloroethyl)-1-nitrosourea)

#### *Incidence*

Interstitial pneumonitis and fibrosis is a relatively frequent and dose-limiting side effect of carmustine. Even though widely used since 1965, the first well substantiated report of interstitial pneumonitis and fibrosis did not appear until 1976 [157]. A large number of cases have now been reported and reviewed by Weiss, Poster and Penta [5], but only a few large series of patients treated with carmustine have been reviewed. In an early series Durant *et al.* [158] reported an incidence of approximately 1%, nine cases out of 794 patients receiving a variety of chemotherapy regimes which included carmustine. In 1980 Aronin *et al.* [159] reported 19 out of 93, i.e. 20%, and Selker *et al.* [160] 14 out of 47, i.e. 30% with lung damage, thus rating the incidence of lung damage from carmustine as high if not higher than that from bleomycin.

### *Clinical features, investigations and histology*

A dry hacking cough, followed by progressive dyspnoea may develop from 1 to more than 36 months (median 12 months) after the onset of treatment. Although the development of symptoms is usually slowly progressive, it can also be fulminating and rapidly progressive [159,161,162]. Fever is unusual. Coarse crepitations may be heard at the lung bases.

The chest X-ray usually shows bilateral diffuse basal shadowing which tends to be irreversible, but in some histologically proven cases of early lung damage reported by Selker [160] and Aronin [159] the chest X-ray was normal despite abnormal respiratory function tests, the usual respiratory function test abnormality being a restrictive and diffusion defect. Histological examination reveals interstitial pneumonitis and fibrosis. The latter is prominent and may even occur in the apparent absence of an inflammatory cell infiltrate.

### *Factors predisposing to pulmonary toxicity*

The likelihood of developing lung damage is dose-related. In the series from Aronin [159] the average total dose of affected cases was $1146\,mg/m^2$ compared with $777\,mg$ in those who did not develop pulmonary toxicity. The probability increases to over 50% with doses of more than $1500\,mg$ as shown in Figure 17.2 [159]. Selker *et al.* [160] also found the majority of problems in patients who had received over $1500\,mg/m^2$. A dose of $1200$–$1500\,mg/m^2$ should therefore be considered as a dose limit in the same way that $550\,mg/m^2$ is recognized as the

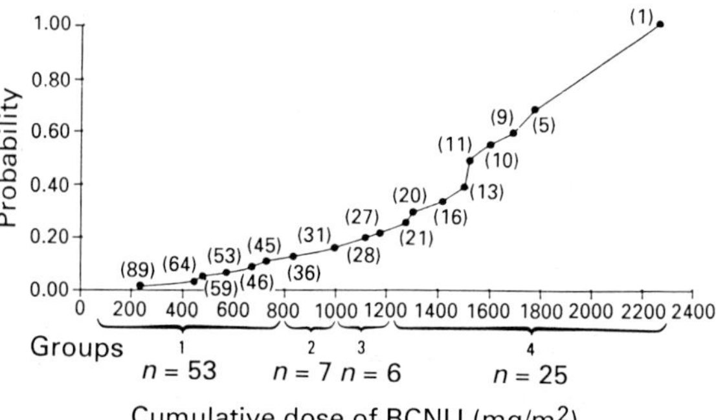


**Figure 17.2** The cumulative probability of lung toxicity based on the cumulative dose of carmustine (BCNU). Mean cumulative toxic dose, $1146\,mg/m^2$; mean cumulative non-toxic dose, $777\,mg/m^2$. The numbers in parentheses indicate the total number of patients at risk at the given dose. Reproduced with permission from ref. [159]

dose limit to minimize the likelihood of cardiac damage from doxorubicin [5]. However, even with low doses toxicity can occur, there being a report of fatal pulmonary toxicity after a single dose of only $400\,mg/m^2$ [163]. Pulmonary toxicity has also proved to be dose-limiting with intensive high-dose chemotherapy when carmustine was used as part of conditioning for autologous bone marrow transplantation. In 63 cases a dose of 1200 mg resulted in a 9.5% incidence of fatal pulmonary toxicity. Even by reducing this dose to $1000\,mg/m^2$ it is not clear that the risk is reduced, though at $600\,mg/m^2$ pulmonary toxicity was not a major problem [6,164].

Other cytotoxic drugs may enhance lung damage. It has been suggested that concurrent cyclophosphamide may reduce the total dose of carmustine at which lung toxicity occurs [158,165]. The evidence is not strong, but increased awareness of the possibility of lung damage may be wise where carmustine is used in combination with other cytotoxic drugs.

Theoretically it seems highly likely that there should be at least an additive increase in pulmonary damage where pulmonary irradiation and carmustine are combined, and it would therefore seem prudent to take particular care in those previously irradiated.

Curiously age *per se* does not appear to be a strong risk factor. There is, however, a higher incidence of history of previous lung disease and tobacco use in those who suffer carmustine lung damage than in comparable patients who are unaffected [159].

### Management and outcome

Of the initial reported cases, 75% died of pulmonary toxicity. Although steroids were used in many of these cases, they were clearly of limited benefit (a transient response has been described in one case report). On the other hand in the later series of Aronin [159] and Selker [160], where perhaps earlier damage was being picked up and carmustine stopped earlier, the mortality was considerably less at 15–35%.

### Pathogenesis

Lung toxicity was reported in the early studies of toxicity of the nitrosoureas, being found in dogs and rhesus monkeys given carmustine [166]. However a satisfactory animal model has been difficult to establish since, unlike bleomycin and cyclophosphamide, the pulmonary toxicity of carmustine in laboratory animals appears to be low. However carmustine has been shown to enhance butylated hydroxytoluene (BHT)-induced lung damage in Sprague Dawley rats when given within 24 h of BHT [167].

## Lomustine (CCNU), semustine (methyl-CCNU), chlorozotocin

Since the reporting of pulmonary toxicity with carmustine, pulmonary toxicity has also been reported with other nitrosoureas. However the cases are few and sporadic.

The first case with lomustine (CCNU) was reported in 1982 [168] and a further two cases in 1983 [169]. The pattern was of insidious onset of pulmonary fibrosis.

There has been just one report of pulmonary fibrosis with semustine (methyl-CCNU) [170]. The nature was again a progressive irreversible fatal pulmonary fibrosis. Although semustine showed moderate activity in gastrointestinal tumours, this was insufficient to warrant general use. However, should more patients receive a high cumulative dose, more lung damage might be seen.

Chlorozotocin, another nitrosourea with limited clinical application, has also been shown to cause pulmonary fibrosis [171]. Streptozotocin, which has been shown to be active against malignant islet cell tumours and carcinoid tumours, as yet has not been reported to cause pulmonary toxicity [5].

# Antimetabolites

## Methotrexate

### Incidence

Methotrexate was one of the earliest drugs reported to cause pulmonary toxicity [2,172], and in these early reports of patients receiving daily low doses of oral methotrexate regimes, up to 7% developed pneumonitis [20]. However with intermittent intravenous administration and also with high-dose methotrexate it is extremely rare.

### Clinical features and investigations

A dry cough, fever and dyspnoea are usually the presenting symptoms, although prodromal symptoms of headache and malaise may occur. Cyanosis, tachypnoea and basal crepitations may be found on examination. About half of the cases develop eosinophilia [172,173]. The chest radiograph shows bilateral linear or reticulonodular infiltrates at the bases and mid zones in most cases, but a range of appearances from normal to widespread opacification has been reported. Pleural effusions and hilar lymphadenopathy have also been reported [173,174]. Lung function tests may show a diffusion defect and a restrictive and ventilatory defect. Although lung function recovers, a residual defect often persists which notably does not deteriorate when methotrexate is later re-introduced [173].

## Histological features

Histological examination of the lungs reveals diffuse alveolar damage, atypical cells, hyaline membranes and interstitial infiltrates of mononuclear cells, and also of plasma cells and eosinophils in some cases. A granulomatous response with multinucleate giant cells may be seen [172,175]. Occasionally interstitial fibrosis develops and may be associated with progressive respiratory failure and death [173,174,176,177].

## Factors predisposing to pulmonary toxicity

Pulmonary toxicity from methotrexate is difficult to predict. Pneumonitis has occurred after a wide range of doses from 40 mg to 41 g, and from as early as 12 days to 5 years after commencing the drug [173]. The development of pneumonitis appears virtually independent of the dose or duration of treatment, although it has been reported with doses of less than 20 mg per week [173]. There is also no correlation with age, sex or underlying disease. It has occurred in patients receiving concurrent steroids or following leucovorin (folinic acid) rescue, so that neither of these agents appears to prevent pneumonitis. Pneumonitis has mostly occurred in patients receiving the drug orally, but has also been reported following intramuscular [2,178], and intrathecal administration [180,181]. It is therefore probably the frequency rather than the route of administration that is important [173]. Other concurrent cytotoxic drugs may increase the likelihood of lung toxicity [182,183]. However, enhancement of radiation pneumonitis by methotrexate alone has not been reported.

## Diagnosis, management and outcome

Most patients recover whether or not treated with steroids, and whether or not methotrexate is stopped [173]. Once improvement begins, resolution is rapid [172,184]. However, some develop chronic pulmonary changes [179]. This tends to occur in elderly patients, to develop insidiously and progressively, and has been fatal in three out of four cases [176,177]. Although there is no definite evidence that stopping methotrexate improves ultimate recovery, there is evidence that by stopping methotrexate and commencing treatment with corticosteroids recovery time is quartered and mortality may be reduced [173]. It has also been reported that daunorubicin may have a beneficial effect. The administration of daunorubicin in three cases of methotrexate pneumonitis was followed by prompt recovery [185].

Once the patient has recovered, methotrexate can be cautiously re-introduced with apparently no risk of recurrence of pneumonitis [173], unless marked fibrosis is present [176,177].

## Pathogenesis

The nature of pulmonary toxicity from methotrexate differs from that seen with bleomycin and the alkylating agents in three principal ways. Firstly, the histology shows giant cell granulomata and seldom shows any fibrosis. Secondly, patients usually show marked or complete resolution. Thirdly, the drug may be re-introduced after recovery from pulmonary toxicity without causing any apparent further damage. In addition pulmonary toxicity following methotrexate appears to be independent of dose. Indeed, even in a study of adolescents receiving high-dose methotrexate there was no demonstrable dose-related decrease in pulmonary function [186].

The pathogenesis of methotrexate lung damage remains unknown and there are no reports of it being reproduced in experimental animals. An immunological mechanism has been postulated because of the presence of the peripheral eosinophilia and granulomata, and the lack of a dose relationship. However, the anti-inflammatory and immunosuppressive properties of methotrexate, and the lack of a response to a second challenge, mitigate against this. A direct toxic effect has been postulated [173,187] and the moderately high levels of methotrexate found in the lung [188] also support this theory.

## Cytarabine (cytosine arabinoside, Ara-C)

### Incidence

Pulmonary toxicity was first described in 1981 in a retrospective autopsy study [189]. Patients with leukaemia who had recently had cytarabine (in doses of up to 90 mg/kg) had a much higher incidence of pulmonary oedema, with a highly proteinaceous interstitial and intra-alveolar infiltrate. These features correlated with the typical gastrointestinal lesions of cytarabine toxicity. In order to overcome natural and acquired unresponsive leukaemic cells, and thus improve therapeutic efficacy, still higher doses of cytarabine have been used. Willemze *et al.* [190] initially reported worrying pulmonary failure from a high-dose cytarabine regime. In a series of 72 cases receiving 12–36 g/m$^2$, 22% developed subacute pulmonary failure including six out of 19 of those receiving 36 g/m$^2$ [7]. In a further study of 64 patients receiving intermediate dose cytarabine (up to 12 g/m$^2$), diffuse lung disease occurred in 11% of remission induction courses and in 21% of those undergoing consolidation therapy [191].

### *Clinical course and management*

Rather sudden onset of respiratory distress with cough, fever and tachypnoea occur anything from 2 to 21 days (average 6 days) from treatment. This progresses rapidly to pulmonary oedema. Radiographically there are bilateral diffuse interstitial, alveolar or mixed patterns. Patients require vigorous supportive care with transfer to an intensive care unit for monitoring in life-threatening situations. High-dose steroids are probably helpful. With such management, Andersson *et al.* [7] reported 15 out of 18 and Tham *et al.* [191] 13 out of 15 cases recovered.

### *Pathogenesis*

Altered capillary endothelial permeability with impaired production and function of surfactant has been proposed.

### 6-Mercaptopurine (6-MP) and azathioprine

Sostman, Matthay and Putman [20] reported a case of 6-MP induced pneumonitis in a 2-year-old child with acute leukaemia in remission following 3 days treatment with 6-MP. The chest radiograph showed fine nodular infiltrates and an open lung biopsy revealed interstitial pneumonitis with no evidence of fibrosis. The patient recovered completely after discontinuing the drug. Two other cases of pulmonary toxicity have been described in the foreign literature [192,193] and there has been at least one report of 6-MP combined with other therapy resulting in interstitial pneumonitis [183].

There have also been two case reports of similar typical pneumonitis following azathioprine, a drug which is metabolized to 6-MP [194–196]. In all cases resolution followed withdrawal of the drug.

## Other drugs

### Procarbazine

'Hypersensitivity' to procarbazine with pleuropulmonary reactions has been reported in two patients with Hodgkin's disease being treated with mustine, vincristine, procarbazine and prednisone (MOPP) [197,198]. Only a few hours after taking the drug the patients developed nausea, fever, a dry cough and dyspnoea. There was mild peripheral eosinophilia. The chest radiograph showed bilateral interstitial infiltrates and a right pleural effusion. Within 24 h of stopping the procarbazine the syndrome resolved. It recurred with the next course of procarbazine and again cleared on stopping the drug. The diagnosis was then confirmed with a specific challenge dose of procarbazine.

In three further patients with Hodgkin's disease receiving MOPP, symptoms developed over several weeks and the histologically proven interstitial pneumonitis resolved following treatment with prednisone [199,200]. In two more recent cases [201,202] symptoms and signs developed at approximately 24 h after completion of the course of MOPP and resolved on steroids. In another histologically proven case procarbazine may have had an additive effect with other agents, although it was not considered to have been the primary cause of lung damage [120].

### Vinblastine and vindesine

Pulmonary oedema was reported following intravenous vinblastine by Israel and Olson [203]. Acute onset of respiratory distress followed vinblastine given with mitomycin C in two further cases of metastatic breast cancer. The time course suggested an acute process related to vinblastine administration possibly augmented by the known tendency of mitomycin to cause lung damage [204]. In both cases the episodes resolved, though one case died several weeks later with progressive pulmonary failure. Rapid onset of pulmonary symptoms was also described in ovarian cancer patients treated with vinblastine, mitomycin C and progesterone [94]. Two further cases of fatal acute respiratory distress in patients receiving vinblastine and mitomycin have been reported [95].

It seems likely therefore that vinblastine can cause acute pulmonary oedema, particularly when given with mitomycin C, which although well documented itself as a cause of interstitial pneumonitis, has not been reported to produce acute onset of respiratory distress nor to cause pulmonary oedema.

Vindesine has also been reported to lead to acute dyspnoea when given with mitomycin C [205]. On reviewing 126 cases treated with vindesine and mitomycin C, Luedke *et al.* [206] found seven cases of pulmonary toxicity, and in five the onset was abrupt, occurring 1–5 h after the vindesine administration. In most improvement occurred either spontaneously or with bronchodilators. None of these five subsequently developed either clinical or radiological features of subsequent damage.

The mechanism of damage with vindesine and vinblastine appears to be a change in the vascular permeability leading to acute respiratory distress, thus acting on the lung in a similar way to cytarabine.

### Other drugs

Other cytotoxic drugs which on occasion have caused interstitial pneumonitis and fibrosis include uracil mustard [207], thioguanosine [187] and VM-26 [208].

# Combination chemotherapy

Many of the reports of pulmonary damage have been in patients treated with several cytotoxic drugs [120, 151, 158, 165, 175, 182, 197, 198, 200, 207]. One principal drug is usually singled out as the most commonly reported drug to cause lung toxicity, and therefore the most likely culprit. However, combined effects probably do occur, particularly when two or more of the agents have been shown to cause lung damage when given individually. As a result, a higher incidence of lung damage than anticipated might be seen [182] or lung damage may occur at lower drug doses than would otherwise have been anticipated, for example with bleomycin and mitomycin [209], with carmustine and cyclophosphamide [158,165], with bleomycin and doxorubicin (Adriamycin), cyclophosphamide, vincristine and prednisone (BACOP) [210], and with cyclophosphamide, methotrexate and etoposide [211]. Also of interest is the vinca alkaloid-mitomycin combination. Alone the vinca alkaloids hardly ever cause pulmonary oedema, but given with mitomycin C this is now an established side effect as described above.

Such combined effects may occur not only when several drugs are given together or within a short time of each other, but also when one drug is given a considerable time after another drug, such as has been documented with uracil mustard after busulphan [207] and thioguanosine after methotrexate [187]. If the initial damage is subclinical, such combined effects would be difficult to demonstrate and may indeed have occurred undetected in many of these reported cases of drug-induced lung damage attributed to a single drug.

# Cytotoxic drugs and irradiation

Of the drugs described above, only bleomycin [43, 55, 212] and busulphan [114] have been reported to enhance radiation lung damage in man as discussed under their respective drug headings. Enhancement of radiation lung damage has also been described with various combinations of cytotoxic drugs [129, 213, 214]. However, in view of the multiple drugs in various doses, and also varying doses of irradiation, it is difficult to demonstrate any definite interactions. None the less it seems likely that multiple agents given with radiotherapy will increase the risk of lung toxicity.

Several cytotoxic drugs not in themselves apparently toxic to the lung may enhance radiation damage. Actinomycin D was the initial classic drug reported to enhance radiation reactions in a number of tissues including the lung [215, 216]. Doxorubicin was soon noted to have a similar effect [129, 130, 217]. Of particular interest is the so-called 'radiation recall reaction'. This describes the situation when symptomatic pneumonitis (or some other radiation reaction) has occurred with irradiation and then settled. The 'radiation' reaction then recurs or is 'recalled' following a subsequent challenge from the drug in question. This 'recall reaction' has been reported with both actinomycin D and doxorubicin [130, 218, 219]. The pneumonitis responds to steroids and is transient. Cisplatin may also enhance radiation lung damage, though the clinical evidence is anecdotal [220]. A study of carboplatin and irradiation used in the treatment of small cell lung cancer showed no significant increase in the enhancement of radiation lung toxicity [221].

A number of drugs have been assessed in experimental animals for interaction with irradiation. In CBA mice, assessing a range of cytotoxic drugs, radiation-induced lung damage was found to be increased by bleomycin [49], cyclophosphamide [137] and doxorubicin [222]. The degree of enhancement was markedly time-dependent with cyclophosphamide. Von der Maase [58] assessed a similar range of drugs in $C_3D_2F_1$/BOM mice and also found enhancement by these drugs and in addition found increased damage with mitomycin C. He reported cisplatin had no significant effect as was also found by Peckham and Collis [222], but Tanabe, Godat and Kallman [223] have reported high enhancement ratios for the lung in $C_3$ H/KM mice when cisplatin was given within 72 h of irradiation. In general maximal enhancement usually occurs when drugs and irradiation are given concurrently, but there can be considerable variation in the resultant damage with different time intervals, particularly within 72 h of irradiation. Applying any individual result to humans is probably totally fallacious, since even between animal strains variation is seen, but the principle that excessive toxicity may occur when radiation and chemotherapy are given close together is important.

# An overview of the pathogenesis of cytotoxic drug-induced lung damage

## Evidence for direct cytotoxic damage

Most of the cytotoxic drugs described in this chapter are thought to act by a direct toxic effect on the lung parenchyma. The direct toxic effect of these cytotoxic drugs is proposed largely on the basis of the lung morphology. The histology of bleomycin-induced lung damage has been carefully examined in man [34,35,37] and in experimental animals [77–79,83]. There are also extensive reports of busulphan lung histology in man [110,116] and of cyclophosphamide-induced lung damage in man [117] and in the mouse [134]. In all these cases and in most of the case reports of other drug-induced lung damage there is early pneumonitis with interstitial oedema, degeneration of type I cells, hyperplasia of the type II cells and vascular damage followed by progressive fibrosis. These changes are thought to represent a direct general reaction of the lung to noxious agents, also being seen with radiation damage and oxygen toxicity. The histological features of methotrexate-induced lung damage, although slightly different, can also be ascribed to a direct drug-induced alveolitis [173].

The direct cytotoxic effect of the drugs on the lung is also supported by the fact that the occurrence of lung damage is related to dose, as has been demonstrated with bleomycin, busulphan and carmustine. With other drugs there is little or no evidence of a dose relationship, but this apparent sporadic nature may be because the doses used in man are so low on the dose-effect plot. If higher doses could be tolerated in man a more definite relationship of dose to the development of lung damage might be seen. Further evidence for such dose dependency comes from animal studies. Reproducible and dose-dependent lung damage occurs following administration of bleomycin and cyclophosphamide to rodents [49,50,134,137].

## Other mechanisms of pulmonary toxicity

Although most drugs act by a direct toxic effect on the parenchyma, some drugs act differently. Procarbazine produces a typical allergic pulmonary eosinophilic response [197,198]. High-dose cytarabine produces a change in the endothelial permeability leading to pulmonary oedema and the combination of vindesine or vinblastine with mitomycin C appears to act similarly.

Other pulmonary complications reported include pulmonary veno-occlusive disease following combination chemotherapy with bleomycin, mitomycin C and cisplatin resulting in death from pulmonary hypertension [224]. Pleurisy may occur following methotrexate [11] and also with mitomycin C. Even pneumothorax has been attributed to chemotherapy [10].

## Characteristic responses to individual drugs

The various types of response can be summarized as shown in Table 17.3. The drugs are listed in order

**Table 17.3 The responses of the lungs to cytotoxic drugs**

| *Type of response* | *Characteristics* | *Drugs* |
|---|---|---|
| Pulmonary oedema | Abrupt onset | Cytarabine<br>Vinblastine or vindesine<br>(+ mitomycin C) |
| Acute reactive | Rapid development,<br>eosinophilia, granulomata<br>reversible,<br>responsive to steroids | Procarbazine<br>Methotrexate<br>(Thioguanosine)<br>(Bleomycin)<br>(6-mercaptopurine)<br>(Azathioprine)<br>(Busulphan) |
| Subacute | Intermediate | Bleomycin<br>Mitomycin C<br>(Peplomycin)<br>(Neocarcinostatin)<br>(Uracil mustard)<br>(VM-26) |
| Chronic fibrotic | Insidious onset,<br>predominant fibrosis,<br>progressive,<br>no response to steroids | (Methotrexate)<br>(Melphalan)<br>Chlorambucil<br>Cyclophosphamide<br>(Semustine)<br>(Lomustine)<br>Carmustine<br>Busulphan |

Underlined, major responses; in brackets, rare responses

from those producing acute pulmonary oedema, through the 'acute reactive' hypersensitivity allergic response of procarbazine to the 'chronic fibrotic' progressive fibrosis of the busulphan lung syndrome. The term 'acute reactive' is used in preference to hypersensitivity, since as has already been discussed with methotrexate, an allergic mechanism may not be involved [173]. Drugs are shown in brackets in the table if there are only one or two case reports or also to indicate unusual responses that have been reported from bleomycin, methotrexate and busulphan [39,109,176,177]. The nature of the response does not appear to depend on dose or schedule, appearing to be a characteristic of the drug itself and is presumably related to qualitative differences in the metabolism of the drugs by the lung parenchyma.

## References


1. Oliner, H., Schwartz, R., Rubio, F. and Dameshek, W. Interstitial pulmonary fibrosis following busulfan therapy. *American Journal of Medicine*, **31**, 134–139 (1961)
2. Acute Leukaemia Group B. Acute lymphocytic leukaemia in children. *Journal of the American Medical Association*, **207**, 923–928 (1969)
3. Ichikawa, T., Katano, I. and Hirokawa, I. Bleomycin treatment of the tumors of penis and scrotum. *Journal of Urology*, **102**, 697–707 (1969)
4. Collis, C.H. Lung damage from cytotoxic drugs. *Cancer Chemotherapy and Pharmacology*, **4**, 17–27 (1980)
5. Weiss, R.B., Poster, D.S. and Penta, J.S. The nitrosoureas and pulmonary toxicity. *Cancer Treatment Review*, **8**, 111–125 (1981)
6. Phillips, G.L., Fay, J.W., Herzig, G.P. *et al.* Intensive 1,2-bis(2-chloroethyl)-1-nitrosourea (BCNU), NSC-4366650 and cryopreserved autologous marrow transplantation for refractory cancer. A phase I–II study. *Cancer*, **52**, 1792–1802 (1983)
7. Andersson, B.S., Cogan, B.M., Keating, M.J. *et al.* Subacute pulmonary failure complicating therapy with high-dose Ara-C in acute leukaemia. *Cancer*, **56**, 2181–2184 (1985)
8. Thalinger, A.R., Rosenthal, S.N., Borg, S. and Arseneau, J.C. Cavitation of pulmonary metastases as a response to chemotherapy. *Cancer*, **46**, 1329–1332 (1980)
9. Murray, G.B. and Greenberg, D.B. Respiratory dyskinesia associated with hexamethylmelamine (letter). *Cancer Treatment Reports*, **64**, 355–356 (1980)
10. Lote, K., Dahl, O. and Vigander, T. Pneumothorax during combination chemotherapy. *Cancer*, **47**, 1743–1745 (1981)
11. Urban, C., Nirenberg, A., Caparros, B. *et al.* Chemical pleuritis as the cause of acute chest pain following high dose methotrexate treatment. *Cancer*, **51**, 34–37 (1983)
12. Steel, G.G. and Adams, K. Enhancement by cytotoxic agents of artificial pulmonary metastases. *British Journal of Cancer*, **36**, 653 (1977)
13. Orr, F.W., Adamson, I.Y. and Young, L. Quantification of metastatic tumour growth in bleomycin-injured lungs. *Clinical and Experimental Metastasis*, **4**, 105–116 (1986)
14. Ellis, J.H. Transbronchial lung biopsy via the fibre-optic bronchoscope. *Chest*, **68**, 524–532 (1975)
15. Boyd, D.B., Coleman, M., Papish, S.W. *et al.* Copblam III: infusional combination chemotherapy for diffuse large-cell lymphoma. *Journal of Clinical Oncology*, 6, 425–433 (1988)
16. De Lena, M., Guzzon, A., Monfardini, S. and Bonadonna, G. Clinical, radiologic and histopathologic studies on pulmonary toxicity induced by treatment with bleomycin. (NSC-125066) *Cancer Chemotherapy Reports*, **56**, 343–356 (1972)
17. Blum, R.H., Carter, S.K. and Agre, K. A clinical review of bleomycin – a new anti-neoplastic agent. *Cancer*, **31**, 903–914 (1973)
18. Van Barneveld, P.W., van der Mark, T.W., Sleijfer, D.T. *et al.* Predictive factors for bleomycin-induced pneumonitis. *American Review of Respiratory Diseases*, **130**, 1078–1081 (1984)
19. Srensen, P.G., Rossing, N. and Rorth, M. Carbon monoxide diffusing capacity: a reliable indicator of bleomycin-induced pulmonary toxicity. *European Journal of Respiratory Diseases*, **66**, 333–340 (1985)
20. Sostman, H.D., Matthay, R.A. and Putman, C.E. Cytotoxic drug-induced lung disease. *American Journal of Medicine*, **62**, 608–615 (1977)
21. Yagoda, A., Mukherji, B., Young, C. *et al.* Bleomycin, an antitumour antibiotic. *Annals of Internal Medicine*, **77**, 861–870 (1972)
22. Balikian, J.P., Jochelson, M.S., Bauer, K.A. *et al.* Pulmonary complications of chemotherapy regimens containing bleomycin. *American Journal of Roentgenology*, **139**, 455–461 (1982)
23. Richman, S.D., Levenson, S.M., Bunn, P.A. *et al.* 67-Ga accumulation in pulmonary lesions associated with bleomycin toxicity. *Cancer*, **36**, 1966–1972 (1975)
24. Bellamy, E.A., Husband, J.E., Blaquiere, R.M. and Law, M.R. Bleomycin related lung damage: CT evidence. *Radiology*, **156**, 155–158 (1985)
25. Goddard, P., Goodman, S. and Bell, J. Bleomycin pulmonary toxicity. *British Journal of Cancer*, **54**, 198 (1986)
26. Rimmer, M.J., Dixon, A.K., Flower, C.D. and Sikora, K. Bleomycin lung: computed tomographic observations. *British Journal of Radiology*, **58**, 1041–1045 (1985)
27. Lien, H.H., Brodahl, U., Telhaug, R. *et al.* Pulmonary changes at computed tomography in patients with testicular carcinoma treated with *cis*-platinum, vinblastine and bleomycin. *Acta Radiologica* (Diagn) (Stockholm), **26**, 507–510 (1985)
28. McCrea, E.S., Diaconis, J.N., Wade, J.C. and

Johnson, C.A. Bleomycin toxicity simulating metastatic nodules to the lungs. *Cancer*, **48**, 1096–1100 (1981)

29. Nachman, J.B., Baum, E.S., White, H. and Cruissi, F.G. Bleomycin-induced pulmonary fibrosis mimicking recurrent metastatic disease in a patient with testicular carcinoma: case report of the CT scan appearance. *Cancer*, **47**, 236–239 (1981)

30. Bellamy, E.A., Nicholas, D. and Husband, J.E. Quantitative assessment of lung damage due to bleomycin using computed tomography. *British Journal of Radiology*, **60**, 1205–1209 (1987)

31. Comis, R.L., Kuppinger, M.S., Ginsberg, S.J. *et al.* Role of single-breath carbon monoxide-diffusing capacity in monitoring the pulmonary effects of bleomycin in germ cell tumour patients. *Cancer Research*, **39**, 5076–5080 (1979)

32. Bell, M.R., Meredith, D.J. and Gill, P.G. Role of carbon monoxide diffusing capacity in the early detection of major bleomycin-induced pulmonary toxicity. *Australian and New Zealand Journal of Medicine*, **15**, 235–240 (1985)

33. Lewis, B.M. and Izbicki, R. Routine pulmonary function tests during bleomycin therapy: tests may be ineffective and potentially misleading. *Journal of the American Medical Association*, **243**, 347–351 (1980)

34. Luna, M.A., Bedrossian, C.W.M., Lichtiger, B. and Salem, P.A. Interstitial pneumonitis associated with bleomycin therapy. *American Journal of Clinical Pathology*, **58**, 501–508 (1972)

35. Rudders, R.A. and Hensley, G.T. Bleomycin pulmonary toxicity. *Chest*, **63**, 626–628 (1973)

36. Bedrossian, C.W.M. and Corey, B.J. Abnormal sputum cytopathology during chemotherapy with bleomycin. *Acta Cytologica*, **20**, 586 (1976)

37. Bedrossian, C.W.M., Luna, M.A., Mackay, B. and Lichtiger, B. Ultrastructure of pulmonary bleomycin toxicity. *Cancer*, **32**, 44–51 (1973)

38. Daskal, Y., Gyorkey, F., Gyorkey, P. and Busch, H. Ultrastructural study of pulmonary bleomycin toxicity. *Cancer Research*, **36**, 1267–1272 (1976)

39. Holoye, P.Y., Luna, M.A., Mackay, B. and Bedrossian, C.W.M. Bleomycin hypersensitivity pneumonitis. *Annals of Internal Medicine*, **88**, 47–49 (1978)

40. Yousem, S.A., Lifson, J.D. and Colby, T.V. Chemotherapy-induced eosinophilic pneumonia. Relation to bleomycin. *Chest*, **88**, 103–106 (1985)

41. Khansur, T., Little, D. and Tavassoli, M. Fulminant and fatal angioedema caused by bleomycin treatment. *Archives of Internal Medicine*, **144**, 2267 (1984)

42. Ginsberg, S.J. and Comis, S.L. The pulmonary toxicity of antineoplastic agents. *Seminars in Oncology*, **9**, 34–51 (1982)

43. Samuels, M.L., Johnson, D.E., Holoye, P.Y. and Lanzotti, V.J. Large-dose bleomycin therapy and pulmonary toxicity. *Journal of the American Medical Association*, **235**, 1117–1120 (1976)

44. Crook, S.T., Einhorn, L.H., Comis, R.C. *et al.* The effects of prior exposure to bleomycin on the incidence of pulmonary toxicities in a group of patients with disseminated testicular carcinomas. *Medical Paediatrics and Oncology*, **5**, 93–98 (1978)

45. Hass, C.D., Coltman, C.A., Gottlieb, J.A. *et al.* Phase II evaluation of bleomycin – a Southwest Oncology Group study. *Cancer*, **38**, 8–12 (1976)

46. Wilson, K.S., Worth, A., Richards, A.G. and Ford, H.S. Low-dose bleomycin lung. *Medical and Pediatric Oncology*, **10**, 283–288 (1982)

47. Iacovino, J.R., Leitner, J., Abbas, A.K. *et al.* Fatal pulmonary reaction from low doses of bleomycin. *Journal of the American Medical Association*, **235**, 1253–1255 (1976)

48. Quigley, M., Brada, M., Heron, C. and Horwich, A. Severe lung toxicity with a weekly low dose chemotherapy regime in patients with non-Hodgkin's lymphoma. *Hematological Oncology*, **6**, 319–324 (1988)

49. Collis, C.H., Down, J.D., Pearson, A.E. and Steel, G.G. Bleomycin and radiation-induced lung damage in mice. *British Journal of Radiology*, **56**, 21–26 (1983)

50. Sikic, B.I. Collins, J.M., Minaugh, E.G. and Gram, T.E. Improved therapeutic index of bleomycin when administered by continuous infusion in mice. *Cancer Treatment Reports*, **62**, 2011–2017 (1978)

51. Krakoff, I.H. Pharmacology and therapeutic efficacy of bleomycin administered by continuous infusion. In *Clinical Applications of Continuous Infusion Chemotherapy and Concomitant Radiation Therapy*, (eds C.J. Rosenthal and M. Rotman), Plenum Press, New York, pp. 13–17 (1986)

52. Miyamoto, T. Antitumour effects and pulmonary toxicity of bleomycin administered by continuous subcutaneous infusion in patients with advanced cervical cancer. *Gan To Kagaku Ryoho*, **14**, 1830–1835 (1987)

53. Svanberg, L.E. Bleomycin and lung cancer. In *Gann Monograph on Cancer Research No. 19. Fundamentals and Clinical Studies of Bleomycin* (eds S.K. Carter, T. Ichikawa, G. Mathe and H. Umezawa), University of Tokyo Press, Japan, pp. 193–220 (1976)

54. Yagoda, A. and Krakoff, I.H. Observations on the use of bleomycin in the treatment of malignant lymphoma in the USA. In *Gann Monograph on Cancer Research No. 19. Fundamental and Clinical Studies of Bleomycin* (eds S.K. Carter, T. Ichikawa, G. Mathe and R. Umezawa), University of Tokyo Press, Japan, pp. 255–268 (1976)

55. Einhorn, L., Krause, M., Hornback, N. and Purnas, B. Enhanced pulmonary toxicity with bleomycin and radiotherapy in oat cell lung cancer. *Cancer*, **37**, 2414–2416 (1976)

56. Chan, P.Y.M., Kagan, A.R., Byfield, J.E. *et al.* Pulmonary complications of combined chemotherapy and radiotherapy in lung cancer. In *Frontiers of Radiation Therapy and Oncology* (ed J.M. Vaeath), **13**, Karger, Basel, pp. 136–144 (1979)

57. Catane, R., Schwade, J.G., Turrisi, A.T. *et al.*

Pulmonary toxicity after radiation and bleomycin: a review. *International Journal of Radiation Oncology, Biology, Physics*, **5**, 1513–1518 (1979)

58. Von der Maase, H., Overgaard, J. and Vaeth, M. Effect of cancer chemotherapeutic drugs on radiation-induced lung damage in mice. *Radiotherapy and Oncology*, **5**, 245–247 (1986)

59. Comis, R.L. Bleomycin pulmonary toxicity. In *Bleomycin: Current Status and New Developments* (eds S.K. Carter, S.T. Crooke and H. Umezawa), Academic Press, New York, pp. 279–291 (1978)

60. Bauer, K.A., Skarin, A.T., Balikian, J.P. *et al.* Pulmonary complications associated with combination chemotherapy programs containing bleomycin. *American Journal of Medicine*, **74**, 557–563 (1983)

61. Greenberg, B.R., Hannigan, J., Gerretson, L. *et al.* Sequential combination of bleomycin and mitomycin in advanced cervical cancer – an American experience. A Northern California Oncology Group Study. *Cancer Treatment Reports*, **66**, 163–165 (1982)

62. Trope, C., Johnsson, J.E., Simonsen, E. *et al.* Bleomycin-mitomycin C in advanced carcinoma of the cervix: a third look. *Cancer*, **51**, 591–593 (1983)

63. Schurig, J.E., Farwell, A.R. and Bradner, W.T. The pulmonary toxicity of bleomycin in combination with other anticancer agents in mice (abstract). *First International Symposium on Organ-Directed Toxicities of Anticancer Drugs*, June 4–6 1987, The Vermont Regional Cancer Centre, Burlington, Vermont, p. 58 (1987)

64. Bennett, W.M., Pastore, L. and Houghton, D.C. Fatal pulmonary bleomycin toxicity in cisplatin-induced acute renal failure. *Cancer Treatment Reports*, **64**, 921–924 (1980)

65. Goldiner, P.L., Carlon, G.C., Cvitkovic, E. *et al.* Factors influencing postoperational morbidity and mortality in patients treated with bleomycin. *British Medical Journal*, **i**, 1664–1667 (1978)

66. Eigen, H. and Wyszomierski, D. Bleomycin lung injury in children. Pathophysiology and guidelines for management. *American Journal of Pediatric Hematology/Oncology*, **7**, 71–78 (1985)

67. Cersosimo, R.J., Matthews, S.J. and Hong, W.K. Bleomycin pneumonitis potentiated by oxygen administration. *Drug Intelligence and Clinical Pharmacy*, **19**, 921–923 (1985)

68. Gilson, A.J. and Sahn, S.A. Reactivation of bleomycin lung toxicity following oxygen administration. A second response to corticosteroids. *Chest*, **88**, 304–306 (1985)

69. Tryka, A.F., Godleski, J.J. and Brain, J.D. Differences in effects of immediate and delayed hyperoxia exposure on bleomycin-induced pulmonary injury. *Cancer Treatment Reports*, **68**, 759–764 (1984)

70. McCleod, B.F., Lawrence, H.J., Smith, D.W. *et al.* Fatal bleomycin toxicity from a low cumulative dose in a patient with renal insufficiency. *Cancer*, **60**, 2617–2620 (1987)

71. Scheulen, M.E. Pulmonary toxicity reduction (abstract). *Anticancer Drugs: Therapeutic Index Improvement by Toxicity Reduction*, April 6–7 1987, London Westminster Hospital, Imperial Cancer Research Fund and Deutsches Krebsforschungszentrum, abstract 2.4 (1987)

72. Chandler, D.B., Butler, T.W., Briggs, D.D. *et al.* Modulation of the development of bleomycin-induced fibrosis by deferoxamine. *Toxicology and Applied Pharmacology*, **92**, 358–367 (1988)

73. Jamieson, D.D., Kerr, D.R. and Unsworth, I. Interaction of *N*-acetylcysteine and bleomycin on hyperbaric oxygen-induced lung damage in mice. *Lung*, **165**, 239–247 (1987)

74. Merrin, C.E. Prevention of bleomycin-induced lung fibrosis with simultaneous administration of prednisone. *Proceedings of the American Society of Clinical Oncology*, **19**, 382 (1978)

75. Thrall, R.S., McCormick, J.R., Jack, R.M. *et al.* Bleomycin-induced pulmonary fibrosis in the rat: inhibition by indomethacin. *American Journal of Pathology*, **95**, 117–130 (1979)

76. Fleishman, R.W., Baker, R.J., Thompson, G.R. *et al.* Bleomycin induced interstitial pneumonia in dogs. *Thorax*, **26**, 675–682 (1971)

77. Adamson, I.Y.R. and Bowden, D.H. The pathogenesis of bleomycin induced pulmonary fibrosis in mice. *American Journal of Pathology*, **77**, 185–190 (1974)

78. Aso, Y., Yoneda, K. and Kikkawa, Y. Morphologic and biochemical study of pulmonary changes induced by bleomycin in mice. *Laboratory Investigation*, **35**, 558–567 (1976)

79. Jones, A.W. Bleomycin lung damage: the pathology and nature of the lesion. *British Journal of Diseases of the Chest*, **72**, 321–326 (1978)

80. Snider, G.L., Hayes, J.A. and Korthy, A.L. Chronic interstitial pulmonary fibrosis produced in hamsters by endotracheal bleomycin. *American Review of Respiratory Diseases*, **117**, 1099–1108 (1978)

81. Starcher, B.C., Kuhn, C. and Overton, J.E. Increased elastic and collagen content in the lungs of hamsters receiving intratracheal injection of bleomycin. *American Review of Respiratory Diseases*, **117**, 299–305 (1978)

82. McCullough, B., Collins, J.F., Johanson, W.G. and Grover, F.L. Bleomycin-induced diffuse interstitial pulmonary fibrosis in baboons. *Journal of Clinical Investigation*, **61**, 79–88 (1978)

83. Bedrossian, C.W.M., Greenberg, S.D., Yawn, D.H. and O'Neal, R.M. Experimentally induced bleomycin sulfate pulmonary toxicity. *Archives of Pathology and Laboratory Medicine*, **101**, 284–254 (1977)

84. Lazo, J.S. Pulmonary metabolism of bleomycin and its role in drug-induced lung injury (abstract). *First International Symposium on Organ-Directed Toxicities of Anticancer Drugs*, June 4–6, The Vermont Regional Cancer Centre, Burlington, Vermont, p. 39 (1987)

85. Cutroneo, K.R., Cockayne, D. and Sterling, K.M.

Jr. Biochemical and molecular bases of bleomycin-induced pulmonary fibrosis: glucocorticoid intervention (abstract). *First International Symposium on Organ-Directed Toxicities of Anticancer Drugs*, June 4–6, The Vermont Regional Cancer Centre, Burlington, Vermont, p. 41 (1987)

86. Watanabe, I., Yokobayashi, T., Nakajima, T. *et al.* Peplomycin-induced pneumonitis resulting in death. *Journal of Maxillofacial Surgery*, **12**, 114–117 (1984)

87. Takahashi, K., Nakatani, T., Takita, T. *et al.* Liblomycin, a new analog of bleomycin (abstract). *Anticancer Drugs: Therapeutic Index Improvement by Toxicity Reduction*, 6–7 April 1987, London, Westminster Hospital, Imperial Cancer Research Fund and Deutsches Krebsforschungszentrum, abstract 1.3 (1987)

88. Newman, R.A., Siddik, Z.H., Ayele, W. *et al.* Assessment of pulmonary and hematologic toxicities of liblomycin (LIB): a novel bleomycin (BLM) analog (abstract). *Proceedings of the Annual Meeting of the American Association of Cancer Research*, **29**, A1287 (1988)

89. Fielding, J.W.L., Stockley, R.A. and Brookes, V.S. Interstitial lung disease in a patient treated with 5-fluorouracil and mitomycin C. *British Medical Journal*, **ii**, 602 (1978)

90. Phillips, F.S., Schwarts, H.S. and Sternberg, S.S. Pharmacology of Mitomycin C. I. Toxicity and pathological effects. *Cancer Research*, **20**, 1354–1361 (1960)

91. Andrews, A.T., Bowman, H.S., Patel, S.B. and Anderson, W.M. Mitomycin and interstitial pneumonitis. *Annals of Internal Medicine*, **90**, 127 (1979)

92. Buzdar, A.U., Legha, S.S., Luna, M.A. *et al.* Pulmonary toxicity of mitomycin. *Cancer*, **45**, 236–244 (1980)

93. Orwoll, E.S., Kiessling, P.J. and Patterson, J.R. Interstitial pneumonia from mitomycin. *Annals of Internal Medicine*, **89**, 352–355 (1978)

94. Ozols, R.F., Hogan, W.M., Ostchega, Y. and Young, R.C. MVP (mitomycin, vinblastine, and progesterone): a second-line regimen in ovarian cancer with a high incidence of pulmonary toxicity. *Cancer Treatment Reports*, **67**, 721–722 (1983)

95. Rao, S.X., Ramaswamy, G., Levin, M. and McCravey, J.W. Fatal acute respiratory failure after vinblastine-mitomycin therapy in lung carcinoma. *Archives of Internal Medicine*, **145**, 1905–1907 (1985)

96. Spain, R., Cullen, S., Berthrong, M. *et al.* Dexamethasone prophylaxis of mitomycin-C (M), *cis*-platinum (P), and continuous vinblastine (V) infusion (M-PV) induced pulmonary toxicity in stage III non-small cell lung cancer (NSCLC) (abstract). *Oncology: Surviving the 80s. Advances in Cancer Control III*, 13–17 March 1985, Association of Community Cancer Centres/Association of American Cancer Institutes, Washington DC, p. 46 (1985)

97. Letendre, F., Latreille, J., Neemeh, J. *et al.* Combination chemotherapy with continuous infusion of 5FU and bolus IV injections of mitomycin-C (MI) and methotrexate (MTX) in patients (PTS) with advanced colorectal carcinoma (abstract). *Proceedings of the Annual Meeting of the American Society of Clinical Oncology*, **6**, A287 (1987)

98. Gunstream, S.R., Seidenfeld, J.J., Sobonya, R.E. and McMahon, L.J. Mitomycin-associated lung disease. *Cancer Treatment Reports*, **67**, 301–304 (1983)

99. Friedman, S. Pulmonary toxicity of mitomycin C (MMC) – an underestimated toxicity? (abstract). *Proceedings of the Annual Meeting of the American Society of Clinical Oncology*, **2**, C-73 (1983)

100. Laufman, L., Courter, S. and Pritchard, J. Fatal mitomycin C (MMC) syndrome heralded by pulmonary symptoms (abstract). *Proceedings of the Annual Meeting of the American Society of Clinical Oncology*, **2**, C-768 (1983)

101. Spain, R., Jost, J. and Kircher, T. Reduction of lung toxicity induced by neoadjuvant mitomycin, cisplatin, and vinblastine infusion (M-PV) for limited stage III non-small lung cancer (NSCLC) (abstract). *Fifth International Conference on the Adjuvant Therapy of Cancer*, 11–14 March 1987, Tucson, Arizona, p. 39 (1987)

102. Von Roemeling, R., Sothern, R.B., Langevin, T.R. *et al.* Mitomycin C toxicity depends upon the time of day of injection (abstract). *Proceedings of the Annual Meeting of the American Association of Cancer Research*, **29**, A2028 (1988)

103. Seltzer, S.E., Griffin, T., O'Orsi, C. *et al.* Pulmonary reaction associated with neocarcinostatin therapy. *Cancer Treatment Reports*, **62**, 1271–1272 (1978)

104. Calvo, D.B., Legha, S.S., McKelvey, E.M. and Bodey, G.P. Zinostatin-related pulmonary toxicity. *Cancer Treatment Reports*, **65**, 165–167 (1981)

105. Rosenow, E.C. The spectrum of drug induced pulmonary disease. *Annals of Internal Medicine*, **77**, 977–991 (1972)

106. Kirschner, R.H. and Esterly, J.R. Pulmonary lesions associated with busulfan therapy of chronic myelogenous leukaemia. *Cancer*, **27**, 1074–1080 (1971)

107. Heard, B.E. and Cooke, R.A. Busulphan lung. *Thorax*, **23**, 187–193 (1968)

108. Littler, W.A. and Ogilvie, C. Lung function in patients receiving busulphan. *British Medical Journal*, **iv**, 530–532 (1970)

109. Gyger, M., Legresley, L.P., Boulianne, P. *et al.* Reterogeneité clinique de la pneumopathie au myeleran. *Union Medicale du Canada*, **106**, 1522–1528 (1977)

110. Podoll, L.N. and Winkler, S.S. Busulfan lung: report of two cases and review of the literature. *American Journal of Roentgenology*, **120**, 151–156 (1974)

111. Harrold, B.P. Syndrome resembling Addison's disease following prolonged treatment with busulphan. *British Medical Journal*, **i**, 463–464 (1966)

112. Smalley, R.V. and Wall, R.L. Two cases of busulfan toxicity. *Annals of Internal Medicine*, **64**, 154–164 (1966)

113. Schallier, D., Impens, N., Warson, F. *et al.* Additive pulmonary toxicity with melphalan and busulfan therapy. *Chest*, **84**, 492–493 (1983)

114. Soble, A.R. and Perry, H. Fatal radiation pneumonia following sub-clinical busulfan injury. *American Journal of Roentgenology*, **128**, 15–18 (1977)

115. Dalri, P., Piscioli, F. and Detassis, C. Busulfan lung: cytologic diagnosis. *Haematologica (Pavia)*, **65**, 469–474 (1980)

116. Littler, W.A., Kay, J.M., Hasleton, P.S. and Heath, D. Busulphan lung. *Thorax*, **24**, 639–655 (1969)

117. Patel, A.R., Shah, P.C., Rhee, H.L. *et al.* Cyclophosphamide therapy and interstitial pulmonary fibrosis. *Cancer*, **38**, 1542–1549 (1976)

118. Andre, R., Rochant, H., Dreyfus, B. *et al.* Fibrose interstitielle diffuse du poumon au cours d'une maladie de Hodgkin traitée par des doses elevés d'endoxan. *Bulletin de la Société de Médecine Paris*, **118**, 1133–1141 (1967)

119. Rodin, A.E., Haggard, M.E. and Travis, L.B. Lung changes and chemotherapeutic agents in childhood. *American Journal of Diseases of Children*, **120**, 337–340 (1970)

120. Dohner, V.A., Ward, H.P. and Standord, R.E. Alveolitis during procarbazine, vincristine and cyclophosphamide therapy. *Chest*, **62**, 636–639 (1972)

121. Topilow, A.A., Rothernberg, S.P. and Cottrell, T.S. Interstitial pneumonia after prolonged treatment with cyclophosphamide. *American Review of Respiratory Diseases*, **108**, 114–117 (1973)

122. Tucker, A.S., Newman, A.J. and Alvorado, C. Pulmonary pleural and thoracic changes complicating chemotherapy. *Radiology*, **125**, 805–809 (1977)

123. Mark, G.J., Lehimgar-Zadeh, A. and Ragsdale, B.D. Cyclophosphamide pneumonitis. *Thorax*, **33**, 89–93 (1978)

124. Spector, J., Zimbler, H. and Ross, J.S. Early onset cyclophosphamide-induced pneumonitis. *Journal of the American Medical Association*, **242**, 2852–2854 (1979)

125. Burke, D.A., Stoddart, J.C., Ward, M.K. and Simpson, C.G. Fatal pulmonary fibrosis occurring during treatment with cyclophosphamide. *British Medical Journal*, **285**, 696 (1982)

126. Buckner, C.D., Rudolph, R.H., Fefer, A. *et al.* High-dose cyclophosphamide therapy for malignant disease. *Cancer*, **29**, 357–365 (1972)

127. Skarin, A., Lokich, J., Goodman, R. *et al.* Combined intensive chemotherapy and radiotherapy in oat cell carcinoma of the lung. *Proceedings of the American Society of Clinical Oncology*, **16**, 264 (1975)

128. Littman, P., Davis, L.W., Nash, J. *et al.* The hazard of acute radiation pneumonitis in children receiving mediastinal irradiation. *Cancer*, **33**, 1520–1525 (1974)

129. Rosen, G., Tefft, M., Martinez, A. *et al.* Combination chemotherapy and radiation therapy in the treatment of metastatic osteogenic sarcoma. *Cancer*, **35**, 622–630 (1975)

130. Cassady, J.R., Richter, M.P., Piro, A.J. and Jaffe, N. Radiation–Adriamycin interaction: preliminary clinical observations. *Cancer*, **36**, 946–949 (1975)

131. Trask, C.W.L., Joannides, T., Harper, P.G. *et al.* Radiation-induced lung fibrosis after treatment of small cell carcinoma of the lung with very high-dose cyclophosphamide. *Cancer*, **55**, 57–60 (1985)

132. O'Connell, T.X. and Berenbaum, M.C. Cardiac and pulmonary effects of high doses of cyclophosphamide and isophosphamide. *Cancer Research*, **34**, 1586–1591 (1974)

133. Berenbaum, M.C. The production of pulmonary oedema in mice by cyclophosphamide and iodide. *Agents and Actions*, **4**, 7–14 (1974)

134. Gould, V.E. and Miller, J. Sclerosing alveolitis induced by cyclophosphamide. *American Journal of Pathology*, **81**, 513–530 (1975)

135. Collis, C.H., Wilson, C.M. and Jones, J.M. Cyclophosphamide-induced lung damage in mice: protection by a small preliminary dose. *British Journal of Cancer*, **41**, 901–907 (1980)

136. Allalunis-Turner, M.J. and Siemann, D.W. Modification of cyclophosphamide-induced pulmonary toxicity in normal mice. *National Cancer Institute Monographs*, **6**, 51–53 (1988)

137. Collis, C.H. and Steel, G.G. Lung damage in mice from cyclophosphamide and thoracic irradiation: the effect of timing. *International Journal of Radiation Oncology, Biology, Physics*, **9**, 685–689 (1983)

138. Lockhart, S.P., Down, J.D. and Steel, G.G. The effects of low dose-rate and cyclophosphamide on the radiation tolerance of the mouse lung. *International Journal of Radiation Oncology, Biology, Physics*, **12**, 1437–1440 (1986)

139. Varekamp, A.E., de-Vries, A.J., Zurcher, C. and Hagenbeek, A. Lung damage following bone marrow transplantation: II. The contribution of cyclophosphamide. *International Journal of Radiation Oncology, Biology, Physics*, **13**, 1515–1521 (1987)

140. Rubio, F.A. Possible pulmonary effects of alkylating agents. *New England Journal of Medicine*, **287**, 1150–1151 (1972)

141. Jacobs, S. The Hamman-Rich syndrome following treatment of lymphoma with chlorambucil. *Journal of the Louisiana State Medical Society*, **127**, 311–315 (1975)

142. Rose, M.S. Busulphan toxicity syndrome caused by chlorambucil. *British Medical Journal*, **ii**, 123 (1975)

143. Crofton, J. and Douglas, A. (eds). *Respiratory Disease*, 2nd edn, Blackwell Scientific Publications, Oxford, p. 613 (1976)

144. Refvem, O. Fatal intra-alveolar and interstitial lung fibrosis in chlorambucil-treated chronic lymphocytic leukaemia. *Mount Sinai Journal of Medicine*, **44**, 847–851 (1977)

145. Cole, S.R., Myers, T.J. and Klatsky, A.U. Pulmonary disease with chlorambucil therapy. *Cancer*, **41**, 455–459 (1978)

146. Lane, S.D., Besa, E.C., Justh, G. and Joseph, R.R. Fatal interstitial lung disease following high dose

chlorambucil therapy. *Proceedings of the American Association for Cancer Research*, **20**, 313 (1979)

147. Godard, P.H., Marty, J.P. and Michel, F.B. Interstitial pneumonia and chlorambucil. *Chest*, **76**, 471–473 (1979)

148. Grand, M., Spector, J.I., Zimbler, H. and Ross, J.S. Pulse dose chlorambucil-induced interstitial pneumonitis (abstract). *Proceedings of the Annual Meeting of the Society of Clinical Oncology*, **2**, C-85 (1983)

149. Hagmann, S.G. Alveolitis and lung fibrosis following therapy with chlorambucil. *Praxis und Klinik der Pneumologie*, **38**, 108–111 (1984)

150. Carr, M.E. Jr. Chlorambucil induced pulmonary fibrosis: report of a case and review. *Virginia Medical*, **113**, 677–680 (1986)

151. Codling, B.W. and Chakera, T.M.H. Pulmonary fibrosis following therapy with melphalan for multiple myeloma. *Journal of Clinical Pathology*, **25**, 668–673 (1972)

152. Taetle, R., Dickman, P.S. and Feldman, P.S. Pulmonary histopathologic changes associated with melphalan therapy. *Cancer*, **42**, 1239–1245 (1978)

153. Westerfield, B.T., Michalski, J.P., McCombs, C. and Light, R.W. Reversible melphalan-induced lung damage. *American Journal of Medicine*, **68**, 767–771 (1980)

154. Goucher, G., Rowland, V. and Hawkins, J. Melphalan-induced pulmonary interstitial fibrosis. *Chest*, **77**, 805–806 (1980)

155. Major, P.P., Laurin, S. and Bettez, P. Pulmonary fibrosis following therapy with melphalan: report of two cases. *Canadian Medical Association Journal*, **123**, 197–198, 201–202 (1980)

156. Giles, F.J., Singer, C.R.J., Goldstone, A.H. and Tobias, J.S. Lung toxicity of melphalan and steroid combination therapy in multiple myeloma (abstract). *Third Meeting of the British Oncological Association*, 3–5 July 1988, pp. 60–61 (1988)

157. Holoye, P.Y., Jenkins, D.E. and Greenberg, S.D. Pulmonary toxicity in long-term administration of BCNU. *Cancer Treatment Reports*, **60**, 1691–1694 (1976)

158. Durant, J.R., Norgard, M.J., Murad, T.M. *et al.* Pulmonary toxicity associated with bischloroethylnitrosourea (BCNU). *Annals of Internal Medicine*, **90**, 191–194 (1979)

159. Aronin, P.A., Mahaley, M.S., Rudnick, S.A. *et al.* Prediction of BCNU pulmonary toxicity in patients with malignant gliomas. An assessment of risk factors. *New England Journal of Medicine*, **303**, 183–188 (1980)

160. Selker, R.G., Jacobs, S.A., Moore, P.B. *et al.* 1,3-Bis(2-chloroethyl)-1-nitrosourea (BCNU)-induced pulmonary fibrosis. *Neurosurgery*, **7**, 560–565 (1980)

161. Patten, G.A., Billi, J.E. and Rotman, H.H. Rapidly progressive fatal pulmonary fibrosis induced by carmustine. *Journal of the American Medical Association*, **244**, 687–688 (1980)

162. Mitsudo, S.M., Greewald, E.S., Banerji, B. and Koss, L.E. BCNU (1,3-bis-(2-chloroethyl)-1-nitrosourea) lung. Drug-induced pulmonary changes. *Cancer*, **54**, 751–755 (1984)

163. Lieberman, A., Ruoff, M., Estey, E. *et al.* Irreversible pulmonary toxicity after single course of BCNU. *American Journal of Medical Sciences*, **279**, 53–56 (1980)

164. Litman, J.P., Dail, D.H., Spitzer, G. *et al.* Early pulmonary toxicity after administration of high-dose BCNU. *Cancer Treatment Reports*, **65**, 39–44 (1981)

165. Schreml, W., Bargon, G., Anger, B. *et al.* Progrediente lungfibrose unter kombinations therapie mit BCNU. *Blut*, **36**, 353–356 (1978)

166. Carter, S. and Newman, J.W. Nitrosoureas 1,3-bis(2-chloroethyl)-1-nitrosourea (BCNU) and 1-(2-chloroethyl)-3-cyclohexyl-1-nitrosourea (CCNU) – clinical brochure. *Cancer Chemotherapy Reports*, **1**, 115–151 (1968)

167. Kehrer, J.P. and Klein-Szanto, A.J. Enhanced acute lung damage in mice following administration of 1,3-bis(2-chloroethyl)-1-nitrosourea. *Cancer Research*, **45**, 5707–5713 (1985)

168. Dent, R.G. Fatal pulmonary toxic effects of lomustine. *Thorax*, **37**, 627–629 (1982)

169. Cordonnier, C., Vernant, J.P., Mital, P. *et al.* Pulmonary fibrosis subsequent to high doses of CCNU for chronic myeloid leukemia. *Cancer*, **51**, 1814–1818 (1983)

170. Lee, W., Moore, R.P. and Wampler, G.L. Interstitial pulmonary fibrosis as a complication of prolonged methyl-CCNU therapy. *Cancer Treatment Reports*, **62**, 1355–1258 (1978)

171. Ahlgren, J.D., Smith, F.P., Kerwin, D.M. *et al.* Pulmonary disease as a complication of chlorozotocin chemotherapy. *Cancer Treatment Reports*, **65**, 223–229 (1981)

172. Clarysse, A.M., Cathey, W.J., Cartwright, G.E. and Wintrobe, M.W. Pulmonary disease complicating intermittent therapy with methotrexate. *Journal of the American Medical Association*, **209**, 1861–1864 (1969)

173. Sostman, H.D., Matthay, R.A., Putman, C.E. and Walker Smith, G.J. Methotrexate-induced pnuemonitis. *Medicine*, **55**, 371–388 (1976)

174. Everts, C.S., Westscott, J.L. and Bragg, D.G. Methotrexate therapy and pulmonary disease. *Radiology*, **107**, 539–543 (1973)

175. Rawbone, R.G., Shaw, M.T., Jackson, J.G. and Bagshawe, K.D. Complications of methotrexate-maintained remission in lymphoblastic leukaemia. *British Medical Journal*, **iv**, 467–468 (1971)

176. Kaplan, R.L. and Waite, D.H. Progressive interstitial lung disease from prolonged methotrexate therapy. *Archives of Dermatology*, **114**, 1800–1802 (1978)

177. Bedrossian, C.W.M., Miller, W.C. and Luna, M.A. Methotrexate-induced diffuse interstitial pulmonary fibrosis. *Southern Medical Journal*, **72**, 313–318 (1979)

178. Robertson, J.H. Pneumonia and methotrexate. *British Medical Journal*, **ii**, 156 (1970)

179. Nesbit, M., Krivit, W., Heyn, R. and Sharp, H. Acute and chronic effects of methotrexate on hepatic, pulmonary and skeletal systems. *Cancer*, **37**, 1048–1054 (1976)

180. Gutin, P.H., Green, M.R., Bleyer, W.A. *et al.* Methotrexate pneumonitis induced by intrathecal methotrexate therapy. *Cancer*, **38**, 1529–1534 (1976)

181. Lascari, A.D., Strano, A.J., Johnson, W.W. and Collins, G.P. Methotrexate-induced sudden fatal pulmonary reaction. *Cancer*, **40**, 1393–1397 (1977)

182. Stutz, F.H., Tormey, D.C. and Blom, J. Nonbacterial pneumonitis with multidrug anti-neoplastic therapy in breast carcinoma. *Canadian Medical Association Journal*, **108**, 710–714 (1973)

183. Bhat, K.S.S., Anderson, K.R. and Stewart, R.D.H. Lung disease associated with methotrexate therapy. *Australian and New Zealand Journal of Medicine*, **4**, 277–280 (1974)

184. Manni, J.J. and Van den Broek, P. Pulmonary complications of methotrexate therapy. *Clinical Otolaryngology*, **2**, 131–137 (1977)

185. Pasquinucci, G., Ferrara, P. and Castellari, R. Daunorubicin treatment of methotrexate pneumonia. *Journal of the American Medical Association*, **216**, 2017 (1971)

186. Wall, M.A., Wohl, M.E.B., Jaffe, N. and Strieder, D.J. Lung function in adolescents receiving high-dose methotrexate. *Pediatrics*, **63**, 741–746 (1979)

187. Filip, D.J., Logue, G.L., Harle, T.S. and Farrar, W.H. Pulmonary and hepatic complications of methotrexate therapy of psoriasis. *Journal of the American Medical Association*, **216**, 881–882 (1971)

188. Anderson, L.L., Collins, G.J., Ojima, Y. and Sullivan, R.D. A study of the distribution of methotrexate in human tissues and tumours. *Cancer Research*, **30**, 1344–1348 (1970)

189. Haupt, H.M., Hutchins, G.M. and Moore, G.W. Ara-C lung: non-cardiogenic pulmonary oedema complicating cytosine arabinoside therapy of leukemia. *American Journal of Medicine*, **70**, 256–261 (1981)

190. Willemze, R., Zwaan, F.E., Colpin, G. and Keuning, J.J. High dose cytosine arabinoside in the management of refractory acute leukaemia. *Scandinavian Journal of Haematology*, **29**, 141–146 (1982)

191. Tham, R.T., Peters, W.G., de-Bruine, F.T. and Willemze, R. Pulmonary complications of cytosine-arabinoside therapy: radiographic findings. *American Journal of Roentgenology*, **149**, 23–27 (1987)

192. Lampert, F. Lungenveranderugen bel der akuten lymphoblastischen leukamie. *Radiologe*, **8**, 308–310 (1968)

193. Okita, H., Ito, K., Taketomi, Y. *et al.* Four patients with leukaemia who showed especially atypical type of interstitial pneumonia, probably caused following the administration of anti-leukaemic drugs. *Japanese Journal of Clinical Haematology*, **15**, 764–773 (1974)

194. Rubin, G., Baume, P. and Vandenberg, R. Azathioprine and acute restrictive lung disease. *Australian and New Zealand Journal of Medicine*, **3**, 272–274 (1972)

195. Weisenberger, D.D. Interstitial pneumonitis associated with azathioprine therapy. *American Journal of Clinical Pathology*, **62**, 181–185 (1978)

196. Krowka, M.J., Breuer, R.I. and Kehoe, T.J. Azathioprine-associated pulmonary dysfunction. *Chest*, **83**, 696–698 (1983)

197. Jones, S.E., Moore, M., Blank, N. and Castellino, R.A. Hypersensitivity to procarbazine manifested by fever and pleuropulmonary reaction. *Cancer*, **29**, 498–500 (1972)

198. Ecker, M.D., Jay, B. and Keohane, M.F. Procarbazine lung. *American Journal of Roentgenology*, **131**, 527–528 (1978)

199. Lokich, J.J. and Moloney, W.C. Allergic reaction to procarbazine. *Clinical Pharmacology and Therapeutics*, **13**, 573–574 (1972)

200. Farney, R.J., Morris, A.H., Armstrong, J.D. and Hammer, S. Diffuse pulmonary disease after therapy with nitrogen mustard, vincristine, procarbazine and prednisone. *American Review of Respiratory Diseases*, **115**, 135–145 (1977)

201. Lewis, L.D. Procarbazine associated alveolitis. *Thorax*, **39**, 206–207 (1984)

202. Cersosimo, R.J., Licciardello, J.T., Matthews, S.J. *et al.* Acute pneumonitis associated with MOPP chemotherapy of Hodgkin's disease. *Drug Intelligence and Clinical Pharmacy*, **18**, 609–611 (1984)

203. Israel, R.H. and Olson, J.P. Pulmonary oedema associated with intravenous vinblastine. *Journal of the American Medical Association*, **240**, 1585 (1978)

204. Konits, P.H., Aisner, J., Sutherland, J.C. and Wiernik, P.H. Possible pulmonary toxicity secondary to vinblastine. *Cancer*, **50**, 2771–2774 (1982)

205. Kris, M.G., Pablo, D., Gralla, R.J. *et al.* Dyspnea following vinblastine or vindesine administration in patients receiving mitomycin plus vinca alkaloid combination therapy. *Cancer Treatment Reports*, **68**, 1029–1031 (1984)

206. Luedke, D., McLaughlin, T.T., Daughaday, C. *et al.* Mitomycin C and vindesine associated pulmonary toxicity with variable clinical expression. *Cancer*, **55**, 542–545 (1985)

207. Hankins, D.G., Sanders, S., MacDonald, F.M. and Drage, C.W. Pulmonary toxicity recurring after a six-week course of busulfan therapy and after subsequent therapy with uracil mustard. *Chest*, **73**, 415–416 (1978)

208. Commers, J.R. and Foley, J.F. Pulmonary hyaline membrane disease occurring in the course of VM-26 therapy. *Cancer Treatment Reports*, **63**, 2093–2095 (1979)

209. Zabbe, C., Bellet-Barthas, M., Clavier, J. *et al.* Preoperative treatment of bronchial epidermoid cancers: study of the pulmonary toxicity of bleomycin. *Colloquium INSERM*, **137**, 519–527 (1986)

210. Schein, P.S., DeVita, V.T., Hubbard, S. *et al.*

Bleomycin, Adriamycin, cyclophosphamide, vincristine and prednisone (BACOP) combination chemotherapy in the treatment of advanced diffuse histocytic lymphoma. *Annals of Internal Medicine*, **85**, 417–422 (1976)

211. Zimmerman, M.S., Ruckdeschel, J.C. and Hussain, M. Chemotherapy-induced interstitial pneumonitis during treatment of small cell anaplastic lung cancer. *Journal of Clinical Oncology*, **2**, 396–405 (1984)

212. Nygaard, K., Smith-Erichsen, N., Hatlevoll, R. and Refsum, S.B. Pulmonary complications after bleomycin, irradiation and surgery for oesophageal cancer. *Cancer*, **41**, 17–22 (1978)

213. Lamoureux, K.B. Increased clinically symptomatic pulmonary radiation reactions with adjuvant chemotherapy. *Cancer Chemotherapy Reports*, **58**, 705–708 (1974)

214. Kun, L.E., DeVita, V.T., Young, R.C. and Johnson, R.E. Treatment of Hodgkin's disease using intensive chemotherapy followed by irradiation. *International Journal of Radiation Oncology, Biology, Physics*, **1**, 619–626 (1976)

215. Margolis, L.W. and Phillips, T.L. Whole-lung irradiation for metastatic tumour. *Radiology*, **93**, 1173–1179 (1969)

216. Wara, W.M., Phillips, T.L., Margolis, L.W. and Smith, V. Radiation pneumonitis: a new approach to the derivation of time-dose factors. *Cancer*, **32**, 547–552 (1973)

217. Willis, N.R., Watring, W.W., Hanskins, L.A. *et al.* Clinical observations on the enhancement of radiation response by Adriamycin in patients with advanced gynaecologic tumours. Presented at the Western Association of Gynaecologic Oncologists Conference, LaJolla, California, May 29–31 (1975)

218. McInerney, D.P. and Bullimore, J. Reactivation of radiation pneumonitis by Adriamycin. *British Journal of Radiology*, **50**, 224–227 (1977)

219. Hill, A.B. and Tattersall, S.F. Recall of radiation pneumonitis after intrapleural administration of doxorubicin. *Medical Journal of Australia*, **1**, 39–40 (1983)

220. Golding, R.P. and van Zanten, T.E.G. Lung destruction after *cis*-platinum radiosensitisation. *British Journal of Radiology*, **56**, 281–282 (1983)

221. Glaholm, J., Repetto, L., Yarnold, J.R. *et al.* Carboplatin (JM8), etoposide (VP16) and thoracic irradiation for small cell lung cancer (SCLC): an evaluation of lung toxicity. *Radiotherapy and Oncology*, **12**, 31–37 (1988)

222. Peckham, M.J. and Collis, C.H. Clinical objectives and normal tissue responses in combined chemotherapy and radiotherapy. *Bulletin of Cancer (Paris)*, **68**(Part 2), 132–141 (1981)

223. Tanabe, M., Godat, D. and Kallman, R.F. Effects of fractionated schedules of irradiation combined with *cis*-diamminedichloroplatinum II on SCC VII/ST tumour and normal tissues of the C3H/KM mouse. *International Journal of Radiation Oncology, Biology, Physics*, **13**, 1523–1532 (1987)

224. Joselson, R. and Warnock, M. Pulmonary venoocclusive disease after chemotherapy. *Human Pathology*, **14**, 88–91 (1983)

# 18

# Radiation morbidity to the gastrointestinal tract and liver

S.R. Smalley and R.G. Evans

Only 2 years elapsed after the discovery of X-rays by William Roentgen before the first description of radiation enteritis and its prevention. Walsh reported in 1897 that diarrhea, abdominal pain, and cramping could result from X-ray exposure and be prevented by shielding [1]. Almost a century later our understanding of the pathophysiology of this entity and its prevention and treatment are much more sophisticated. Nevertheless, radiation bowel damage remains incompletely understood, continues to afflict patients, and bowel tolerance still limits radiation to sometimes suboptimal doses. Therefore, appreciation of our current knowledge of the causes, prevention and treatment of radiation bowel damage is essential to optimize care of patients requiring abdominopelvic radiotherapy.

Two caveats should be noted from the start. Firstly, under-reporting of cancer treatment toxicity has been well documented [2]. Since Rubin and Casarett's landmark work on radiation toxicity in 1966 [3], a voluminous literature has appeared in which radiotherapy (XRT) has been administered to the abdominopelvic structures. Collation of these reports allows a reasonably clear picture of XRT toxicity, but our interpretation must be tempered by an appreciation of the potential bias of under-reporting. Secondly, doses in the abdominopelvic cavity uniformly ignore the potential impact of gas in the path of the beam. The impact of even relatively small quantities of gas may produce substantially higher doses of absorbed radiation in malignant tissue. A 2.5 cm thickness of gas has been calculated to produce a 10% elevation of dose in the pelvis [4,5]. Two groups have measured pelvic doses 10% or more than expected [6,7]. Obviously this is a major potential source of error in our attempts to construct relationships between dose and toxicity. Though it seems likely that the commonplace use of

energies of 6 MeV or greater will minimize the potential impact of bowel gas, few data exist on this point. Caution is again appropriate in light of the interpatient differences in bowel gas, and the variety of treatment energies used in the literature.

## Radiation gastritis, enteritis and proctocolitis

### Pathophysiological changes antecedent to radiation

Malignancy anywhere may be associated with secondary abnormalities in the small intestinal mucosa. These abnormalities are independent of, and antecedent to therapy [8–11]. Histologically this condition exhibits a decrease in total mucosal thickness. The mucosa usually has a normal villous weight/ mucosal thickness ratio, is sometimes flattened or has increased convolutions or ridge formations [8,11]. DNA epithelial cell loss rate is decreased [11]. If there is equilibrium between epithelial cell production in the crypts and epithelial cell loss in the villi, then epithelial cell turnover is reduced. Therefore, the architectural changes may be attributed to true mucosal hypoplasia. This hypoplastic mucosa is physiologically abnormal as well [8,11–13]. Patients manifesting this condition usually have substantial weight loss [8,11] and a variety of mucosal functional abnormalities [8,11–13].

Interestingly, these abnormalities are likely to be the result of the nutritional deprivation and cachexia and not vice versa. Barry [11] has demonstrated identical mucosal morphology, epithelial DNA cell loss, and malabsorption in patients with profound weight loss without malignancy. Hypoplastic mucosa has also been demonstrated in starvation, voluntary extreme weight loss, total intravenous alimentation [14] and anorexia nervosa. Loops of bowel which have been bypassed and therefore receive minimal luminal nutrition exhibit hypoplastic changes, while the remainder of the bowel demonstrates hyperplasia [15]. The enteral availability of nutrients thus assumes great importance because the bowel mucosa, in large part, has been shown to depend upon luminal nutrients for its own nutritional supply [14]. Amino acids, in particular, play a critical trophic role on intestinal mucosa [14].

Diversion colitis, initially described in 1981, is another example of a non-radiation induced problem which can predate radiation and mimic XRT toxicity. Diversion colitis is an inflammatory process occurring in colorectal segments which have been deafferented from the fecal stream by surgical diversion. The incidence may be nearly 100% when examined prospectively [16] though it is usually asymptomatic [16,17]. It may produce bloody fluid, cramping pain with onset between 3 months and 3 years after diversion. Endoscopy shows erythema, friability, edema, aphthous ulcers, exudates and bleeding. The use of topical steroids is usually fruitless. The colitis may progress to stricture formation unless proper therapy is initiated [16,17]. Though reanastomosis is almost uniformly curative, diversion colitis is caused by depletion of short-chain fatty acids (SCFA) which are the major solutes of the aqueous phase of colonic contents and the major energy source of the human colonic epithelium. This SCFA dependence, which is greater in the distal than proximal colon, is important since the major colonic SCFA are produced by anaerobic bacterial metabolism, are not produced by mammalian cells, and are present in only negligible concentration in plasma. Thus while instillation of SCFAs intraluminally will correct the condition [16], diversion colitis could easily be confused with radiation toxicity in patients who have received XRT to deafferented segments of colorectum.

In summary, though a true 'malignant enteropathy' probably does not exist (or if it does, is exceedingly rare), the intestinal mucosa is frequently abnormal prior to XRT. Though this enteropathy results from luminal nutritional deficiency, it nevertheless may produce absorption problems on its own, and exacerbate nutritional problems already present. These principles are an important prerequisite to an understanding of the role of elemental diets in the prevention and treatment of XRT radiation enteropathy.

## Acute pathological changes from radiation

The acute and chronic pathological changes of the gut have been well described in both animals and humans [3,18–36]. Acute morphological changes in the mucosa are, in large part, due to interruption of the homeostatic cell renewal system. The pattern of human epithelial renewal in the intestine and colorectum is similar qualitatively to, though quantitatively 2–3 times longer than, laboratory animals [37,38]. The normal migration time of tritiated labeled cells from the base of the crypts to the surface is approximately 5–6 days. Though there is some recruitment of non-cycling cells into proliferation and possibly some reduction in generation time of cycling cells [35], these responses are inadequate to compensate for the cell loss induced by most clinically utilized radiation schemes. Morphological changes are therefore seen relatively quickly after initiation of XRT since cell turnover in this actively proliferating system is so rapid.

Mucosal morphological changes have been evaluated by sequential biopsies in three studies [22,23,34]. Trier and Browning [34] studied nine patients treated with 1 MeV X-rays, 5–6 days per week, at fractional skin doses of 150–300 cGy, to total doses of 2000–3000 cGy. Sequentially, a total of 114 peroral biopsies were taken both within and outside the irradiated area. The villous architecture was normal at low magnification during the first week, but exhibited significant changes at higher power. Within 12 h, the number of mitotic figures was greatly reduced in the crypts. This mitotic reduction progressed during the first week and persisted at low levels until discontinuation of treatment. Mitoses during therapy showed morphological abnormalities such as chromosomal bridging and clumping. Small, spherical inclusion bodies which stained intensely by the Feulgen technique, consistent with fragments of disintegrating epithelial cells, were seen during the first week and were uncommon thereafter. The second week characteristically showed villous shortening which progressed. At the completion of therapy the villi were markedly shortened and mucosal thickness considerably reduced. Cellular elements within the lamina propria were more marked by the second week and also increased during therapy. Infiltration by plasma cells, eosinophils, histiocytes and homogeneous eosinophilic material consistent with edema fluid was characteristic. Lymphocytes were uncommon. The cellular elements progressed to exhibit accumulations of polymorphonuclear leukocytes, in some cases sufficiently severe to produce crypt abscess formation with microabscesses composed of polymorphonuclear leukocytes and cellular debris. The epithelium exhibited transformation of the pretreatment columnar histology to a cuboidal or even a squamous appearance. Megalocytosis, with large hyperchromatic nuclei, were common. Paneth cells were diminished quantitatively but normal in appearance. Goblet cells were normal quantitatively, but also exhibited decreased height and increased width during therapy. Electron microscopy showed severe changes which were most marked in crypt cells and spotty and less consistent in other cell types (Paneth, enterochromaffin and goblet cells). Microvilli became short and irregular. There was dilatation of mitochondria and endoplasmic reticulum and reduction of undifferentiated secretory granules. Nuclei displayed a scalloped appearance at the periphery and huge nucleoli. The number of mitoses per crypt decreased rapidly to 50–75% of pretreatment levels and preceded reduction of epithelial thickness. Mitoses per crypt increased to normal within a few days and preceded return of epithelium to normal. At these moderate doses, all light microscopic and ultrastructural changes in the epithelium reverted to normal by 2–3 weeks. If larger doses are delivered, epithelial changes can progress to frank ulceration. These doses are often associated with more severe vascular and connective tissue stromal changes. This marked damage can produce alteration and disorganization of mucosa as described under chronic changes.

## Vascular and connective tissue stromal changes

Vascular and connective tissue changes also occur acutely during treatment and are especially important since the host response to these acute changes often produces late toxicity. Acute changes in the connective tissue of the mucosa, muscular tissues and serosa includes edema, hemorrhage, inflammation and vascular spasm. Edema, with exudative fibrin, is often the dominant acute process. The normal fibrillar appearance of collagen is disrupted by the swelling and edema. Non-proliferating, non-collagen-producing fibroblasts appear. Edema is also seen in blood vessels. Bosniak *et al.* [19] have analyzed vascular changes after high dose (1500, 3000 R single fraction) XRT. The first stage was that of marked vascular spasm, almost completely relieved by papaverine and procaine hydrochloride. Relief of spasm uncovered hyperemia and a mucosal capillary blush. The vascular spasm occurred as early as 1 day after radiation, peaked in 1–2 weeks and became minimal after 5 weeks. The second stage, from 4–12 weeks, showed endarteritis, thrombosis and arteriographic evidence of arterial occlusion, atrophy and dropout. Finally, the third stage beginning about 12 weeks showed some repair and revascularization. The revascularization was supplied from side-branches of arteries in adjacent non-irradiated bowel. This report is consistent with a similar study by Spratt, Heinbecker and Saltzstein [39] who also angiographically demonstrated mucosal capillary blush, followed by vascular occlusion and then side-branch revascularization from adjacent non-irradiated bowel. Zweifach and Kivy-Rosenberg [40] also have noted changes in enhance-

ment of vascular reactivity to a variety of stimuli, including epinephrine (adrenaline) and norepinephrine (noradrenaline) beginning 1 day after irradiation. These reports are intriguing since they demonstrate physiological changes (spasm) preceding histological evidence of cell death. The etiology of this rapid expression of spasm is not known.

The initial vascular injury is predominantly endothelial and may be reversible. Damage to the media and adventitia consists initially of edema, progresses to hyalinization of the wall, hypertrophy and distortion of muscle, thrombosis and finally obliterative endarteritis and endophlebitis.

## Chronic pathological changes from radiation

The precise target(s) of late radiation damage and the exact mechanism(s) by which radiation exerts its deleterious effect is unknown. Some experimental and clinicopathological observations suggest the probability that events occurring in the vascular and stromal tissues are critical.

Grossly, bowel segments with chronic changes exhibit thickening and induration. Stenosis, due either to diffuse sclerosis with generalized constriction or a stricture at a site of ulceration, is frequent. The serosa is thickened with prominent telangiectasia, as is the mesentery. The mucosa is often ulcerated or atrophic. Inflammatory reactions, characterized by adhesions, fibrinopurulent membranes, or fibrin exudates, are frequent. These reactions are secondary to either a generalized non-specific inflammation or to perforating ulcers or fistulae and often obliterate tissue planes.

Histologically, vascular changes are impressive. Arteries show early edema of the wall followed by hyaline thickening, muscle hypertrophy, distortion and vessel sclerosis. Venous endophlebitis with lymphatic and venous ectasia is striking. Fonkalsrud *et al.* [20] reported large vessel endothelial damage within 48 h of completion of fractionated XRT. Though endothelial change peaked 1–3 weeks post-therapy, these changes were nearly completely gone by 4 months. On the other hand, the media and adventitia first showed changes 1–3 weeks post-therapy which progressed to produce vascular narrowing by 4 months. Decreased muscle cellularity was followed by fibrosis in the media, and adventitial edema, with focal hemorrhage followed by chronic inflammation. The authors interpreted these changes to be possibly due to vasa vasorum injury. The gut epithelium is frequently ulcerated with chronic toxicity, but can show marked atrophy or metaplasia to a flattened epithelium. Goblet cells are large, numerous, full and sometimes distorted. The muscle layer of the bowel is also altered. Interstitial fibrosis, edema and hyalinization of connective tissue is prominent. Muscle fiber degeneration and atrophy is not uncommonly widespread. Both Sugg and others [41] and Wood, Ralston and Kurrle [42] have observed that chronic epithelial changes do not occur unless chronic vascular changes become manifest.

Goldgraber and colleagues [43] and Doig, Funder and Weiden [44] performed serial biopsies in patients undergoing gastric XRT. The earliest change on day 10 of treatment was eosinophilic changes in cells associated with loss of cytoplasmic detail which they termed coagulation necrosis. These abnormalities occurred in the depths of the fundal glands and involved both chief and parietal cells and progressed toward the pits. The peak reaction occurred 3 weeks after XRT, at which time mucosal thinning, interstitial edema with chronic inflammation, and marked epithelial changes (such as parietal cell vacuolization and cell flattening) were evident. These changes were patchy with some alternating nearly normal mucosa. The mucosa reverted completely to normal at 5–12 weeks post-therapy.

## Functional changes (Figure 18.1)

### *Altered glycocalyx and barrier protection*

The intestinal glycocalyx is a glycoprotein extending from the tips of the microvilli. It is composed of the carbohydrate component of disaccharidases, aminopeptidases and other digestive enzymes while the protein component penetrates the lipid bilayer of the membrane. This glycocalyx facilitates digestive

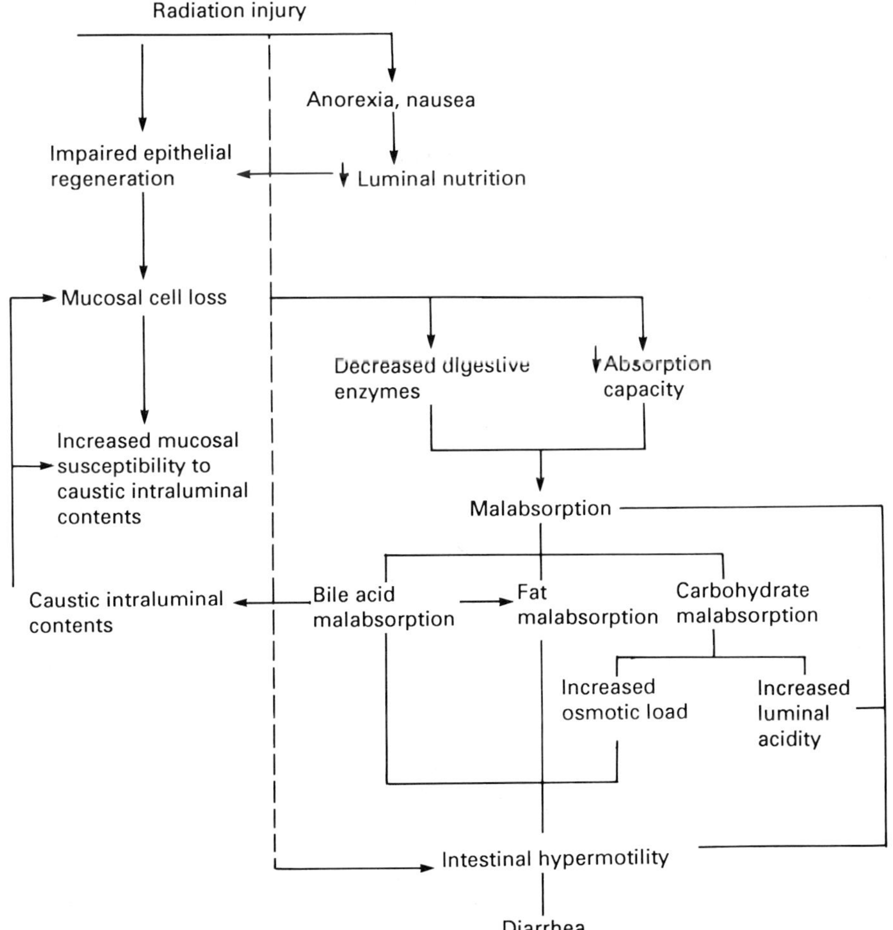


**Figure 18.1** Pathophysiology of acute radiation enteritis

function enzymatically, but also provides the entero-cyte protection against the erosive action of trypsin and other luminal irritants [14]. The glycocalyx is markedly reduced or removed altogether during XRT [22]. Depletion of the glycocalyx thus may explain in part the XRT-induced reduction of disaccharidases and aminopeptidases. Moreover, the corrosive action of pancreaticobiliary secretions may produce greater damage on intestinal epithelial cells in the absence of the glycocalyx barrier. This assault by pancreaticobiliary secretions has been documented to play an important role in other forms of gut injury [14].

## Malabsorption

The absorptive function of the intestine is diminished during and after XRT. This malabsorption is multifactorial in cause, resulting from diminution of intestinal glycocalyx (see above), epithelial cell mass loss with its associated decrease in absorptive surface area, and other poorly characterized abnormalities. The significance of the problem is proportional to the volume, dose and site of radiation. The incidence of absorption abnormalities is grossly underestimated, since the majority of patients with detectable abnormalities are asymptomatic.

Protein deficiency can result from radiation induced malabsorption as demonstrated by Duncan and Leonard [45]. A reduction in gut epithelial uptake of $^{14}$C-labeled leucine occurs within 2–3 days of exposure to 2500 R [46]. Moreover, Vatistas and Hornsey documented that fecal loss of inoculated $^{131}$I-labeled polyvinylpyrrolidone increased from 4%/24 h in normal mice to 30%/24 h in radiated mice. These changes were induced by only 300 R [47]. Irradiated gut can also produce albumin loss in the rabbit [48].

Fat absorption abnormalities were well established by Reeves and colleagues [49,50]. Patients with a decrease in normal blood levels and high fecal fat levels of ingested $^{131}$I-labeled glycerol triolate developed clinical diarrhea. Abnormal absorption of $^{131}$I-labeled neutral fat occurred in fully three-quarters of patients undergoing abdominopelvic radiotherapy usually by the second to third week of therapy.

Sugar, vitamin and electrolyte absorption are also adversely affected [3,51,52]. Anderson, Bosaeus and Nystrom and Stryker, Mortel and Hepner both have documented lactose absorption impairment [51,52]. Carbohydrase histochemical assays have been developed for lactase, sucrase and maltase. A wide variety of sugars exhibit absorption problems within hours to a few days after radiation indicating that the onset of enzymatic abnormalities may in some cases precede the histological changes. Tarpila [22] found decreased carbohydrase levels in biopsies

from patients receiving more than 3000 cGy. He also administered D-xylose absorption tests which screen for malabsorption of carbohydrates in patients with normal liver and renal function, since this 5-carbon sugar does not require pancreatic enzymes for digestion [53]. Patients treated with <1000 cGy showed normal urinary excretion, while those receiving >1000 cGy had slightly diminished D-xylose urinary excretion. Carbohydrate malabsorption is important since unabsorbed mono- and oligosaccharides exert within the small bowel lumen a marked osmotic effect. The increased intraluminal fluid causes bowel distension and increases peristalsis. Furthermore, the unabsorbed carbohydrates are metabolized by colonic bacteria whose fermentation products include organic acids and gases. These increase the acidity of the colonic contents which subsequently further impairs water and electrolyte transport [54]. Kinsella and Bloomer [35] administered $^{14}$C-glycine glycocholate breath tests and either lactose or hydrogen breath tests to 34 patients receiving ≥50 Gy to the pelvis. Abnormal results during week 2 of therapy were present in 36% (18% had abnormalities of both tests); 2–4 weeks post-therapy 21% had abnormalities (usually bile acid breath test only) and 3 months post-therapy only 6% had bile acid breath test abnormalities. Overgaard and Matsui [55] have demonstrated a well defined dose-response glucose absorption abnormality in mouse jejunum which was present only acutely.

## Bile acid malabsorption – cholerheic enteropathy

Bile acids are normally reabsorbed in the terminal ileum. Diseases of the terminal ileum can produce cholerheic enteropathy in which decreased bile acid reabsorption in the terminal ileum allows passage of bile acids into the colon where they induce secretion of water and electrolytes by the colonic mucosa. The precise mechanism by which the increased bile acid concentration mediates diarrhea is not completely understood, but the phenomenon has been clearly defined in patients undergoing abdominopelvic XRT. In rat experiments, Sullivan utilized bile duct cannulation with diversion to prevent radiation-induced diarrhea [56]. Furthermore he showed this prevention of diarrhea was associated with preservation of colonic mucous coating [57]. Impaired ileal bile salt absorption has been clearly documented [51,58,59] in clinical abdominopelvic XRT. Moreover, it occurs frequently. Newman and colleagues [58] studied 17 women following pelvic radiotherapy; 12 had noted a permanent change in bowel habits. Abnormal cholyl-glycine breath tests indicating abnormal deconjugation of bile acids by bacteria occurred in 16/17 studied and in all 12 with symptoms. These women had usually been treated more than 1 year prior to testing, suggesting chronic ileal dysfunction occurs more frequently than does clinical evidence of chronic enteropathy. Stryker, Hepner and Mortel [59] serially tested 33 women, again utilizing the cholyl-glycine breath test during weeks 1 and 5 of therapy and, in 19, 3 months post-treatment. Abnormal tests were obtained in 3/33 (9%) in week 1; 15/33 (45%) in week 5; 4/19 (21%) 3 months post-therapy; and 0/8 1 year post-therapy. This study indicated that bile salt malabsorption occurred frequently but was not universal, usually completely disappeared, was present after histological changes of acute radiation enteropathy have recovered, and correlates imperfectly with diarrhea. Thus, while cholerheic enteropathy is not the sole cause of diarrhea, its frequency is substantial and an understanding of its pathophysiology is critical in the dietary and medical management of radiation enteropathy.

### Radiation-induced emesis and anorexia

Vomiting, nausea and loss of appetite are among the most important concerns of patients receiving abdominal radiation. Paradoxically, our understanding of their etiology is pathetically limited. Emesis can follow upper abdominal radiation within hours of doses of 1.5–2.0 Gy. The vomiting, anorexia and nausea is more frequently observed when larger volumes of stomach are irradiated. Wang, Renzi and Chinn performed a series of animal experiments in dogs and cats [60] in which they tested the impact of either chemoreceptor trigger zone (CTZ) ablation in the area postrema of the medulla, and/or abdominal vagotomy and/or abdominal sympathectomy. These studies show that acute radiation emesis is mediated via the CTZ since ablation will eliminate emesis. Visceral deafferentation may delay acute emesis but will not prevent it. Thus while visceral afferents appear to possibly mediate some of the acute emetogenic effects of radiation, other unknown factors, possibly chemical in nature, appear to be more important. Attempts to prevent or control emesis must be directed at the CTZ level until the etiology of this problem is more fully elucidated.

### Motility disturbances

Intestinal motility is increased almost immediately after exposure to doses of 100 cGy or more in animal systems [61], long before the earliest evidence of histological change. Likewise, motility is increased in human intestinal radiotherapy. Reeves *et al.* [50] noted hypermotility in 42% with 21% showing an increased transit time. Hypermotility with associated hypersecretion increased fold thickness, and erosions were present in 36% of patients following

whole abdominal XRT in Wittich's series [62]. In contrast to the intestinal hypermotility, gastric emptying time in animals appears to be markedly prolonged immediately after XRT [63]. Though animal models of altered gastric [63–66] and intestinal motility [61] occurring within hours of radiation suggest that radiation may have a direct effect on gut motility, many other factors are present by the time clinical diarrhea becomes manifest. It is, therefore, impossible to determine how much, if any, of the observed hypermotility is due to a direct radiation effect *per se*.

In contrast to the hypermotility of acute XRT changes, late effects frequently include segments of gut with diminished or absent mobility. These segments of bowel with diminished motility can allow bacterial overgrowth with ensuing malabsorption and/or diarrhea. Two cases of intestinal pseudo-obstruction have also been reported from late XRT damage presumably mediated by damage to the smooth muscle [67] of the bowel wall.

### Gastric secretions

Bruegel first utilized radiation to depress gastric acid secretion for peptic ulcer disease in 1917 [68]. Since then many reports have confirmed the hydrochloric acid and pepsin reduction by modest doses of radiation [3,43,69,70]. Though no longer utilized as peptic ulcer disease therapy because more effective therapy exists, data obtained during the XRT era of peptic ulcer disease provide insights into the physiological impact of X-rays on the gut. Carpender *et al.* [70] reported on 116 patients with gastric ulcers and 113 with duodenal ulcers usually treated with 16–17 Gy in ten fractions. The gastric ulcers healed in 93%, though subsequently 40% recurred. Achlorhydria was induced in 35% and in 23% this achlorhydria lasted from 7 months to over 10 years. In 29% a permanent reduction of gastric secretion of 50% was obtained. Among duodenal ulcer patients achlorhydria was induced in 23%, and a 50% reduction in free hydrochloric acid was achieved in 35%. The decrease in acid production lasted 1–6 months in two-thirds and persisted for 1–5 years in one-quarter. Palmer and Templeton [69] studied 88 cases of peptic ulcer disease treated with 3000–3600 R. Some gastric acid decrease was seen in all cases, but the extent and duration was variable. Complete achlorhydria developed in 40% lasting a few days to over 1 year. Suppression of acid production without achlorhydria similarly lasted from days to many months [69]. Pepsin secretion follows a similar reduction to that of hydrochloric acid [3]. Reduction of both pepsin and hydrochloric acid secretion initially paralleled the histological changes observed by Goldgraber *et al.* [43] and Doig, Funder and Weiden [44]. However, a substantial percentage exhibited acid reduction long after

12 weeks when the gastric mucosal histology had reverted to normal. Thus, there appears to be a physiological effect on gastric secretion not completely explained by histological changes.

## Clinical presentation

### Acute period

The symptoms occurring during abdominopelvic radiation are common and well known. Nausea, vomiting, early satiety and anorexia can be the earliest sequelae of therapy. These symptoms may occur within several hours of the first treatment if substantial volumes of stomach are within the field [70]. In Palmer and Templeton's series [69], discussed earlier, nausea and vomiting were present during the first several treatments as a rule and thereafter diminished in severity. Others tolerate the initial portion of therapy with minimal problems, but experience increasing nausea, vomiting and anorexia after variable periods of treatment. Volume of stomach included and fraction size appear to be important determinants of these side effects. Patients may tolerate upper abdominal XRT better following gastrectomy [71] and with individually shaped fields [71].

The Gastrointestinal Tumor Study Group randomized locally advanced gastric cancer to receive either 5-FU and semustine (methyl-CCNU) alone or two courses of 25 Gy in 15 fractions, one fraction/day, with intravenous bolus of 5-FU 500 mg/m$^2$ on days 1–3 separated by a 2-week break followed by 5-FU and semustine. Toxicity in the combined modality arm was substantially increased with nutritional deaths occurring in 7% and septic deaths in 7% [72]. The profound nutritional problems observed in this study increased awareness of the potentially devastating gastrointestinal toxicity associated with this type of therapy. More recent studies have emphasized tightly contoured fields and rigorous nutritional support. Smith and colleagues [73] treated 56 locally advanced gastric or pancreatic malignancies with 5-FU, doxorubicin, mitomycin C chemotherapy before and after combined XRT and 5-FU. Radiation was given in two cycles of 22.5 Gy in ten fractions separated by a 2-week break. Each XRT cycle was given with 5-FU, 350 mg/m$^2$/day intravenous bolus on days 1–3. Nausea and vomiting were encountered in 70% but was manageable with antiemetic therapy. Mean weight change was a 5 kg loss with no nutritional deaths, though non-gastrointestinal toxicity was formidable (16% with life-threatening myelosuppression, 5% treatment-related mortality). Gunderson and others [74] treated 40 locally advanced gastric cancers with chemotherapy and doses $\geq$50 Gy, but utilizing carefully shaped portals and fractions of $\leq$1.8 Gy per day.

Though acute nausea, vomiting and anorexia occurred, it was easily controlled by antiemetics, no severe or life-threatening nutritional complications were noted, and average weight loss was only 2 kg. Further supporting the concept that volume of stomach is important in the acute nausea and vomiting syndrome are the numerous biliary and pancreatic series which report quantitatively far less frequent and severe toxicity. Though doses of 50–60+ Gy are used, these fields are shaped to exclude major portions of the stomach and are better tolerated.

Though tightly contoured portals and fraction sizes of $\leq$1.8 Gy allow gastric XRT to be tolerated relatively safely, we are approaching acute tolerance limits with available combined modality approaches. Preliminary data indicate full dose upper abdominal radiation (tumor-nodal volume 45–50 Gy; boost 10–15 Gy) with concomitant continuous infusion of 5-FU (200–300 mg/m$^2$/day) can be tolerated but requires vigorous nutritional support (Tyvin Rich, personal communication). The Mayo Clinic piloted hyperfractionated gastric radiation, 1.5–1.7 Gy twice daily to a tumor-nodal dose of 40 Gy and boost dose of 45 Gy. 5-FU and doxorubicin were given before and after radiotherapy. Hyperfractionated radiation with concomitant 5-FU by intravenous bolus was not tolerated despite aggressive nutritional support. Hyperfractionated radiation alone was somewhat better tolerated, though again anorexia and nausea was universal, often severe and associated with substantial weight loss [75].

Fatigue is a nearly universal sequel of XRT to virtually all gastrointestinal sites. The cause is unknown. Patients can develop fatigue as the only predominant symptom of radiation if moderate doses and volumes are used. Advising people of this side effect and reassuring them of its gradual resolution a few months following treatment will usually provide some solace.

The majority of patients undergoing pelvic radiation experience acute proctocolitis. Sigmoidoscopy during treatment may reveal an inflamed, edematous, friable mucosa. Symptoms of frequent loose to watery stools associated with rectal urgency and tenesmus are characteristic. Though complaints of frequent small loose stools may occur in anyone with proctitis, these complaints are particularly common following a low anterior resection since the rectal vault capacity is markedly diminished and stool frequency exists even before therapy begins [76]. Hematochezia is infrequent and occasionally due to hemorrhoidal irritation or anal fistulae produced by the diarrhea. History and physical examination with proctoscopy are sufficient to discern the etiology of hematochezia.

Radiation enteritis occurs if significant volumes of small bowel are radiated to even low doses. The duration between initiation of treatment and symptom onset depends upon volume of small bowel treated and fraction size. Symptoms of radiation enteritis usually become manifest after 2–3 weeks of conventional pelvic treatment. Once enteritis becomes manifest, it increases in severity until several days after discontinuing treatment. Patients may complain of nausea and anorexia but vomiting is uncommon. Loose to watery diarrhea with voluminous frequent stools and cramping abdominal pain is characteristic of fully developed enteritis. Acute radiation enteritis is self-limited with the onset and resolution of symptoms closely following the histological changes, previously described in the epithelium.

## Chronic period

Different sites within the gut, when they develop chronic late effects, have characteristic clinical presentations. It is important to understand these differences. However, frequently late damage affects multiple gastrointestinal sites. Several reports [31,41,77–82] of late effects report multiple gastrointestinal organs damaged in 28–60%. Galland and Spencer [80] and Cram, Pearlman and Jochimsen [82] report that about half with multiple site damage had all affected sites identified at the time of initial clinical presentation; the remainder developed additional sites subsequently. Genitourinary and other intra-abdominal sites are also frequently involved [29,41,80,81,83].

### *Stomach*

The Walter Reed Army Hospital group [84,85] classified late gastric injury into four types:

1. Radiation dyspepsia: patients with unremarkable radiographic and physical examinations who had complaints of epigastric pain, heartburn, belching, flatulence and other vague abdominal complaints. It was recognized that some of these complaints were functional.
2. Radiation gastritis: radiographic evidence of antral narrowing, mucosal thickening and spasm. These patients usually were symptomatic and gastroscopy showed antral narrowing and loss of rugae, sometimes with mucosal atrophy.
3. Radiation ulcer.
4. Radiation ulcer with perforation.

Gastric late effects usually become manifest shortly after completion of therapy [86]. In the Walter Reed cohort [84,85] the median time to onset of symptoms from completion of therapy was: ulcer with perforation, 2 months (range 1–30 months); ulcer, 4 months (range 1–72 months);

gastritis, 2 months (range 1–48 months); and dyspepsia, 6 months (range 2–60 months). Radiation-induced ulcers resemble benign peptic ulcer disease [30,85,87] radiographically and are usually not associated with gastric outlet obstruction. These ulcers can be extremely difficult to heal [30,85–89], and with serial examinations can show progressive deformity [30,86]. Another radiographic pattern is of fixed narrowing of the antral-pyloric region without ulcers [3,30,84,89]. Peristalsis is minimal and the stomach rigid on fluoroscopy [30,87,89]. Multiple, small, superficial ulcerations are seen and mucosal folds are either prominent or markedly effaced [30,87]. Though radiation suppresses gastric secretions acutely, secretions recover with time [3,69,70], and significant depression of gastric acid production a few years after even large doses of antral radiation is uncommon [90].

Symptoms of ulcers and gastritis are those of epigastric discomfort. Though symptoms may respond to anti-ulcer therapy, they characteristically may not be alleviated by food [3,85,89]. If progressive contracture of the stomach occurs, early satiety, anorexia, vomiting and weight loss ensues. Anemia can be seen due to blood loss [3,84,88]. Vitamin $B_{12}$ deficiency, though theoretically possible due to insufficient intrinsic factor elaboration in the stomach, is uncommon [3].

### *Small bowel*

The clinical picture of small intestinal late radiation effects is shown in Table 18.1. Though small bowel injury can occur within the first few months following therapy, its median onset is 1–5 years. Moreover, extremely long latent periods of over 20–30 years are not unusual [29,80,81,91,92]. The onset of late effects may be hastened by use of concomitant chemotherapy [93]. Obstruction is clearly the most common manifestation of late small bowel damage. Diagnosis sometimes is preceded by either sporadic or gradually more frequent episodes of acute, colicky abdominal discomfort which spontaneously resolve. Perforation will often be unheralded by prior symptoms and presents with the catastrophic picture of an acute abdomen [3,33,80–82,86,91–94]. Occasionally patients can present with massive bleeding as the only manifestation of late bowel damage [27,33,80,95]. Intestinal pseudo-obstruction has also been reported as a late radiation effect [67].

Radiographic evaluation shows straightening and thickening of the valvulae conniventes, nodular filling defects and/or thumbprinting as a result of edema and fibrosis in addition to the areas of narrowing [3,30,62]. Separation of bowel loops can result from the intestinal wall thickening. Occasionally, small ulcers are visible but this is difficult to

**Table 18.1 Clinical presentation of small bowel injury**

| Series [ref.] | Interval from radiation to injury | No. of patients | No. with obstruction | No. with perforation | No. with fistula | No. with malabsorption |
|---|---|---|---|---|---|---|
| DeCosse [81] | 6.5 years[a] (1 month–31 years) | 25 | 14 | 8 | 3 | |
| Kwitko [29] | 5.1 years[a] (4 months–22 years) | 31 | 25[d] | 1 | 5 | 11 |
| Galland [80] | 35 months[b] (0–18 years) | 28[c] | 19 | 4 | 4 | |
| Miholic [93] | 10 months[b] (2 months–10 years) | 34 | 30 | 3 | 4 | |
| Sugg [41] | – | 11 | 10 | | 1 | |
| Lillemoe [91] | 12 months[b] (2 months–27 years) | 17 | 13 | | 4 | |
| Cochrane [94] | 11 months[b] (2 months–39 months) | 13 | 7 | | 6 | |
| Wellwood [31] | | 21 | 11 | 6 | 2 | 9 |
| Total | | 180 | 129 (72%) | 22 (12%) | 29 (16%) | |

[a]Mean time from completion of radiotherapy to injury.
[b]Median time from completion of radiotherapy to injury.
[c]One had small intestinal bleeding as only late sequel.
[d]Nineteen had obstruction at initial onset of small bowel disease; six developed obstruction subsequently.
Note: Some patients had more than one lesion; malabsorption not always reported.

demonstrate because of their small size [30,62]. Small bowel series also can reflect the marked mesenteric adhesion, thickenings and contractures which so frequently accompany luminal changes. In this instance, loops are fixed, matted, sometimes sharply angulated and displaced fluoroscopically en masse by palpation. These mesenteric changes can be confused with recurrent disease since it can produce a mass effect on the bowel with traction of adjacent loops [3,30,62]. Mesenteric angiography will show vessel crowding, tortuosity, angulations and narrowing in the mid-arterial phase while the late arterial phase may reveal a vascular blush in the affected bowel wall [3]. Small bowel double contrast studies utilizing methylcellulose and duodenojejunal intubation has been more definitive in the evaluation of post-therapy small bowel obstruction in several series [62,96,97]. Patients presenting with a clinical picture of an acute abdomen from either sudden obstruction or perforation will not allow the luxury of a detailed radiographic evaluation. Plain abdominal films, supine and upright with clinical evaluation, may have to suffice.

Malabsorption is probably more common than is clinically appreciated. The experience of Newman *et al.* [58] in which 16/17 women tested usually a year or more following radiation had abnormal cholylglycine breath test has been previously discussed. Other studies indicate malabsorption is much less common [35,59]. Nevertheless, malabsorption can exist without clinical symptoms [58] and frequently accompanies other late effects [3,27,31,33,86,98, 99]. Patients with weight loss, fatigue, diarrhea or other gastrointestinal symptomatology should be carefully evaluated. Mechanisms by which malabsorption is produced from chronic late effects are numerous. Extensive ileal involvement produces bile salt wasting with diarrhea and steatorrhea. If sufficient segments of small bowel lose peristaltic tone with partial narrowing and fibrosis, then the resulting stasis can predispose to bacterial overgrowth and malabsorption on this basis. Enterocolonic fistulae, likewise, can cause massive intraluminal bacterial overgrowth with severe steatorrhea and $B_{12}$ deficiency.

## *Large bowel*

The clinical picture of large bowel late effects is shown in Table 18.2. Though the types and mechanisms of radiation injury are similar to those of the small bowel, there are important differences. Large bowel injury characteristically becomes manifest earlier than small bowel injury – within 2 years of treatment (median 6–18 month latency) – though can present immediately after XRT. Extremely long latency periods of 5 years or more are distinctly unusual in the large bowel in contrast to the small intestine. Fistulae occur much more frequently in the rectum than anywhere else in the gut. Fistulae are confined almost exclusively to cases where brachytherapy has been utilized. Fistulae and ulcerations usually occur along the anterior rectal wall, posterior to the vaginal fornix. Here the brachytherapy dose is highest and blood supply poorest. Mucosal injuries are more frequently reported in the large bowel for a variety of reasons including the greater accessibility of the mucosa to inspection, as well as the different sensory innervation of the rectum.

Symptoms of fistulae, perforation and obstruction are obvious. Interestingly, when radiographic evaluations are performed prospectively, a surprisingly high frequency of strictures are asymptomatic but radiographically unequivocal. This can be seen in as many as 25% of strictures [84,85]. Mucosal injury

**Table 18.2 Clinical presentation of large bowel injury**

| Series [ref.] | Interval from radiation to injury | No. of patients | No. with obstruction | No. with perforation | No. with fistula | No. with mucosal injury[c] |
|---|---|---|---|---|---|---|
| Warren [100] | 5 months[a] (0–20 months) | 25 | | | 5 | |
| Brick [84][d] | 18 months[b] (2–60 months) | 31 | 28[e] | 3 | | |
| Dirksen [101][f] | 12 months[a] (6–84 months) | 9 | 5 | | 3 | 1 |
| Wellwood [31] | – | 25 | 13 | 3 | 3 | 25[g] |
| Cochrane [94][f] | 9 months[a] (0–24 months) | 16 | 8 | 3 | 2 | 3 |
| DeCosse [81] | – | 81 | 19 | | 29 | 54 |
| Galland [80] | 16 months[a] (0–13 years) | 23 | 9 | 4 | 7 | 6 |
| Total | | 210 | 82 (39%) | 13 (6%) | 49 (23%) | 89 (42%) |

[a]Median.
[b]Mean.
[c]Bleeding, ulcer, mucositis, 'sclerosis'.
[d]External beam therapy only.
[e]Seven asymptomatic.
[f]All with intracavitary brachytherapy as component of treatment.
[g]Eighteen proctocolitis, seven rectal ulcer, three necrosis.
Note: Some patients may have had more than one lesion; mucosal injury not reported consistently in all series.

can be debilitating even in the absence of stricture, perforation or fistula. Tenesmus, bleeding, cramps, obstipation, diarrhea, and rectal urgency, if severe, can require surgical intervention.

Radiographically the most frequent appearance is a smooth elongated narrowing. These segments are often straightened and elevated out of the pelvis because of thickening of both the bowel wall and adjacent pelvic tissues [3,17,30,31,102]. Alternatively, submucosal changes may give rise to a nodular or thumbprinting effect on the wall [3,30]. Mesenteric shortening can produce traction of the transverse colon cephalad and produce sharp angulation. Ulceration is frequent and may be superficial or deep, at times simulating diverticulitis [30,103]. When this ulcerated, narrowed appearance has abrupt margins it requires careful differentiation from carcinoma. This can be particularly difficult if these mucosal findings occur with enlargement of the retrorectal space. Retrorectal space enlargement can occur with either recurrent neoplasm or radiation effect. It is often part of a clinical syndrome in which the pelvic soft tissues become indurated, swollen, and firm or hard. This condition is sometimes called 'pseudotumor'. CT scans and MRI are extremely helpful in this important differentiation [103,104]. Serial radiographic examinations, including baseline CT scan 4–6 months after therapy, greatly facilitate follow-up.

# Prevention

The original description of radiation enteritis by Walsh in 1897 included the observation that shielding from the beam would prevent toxicity [1].

Limiting tissues from receiving unnecessary radiation remains the most important component of radiation enteritis prevention almost 100 years later. Limiting tissue exposure is a multifaceted procedure and includes:

1. Communication between surgeons, pathologists and radiation oncologists.
2. Optimization of dose homogeneity.
3. Optimization of dose fractionation schedule.
4. Small bowel mobilization.

## *Communication between surgeons, pathologists and radiation oncologists*

Operative notes should carefully delineate the boundaries of resected and residual disease. Areas of concern to the surgeon should be marked with small vascular clips which will not interfere with follow-up CT scans but will allow precise tailoring of radiotherapy fields. It is encumbent upon the radiation oncologist to avail her or himself of all pertinent information so that tissues at lower risk are spared from unnecessary dose. Tissues should be routinely spared by custom blocking and shrinking field technique.

## *Optimization of dose homogeneity*

The Walter Reed experience, which encountered higher than expected rates of radiation late effects, may have been in part due to the exclusive use of AP:PA fields and 1 MeV energy photons [84–86].

This treatment results in inhomogenous dose distribution with substantial volumes receiving ≥10% of the prescribed midline dose. Kwitko *et al.* [29] and the RTOG in two trials [105,106] also reported higher complications when AP:PA fields alone are used. Homogeneity is improved by higher energy machines, multifield technique and computerized treatment planning with liberal use of beam aids such as wedges and compensating filters.

## Optimization of dose fractionation schedule

Large fraction sizes clearly predispose to late toxicity. Therefore, when doses at or approaching tolerance are required, utilization of fraction sizes of 1.8–2.0 Gy is mandatory. A corollary of this is the principle of treating multiple fields per day. Treating more than one field per day decreases the daily fraction size of the dose deposited in tissues outside the target volume. This reduction in daily fraction size occurs because:

1. The dose which is delivered through the other fields may block non-target tissue treated via the other fields completely and therefore spare them this proportion of dose. Lateral pelvic and para-aortic fields, for example, routinely spare some small bowel anterior to the lateral fields which are treated via the AP:PA fields; and
2. Because delivery of radiation through multiple field reduces the daily given dose from each field.

## Small bowel mobilization

Green, Iba and Smith reported in 1975 that small bowel radiographs could be superimposed on simulated treatment fields. This permitted a semi-quantitative method of estimating the volume of small bowel radiated, assessment of techniques displacing small bowel from the XRT field, and modification of fields to exclude small bowel from the high-dose volume [107]. Several reports have subsequently explored small bowel radiographs in radiotherapy [108–116,123]. Because the volume of small bowel radiated is directly related to the risk of acute and chronic toxicity [107–109,114], mobilization of small bowel is of great concern.

Fixation of small bowel in the pelvis is markedly increased following surgery [107,109,114]. Green noted fixation in only 18% without prior surgery versus 65% with prior surgery [109]. The volume of small bowel irradiated is also markedly increased. Gallagher *et al.* performed a quantitative estimate of the small bowel volume in the treatment field as shown in Table 18.3, which confirms that there is substantially more small bowel irradiated after surgery, especially abdominoperineal resection [114,123].

Treatment in the prone position allows displacement of intestines out of the radiation field [107,109,114,116–119]. Green found a 15% average reduction of small bowel volume in the treatment field when in the prone versus the supine position [109] with an average 2 cm displacement superiorly [107]. Gallagher, utilizing a quantitative estimate of small bowel volume exposed to radiation (Table 18.3), documented that prone positioning produced an average reduction of 35% (when treatment followed APR) to 70% (with no prior surgery). Treatment with a full bladder also displaces small intestine superiorly and anteriorly [109,114–119]. The decrease in irradiated bowel is greatest from lateral fields. Nevertheless, Caspers *et al.* [115] documented a 33% volume reduction with a median upward shift of 1.2 cm within AP:PA fields alone with bladder distension. Utilization of an anterior abdominal compression device, whether alone or in combination with other small bowel mobilization techniques [114], can also be effective. Elman, in a group of 12 patients from the University of Utah, felt that this technique was of greater value than bladder distension [117,120]. Trendelenburg position has provided superior displacement compared

**Table 18.3 Association of treatment position and prior surgery on average pelvic small bowel volume (in cm³)**

| | No prior surgery (n = 75) | | Non-APR[a] surgery (n = 50) | | APR (n = 25) | |
|---|---|---|---|---|---|---|
| | *Two-field*[b] | *Four-field*[c] | *Two-field* | *Four-field* | *Two-field* | *Four-field* |
| Supine | 425 | 165 | 620 | 370 | 1010 | 600 |
| Prone[d] | 165 | 50 | 190 | 145 | 565 | 385 |

[a]Abdominopelvic resection.
[b]AP:PA.
[c]AP:PA and opposed laterals.
[d]Prone with abdominal wall compression or bladder distension.
From Gallagher *et al.* [ref. 114].

with prone positioning alone [116], though Green [107] did not find any advantage to Trendelenburg which is cumbersome and time-consuming. A 'false table top' [117] allows the anterior abdominal wall and small bowel to fall anteriorly. It is rarely of major benefit in pelvic treatment, but can be extremely helpful when para-aortic nodes are treated via laterals. Finally, Gunderson has described the use of lateral decubitus position for extrapelvic colon cancer [117,118,121,122]. Utilizing lateral decubitus position for right or left-sided colon lesions [122] resulted in complete shift of all small bowel outside XRT field in 16/53 (30%) and no more than one or two loops 'stuck' within the tumor bed in an additional 21/53 (40%).

A variety of surgical procedures can also be used to displace intestine. Reperitonealizing the pelvic floor may diminish fixation of small bowel by minimizing the surface area of granulating abraded tissue and decreasing the pelvic cul-de-sac size [118,121]. There are several techniques to physically prevent small bowel from entering the pelvis. The bladder or uterus and broad ligament can be sutured to the posterior and lateral pelvic side walls. This fills the pelvis with an endogenous space-occupying mass displacing bowel out of the treatment volume [108,117,121]. Alternatively, an omental pedicle flap can be placed in the pelvis which prevents small intestine from entering the radiation field. Two approaches have utilized exogenous material to limit small bowel exposure. Sugarbaker [124], Edington, Hancock and Coe [125] and Durig *et al.* [126] have advocated use of pelvic prostheses to displace bowel. This technique, though effective, requires the placement of a foreign body in the pelvis indefinitely with the attendant risk of adjacent tissue erosion from the prosthesis, or a second operation to remove the device. Recently, an absorbable polyglycolic acid mesh (PGAM) sling has been utilized to suspend the intestine out of the pelvis [110–113]. The PGAM is hydrolyzed by the body and disappears 3–6 months after placement [112]. Utilizing the PGAM sling effectively excluded the small bowel from the lateral field in ≥80% [113].

## Dietary prevention

Elemental diets (ED) are chemically defined products that contain nutrients in their simple molecular form, without lactose or fiber. Bile and pancreatic proteases are noxious to the intestinal epithelium and adversely affect the intestinal lesion and survival of irradiated animals [127–130]. ED reduces the concentration of these noxious substances while providing the intestinal epithelium with a readily absorbable form of nutrient [127]. Therefore it was logical to test the value of these diets in abdomino-pelvic XRT. Mice [127,131], rats [127,132] and dogs [127] undergoing XRT all experimentally benefited from ED. Several clinical reports suggest ED may benefit humans as well. Bounous *et al.* [127,133] conducted a prospective randomized trial of ED in the context of abdominal radiotherapy, 39–40.4 Gy. The ED allowed weight and serum proteins to remain stable while XRT was completed without interruption. Controls on an isocaloric hospital diet suffered decreases in weight, serum protein levels and importantly required treatment breaks in 33%. McArdle and colleagues [134], in a non-randomized trial, compared ED in 24 patients with 32 controls on a hospital diet or total parenteral nutrition. All received 4 Gy × 5 precystectomy. Control patients developed nausea, vomiting, diarrhea, and biopsy evidence of mild to moderate radiation enteropathy and required longer for bowel function to return postoperatively. Finally, since the Institut Gustave-Roussy instituted ED in children receiving whole or hemiabdominal radiotherapy, there have been no cases of either severe acute or late radiation enteritis. Prior to institution of ED, the incidence of acute radiation enteritis was 70% and delayed enteritis 36% [135]. ED clearly deserves further clinical testing.

Simple dietary restrictions have also been evaluated. Booth, McIntyre and Mollin [136] and Bosaeus, Andersson and Nystrom [137] have reported that diarrhea associated with small bowel radiation is reduced by a low-fat diet. Stryker and Bartholomew [138] randomized 64 patients receiving pelvic radiation to a regular diet, a regular diet including lactase enzyme, or a lactose-restricted diet. No significant advantage was seen for the diet-restricted groups in terms of either diarrhea, stool frequency or diphenoxylate usage.

## Drug therapy

Rachootin, Shapiro and Yamakawa [139] have attempted to neutralize the effect of proteases pharmacologically. Potent antiproteases from the nematode *Ascaris lumbricoides* appeared in early observations to be efficacious in the prevention of radiation enteropathy. Further work is necessary with this very interesting approach.

Chary and Thomson [140] conducted a prospective randomized trial of the value of cholestyramine during pelvic radiotherapy. Thirty-five patients receiving pelvic XRT were placed on a 40 g fat diet. The low-fat diet had previously been reported to decrease diarrhea and bile salt excretion [132,136]. Patients were then randomized at the end of the second week to either cholestyramine (a non-absorbable ion exchange resin which binds bile salts) 4 g twice daily orally or placebo. Diarrhea ensued in 38% of the placebo group compared with 6% of the cholestyramine-treated cohort. The placebo group manifested greater diarrhea and diarrhea scales throughout the entire observation period. Though cholestyramine was effective, adverse effects associated with cholestyramine were noted and its use was not recommended. Stryker, Chung and Layser reported a study utilizing colestipol hydrochloride, a bile sequestering resin, without dietary modification. They concluded colestipol, by itself, was ineffective [141]. Bile salt binding resins, while not of sufficient benefit at this point to justify their routine use, can be given an empirical trial in the individual patient who does not respond to more conservative therapy.

Antibiotic prophylaxis with succinylsulfathiazole proved useful in an animal model by decreasing radiation lethality and improving the granulation of radiation ulcers [39]. It is unclear what significance this has clinically. Finally, Mennie and others presented a report of acetylsalicylate controlling radiation-induced diarrhea. They postulated that this diarrhea was, in part, mediated by tissue prostaglandins [142]. This report is unconfirmed.

Alkoxyglycerols have also been administered prophylactically to prevent XRT damage [143]. These substances are found in human milk, mammalian hematopoietic tissue, and most abundantly in the liver oil of certain shark species. Brohult has performed a retrospective review and one prospective double blind trial of its use in cervical carcinoma. Patients who received alkoxyglycerols had a lower incidence of both mild symptomatic toxicity as well as a lower rate of fistulization. These fascinating observations will require confirmation by others.

# Etiology

The most important determinants of radiation toxicity in the gut are the time-dose fractionation (TDF) scheme utilized and volume of bowel treated. Other biological variables may also play a role though not infrequently mediate their influence by impacting the volume of bowel treated. Definition of tissue tolerance is exclusively an empirical exercise. Though animal models are helpful in the elucidation of pathophysiology of injury, they only provide general concepts [26,144,145] about the tissue tolerance of various time-dose fractionation schemes. The difficulty with defining tissue tolerance on an empirical basis is obvious. No investigator has conducted a prospective dose escalation experiment of gut tolerance in humans. Doses have generally been chosen based upon the clinical experience of the treating physician, the collective wisdom of the radiation oncology community, and a few imperfect retrospective reviews. Certainly, these experiences

transmitted pearls of wisdom, and retrospective reviews are far from perfect. Nevertheless, they do rely on observations of perceptive, intelligent clinicians with considerable experience. Analysis of these observations provides a somewhat consistent picture. The Walter Reed Army Hospital experience provides a convenient beginning point in the discussion of dose tolerance of various portions of the gut. A caveat regarding this experience is necessary however. The Walter Reed cohort was treated via AP:PA portals only with 1 MeV (3 mm tungsten filter, 3.9 mm lead half-value layer), 70 cm target-skin distance or 200 keV photons, and usually to only one field each day often with extremely high daily doses. Approximately 300 cGy per day was delivered to midplane with daily skin doses of 400–600 cGy per day [146], thus the overlying stomach and small bowel may have received 300–600 cGy per day [84–86,88,90,146]. This fractionation scheme is far from typical radiotherapy by today's standards and the fractionation scheme almost certainly produced more late toxicity. However, the cohort studied was large, had good follow-up and was analysed in detail. Approximately 230 testicular cancers were treated from 1942 to 1946 of whom 72 had autopsies, and almost 100 of the 135 patients surviving 5 years were restudied in detail in 1951. Those living but not examined (48) or dead without autopsy (37) were evaluated from clinical records and correspondence.

## Stomach

### *Time-dose fractionation (TDF)*

The Walter Reed group [84–86] categorized gastric damage into either gastric ulcer with perforation or obstruction, uncomplicated gastric ulcer, radiation gastritis, or dyspepsia (see above). The relationship between dose and these gastric late effects is described in Table 18.4. Gastric toxicity was uncommon below 40 Gy, but doses of 45–59 Gy were associated with a 20–30% incidence of ulceration which was complicated by perforation or ulceration in 30–50%. Doses of 60 Gy carried a 50% risk of ulceration which was usually complicated. Virtually all the ulcerations were unresponsive to conservative therapy and required surgery [85,86,88,89].

The Walter Reed data are supported by a myriad of other para-aortic radiation series (Table 18.5). Para-aortic radiation data sets from lymphoma [147–150] and seminoma [151–154] cohorts and low-dose (35–40 Gy) locally unresectable gastric trials [155] and pancreatic trials [156,157] confirm the safety of doses of 40 Gy or less. However, the data summarized in Table 18.5 are somewhat at odds with the Walter Reed experience in terms of the safety of doses in the 45–55 Gy range. As can be seen from Table 18.5, it is quite uncommon for

**Table 18.4 Relationship between dose and radiation late effects in the stomach: Walter Reed experience**

| Dose (Gy) | No. of[b] patients | Radiation late effect (%)[a] | | | |
|---|---|---|---|---|---|
| | | Dyspepsia | Gastritis | Ulcer | Complicated ulcer[c] |
| <40 | 111 | 5 | 2 | 3 | 0 |
| 40–44.9 | 23 | 0 | 22 | 0 | 0 |
| 45–49.9 | 27 | 4 | 19 | 11 | 11 |
| 50–54.9 | 34 | 0 | 24 | 18 | 12 |
| 55–59.9 | 14 | 0 | 50 | 14 | 7 |
| >60 | 8 | 0 | 0 | 13 | 38 |

[a]Percentage injured in each type of injury is no. with injury/no. treated with this dose.
[b]Total number of patients treated at this dose.
[c]Ulcers complicated by either obstruction or perforation.

**Table 18.5 Late complications of para-aortic radiation**

| Series [ref.] | Diagnosis | No. of patients | Site | | Total/fraction dose (Gy) | Comments (see key) |
|---|---|---|---|---|---|---|
| | | | Gastric | Small bowel | | |
| Piver [158] | Cx | 21 | 3 | 7 (33%) | 60/2.0 | 2,A,ii,4 |
| Nelson [159] | Cx | 23 | 1 | 2 (9%) | 60/2.0 | 1,A,i,3 |
| Tewfik [160] | Cx | 23 | 0 | 8 (35%) | 50–55/1.8 | 1,A,i,3 |
| Fletcher [161,277] | Cx | 54 | – | 11 (20%) | 45–55/1.7–2.0 | 1,A,i,3,5 |
| Goldstein [87] | Cx | 121 | 11 | – | 45–55/1.7–2.0 | 1,A,i,3,5 |
| Rubin [162,163] | Cx | 16 | 0 | 3 (19%) | 40–50/1.7–2.0 | 1,A,i,4 |
| Piver [158] | Cx | 10 | 0 | 1 (10%) | 44–50/2.0 | 1,A,i,4 |
| Welander [164] | Cx | 26 | 0 | 6 | 44/1.8–2.0 | 1,2,A,i |
| Hughes [165] | Cx | 41 | 0 | 2 (5%) | 36–51/1.7 | 1,A,i,3,4 |
| Berman [166] | Cx | 11 | 0 | 1 | 40–52/– | 1,A – 4 (1 SBO), B – 7 |
| Potish [167,205] | Cx | 104 | 0 | 2 | 45–50/1.8–2.0 | 1,3,B – 21, C – 83,4,5,i |
| LaPolla [168] | Cx | 16 | 0 | 1 | 40–50/1.8–2.0 | 1,A – 8, B – 8,i |
| Ballon [169] | Cx | 18 | 0 | 0 | 43–51/– | 1,B,3,4,i |
| Jolles [170] | Cx | 11 | 0 | 0 | 45–50/1.8 | 1,C,5 |
| Emami [171] | Cx | 36 | 0 | 2 | 45–50/1.75 | 1,C,i |
| Rotman [172] | Cx | 42 | 0 | 1 | 45/1.8 | 2,C,3,i |
| Potish [173] | Endo | 48 | 0 | 0 | 45–51/1.5–1.7 | 1,A – 30, C – 18,4,5,i |
| Goldstein [87] | Testes | 52 | 1 | – | 40–50/– | – |

Key: 1, AP:PA only; 2, AP:PA with rotational or lateral fields; 3, Co-60; 4, 2–6 MeV; 5, >6 MeV: A, intraperitoneal staging; B, extraperitoneal staging; C, radiographic staging; i, continuous course; ii, split course. Cx, cervix; Endo, endometrium

doses of 45–55 Gy to produce gastric ulceration when fraction sizes of 1.5–2.0 Gy are used. Only the M.D. Anderson series reported significant toxicity from these doses and only in the subset of patients treated for cervical carcinoma was this observed. Testicular and retroperitoneal tumors had less than a 2% incidence of ulceration when treated similarly [87]. The para-aortic series do confirm that 60 Gy doses carry substantial risk of late gastric toxicity.

The impression from the para-aortic data that doses in the 45–55 Gy range are reasonably well tolerated is also corroborated by several upper abdominal series. Gunderson *et al.* [74] treated whole or partial gastric volumes in 36 of 46 patients with gastric cancer. Usual doses were 45–52 Gy in 1.8 Gy fractions, though four received 53–59 Gy and two an $^{125}$I implant to gross residual disease. All were treated with tightly contoured fields and almost all with chemotherapy before and/or after XRT. No late effects were observed. Similarly, four locally unresectable gastric cancer trials including the GTSG study [72] previously mentioned (25 Gy in 3 weeks, 2-week rest, 25 Gy in 3 weeks with concomitant 5-FU and post-radiotherapy 5-FU and semustine), the Mid-Atlantic Oncology Program [73] trial (22.5 Gy per 10 fractions, 2-week break,

22.5 Gy per 10 fractions with concomitant 5-FU and sandwich 5-FU, doxorubicin, mitomycin C chemotherapy), the Southwest Oncology Group [174] trial (15 Gy in 1.8–2.0 Gy fractions × 3 on days 8, 36 and 64 to a total dose of 45 Gy and sandwich 5-FU, doxorubicin and mitomycin C), and Thirlwell and colleagues [175] report (46 Gy, 2 Gy fractions with concurrent 5-FU and post-radiation 5-FU and semustine) report no gastric late effects in a total of 115 patients. Likewise, high-dose (55–60 Gy) locally unresectable pancreatic trials and biliary series which by necessity universally treat a portion of stomach, often with concurrent 5-FU, report less than a 5% incidence of gastric ulceration [176–187].

In summary, using high energy, conventionally fractionated radiation, the incidence of gastric late effects is less than 5% at or below 45 Gy, is probably in the range of 5% with 50–55 Gy, and is probably 5–15% or more with 60 Gy and greater.

## Small intestine

Small bowel tolerance is also defined primarily by TDF scheme and the volume and mobility of small bowel. The Walter Reed data are summarized on Table 18.6.

### *Dose*

A substantial incidence of late small bowel damage was seen with doses above 40 Gy. However, the majority of late effects did not significantly impact patients' well-being until higher doses were given [148]. Mild radiation damage was defined as clear roentgenographic or pathological evidence of small bowel damage in which the patients were free of gastrointestinal symptoms ≥4 years after therapy. Though mild damage occurred with doses of 40–61 Gy, moderate damage was noted with doses of 55–104 Gy and severe damage was observed in the 59.5–67.5 Gy range.

The other para-aortic XRT series (Table 18.5) and whole abdominal XRT experiences (Table 18.7) again provide deeper insight into small bowel tolerance. The para-aortic series confirm that doses of 45–50 Gy carry at least a 5% risk of late small bowel damage [158,162–165] if the peritoneal cavity has been violated prior to XRT. If doses of 50–60 Gy are delivered following an intraperitoneal procedure [158,159–161] the late effect rate may be 20–35% with substantial morbidity and mortality. However, if 45–50 Gy is delivered without intraperitoneal violation, the small bowel may be expected to experience minimal [171,172] or no [166,167,169,170,173] toxicity.

### *Fractionation*

Small bowel tolerance also appears to be impacted by fraction size. Table 18.5 shows a greater incidence of late effects at doses of 40–50 Gy when fraction sizes of 1.8–2.0 Gy [158,162,164,167,168] were used (late effects in 13/172 or 8%) vs doses of 40–50 Gy when fraction sizes of 1.5–1.8 Gy [165,170–173] were used (late effects in 5/178 or 3%). Though mitigating factors such as the frequency of intraperitoneal procedures make this type of comparison tenuous, fractionation is important in other clinical and experimental data sets. The Patterns of Care Outcome Studies [150] reported toxicity in 855 Hodgkin's and seminoma patients receiving 25–45 Gy to the infradiaphragmatic nodal groups. The 3-year actuarial rate of major bowel complications was 2% (16/789) if the daily fraction size was 2.0 Gy or less compared with 5% for fraction sizes >2.0 Gy. Similarly, Habrand *et al.* [206] reported a cohort of Hodgkin's disease all treated with the same technique and dose (40 Gy ± 1–5 Gy). Fraction sizes of >2 Gy carried a higher risk of bowel complications ($P = 0.03$) and these complications occurred earlier after therapy than when lower fraction sizes were utilized.

**Table 18.6 Relationship between dose and radiation late effects in the small intestine: Walter Reed experience**

| Dose (Gy) | Colon | | | Small bowel[a] | Mesenteric[a] fibrosis |
|---|---|---|---|---|---|
| | Asymptomatic constriction | Partial obstruction | Perforation | | |
| <40 | 0/92 | 1/92 | 0/92 | 2/99 (2%) | 1/99 |
| 40–44.9 | 1/15 | 1/15 | 0/15 | 2/17 (12%) | 0/17 |
| 45–49.9 | 0/10 | 1/10 | 0/10 | 5/14 (36%) | 1/14 |
| 50–54.9 | 1/21 | 1/21 | 0/21 | 7/21 (33%) | 1/21 |
| 55–59.9 | 1/23 | 3/23 | 0/23 | 5/31 (16%) | 2/31 |
| >60 | 4/57 | 14/57 | 3/57 | 11/36 (31%) | 5/36 |

[a] Late effects expressed as no. with injury/no. evaluable at this dose

**Table 18.7 Late complications of whole abdominal radiation**

| Series [ref.] | Diag-nosis | XRT | No. of patients | Small bowel | Liver (Gy) | Comments |
|---|---|---|---|---|---|---|
| | | | | *No. showing toxicity* | | |
| 1. Dembo [188] | O | ABD: 22.5 Gy; 2.25 Gy/fraction; MS PB; 22.5 Gy; 2.25 Gy/fraction | 75 | 1 | 1 (22.5) | A; two with mild sigmoid stenosis |
| 2. Dembo [189] | O | ABD: 22.5 Gy; 2.25 Gy/fraction; MS PB: 22.5 Gy; 2.25 Gy/fraction | 95 | 7 | 0 (22.5) | A; randomized with series no. 3 |
| 3. Dembo [189] | O | ABD: 22.5 Gy; 2.25 Gy/fraction; OF PB: 22.5 Gy; 2.25 Gy/fraction | 139 | 2 | 0 (22.5) | A; randomized with series no. 2 |
| 4. Fazekas [190] | O | ABD: 30 Gy; 3.75 Gy/fraction; MS PB: none | 25 | 0 | 0 (30) | A; randomized with series no. 5 |
| 5. Fazekas [190] | O | ABD: 40 Gy; 1 Gy/fraction; OF PB: none | 25 | 1 | 0 (40) | A; randomized with series no. 4 |
| 6. Van Bunningen [191] | O | ABD: 25 Gy; 1.5 Gy/fraction; OF PB: 25 Gy; 1.75 Gy/fraction | 85 | 6 | 0 (25) | A |
| 7. Macbeth [192] | O | ABD: 22.5 Gy; 1.25 Gy/fraction; OF PB: 22.5 Gy; 2.25 Gy/fraction | 57 | 8 | 0 (22.5) | A; four SBO treated surgically |
| 8. Loeffler [193] | E | ABD: 30 Gy; 1.25 Gy/fraction; OF PB: 15 Gy; 1.8 Gy/fraction | 16 | 1 | 0 (30) | A |
| 9. Greer [194] | E | ABD: 26–28 Gy; –; MS PB: 20 Gy; – | 31 | 7 | 0 (13) | A; only one patient required surgery for complications |
| 10. Potish [195] | E | ABD: 20 Gy; 2 Gy/fraction; OF PB: 20–30 Gy; 1.5–1.75 Gy/fraction | 27 | 1 | 0 (20) | A; 18 received additional brachytherapy boost |
| 11. Fabian [196] | Colon | ABD: 30 Gy; 1 Gy/fraction; OF Boost: 16 Gy: 1.6 Gy/fraction | 36 | 0 | 0 (20) | Surgical adjuvant given with concomitant 5-FU |
| 12. Brenner [197] | Colon | ABD: 20 Gy; 2.5 Gy/fraction; MS Boost: 20–30 Gy; – | 21 | 2 | 0 (20) | Surgical adjuvant given with concomitant 5-FU |
| 13. Hacker [198] | O | ABD: 30 Gy; 1.2 Gy/fraction; OF PB: 20 Gy; 1.8 Gy/fraction | 30 | 10 | 0 (30) | Salvage |
| 14. Hainsworth [199] | O | ABD: 30 Gy; 1–2 Gy/fraction; OF PB:14–20 Gy in 7 pts. | 17 | 0 | 0 (27.5) | Salvage |
| 15. Schray [200] | O | ABD: 25.5–30 Gy; 1.5 Gy/fraction; OF PB:20–24.5 Gy; 1.5–1.8 Gy/fraction | 53 | 21 | 0 (22.5) | Salvage |
| 16. Fuks [201,202] | O | ABD: 30 Gy; 1.5 Gy/fraction; OF PB: 20 Gy; 1.5–1.8 Gy/fraction | 38 | 3 | 0 (22.5) | Consolidative |
| 17. Steiner [203] | O | ABD: 30 Gy; 1.5 Gy/fraction; OF PB: 20 Gy; 2.0 Gy/fraction | 10 | 0 | 0 (15) | Salvage |
| 18. Goldhirsch [204] | O | ABD: 26 Gy; 2.6 Gy/fraction; MS ABD: 30 Gy; 1.3 Gy/fraction; OF | 19 31 | 1 0 | 0 (26) 0 (30) | Salvage |

MS, moving strip technique; OF, open field; ABD, abdominal therapy; PB, pelvic boost therapy; A, primary therapy; O, ovarian cancer; E, endometrial cancer.

The considerable experimental data which exist [28,207,208] suggest that the $\alpha/\beta$ ratio for early effects is rather large, in the range of 7–15 Gy. The $\alpha/\beta$ ratio for late effects is smaller, in the range of 3–5 Gy. This suggests that for the same total dose, a small increase in dose/fraction could significantly increase late toxicity. Several groups have reported preliminary pilot studies of hyperfractionated [209] or accelerated [210] fractionation based on these data. Edsmyr *et al.* [211] reported a prospective trial in bladder cancer in which patients were randomized to 1.0 Gy fractions t.i.d. (4-h intervals) to a total dose of 84 Gy with a 2-week rest after 42 Gy; or 2.0 Gy fractions q.d. to a total dose of 64 Gy with a 2-week rest after 32 Gy. The 84 Gy group had improved survival without a significant increase in bowel complications requiring surgery. Wang [212] reported use of 1.5 Gy b.i.d. to the pelvis with a planned interruption at 10–14 days. Late effects were no greater in frequency or severity than after common fractionation.

In summary, the available clinical information seems to confirm the experimental data suggesting fractionation is of major importance as far as late small bowel damage is concerned. Fraction sizes of >2.0 Gy should probably be avoided unless the total dose is correspondingly reduced. Doses of ≤1.8 Gy may be even better tolerated but few data exist on this point.

## Volume

The volume of small bowel irradiated is perhaps the greatest determinant of acute effects and a major factor in late toxicity. The most definitive work in this regard was reported by Gallagher and colleagues [116,125] who performed small bowel radiographs at the time of simulation in 150 consecutive patients receiving pelvic radiotherapy. Virtually all were treated with 15 MeV photons, 1.8–2.0 Gy per day, two or more fields per day to a total dose of 45–50 Gy, thus suggesting that observed differences in toxicity resulted from volume of bowel irradiated instead of technique, dose or fraction size differences. Quantitative estimates of pelvic small bowel (PSB) volume in three dimensions was determined by dividing the area of opacification in the AP and lateral views into 1 cm segments and summing the products of the opacified lengths in the two projections. Two-field PSB volume included the volume included by an AP:PA field only, whereas the four-field PSB volume excluded the volume anterior to a plane from 1 cm anterior to the inferior margin of L5 to a point 1 cm cephalad to the pubic ramus. The actual irradiated volume was defined as the PSB receiving the prescribed dose and excluded bowel shielded in the AP:PA or lateral fields. The average PSB volume was reduced by prone positioning, bladder distension and anterior abdominal compression (Table 18.3). However, prior surgery especially abdominopelvic resection (APR) markedly increased the volume of PSB. Moreover, the volume of bowel irradiated correlated extremely well with both acute and late bowel toxicity (Table 18.8). Patients with no prior surgery had no significant volumes irradiated to high dose and no late effects.

Other small bowel volumetric data sets lend credence to the importance of the relationship between bowel volume and late effects. Caspers *et al.* [213] also performed two-field PSB volumetrics in those receiving pelvic XRT. They also found a significant correlation between PSB volume irradiated and acute toxicity. Letschert, Lebesque and de Boer [214] performed a true three-dimensional volumetric analysis of PSB utilizing CT scans. They found a late effect incidence of <5% with up to 500 cm³ compared with 30% with >500 cm³ for 45 Gy in 5 weeks.

Clinical series also substantiate the critical role of treated bowel volume on acute and late toxicity. Perhaps the most obvious example of this is whole abdominal radiation (WAR) experience (Table

**Table 18.8 Average volume irradiated small bowel compared with acute and late gastrointestinal effects**

| Degree of symptoms | Acute[d] | | Chronic | | | | | |
|---|---|---|---|---|---|---|---|---|
| | No. of patients | Average volume (cm³) | No. of patients | Average volume (cm³)[f] | | | | |
| | | | | 45 Gy | 50 Gy | 55 Gy | 60 Gy | 65 Gy |
| No diarrhea | 43 | 58 | 90 | 78 (90) | 17 (72) | 14 (44) | 0.5 (29) | 0 (24) |
| Mild diarrhea[a] | 30 | 116 | 17 | 105 (17) | 34 (13) | 22 (10) | 22 (10) | 17 (8) |
| Responsive diarrhea[b] | 29 | 342 | 5 | 473 (5) | 225 (4) | 225 (4) | 138 (1) | 138 (1) |
| Unresponsive diarrhea[c] | 5 | 485 | 0 | – | – | – | – | – |
| Treatment interruption | 0 | – | – | – | – | – | – | – |
| Small bowel obstruction (SBO) | – | – | 5[e] | 664 (5) | 380 (5) | 317 (2) | – | – |

[a]Not requiring diet change or diphenoxylate.
[b]Responding to diet and/or diphenoxylate.
[c]Not responding to diet or diphenoxylate.
[d]Difference in acute effects by volume irradiated (*P* < 0.001).
[e]SBO in 0/75 without pelvic surgery; 2/50 (4%) with prior non-APR pelvic surgery; 3/25 (12%) with prior APR. All SBOs corrected surgically and alive without late effects.
[f]Figures in parentheses are nos. of patients.
Note: Acute effects – surgery versus no surgery and non-APR surgery versus APR, both *P* < 0.01. Late effects surgery versus no surgery, *P*. < 0.01.
From Gallagher *et al.* [114,123]

18.7). Doses of only 20–35 Gy are used, often with fraction sizes of 1.0–1.5 Gy. Acute toxicity, often profound, is present in 80% or more [192,193,196,198,200,201]. The cumulative late effects reported are 71 of 830 or 9%. This illustrates that WAR by virtue of its huge small bowel treatment volume produces early and late toxicity far in excess of pelvic or para-aortic techniques at similar doses.

Finally, progressive reduction in field size and corresponding PSB irradiation has resulted in progressively diminishing incidence of small bowel obstruction requiring operation. The M.D. Anderson using AP:PA techniques reported a 17.5–25% incidence of SBO requiring surgery with fields above L5 compared with 11% with the superior margin of the field at or below this level [119,215]. This is similar to the 10% incidence using AP:PA techniques reported by Gunderson *et al.* [119] at the Latter Day Saints Hospital in Utah. In contrast, the Massachusetts General Hospital [121] and Mayo [216] reports both utilized a four-field box technique which decreases PSB volume irradiated. They both reported approximately a 5% incidence of small bowel obstruction requiring operation in a total of 236 patients. This compares favorably with the 5% reported incidence of small bowel obstruction from surgery alone (no XRT) in both the M.D. Anderson [119] and Massachusetts General Hospital series [121].

## Biological variables

A wide range of biological variables have been reported as important in the production of late gut damage. These include pelvic inflammatory disease [109,218], hypertension [27,83,109,219], diabetes mellitus [83,109,218,219], body habitus [109,219], age [116,217,220] and sex [109]. Conflicting data exist concerning the importance of all of these factors [217,221,222]. This inconsistency suggests that these variables are less powerful predictors than dose fractionation and volume. Four biological factors – previous surgery, particle therapy, chemotherapy and circadian rhythm – are of sufficient interest to mention briefly.

Previous surgery is acknowledged as clearly increasing the risk for late gut toxicity [116,217,221–223]. Potish in several publications has performed multivariable analyses in which previous surgery carries significant independent predictive power for the development of small bowel obstruction [217,221]. LoIudice, Baxter and Balint [222] performed a retrospective, controlled study comparing patients with radiation enteropathy with a controlled matched group surviving radiation without enteropathy. The group developing enteropathy was seven times more likely to have had prior surgery and surgery was highly statistically associated with the development of late gut toxicity. Izar and others [223] found a near linear association with a number of prior laparotomies and chronic ileal dysfunction incidence. Gallagher's work mentioned previously [116] showed a much higher small bowel obstruction rate in surgically treated patients. Finally, the WAR series in Table 18.7 indicates late effects are much more frequent when WAR is used as salvage after chemotherapy and two or more laparotomies. Series 13–18 in Table 18.7 utilized WAR as salvage with small bowel obstruction in 35/198 (18%). In contrast, series 1–12 used WAR as primary therapy usually after only one laparotomy and reported small bowel obstruction in only 36/632 (6%). The polemic is whether prior surgery exerts its adverse effects purely by increasing the volume of PSB irradiated or via another mechanism. Prior surgery has also been reported to increase the risk of rectal late effects [223]. This suggests that the mechanism may be more complicated than simply volume or mobility alone since the rectum is immobile and one would not expect a change in volume irradiated after surgery. More data on this point are required, but regardless of mechanism, extra caution is warranted when XRT follows surgery.

The radiobiology and rationale for use of particle therapy has been extensively reviewed [28,220,224,225]. Its use remains experimental at present but three groups have reported bladder trials comparing photon irradiation with neutron therapy [225–228]. These trials have all noted a marked increase in serious late bowel toxicity with neutron therapy. Subsequent editorial commentary by Drs Ellis and Weatherburn called attention to the fact that the relative biological effectiveness (RBE) of neutrons relative to photons increases as the neutron dose is lowered. Because of this, a constant RBE of 3.0 cannot be utilized since neutron deposition decreases along the beam path and as the neutron dose decreases its RBE increases. Therefore, 'equivalent photon' isodose plans should be developed for neutron therapy to prevent against overdosing. Pion therapy and helium ion irradiation also has been reported to cause substantial late gut toxicity [220,229]. It is perhaps important to note that helium ions also exhibit substantial change in RBE from plateau to peak of their spread out Bragg peak in intestinal crypt cells [224]. Though the radiobiological and physical properties of particles make them interesting for clinical investigation, the substantial gut toxicity experienced thus far will warrant close monitoring.

Chronotropic effects of antineoplastic therapy are actively being investigated. In this regard, the diurnal cycle of jejunal crypt cells, which have a peak and nadir of mitotic and synthetic activity approximately 12 h apart, may be relevant. Animal experiments by several groups demonstrated the greatest gastrointestinal lethality when animals were irradiated at the peak of jejunal crypt cell activity [230]. The significance of these observations in humans is unknown.

The use of concomitant radiation–chemotherapy is increasingly being utilized for pelvic and gastrointestinal malignancies. It is surprising that there are relatively few data which address the issue of whether these two modalities synergistically promote late effects. A variety of animal experiments have suggested [35] that chemotherapy, especially actinomycin D [230,231] and doxorubicin [232], may exacerbate late effects. Donaldson *et al.* [233] reported a greater likelihood of late gut toxicity among children receiving actinomycin D and WAR. However, several investigators have reported no excessive late effects with high-dose conventionally fractionated XRT and concomitant constant infusion of 5-FU [234–238] or bolus 5-FU [238]. Danjoux and Calton have reported a 30% incidence of late toxicity with split-course high-dose radiation and 5-FU for inoperable rectal cancer [238]. However, the high fraction size and lack of control receiving XRT alone make conclusions tenuous. Two prospective randomized trials [240,241] have compared pelvic radiotherapy alone with pelvic XRT plus concomitant 5-FU with 5-FU and semustine as sandwich chemotherapy. The GTSG using AP:PA fields to 40–48 Gy reported that 2/46 in the combined modality arm compared with 0/50 in the XRT alone experienced lethal late radiation enteritis. The NCCTG trial using similar chemotherapy but a four-field pelvic box technique to approximately 50 Gy found no difference between the XRT alone arm (4/92 with serious enteritis) compared with the combined modality arm (3/96 with serious enteritis). The GTSG unresectable pancreas trial comparing 60 Gy alone with 60 Gy plus 5-FU or 40 Gy plus 5-FU found a greater incidence of nausea, vomiting, diarrhea and late life-threatening gastrointestinal haemorrhage in the combined modality arms [178]. The GTSG follow-up study compared 60 Gy plus 5-FU with 40 Gy doxorubicin in unresectable pancreatic cancer [242]. Severe or worse toxicity was more frequent ($P < 0.02$) with doxorubicin than 5-FU.

In summary, chemotherapy may increase toxicity somewhat but both modalities can be given with acceptable toxicity in several schedules. The schedule dependency, dose effect and other important issues require further study.

## Extrapelvic colon and mesentery

The Walter Reed dose response data are shown in Table 18.6. Colonic constriction and mesenteric fibrosis were quite uncommon below 55 Gy, and were not frequent until $\geqslant$60 Gy. This dose far exceeds small bowel and gastric tolerance and

explains why their experience is unique. Other series in which extrapelvic colon cancer has been treated adjuvantly [196,238,242,243] usually have not exceeded doses of 50–55 Gy $\pm$ 5-FU and have not reported this complication.

## Rectum

### *External beam alone*

External beam alone may cause acute mild to moderate proctocolitis at doses of 40–55 Gy at fractions of 1.8–2.0 Gy. Symptoms include frequency, urgency and burning with bowel movements and rarely bleeding. Acute proctocolitis usually abates within 2–3 weeks of finishing therapy though minor symptoms can persist for several months.

Serious late toxicity from external beam radiotherapy alone is unusual below 60 Gy. Fistula formation is extremely rare with external beam alone. Late toxicity usually consists of mucosal manifestations such as bleeding, friable, tender mucosa which produces pain, urgency and frequency. Luminal narrowing can produce stenosis with tenesmus or obstruction. The pelvis can become densely fibrotic and produce a 'frozen pelvis' picture sometimes termed pseudocarcinoma. Table 18.9 summarizes a variety of pelvic external beam series which have described late toxicity. Rectal adjuvant XRT at doses of 46–50 Gy in 1.8–2.0 Gy fractions (first six series in Table) rarely cause late toxicity and the condition usually resolves without a surgical procedure. Daily fraction sizes above 2.0 Gy may increase rectal late effects at doses of 50–60 Gy as exemplified in the series of Cummings *et al.* [248] and Quilty and Duncan [252]. Interpretation of the Cummings data is difficult since these patients also received concomitant continuous infusion 5-FU and mitomycin C. Doses of 50–60 Gy are also reasonably well tolerated if fraction sizes of 1.8–2.0 Gy are implemented. Rich *et al.* [247] reported 26 patients treated with adjuvant XRT after local excision of rectal cancer. He noted rectal complications in 1/16 receiving <60 Gy versus 5/10 with $\geqslant$63 Gy.

difficult to assess since these doses are rarely delivered to the entire rectal circumference unless it is involved by tumor. The majority of experience with doses of this magnitude comes from prostate or bladder series. These series usually use techniques which treat only a partial rectal circumference. Animal experiments [257] show that partial circumference XRT, even in extremely high doses, will not cause obstruction of the colon, suggesting that bladder and prostate series underestimate the rectal risk of a given dose fractionation scheme. Glimelius and Pahlman [249] treated 19 cases of anal cancer with definitive XRT at doses of 60–65 Gy, 2 Gy per

**Table 18.9 Pelvic external radiotherapy and late effects**

| Series [ref] | No. of patients | Primary | Dose/fraction (Gy) | Small bowel | Rectum | Comments (see key) |
|---|---|---|---|---|---|---|
| | | | | *Complication site* | | |
| Fisher [244] | 184 | Rectum | 46/1.8 | 0 | 0/40 | B,i |
| Schild [216] | 139 | Rectum | 50/1.8–2.0 | 8 (6%) | 1 (1%) | B,i |
| Balslev [245] | 207 | Rectum | 50/2.0 | 21 (10%) | 0/138 | B,i,lethal complications in 1.5% |
| O'Connell [246] | 44 | Rectum | 50/2.0 | 7 (16%) | 0/44 | A,ii,2% required surgery due to XRT alone |
| Vigliotti [215] | 105 | Rectum | 40–50/2.0 | 14 (13%) | 0/33 | A,i |
| Tepper [76] | 165 | Rectum | ≥50.4/1.8 | 12 (7%) | 4/70 (6%) | B,i,lethal SBO – 1 |
| Rich [247] | 26 | Rectum | 50–70+/1.8–2.0 | — | 6/26 (23%) | A – 5;B/C – 21,5/10 complications ≥ 63 Gy; 1/16 complications <60 Gy |
| Cummings [248] | 30 | Anus | 50/2.5 | — | 4/30 (13%) | B,i – 16;ii – 14 Includes anal complications |
| Glimelius [249] | 19 | Anus | 60–65/2.0 | 0 | 9/19 (47%) | A,C,ii All resolved without surgery |
| Yu [250] | 309 | Bladder | 60–66/2.0 | 3 (1%) | 3/309 (1%) | B,i |
| Marcial [251] | 48 | Bladder | 55/2.75 | 1 (2%) | 0 | A,B,C,ii |
| Marcial [251] | 48 | Bladder | 60/2.0 | 0 | 0 | A,B,C,i |
| Quilty [252] | 161 | Bladder | 50–58/2.75 | — | 10/161 (6%) | B,i,complications all RTOG grade 3 or > |
| Forman [253] | 240 | Prostate | 65/1.8–2.0 | 2 (1%) | 17/240 (7%) | C,i,4/17 rectal complications required surgery. |
| Rangala [254] | 128 | Prostate | 65/1.8–2.0 | — | 14/128 (11%) | B,C,i |
| Zagars [255] | 113 | Prostate | 62–71/2.0 | — | 23/113 (20%) | B,i; all resolved spontaneously |
| Pilepich [256] | 267 | Prostate | 65–70+/2.0 | 3/267 (1%) | 16/267 (6%) | A – 82%;B/C – 18%,two SBO and one proctitis required surgery |

A, AP:PA, B, 3- or 4-field technique; C, rotational technique or multifield; i, continous course; ii, split course.

fraction, and noted 47% with chronic proctitis, all of which resolved without surgery. Prostate series utilizing 60–70 Gy report proctitis in 5–20%, but the overwhelming majority resolve without surgery [253,255,256]. The report of complications by Pilepich *et al.* [256] is of considerable interest since 82% of these patients were treated with AP:PA fields only, the boost being delivered via AP fields with 22 MeV photons. Dosimetric data provided [256,258] indicated that the anterior rectal wall routinely received doses >65 Gy while the posterior rectum received ≥60 Gy. Even with these substantial doses, proctitis was reported in only 5% and only 1/267 required surgical intervention. Pilepich has also reported results of two prospective prostate trials [105,106] in which detailed complication rate information and prostate dose data are available in 749 patients. The overall rectal complication rates were almost identical between the two trials with

ulcers in 1–2%, bleeding in 9–10%, stricture in 4–5% and proctitis in 10%. However, no consistent relationship is evident between prostate doses (analyzed at 62.5–65, 65–67.5, 67.5–70 and >70 Gy intervals) and these complications. Helle, Smit and van Patten [259] reported correlations between anterior rectal wall dose above 70 Gy in 153 patients with CT treatment planning and three-field technique. Only 41% had any rectal toxicity even at these high doses. Colostomy was required in 0/37 receiving 70 Gy to the anterior rectal wall; 3/85 (4%) receiving 71–75 Gy; and in 3/31 (10%) with ≥75 Gy. Multivariate Cox regression analysis revealed that only previous pelvic surgery and dose influenced incidence of moderate or severe proctitis. Miller [260] reported rectal toxicity by TDF in 533 bladder cancer patients. Miller's findings by TDF, 2.0 Gy fraction total dose equivalent, and late rectal complications are as follows: TDF 90–99 (approximately

55–60 Gy; 2.0 Gy/fraction), 2/93 (2%) rectal complications; TDF 100–109 (approximately 60–67 Gy; 2.0 Gy/fraction), 1/81 (1%) rectal complication; TDF 110–119 (approximately 68–72 Gy; 2.0 Gy/fraction), 7/122 (6%) rectal complications; TDF >120 (>72 Gy; 2.0 Gy/fraction), 24/38 (63%) rectal complications.

In summary, doses of 45–50 Gy (1.8–2.0 Gy/fraction) will not uncommonly produce acute toxicity but late toxicity is rare [216,244–246]. Doses in the 50–60 Gy range (1.8–2.0 Gy/fraction) may have a 5% incidence of late toxicity but will usually resolve without surgery [76,247]. Doses of 60–65 Gy (1.8–2.0 Gy/fraction) will produce late toxicity in 5–50% [247,249,253,254–256], requiring surgical correction in 5–24% [249,253,256]. Insufficient data exist regarding whole circumference rectal radiation doses above 65 Gy. Partial rectal circumference doses of 65–70 Gy may produce a 5–10% late effect rate, while partial circumference doses of 70–75 Gy may have as much as a 20–60% late effect rate and a colostomy rate approaching 10%.

## External beam and brachytherapy

Cervical carcinoma is overwhelmingly the most frequent indication for brachytherapy and external beam radiation therapy. Rectal complications are reported in all large series with incidences ranging from 2% to 15% [261–267]. Rectal injuries are frequently serious with fistula rates accounting for 12–60% of all rectal injuries.

It is unfortunate that, while rectal complications are a paramount concern, only a few somewhat tentative generalizations can be made regarding their etiology. Part of the problem is the cornucopia of 'systems' utilized to administer the brachytherapy and external beam. Though all give external beam and an implant, both components are prescribed accordingly to widely heterogeneous philosophies. The external beam varies in dose, fraction size, field arrangement, use of midline blocks and sequencing with the implant. Many implant devices exist and prescriptions vary in terms of units (Gy versus mg/h), points of prescription, applicator system, dose rate and in many other respects.

The most consistent risk factor for development of late rectal complications is a prior history of abdominal or pelvic surgery [266]. Bourne *et al.* [266] in a carefully reviewed experience with 784 cervical cancer patients found a 2.5% complication rate in those without prior surgery compared with a 5.3% complication rate in those with prior surgery ($P < 0.05$). In this series no other factor was associated with late effects, with the exception of the development of early complications (see below). Powel-Smith studied 318 cervical carcinoma cases treated by external beam and brachytherapy. While

dose expressed as either overall dose or time-dose equivalents did not correlate with late effects, prior abdominal surgery or non-surgical abdominal disease was associated with a 2.6 increase in relative risk [268]. Several other groups [218,269–271] have documented an increased risk of late complications with prior abdominal surgery or inflammatory abdominopelvic processes (diverticulitis, pelvic inflammatory disease, etc.). van Nagell *et al.* [218] observed this increased risk and found a significantly increased incidence of serosal vessel endarteritis, fibrin thrombosis and perivascular fibrosis in patients with non-irradiated bowel after pelvic inflammatory disease alone compared with age-matched controls. They postulated this was important etiologically.

Dose is another possible factor, though there have been several reports, some of which included direct dosimeter readings of the anterior rectal wall, which show no correlation of dose and complications [266,268,272]. However, the preponderance of experience is that dose is important. Several investigators have reported a correlation of dose to point A (or permutation of point A) with rectal late effects [264,265,269,273,274]. Stryker *et al.* [267] measured rectal dose via computer modeling in 132 patients and found rectal dose with the implant delivered a mean dose of 39.2 Gy in those with severe rectal injury compared with 31.3 Gy in those with no or mild toxicity ($P = 0.03$). Orton and Wolf-Rosenblum [262] compared TDFs from data derived by direct intracavitary dosimetric measurements among patients with severe rectal injury and randomly selected controls. The incidence as well as the severity of rectal toxicity was directly related to the TDF. Perez *et al.* [275] have also found a slightly higher rate of rectal complications when the total dose (external + implant) is >80 Gy. The Perez and Orton series are both flawed by the fact that significant numbers of actual patient data or implant films were not available and doses in these cases were estimated. Overall, the literature supports some association between dose and rectal toxicity, though admittedly the association is not extraordinarily powerful or completely consistent from series to series. One major problem in seeking a correlation of dose with toxicity is the substantial heterogeneity of dose three-dimensionally and the marked variation of dose-limiting structure location within this heterogeneous volume. Also, computerized dose distributions around shielded ovoids are in error by 10–20% since treatment planning software is unable to account for the shields [276,277]. Ling and others [277] studied eight patients with Fletcher-Suit applicators with CT-assisted three-dimensional treatment planning. The maximum organ doses were, on average, two times higher with CT planning than with the orthogonal film pair method. These differences were highly variable from patient to patient. Hopefully, the advent of three-dimensional treatment planning will allow future investigators to address this issue more completely.

Finally, geometric problems with placement of the implant exacerbate toxicity. It is difficult to generalize because of the plethora of implant applicators and philosophies. Some groups routinely allow the use of protruding sources from the tandem with acceptable morbidity, but others operating under different systems and philosophies utilize protruding sources only in difficult situations and experience increasing rates of rectal ulcers [278]. Narrow vaginal vaults [278] and retroflexed uteri [268,275] are also associated with higher complication rates. The Ernst application has, in some hands, been associated with higher complication rates [265,279]. We are still practising in an era where the therapy of cervical carcinoma is largely empirical. It is, therefore, not surprising that implementation of non-standard loading or geometry [266] which is not empirically tested is associated with higher complication rates.

## Association of early versus late effects

The relationship between acute and late effects is not well understood. The majority who develop late effects have no acute complications [209,264]. This has prompted some to comment that acute and late effects do not necessarily share the same etiological factors [280]. Nevertheless, several recent laboratory [14,28] and clinical [32,114,123,135,266,281] experiences suggest that early and late effects are linked. Bourne *et al.* [266] reported among 1390 consecutive cervix cancer patients an 8.2% late complication rate in those who had early complications compared with 3.0% late complications in those who had not (increased relative risk of 2.7; $P < 0.05$). However, 75% with late complications did not have a severe acute one. Thames [280] has pointed out that while there appeared to be an association between late and early toxicity, the factors predicting for either early or late toxicity were different. Moreover, since fractionation schedule was constant in Bourne's data, it does not address the potential differential impact of fractionation on early versus late effects. This is especially important since the $\beta/\alpha$ ratio is larger for late effects in experimental systems [28,207,208,280] predicting that, for the same total dose, a decrease in dose/fraction could reduce late effects. Gallagher has reported that irradiated small bowel volume predicts for both acute and late toxicity [114], but again fractionation scheme was constant in his material. In summary, while early and late effects seem associated by volume of bowel irradiated and other factors, they may still be influenced by different pathophysiological mechanisms which could be amenable to therapeutic exploitation.

# Treatment
## Acute toxicity

Toxicity occurring during and shortly after radiation is managed symptomatically. Though there are few hard scientific data available, these remedies are sufficient to allow completion of prescribed therapy in the overwhelming majority. No prospective data exist regarding the optimal use of antiemetics. If significant stomach or small bowel volumes are within the treatment field, prophylactic use of antiemetics should be considered. If nausea and vomiting persist, lower daily fraction sizes will often reduce symptoms and total doses can be modified so as not to compromise tumor control [35]. Diarrhea is managed initially with antispasmodic, anticholinergic and opiate analogues. Nutritional considerations are important to address by careful monitoring of weight, caloric intake and stools during therapy. A defined diet low in fiber, milk, fat and lactose may decrease the severity of enteritis [14]. If diarrhea becomes severe despite these interventions, a treatment interruption is required. Proctitis is treated initially by control of diarrhea which often accompanies it. Sitz baths and perineal compresses have also been used if simple analgesics fail. Steroid enemas or suppositories are also often employed though no data exist regarding their efficacy. Several studies have recently utilized sulfasalazine (Salazopyrin) [282,283] or formalin [284] with favorable early results. Symptoms of acute gastrointestinal toxicity will usually begin to resolve within 7–10 days after discontinuing treatment and abate within 2–3 weeks.

## Chronic toxicity
### *Conservative therapy*

Gastric late effects of gastritis, duodenitis or uncomplicated ulcers can be initially managed by $H_2$-receptor blockers possibly with sucralfate in addition. The majority of patients will heal with conservative therapy [85,88,89]. In Hamilton's series [89], 35 ulcers were proven radiographically of which eight required subtotal gastrectomy and eight died with autopsy. The high mortality may have been due to undue surgical delay [85]. These patients need extremely careful endoscopic and radiographic follow-up. In general, the indications for surgery are similar to those of benign peptic ulcer disease [88,89]. Failure to heal with conservative therapy, perforation, hemorrhage or obstruction provide justification for surgery unless extenuating circumstances exist. Gastric ulcers were complicated by perforation or hemorrhage in about 40% of the Walter Reed series [84,85] and were fatal in 8/35 in Hamilton's report [89]. The fact that subtotal gastrectomy appears curative in the majority argues strongly for close follow-up with surgical intervention judiciously employed.

Small intestinal late effects present in many forms. Malabsorption, obstruction, fistula, hemorrhage or perforation all require somewhat different therapeutic approaches. Barring catastrophic presentations, patients require thorough evaluation of other potential nutritional or anatomical problems. Though precise definition of etiology and specific therapy are the goal, in practice many of these patients have had numerous surgeries present with extremely complex problems and sometimes require empirical therapy.

Malnutrition following radiation requires thoughtful and complete clinical, laboratory and radiographic evaluation. Potential causes of malnutrition are myriad. Recurrent neoplasm and anatomical-physiological complications of previous surgery must be ruled out. Even when radiation enteropathy seems most likely, the potential mechanisms by which radiation damage can produce malnutrition must all be considered. Diminished absorptive capacity of the terminal ileum for bile salts is a well recognized cause of chronic diarrhea, as previously discussed. When limited portions of ileum are dysfunctional, cholestyramine (a bile salt anion-exchange resin) can ameliorate diarrhea. Heusinkveld, Manning and Aristizabal [285] documented resolution of diarrhea with cholestyramine in four patients with late toxicity from radiation enteropathy. Extensive ileal dysfunction produces diarrhea because of both bile salt and fat malabsorption. Therefore cholestyramine may be inadequate to abate the diarrhea. Bosaeus, Andersson and Nystrom [137] reported control of diarrhea with a low-fat diet (without medium chain triglycerides added) in all but one of nine patients with radiation enteropathy. The ninth patient required cholestyramine plus the low-fat diet to control diarrhea. More diffuse absorptive defects are probably best managed by dietary intervention with elemental enteral or parenteral feedings.

Malabsorption can also result from bacterial overgrowth due to fistula(e) or to defunctionalized loops of small bowel (which diminish peristalsis and allow segments of bowel in which bacteria propagate excessively). Fistulae often are amenable to definitive surgical correction. Medical therapy with broad-spectrum antibiotics for bacterial overgrowth is often efficacious as well [33,286,287].

Obstruction following XRT similarly has several potential etiologies including recurrent tumor, post-operative adhesions and radiation enteropathy. A substantial percentage of radiation-induced small bowel obstructions are partial [62] and amenable to conservative therapy. The majority of small bowel obstructions will eventually require surgery [76,114,122,150,216,241,288]. However, 20–60% may resolve with decompression and conservative therapy making this the initial management policy in uncomplicated obstruction [150,216,241,288]. A trial of conservative decompression will allow a substantial percentage to avoid surgery, provide time to thoroughly evaluate the patient, and allow institution of total parenteral nutrition which will facilitate surgery should it become necessary.

Medical therapy can be considered in patients with radiation small bowel damage who do not require surgery or decompression. Goldstein, Khoury and Thornton [289] provided long-term follow-up on four patients with severe well documented radiation enteritis and colitis. All were treated with sulfasalazine and demonstrated clear clinical improvement with complete or near-complete radiographic regression of abnormalities in three cases and incomplete regression in one. Donaldson *et al*. [233] reported the use of elemental diets in five children with severe laparotomy-confirmed radiation enteropathy. All five had resolution of obstruction, malabsorption, radiographic changes and histological abnormalities and were able to resume a normal diet after 1–2 years. These reports of reversal of late toxicity with medical therapy are, obviously, fragmentary though optimistic. More investigation is required.

Radiation proctitis is usually a self-limited, often subclinical process [32,290,291]. Gilinsky and colleagues [291] in 88 proctosigmoiditis cases found a high rate of spontaneous remission with conservative therapy in those without transfusion requirements and little bowel disturbance or pain. Those with transfusion-dependent bleeding and substantial bowel disturbance or pain rarely underwent spontaneous remission. Conservative management with soft softeners, sitz baths, perianal hygiene and analgesics are simple, non-morbid modalities which are often employed. Steroid retention enemas are often administered though no documentation of their efficacy exists. Two recent reports [282,283] suggest sulfasalazine enemas may be of substantial benefit in both mild and severe cases of XRT-induced proctitis. Recently, endoscopic laser therapy for severe radiation-induced rectal bleeding has been demonstrated in a few reports to be highly effective [292,293] and should be strongly considered in patients with this presentation.

## Surgical therapy

Surgical therapy applies general surgical principles to the specific pitfalls of operating on radiation damaged bowel. When possible the extent of radiation damage should be delineated radiographically. The prior radiation portals should be carefully reviewed to define all irradiated tissues and to allow non-irradiated, non-damaged sites to be identified preoperatively. Biochemical and nutritional problems are common since many have malabsorption preceding their surgical problem. Several series document improved surgical results with total parenteral nutrition (TPN) [77,93,98,99]. Optimal surgical results will require correction of existing abnormalities and a positive nitrogen balance. It is difficult, however, to ascribe all of the improved results to nutrition alone because other diagnostic and therapeutic modalities became available during the period when TPN was introduced.

Patients with obstruction require either resection of affected bowel or bypass. Adhesiolysis of obvious radiation-induced obstruction is ill advised [27,78,81,82]. Radiated bowel has limited vascularity and adhesiolysis may further impair blood supply increasing the risk of fistula or perforation. Nevertheless, a subset of intestinal obstructions following combined modality therapy will be due to an isolated band of adhesion resulting from the surgery. In these instances, lysis of adhesions can be cautiously employed [77,98].

Bowel complications requiring surgery will require either a resection or bypass procedure. There are numerous advocates of both procedures. Table 18.10 summarizes the surgical complications and mortality with each procedure. Swan, Fowler and Boronow [294] reviewed the literature and selected 199 patients treated for radiation enteropathy with either a resection or bypass. Though no bibliographical sources were cited, they found a postoperative mortality of 21% and anastomotic dehiscence rate of 21% in the resection group. The bypass group, in comparison, had only a 10% mortality and a 6% dehiscence rate. Unfortunately, bypass procedures leave diseased bowel behind and these segments can cause problems such as hemorrhage, perforation, fistulization or development of a blind loop syndrome. In Swan's own series, 56% of the bypass group had chronic significant intestinal problems. Galland and Spencer [80] reported persistent bleeding, fistulization or perforation in 32% of 22 bypassed. DeCosse *et al.* reported almost half of their sigmoid colostomies developed complications requiring refashioning [81]. Despite these objections, bypass procedures have documented efficacy and will be required in patients with rectovaginal fistula, massively damaged bowel precluding more extensive operations, or patients too ill to tolerate lengthy operations. If a bypass procedure is performed for rectovaginal fistula, it should be constructed so that future repair of the fistula is possible [32,79,81]. Either a loop ileostomy [79] or a colostomy in the right transverse colon [32] have been suggested if future repair is contemplated. Sigmoid colostomies seem ill-advised since the sigmoid colon's location near or within the previous XRT field makes it susceptible to XRT damage [81].

Resection, as shown in Table 18.10, carries a substantial risk of morbidity and mortality. It is difficult to directly compare resection with bypass, since different selection criteria for the two procedures exist from series to series. Nevertheless, resection of bowel damaged by irradiation is a formidable procedure which should be reserved preferably for surgeons experienced in its management. Several data sets demonstrate improved outcome with resection as a result of modern antibiotics, TPN [77,93,98,99], tube decompression [41,78,99], and experience [32,93,99]. Galland and Spencer [32] reported that with the implementation of terminal ileal resection followed by ileo-transverse anastomosis and/or rectosigmoid resection followed by mobilization of the splenic flexure for anastomosis, no clinically apparent anastomotic leaks or operative deaths have occurred in 14

**Table 18.10 Surgical management of late gastrointestinal complications**

| Series [ref.] | Bypass[a] complication | Mortality[b] | Resection complication | Mortality[b] |
|---|---|---|---|---|
| Localio [92] | 1/1 | 1 | 0/11 | 0 |
| Sugg [41] | 3/4 | 1 | 7/27 | 4 |
| Swan [294] | 3/28 | 2 | 13/17 | 9 |
| Makela [295] | 11/26 | 2 | 9/17 | 4 |
| Miholic [95] | 7/17 | ? | 5/15 | ? |
| Cram [82] | 7/19 | 2 | 2/7 | 1 |
| Dirksen [101] | 6/11 | 2 | 5/15 | 0 |
| Galland [80] | 5/13 | 1 | 11/24 | 10 |
| Galland [32] | | | 0/14 | 0 |
| Cochrane [94] | 7/15 | 5 | 3/6 | 3 |
| Lillemoe [91] | 3/11 | 1 | 3/6 | 3 |
| Total | 53/145 (37%) | 17/128 (13%) | 58/159(36%) | 34/144(24%) |

[a]Diverting colostomy considered bypass procedure.
[b]Mortality includes deaths from complications of surgery or any deaths in postoperative period.

patients. Prior to implementation of these techniques, 14 of 27 anastomoses leaked and 10 of 24 died [80]. Marks and Mohiuddin described no leaks in intraperitoneal anastomoses and only four in 52 extraperitoneal anastomoses [296]. Optimal results require anastomoses to be performed in healthy bowel. Frozen sections have been advocated [27,41,78,81,82,101] in this regard, though some [32] find them of little benefit. Omental pedicles can be sutured around an anastomosis to further decrease dehiscence [78,98]. Palmer and Bush [297] reported only two leaks in 31 resections using an omental pedicle wrap.

Rectovaginal fistulae are notoriously difficult management problems prompting many to abandon attempts at repair and relegate management to diverting colostomy [27]. More recently several groups have successfully repaired these lesions. A proximal diverting colostomy is initially performed and reconstruction utilizing non-irradiated tissue is attempted after a prolonged period (usually 1 year or more) to allow full resolution of inflammation and maximal healing. A Martius technique (using a bulbocavernous-labial flap) has been used to successfully repair radiation-induced rectovaginal fistula in 16/19 by Boronow [298] and in 11/12 by White et al. [299]. However, Aartsen and Sindram [300] reported that while successful initial closure was achieved with the Martius procedure in 14/14 cases, subsequent progression of radiation damage was significant and with follow-up only 6/14 remained colostomy-free and vaginal intercourse was exceedingly uncommon. These authors favor use of gracilis muscle repair over the Martius technique [293,300]. Graham utilized gracilis flaps successfully in 16/21 vaginal fistulae [301]. An alternative to these techniques is the colo-anal pull-through. Cooke and DeMoor [302] and Cooke and Wellsted [303] achieved continence in approximately 75% of 28 patients at 1 year. Though these series attest to the value of surgical repair in rectovaginal fistulae, it should be emphasized that these repairs should be performed only in selected cases after optimal preoperative evaluation and preparation by experienced surgeons.

## Hepatic radiation toxicity

The sensitivity of the liver to radiation and the striking clinical syndrome of radiation toxicity has been described only since the mid 1960s. There are several explanations for the surprisingly long delay before this entity was first described. In the first place, animal models often fail to mimic the characteristic human pattern of radiation toxicity [304,305]. Secondly, initial animal experiment results indicated marked radiation resistance [394]. Finally, in Case and Warthin's initial pathological

description of radiation toxicity in humans they focused their attention largely on bile duct changes while minimizing hepatic parenchymal effects [304]. The report by Ingold et al. in 1965 was the first and remains the quintessential report of radiation hepatitis [306].

The clinicopathological description of acute and chronic radiation-induced hepatic toxicity is well known [305–309]. The liver will manifest enzyme elevation and decreased radioisotopic uptake after modest doses of radiation. These findings are rarely symptomatic until the entire liver (or at least a substantial portion of its volume) receives therapy [310,312]. Acute radiation toxicity usually presents 2–6 weeks after completion of therapy [306,308] though it may not become manifest for 6 months or longer [308,312]. Severity of acute toxicity varies markedly but generally symptoms include rapid weight gain, increase in abdominal girth, fatigue and anorexia [306,308]. Physical examination shows hepatomegaly, ascites and sometimes pleural effusions and laboratory findings of elevated serum alkaline phosphatase out of proportion to the elevations of SGOT and SGPT are characteristic [306,308]. Occasionally transient thrombocytopenia has been observed [305,310]. Liver scanning during this period will show decreased uptake in the XRT portal if partial liver volumes were given [310,312–314]. Biopsy findings during this period are those of veno-occlusive liver disease (VOD). VOD is characterized by obstruction of the central veins by loose, edematous fibrous tissue associated with variable centrilobular congestion and liver cell atrophy. Many red blood cells are present within a mesh of collagen and reticulin fibers. Necrosis of liver cells is present around the central vein. Portal veins are occasionally involved in a similar process. Electron microscopy confirms the above and also reveals fibrin in the central veins, usually abundantly. This morphological picture is strongly reminiscent of VOD which occurs with the pyrrolizidine alkaloids of 'bush tea' in the West Indies, as well as the VOD described with cytarabine, 6-thioguanine, graft-versus-host disease, etc.

The majority of patients in Ingold's series recovered uneventfully. Three died from widespread tumor, three from VOD, and seven were alive at 1 year with five of these achieving complete recovery of all abnormalities. However, Wharton's group fared less well with 10 of 14 succumbing to their acute toxicity. Tefft et al. found only seven of 37 with acute toxicity to have complete normalization with follow-up [310]. The management of acute toxicity is that of hepatic insufficiency of any cause. Remarkably, when patients recover from VOD their histological changes can revert entirely to normal. The centrilobular congestion is alleviated by recanalization of the occluded central vein, or by development of collateral circulation [308,310].

When radiation damage is more severe and the centrilobular zone fails to reconstitute and becomes fibrosed, the deleted hepatic cells are not replaced. There can be progressive sclerosis of arterioles and development of portal and trabecular fibrosis [306–310]. Fully expressed, this damage closely resembles finely nodular cirrhosis both pathologically and clinically.

The incidence of radiation VOD is influenced by volume of liver treated, total dose, chemotherapy, age and probably fraction size and technique. The liver frequently receives moderate dose radiation to half or more of its volume in a variety of upper abdominal malignancies without clinical sequelae of hepatic insufficiency. This is undoubtedly due to the functional reserve of the organ. Though substantial liver volumes can be safely included to doses of 45–55 Gy, great caution should be exercised when therapy to more than 0.5–0.6 of the volume is contemplated. The relationship between the incidence of acute VOD hepatitis and dose utilizing open field technique is shown in Table 18.11. The

**Table 18.11 Relationship between the incidence of radiation hepatitis and dose**

| Dose | Ingold [306] | Tefft [319][a] | Phillips [316] | Total |
|---|---|---|---|---|
| ≤30 | 1/9 | 0/12 | 0/14 | 1/35 (3%) |
| ≥30–35 | 2/9 | 0/4 | 1/25 | 2/38 (5%) |
| >35–40 | 7/18[b] | 0/3 | 0/6 | 7/27 (26%) |
| >40 | 3/4[c] | – | – | 3/4 (75%) |

[a]Includes only patients treated to whole liver without resection.
[b]One death.
[c]Two deaths.

data regarding safety of whole organ doses of >30 Gy are quite limited, though doses of 25–30 Gy appear to be reasonably safe. Doses of ≥30 Gy were delivered to a total of 102 patients via open field technique in Table 18.7 as part of whole abdominal therapy [190,193,198,204]. None developed acute radiation hepatitis. Kim *et al.* treated whole abdomen to 30 Gy in 1 Gy fractions in 117 consecutive lymphoma cases [314] with only two instances of acute hepatitis which was reversible in both. Though 30 Gy is reasonably safe if conventionally fractionated, occasional reports of severe, sometimes fatal acute toxicity with doses less than 30 Gy have appeared [305,312,315]. Finally, acute toxicity rises quickly from >30 Gy to 40 Gy, and Ingold reported three fatalities with doses of 38 Gy and above.

Chemotherapy has been utilized with radiation safely in several trials [317,318] though fragmentary data suggest its use may increase the risk of acute toxicity. Actinomycin D [310,312] and vincristine [319] both have been implicated in this regard.

However, several multimodality trials have documented the feasibility and safety of this approach. In combination with 21 Gy (seven fractions), doxorubicin and intra-arterial 5-FU (13 patients), doxorubicin, 5-FU, intra-arterial methotrexate, and leucovorin (folinic acid) (11 patients), doxorubicin, intra-arterial methotrexate and mitomycin C (eight patients), and doxorubicin, intravenous 5-FU and mitomycin C (12 patients) have all been well tolerated from a hepatic standpoint [317]. Concomitant infusional 5-FU (25 mg/kg/day, days 1–5, weeks 1, 3, 5) has been administered with 27.75 Gy (1.8–2.0 Gy/fraction) without hepatic toxicity in 23 patients [320]. Continuous infusion doxorubicin (12 mg/m$^2$/day, days 1–5) with concomitant radiation (1.5 Gy, days 1–5) every 4 weeks for 3–4 cycles or 22.5–30 Gy also produced no acute hepatic toxicity in 11 patients [321].

Children have developed acute VOD at doses below 25 Gy [310,312,313] suggesting that the pediatric age group may be at greater risk. Finally, patients treated with moving strip technique have developed VOD at doses below 30 Gy [188,308] as have some treated with high daily fractions [305] or immediately following hepatic resection [310]. Caution is therefore appropriate when utilizing these regimens.

# References


1. Walsh, D. Deep tissue traumatism from roentgen ray exposure. *British Medical Journal*, **ii**, 272 (1897)
2. Parliament, M., Danjoux, C. and Clayton, T. Is cancer treatment toxicity accurately reported? *International Journal of Radiation Oncology, Biology, Physics*, **11**, 603–608 (1985)
3. Rubin, P. and Casarett, G. *Clinical Radiation Pathology*, W.B. Saunders, Philadelphia, pp. 153–292 (1968)
4. Young, E. and Gaylord, J. Experimental tests of corrections for tissue inhomogeneities in radiotherapy. *British Journal of Radiology*, **43**, 349–355 (1970)
5. Batho, H. Lung corrections in cobalt-60 beam therapy. *Journal of the Canadian Association of Radiologists*, **15**, 79–83 (1964)
6. Ryall, R. and Rapley, L. A source of error in pelvic dosimetry. *South African Medical Journal*, **43**, 1493–1495 (1969)
7. Dische, S. and Zanelli, J. Bowel gas – a cause of elevated dose in radiotherapy. *British Journal of Radiology*, **49**, 148–150 (1976)
8. Creamer, B. Malignancy and the small-intestinal mucosa. *British Medical Journal*, **ii**, 1435–1436 (1964)
9. Wengell, A. and Deller, D. Malabsorption syndrome associated with carcinoma of the bronchus. *Gut*, **6**, 73–76 (1965)
10. Loehry, C. and Creamer, B. Post-mortem study of

small intestinal mucosa. *British Medical Journal*, **i**, 827–829 (1966)

11. Barry, R. Malignancy, weight loss, and the small intestinal mucosa. *Gut*, **15**, 562–570 (1974)

12. Dymock, I., Mackay, N., Miller, V. *et al*. Small intestinal function in neoplastic disease. *British Journal of Cancer*, **21**, 505–511 (1967)

13. Klipstein, F. and Smarch, G. Intestinal structure and function in neoplastic. *American Journal of Digestive Diseases*, **14**, 887–889 (1969)

14. Bounous, G. The use of elemental diets during cancer therapy. *Anticancer Research*, **3**, 299–304 (1983)

15. Gleeson, M., Cullen, J. and Dowling, R. Intestinal structure and function following small bowel by-pass in the rat. *Clinical Science*, **43**, 731–732 (1972)

16. Harig, J.M., Soergel, K.H., Komorowski, R.A. and Wood, C.M. Treatment of diversion colitis with short-chain-fatty acid irrigation. *New England Journal of Medicine*, **320**, 23–28 (1989)

17. Hochter, W., Kuhner, W. and Ottenjann, R. Rare forms of colitis. *Hepatogastroenterology*, **30**, 211–221 (1983)

18. Montagna, W. and Wilson, J. Cytologic study of intestinal epithelium of mouse after total body X-irradiation. *Journal of the National Cancer Institute*, **15**, 1703–1736 (1955)

19. Bosniak, M., Hardy, M., Quint, J. and Ghossein, N. Demonstration of the effect of irradiation on canine bowel using *in vivo* photographic magnification angiography. *Radiology*, **93**, 1361–1368 (1969)

20. Fonkalsrud, E., Sanchez, M., Zerubavel, R. and Mahoney, A. Serial changes in arterial structure following radiation therapy. *Surgery, Gynecology and Obstetrics*, **145**, 395–400 (1977)

21. Cooling, C. Irradiation damage to the bowel. *Proceedings of the Royal Society of Medicine*, **53**, 650 (1960)

22. Tarpila, S. Morphological and functional response of the human small intestinal mucosa to ionizing radiation. *Scandinavian Journal of Gastroenterology*, **6**, 1 (1971)

23. Wiernik, G. Radiation damage and repair in the human jejunal mucosa. *Journal of Pathology*, **91**, 389 (1966)

24. Warren, S. and Friedman, N. Pathology and pathologic diagnosis of radiation lesions in the gastrointestinal tract. *American Journal of Pathology*, **18**, 499–513 (1942)

25. Greenberger, N. and Isselbacher, K. Malabsorption following radiation injury to the gastrointestinal tract. *American Journal of Medicine*, **36**, 450–456 (1964)

26. Hauer-Jensen, M., Poulakos, L. and Osborne, J.W. Effects of accelerated fractionation on radiation injury of the small intestine: a new rat model. *International Journal of Radiation Oncology, Biology, Physics*, **14**, 1205–1212 (1988)

27. Localio, S., Pachter, H. and Gouge, T. The radiation-injured bowel. *Surgery Annual*, **11**, 181–205 (1979)

28. van der Kogel, A., Jarrett, K., Paciotti, M. and Raju, M. Radiation tolerance of the rat rectum to fractionated X-rays and pi-mesons. *Radiotherapy and Oncology*, **12**, 225–232 (1988)

29. Kwitko, A., Pieterse, A., Hecker, R. *et al*. Chronic radiation injury to the intestine: a clinicopathological study. *Australian and New Zealand Journal of Medicine*, **12**, 272–277 (1982)

30. Rogers, L. and Goldstein, H. Roentgen manifestations of radiation injury to the gastrointestinal tract. *Gastrointestinal Radiology*, **2**, 281–291 (1977)

31. Wellwood, J. and Jackson, B. The intestinal complications of radiotherapy. *British Journal of Surgery*, **60**, 814–818 (1973)

32. Galland, R. and Spencer, J. Natural history and surgical management of radiation enteritis. *British Journal of Surgery*, **74**, 742–747 (1987)

33. Earnest, D. and Trier, J. Radiation enteritis and colitis. In *Gastrointestinal Disease*, Volume 2, (eds M. Sleisinger and J. Fordtran), W.B. Saunders, Philadelphia, pp. 1736–1745 (1978)

34. Trier, J. and Browning, T. Morphologic response of the mucosa of human small intestine to X-ray exposure. *Journal of Clinical Investigation*, **45**, 194–204 (1966)

35. Kinsella, T. and Bloomer, W. Tolerance of the intestine to radiation therapy. *Surgery, Gynecology and Obstetrics*, **151**, 273–284 (1980)

36. Moss, W., Brand, W. and Battifora, H. The gastrointestinal tract. In *Radiation Oncology: Rationale, Technique, Results*, 5th edn (eds W. Moss, W. Brand and H. Battifora), C.V. Mosby Company, St Louis, pp. 332–365 (1979)

37. Messier, B. and Leblond, C. Cell proliferation and migration as revealed by radioautography after injection of thymidine-H$^3$ into male rats and mice. *American Journal of Anatomy*, **106**, 247 (1960)

38. MacDonald, W., Trier, J. and Everett, N. Cell proliferation and migration in the stomach, duodenum, and rectum of man: radioautographic studies. *Gastroenterology*, **46**, 405–417 (1964)

39. Spratt, J., Heinbecker, P. and Saltzstein, S. The influence of succinylsulfathiazole (sulfasuxidine) upon the response of canine small intestine to irradiation. *Cancer*, **14**, 862–874 (1961)

40. Zweifach, B. and Kivy-Rosenberg, E. Microcirculatory effects of whole-body X-irradiation and radiomimetic procedures. *American Journal of Physiology*, **208**, 492–498 (1965)

41. Sugg, W., Lawler, W., Ackerman, L. and Butcher, H. Operative therapy for severe irradiational injury in the enteral and urinary tracts. *Annals of Surgery*, **157**, 62–70 (1962)

42. Wood, I., Ralston, M. and Kurrle, G. Irradiation injury to the gastrointestinal tract: clinical features, management, and pathogenesis. *Australasian Annals of Medicine*, **12**, 143–152 (1963)

43. Goldgraber, M., Rubin, C., Palmer, W. *et al.* The early gastric response to irradiation, a serial biopsy study. *Gastroenterology*, **27**, 1–20 (1954)

44. Doig, R., Funder, J. and Weiden, S. Serial gastric biopsy studies in a case of duodenal ulcer treated by deep X-ray therapy. *Medical Journal of Australia*, **38**, 828–830 (1951)

45. Duncan, W. and Leonard, J. Malabsorption syndrome following radiotherapy. *Quarterly Journal of Medicine*, **34**, 319–329 (1965)

46. Lipkin, M., Quastler, H. and Muggia, F. Protein synthesis in the irradiated intestine of the mouse. *Radiation Research*, **19**, 227–285 (1963)

47. Vatistas, S. and Hornsey, S. Radiation-induced protein loss into the gastrointestinal tract. *British Journal of Radiology*, **34**, 547–550 (1966)

48. Wetterfors, J., Liljedahl, S., Plantin, L. and Birke, G. The acute radiation syndrome – the importance of the gastrointestinal injury in the catabolism and distribution of serum albumin. *Acta Medica Scandinavica*, **177**, 227–242 (1965)

49. Reeves, R., Cavanaugh, P., Sharpe, K. *et al.* Fat absorption from the human gastrointestinal tract in patients undergoing radiation therapy. *Radiology*, **73**, 398–401 (1959)

50. Reeves, R., Sanders, A., Isley, J. *et al.* Fat absorption studies and small bowel X-ray studies in patients undergoing Co-60 teletherapy and/or radium application. *American Journal of Roentgenology*, **94**, 848–851 (1965)

51. Anderson, H., Bosaeus, I. and Nystrom, C. Bile salt malabsorption in the radiation syndrome. *Acta Radiologica Oncology*, **17**, 312–318 (1978)

52. Stryker, J., Mortel, R. and Hepner, G. The effect of pelvic irradiation on lactose absorption. *International Journal of Radiation Oncology, Biology, Physics*, **4**, 859–863 (1978)

53. Finlay, J., Hogarth, J. and Wightman, K. A clinical evaluation of the D-xylose tolerance test. *Annals of Internal Medicine*, **61**, 411 (1964)

54. Christopher, N. and Bayless, T. Role of the small bowel and colon in lactose-induced diarrhea. *Gastroenterology*, **60**, 845 (1971)

55. Overgaard, J. and Matsui, M. Effect of irradiation on glucose absorption in the mouse jejunum (abstract). *Proceedings of the European Society of Therapeutic Radiation Oncology* p. 279 (1988)

56. Sullivan, M. Dependence of radiation diarrhea on the presence of bile salts in the intestine. *Nature*, **195**, 1217–1218 (1962)

57. Sullivan, M., Hulse, E. and Mole, R. The mucus-depleting action of bile in the small intestine of the irradiated rat. *British Journal of Experimental Pathology*, **46**, 235–244 (1965)

58. Newman, A., Katsaris, J., Blendis, L. *et al.* Small-intestinal injury in women who have had pelvic radiotherapy. *Lancet*, **ii**, 1471–1473 (1973)

59. Stryker, J., Hepner, G. and Mortel, R. The effect of pelvic irradiation on ileal function. *Therapeutic Radiology*, **124**, 213–216 (1977)

60. Wang, S., Renzi, A. and Chinn, H. Mechanism of emesis following X-irradiation. *American Journal of Physiology*, **193**, 335–339 (1958)

61. Conard, R. Effect of X-irradiation on intestinal motility of the rat. *American Journal of Physiology*, **165**, 375 (1951)

62. Wittich, G., Salomonowitz, E., Szepesi, T. *et al.* Small bowel double-contrast enema in stage III ovarian cancer. *American Journal of Roentgenology*, **142**, 299–304 (1984)

63. Dickson, H. Effect of X-irradiation on glucose absorption. *American Journal of Physiology*, **182**, 477–486 (1955)

64. Fenton, P. and Dickson, H. Changes in some gastrointestinal functions following X-irradiation. *American Journal of Physiology*, **177**, 528–530 (1954)

65. Brecher, G., Cronkite, E., Conard, R. and Smith, W. Gastric lesions in experimental animals following single exposures to ionizing radiations. *American Journal of Pathology*, **34**, 105–119 (1958)

66. Bond, V. Effects of radiation on intestinal absorption. *American Journal of Clinical Nutrition*, **12**, 194–204 (1963)

67. Perino, L., Schuffler, M., Mehta, S. and Everson, G. Radiation-induced intestinal pseudo-obstruction. *Gastroenterology*, **91**, 994–998 (1986)

68. Bruegel, C. Die beeinflussung des magenchemismus durch rontgenstrahlen. *Müchener Medizinische Wochenschrift*, **64**, 379 (1917)

69. Palmer, W. and Templeton, F. The effect of radiation therapy on gastric secretion. *Journal of the American Medical Association*, **112**, 1429–1434 (1939)

70. Carpender, J., Levin, E., Clayman, C. and Miller, R. Radiation in the therapy of peptic ulcer. *American Journal of Roentgenology*, **75**, 374–379 (1956)

71. Gunderson, L. Gastric cancer. In *Principles and Practice of Radiation Oncology*, (eds C. Perez and L. Brady), J.B. Lippincott, Philadelphia, pp. 793–800 (1987)

72. Gastrointestinal Tumor Study Group. A comparison of combination chemotherapy and combined modality therapy for locally advanced gastric carcinoma. *Cancer*, **49**, 1771–1777 (1982)

73. Schein, P., Smith, F., Dritschilo, A. *et al.* Phase I–II trial of combined modality FAM (5-fluorouracil, adriamycin and mitomycin C) plus split course radiation (Fam-Rt-Fam) for locally advanced gastric (lag) and pancreatic (lap) cancer (abstract). *Proceedings of the American Society of Clinical Oncology*, **2**, 126 (1983)

74. Gunderson, L., Hoskins, B., Cohen, A. *et al.* Combined modality treatment of gastric cancer. *International Journal of Radiation Oncology, Biology, Physics*, **9**, 965–975 (1983)

75. O'Connell, M., Gunderson, L., Moertel, C. and Kvols, L. A pilot study to determine clinical tolerability of intensive combined modality therapy for locally unresectable gastric cancer. *International Journal of Radiation Oncology, Biology, Physics*, **11**, 1827–1831 (1985)

76. Tepper, J., Cohen, A., Wood, W. *et al*. Postoperative radiation therapy of rectal cancer. *International Journal of Radiation Oncology, Biology, Physics*, **13**, 5–10 (1987)

77. Deitel, M. and Vasic, V. Major intestinal complications of radiotherapy. *American Journal of Gastroenterology*, **72**, 65–70 (1979)

78. Russel, J. and Welch, J. Operative management of radiation injuries of the intestinal tract. *American Journal of Surgery*, **137**, 433–442 (1979)

79. Stuart, M., Failes, D., Killingback, M. and DeLuca, C. Irradiation injuries of the large intestine. *Diseases of the Colon and Rectum*, **23**, 94–97 (1980)

80. Galland, R. and Spencer, J. Surgical aspects of radiation injury to the intestine. *British Journal of Surgery*, **66**, 135–138 (1979)

81. DeCosse, J., Rhodes, R., Wentz, W. *et al*. The natural history and management of radiation induced injury of the gastrointestinal tract. *Annals of Surgery*, **170**, 369–384 (1969)

82. Cram, A., Pearlman, N. and Jochimsen, P. Surgical management of complications of radiation-injured gut. *American Journal of Surgery*, **133**, 551–553 (1977)

83. Klaassen, D., Shelley, W., Starreveld, A. *et al*. Early stage ovarian cancer: a randomized clinical trial comparing whole abdominal radiotherapy, melphalan, and intraperitoneal chromic phosphate: a National Cancer Institute of Canada clinical trials group report. *Journal of Clinical Oncology*, **6**, 1254–1263 (1988)

84. Brick, I. Effects of million volt irradiation on the gastrointestinal tract. *A.M.A. Archives of Internal Medicine*, **96**, 26–31 (1955)

85. Friedman, M. Calculated risks of radiation injury of normal tissue in the treatment of cancer of the testis. *Proceedings of the Second National Cancer Conference*, **1**, 390–400 (1952)

86. Roswit, B., Malsky, S. and Reid, C. Severe radiation injuries of the stomach, small intestine, colon and rectum. *American Journal of Roentgenology, Radium Therapy and Nuclear Medicine*, **114**, 460–475 (1972)

87. Goldstein, H., Rogers, L., Fletcher, G. and Dodd, G. Radiological manifestations of radiation-induced injury to the normal upper gastrointestinal tract. *Radiology*, **117**, 135–140 (1975)

88. Bowers, R. and Brick, I. Surgery in radiation injury of the stomach. *Surgery*, **22**, 20–40 (1947)

89. Hamilton, F.E. Gastric ulcer following radiation. *Archives of Surgery*, **55**, 394–399 (1946)

90. Brick, I.B. The effect of large dosages of irradiation on gastric acidity. *New England Journal of Medicine*, **237**, 48–51 (1947)

91. Lillemoe, K., Brigham, R., Harmon, J. *et al*. Surgical management of small-bowel radiation enteritis. *Archives of Surgery*, **118**, 905–907 (1983)

92. Localio, S., Stone, A. and Friedman, M. Surgical aspects of radiation enteritis. *Surgery, Gynecology and Obstetrics*, **129**, 1163–1172 (1969)

93. Miholic, J., Schlappack, O., Klepetko, W. *et al*. Surgical therapy of radiation-induced small-bowel lesions. *Archives of Surgery*, **122**, 923–925 (1987)

94. Cochrane, J., Yarnold, J. and Slack, W. The surgical treatment of radiation injuries after radiotherapy for uterine carcinoma. *British Journal of Surgery*, **68**, 25–28 (1981)

95. Taverner, D., Talbot, I.C., Carr-Locke, D.L. and Wicks, A.C.B. Massive bleeding from the ileum: a late complication of pelvic radiotherapy. *American Journal of Gastroenterology*, **77**, 29–31 (1982)

96. Herlinger, H. Small bowel. In *Double Contrast Gastrointestinal Radiology – With Endoscopic Correlation* (ed. I. Laufer), W.B. Saunders, Philadelphia, pp. 423–494 (1979)

97. Bruneton, J., Faire, X. and Bourry, J. A radiologic study of chronic radiation-induced injuries of the small intestine and colon. *ROFO*, **136**, 129–132 (1982)

98. Deitel, M. and To, T. Major intestinal complications of radiotherapy. *Archives of Surgery*, **122**, 1421–1424 (1987)

99. Deitel, M., Degani, C. and Alexander, M. Major gastrointestinal problems after radiotherapy, management and nutritional considerations. *International Surgery*, **62**, 334–337 (1977)

100. Warren, S. and Friedman, N. Pathology and pathologic diagnosis of radiation lesions in the gastrointestinal tract. *American Journal of Pathology*, **18**, 499–513 (1941)

101. Dirksen, P., Matolo, N. and Trelford, J. Complications following operation in the previously irradiated abdominopelvic cavity. *American Surgeon*, **43**, 234–241 (1977)

102. Mason, G., Dietrich, P., Friedland, G. and Hanks, G. The radiological findings in radiation-induced enteritis and colitis. A review of 30 cases. *Clinical Radiology*, **21**, 232 (1970)

103. Meyer, J. Radiography of the distal colon and rectum after irradiation of carcinoma of the cervix. *American Journal of Roentgenology*, **136**, 691–699 (1981)

104. Krestin, G.P., Beyer, D. and Steinbrich, W. Computed tomography in the differential diagnosis of the enlarged retrorectal space. *Gastrointestinal Radiology*, **11**, 364–369 (1986)

105. Pilepich, M., Krall, J., Sause, W. *et al*. Correlation of radiotherapeutic parameters and treatment related morbidity in carcinoma of the prostate – analysis of RTOG study 75-06. *International Journal of Radiation Oncology, Biology, Physics*, **13**, 351–357 (1987)

106. Pilepich, M., Asbell, S., Krall, J. *et al*. Correlation of radiotherapeutic parameters and treatment related morbidity – analysis of RTOG study 77-06. *International Journal of Radiation Oncology, Biology, Physics*, **13**, 1007–1012 (1987)

107. Green, N., Iba, G. and Smith, W. Measures to minimize small intestine injury in the irradiated pelvis. *Cancer*, **35**, 1633–1640 (1975)

108. Freund, H., Gunderson, L., Krause, R. and Fischer, J. Prevention of radiation enteritis after abdomino-

perineal resection and radiotherapy. *Surgery, Gynecology and Obstetrics*, **149**, 206–208 (1979)

109. Green, N. The avoidance of small intestine injury in gynecologic cancer. *International Journal of Radiation Oncology, Biology, Physics*, **9**, 1385–1390 (1983)

110. Kavanah, M., Feldman, M., Devereux, D. and Kondi, E. New surgical approach to minimize radiation-associated small bowel injury in patients with pelvic malignancies requiring surgery and high-dose irradiation. *Cancer*, **56**, 1300–1304

111. Devereux, D., Kavanah, M., Feldman, M. *et al.* Small bowel exclusion from the pelvis by a polyglycolic acid mesh sling. *Journal of Surgical Oncology*, **26**, 107–112 (1984)

112. Devereux, D., Thompson, D., Sandhaus, L. *et al.* Protection from radiation enteritis by an absorbable polyglycolic acid mesh sling. *Surgery*, **101**, 123–129 (1986)

113. Feldman, M., Choe, S. and Kavanah, M. New surgical technique to eliminate the complication of radiation enteropathy. *American Journal of Clinical Oncology*, **10**, 101–116 (1987)

114. Gallagher, M., Brereton, H., Rostock, R. *et al.* A prospective study of treatment techniques to minimize the volume of pelvic small bowel with reduction of acute and late effects associated with pelvic irradiation. *International Journal of Radiation Oncology, Biology, Physics*, **12**, 1563–1573 (1986)

115. Caspers, R., Jobsen, J., Gerts, M. *et al.* Irradiation of true pelvis with full bladder to prevent small bowel damage (abstract). *Proceedings of The European Society of Therapeutic Radiation Oncology*, p. 310 (1988)

116. Caspers, R. and Hop, W. Irradiation of true pelvis for bladder and prostatic carcinoma in supine, prone, or Trendelenburg position. *International Journal of Radiation Oncology, Biology, Physics*, **9**, 589–593 (1983)

117. Gunderson, L., Russell, A., Llewellyn, H. *et al.* Treatment planning for colorectal cancer: radiation and surgical techniques and value of small-bowel films. *International Journal of Radiation Oncology, Biology, Physics*, **11**, 1379–1393 (1985)

118. Gunderson, L., Rich, T., Tepper, J. *et al.* Large bowel cancer: utility of radiation therapy. In *Clinical Management of Gastrointestinal Cancer* (eds P. Sherlock and J. DeCosse), Martinus Nijhoff, Boston, pp. 189–219 (1984)

119. Hoskins, R., Gunderson, L., Dosoretz, D. *et al.* Adjuvant postoperative radiotherapy in carcinoma of the rectum and rectosigmoid. *Cancer*, **55**, 61–71 (1985)

120. Elman, A. ASTR and RSNA demonstrations (1979)

121. Minsky, B. Minimizing the toxicity of pelvic radiation therapy in rectal cancer. *Oncology*, **2**, 21–24 (1988)

122. Duttenhaver, J., Hoskins, R., Gunderson, L. and Tepper, J. Adjuvant postoperative radiation therapy in the management of adenocarcinoma of the colon. *Cancer*, **57**, 955–963 (1986)

123. Gallagher, M., Brereton, H., Rostock, R. *et al.* A prospective study of the acute and late small bowel effects in 300 patients receiving pelvic radiation – an update (abstract). *Proceedings of the 29th Annual ASTRO Meeting*, p. 195 (1987)

124. Sugarbaker, P. Intrapelvic prosthesis to prevent injury of the small intestine with high-dose pelvic irradiation. *Surgery, Gynecology and Obstetrics*, **157**, 269–271 (1983)

125. Edington, H., Hancock, S. and Coe, F. Preliminary report of a new treatment strategy for advanced pelvic malignancy: surgical resection and radiation therapy using afterloading catheters plus an inflatable displacement prosthesis in the treatment of advanced primary and recurrent rectal carcinoma. *Surgery*, **100**, 494–498 (1986)

126. Durig, M., Steenblock, U., Heberer, M. and Harder, F. Prevention of radiation injuries to the small intestine. *Surgery, Gynecology and Obstetrics*, **159**, 162–163 (1984)

127. Bounous, G. The use of elemental diets during cancer therapy. *Anticancer Research*, **3**, 299–304 (1983)

128. Archambeau, J., Maetz, M., Jesseph, J. and Bond, V. The effects of bile diversion and pancreatic duct ligation on the gastrointestinal syndrome in dogs receiving 1500 rads whole-body irradiation (abstract). *Radiation Research*, **25**, 173 (1965)

129. Berk, R. and Seay, D. Cholerheic enteropathy as a cause of diarrhea and death in radiation enteritis and its prevention with cholestyramine. *Radiology*, **104**, 153–156 (1972)

130. Morgenstern, L. and Hiatt, N. Injurious effect of pancreatic secretions on postradiation enteropathy. *Gastroenterology*, **53**, 923–929 (1967)

131. Hugon, J. and Bounous, G. Elemental diet in the management of the intestinal lesions produced by radiation in the mouse. *Canadian Journal of Surgery*, **15**, 18–26 (1972)

132. Pageau, R., Lallier, R. and Bounous, G. Systemic protection against radiation. I. Effect of an elemental diet on hematopoietic and immunologic systems in the rat. *Radiation Research*, **62**, 357–363 (1975)

133. Bounous, G., Lebel, E., Shuster, J. *et al.* Dietary protection during radiation therapy. *Strahlentherapie*, **149**, 476–483 (1975)

134. McArdle, A., Freeman, C., Duguib, W. and Reid, C. Protection from radiation injury to the intestine by feeding an elemental diet to patients with invasive bladder cancer. *Journal of Parenteral and Enteral Nutrition*, **2**, 682–686 (1982)

135. Donaldson, S., Jundt, S., Ricour, C. *et al.* Radiation enteritis in children. A retrospective review, clinicopathologic correlation, and dietary management. *Cancer*, **35**, 1167–1178 (1975)

136. Booth, C., MacIntyre, I. and Mollin, D. Nutritional problems associated with extensive lesions of the distal small intestine in man. *Quarterly Journal of Medicine*, **131**, 401 (1964)

137. Bosaeus, I., Andersson, H. and Nystrom, C. Effect of a low fat diet on bile salt excretion and diarrhoea

in the gastrointestinal radiation syndrome. *Acta Radiologica, Oncology*, **18**, 460–464 (1979)

138. Stryker, J. and Bartholomew, M. Failure of lactose-restricted diets to prevent radiation-induced diarrhoea in patients undergoing whole pelvis irradiation. *International Journal of Radiation Oncology, Biology, Physics*, **12**, 789–792 (1986)

139. Rachootin, S., Shapiro, S. and Yamakawa, T. Potent antiproteases derived from *Ascaris lumbricoides*: efficacy in amelioration of post-radiation enteropathy. *Gastroenterology*, **62**, 796 (1972)

140. Chary, S. and Thomson, D. A clinical trial evaluating cholestyramine to prevent diarrhea in patients maintained on low-fat diets during pelvic radiation therapy. *International Journal of Radiation Oncology, Biology, Physics*, **10**, 1885–1890 (1984)

141. Stryker, J., Chung, C. and Layser, J. Colestipol hydrochloride prophylaxis of diarrhea during pelvic radiotherapy. *International Journal of Radiation Oncology, Biology, Physics*, **9**, 185–190 (1983)

142. Mennie, A., Dalley, V., Dinneen, L. and Collier, H. Treatment of radiation induced gastrointestinal distress with acetylsalicylate. *Lancet*, **ii**, 942 (1975)

143. Brohult, A., Brohult, J., Brohult, S. and Joelsson, I. Effect of alkoxyglycerols on the frequency of fistulas following radiation therapy for carcinoma of the uterine cervix. *Acta Obstetricia Gynecologica Scandinavica*, **58**, 203–207 (1979)

144. Hagemann, R. and Concannon, J. Time/dose relationships in abdominal irradiation: a definition of principles and experimental evaluation. *British Journal of Radiology*, **48**, 545–555 (1975)

145. Quastler, H., Bensted, J., Chir, B. *et al.* Adaptation to continuous irradiation: observations on the rat intestine. *British Journal of Radiology*, **32**, 501–512 (1959)

146. Amory, H. and Brick, I. Irradiation damage of the intestines following 1000 kV roentgen therapy. Evaluation of tolerance dose. *Radiology*, **56**, 49–57 (1951)

147. Van Rijswijk, R., Verbeek, J., Haanen, C. *et al.* Major complications and causes of death in patients treated for Hodgkin's disease. *Journal of Clinical Oncology*, **5**, 1624–1633 (1987)

148. Willett, C., Linggood, R., Meyer, J. *et al.* Results of treatment of stage 3A Hodgkin's disease. *Cancer*, **59**, 27–30 (1987)

149. Farah, R., Ultmann, J., Griem, M. *et al.* Extended mantle radiation therapy for pathologic stage I and II Hodgkin's disease. *Journal of Clinical Oncology*, **6**, 1047–1952 (1988)

150. Coia, L. and Hanks, G. Complications from large field intermediate dose infradiaphragmatic radiation: an analysis of the patterns of care outcome studies for Hodgkin's disease and seminoma. *International Journal of Radiation Oncology, Biology, Physics*, **15**, 29–35 (1988)

151. Thomas, G., Rider, W., Dembo, Al *et al.* Seminoma of the testis: results of treatment and patterns of failure after radiation therapy. *International Journal of Radiation Oncology, Biology, Physics*, **8**, 165–174 (1982)

152. Cionini, L., Ciatto, S., Pirtoli, L. *et al.* Radiotherapy of seminoma of the testis. Report on 129 patients. *Tumori*, **64**, 183–192 (1978)

153. Ball, D., Barrett, A. and Peckham, M. The management of metastatic seminoma testis. *Cancer*, **50**, 2289–2294 (1982)

154. Smalley, S., Evans, R., Richardson, R. *et al.* Radiotherapy as initial treatment for bulky stage II testicular seminomas. *Journal of Clinical Oncology*, **3**, 1333–1338 (1985)

155. Moertel, C., Childs, D., Reitimeier, R. *et al.* Combined 5-fluorouracil and supervoltage radiation therapy of locally unresectable gastrointestinal cancer. *Lancet*, **ii**, 865–867 (1969)

156. Kalser, M. and Ellenberg, S. Pancreatic cancer: adjuvant combined radiation and chemotherapy following curative resection. *Archives of Surgery*, **120**, 899–903 (1985)

157. Gastrointestinal Tumor Study Group. Further evidence of effective adjuvant combined radiation and chemotherapy following curative resection of pancreatic cancer. *Cancer*, **59**, 2006–2010 (1987)

158. Piver, S., Barlow, J. and Krishnamsetty, R. Five-year survival (with no evidence of disease) in patients with biopsy-confirmed aortic node metastasis from cervical carcinoma. *American Journal of Obstetrics and Gynecology*, **139**, 575–578 (1981)

159. Nelson, J., Boyce, J., Macasaet, M. *et al.* Incidence, significance, and follow-up of para-aortic lymph node metastases in late invasive carcinoma of the cervix. *American Journal of Obstetrics and Gynecology*, **128**, 336–340 (1977)

160. Tewfik, H., Buchsbaum, H., Latourette, H. *et al.* Para-aortic lymph node irradiation in carcinoma of the cervix after exploratory laparotomy and biopsy-proven positive aortic nodes. *International Journal of Radiation Oncology, Biology, Physics*, **8**, 13–18 (1982)

161. Fletcher, G., Lindberg, R., Caderao, J. and Wharton, J. Hyperbaric oxytgen as a radiotherapeutic adjuvant in advanced cancer of the uterine cervix. *Cancer*, **39**, 617–623 (1977)

162. Rubin, S., Brookland, R., Mikuta, J. *et al.* Para-aortic nodal metastases in early cervical carcinoma: long-term survival following extended-field radiotherapy. *Gynecologic Oncology*, **18**, 213–217 (1983)

163. Brookland, R., Rubin, S. and Danoff, B. Extended field irradiation in the treatment of patients with cervical carcinoma involving biopsy proven para-aortic nodes. *International Journal of Radiation Oncology, Biology, Physics*, **10**, 1875–1879 (1984)

164. Welander, C., Pierce, V., Nori, D. *et al.* Pretreatment laparotomy in carcinoma of the cervix. *Gynecologic Oncology*, **12**, 336–347 (1981)

165. Hughes, R., Brewington, K., Hanjani, P. *et al.*

Extended field irradiation for cervical cancer based on surgical staging. *Gynecologic Oncology*, **9**, 153–161 (1980)

166. Berman, M., Lagasse, L., Watring, W. *et al.* The operative evaluation of patients with cervical carcinoma by an extraperitoneal approach. *Obstetrics and Gynecology*, **50**, 658–664 (1977)

167. Potish, R., Twiggs, L., Prem, K. *et al.* The impact of extraperitoneal surgical staging on morbidity and tumor recurrence following radiotherapy for cervical carcinoma. *American Journal of Clinical Oncology*, **7**, 245–251 (1984)

168. LaPolla, J., Schlaerth, J., Gaddis, O. and Morrow, C. The influence of surgical staging on the evaluation and treatment of patients with cervical carcinoma. *Gynecologic Oncology*, **24**, 194–206 (1986)

169. Ballon, S., Berman, M., Lagasse, L. *et al.* Survival after extraperitoneal pelvic and paraaortic lymphadenectomy and radiation therapy in cervical carcinoma. *Obstetrics and Gynecology*, **57**, 90–95 (1981)

170. Jolles, C., Freedman, R., Hamberger, A. and Horbelt, D. Complications of extended-field therapy for cervical carcinoma without prior surgery. *International Journal of Radiation Oncology, Biology, Physics*, **12**, 179–183 (1986)

171. Emami, B., Watring, W., Tak, W. *et al.* Para-aortic lymph node radiation in advanced cervical cancer. *International Journal of Radiation Oncology, Biology, Physics*, **6**, 1237–1241 (1980)

172. Rotman, M., Moon, S., John, M. *et al.* Extended field para-aortic radiation in cervical carcinoma: the case for prophylactic treatment. *International Journal of Radiation Oncology, Biology, Physics*, **4**, 795–799 (1978)

173. Potish, R., Twiggs, L., Adcock, L. *et al.* Para-aortic lymph node radiotherapy in cancer of the uterine corpus. *Obstetrics and Gynecology*, **65**, 251–256 (1985)

174. Haas, C., Mansfield, C., Leichman, L. *et al.* Combined nonsimultaneous radiation therapy and chemotherapy with 5-FU, doxorubicin, and mitomycin for residual localized gastric adenocarcinoma: a Southwest Oncology Group pilot study. *Cancer Treatment Reports*, **67**, 421–424 (1983)

175. Thirlwell, M., Keable, H., Kost, K. *et al.* Combination of 5-fluorouracil plus semustine with and without radiotherapy in advanced gastric and pancreatic carcinoma (abstract). *Proceedings of the American Society of Clinical Oncology*, p. 449 (1981)

176. Cheung, A. Extended field irradiation for invasive carcinoma of the cervix. *Gynecologic Oncology*, **9**, 280–291 (1980)

177. Flickinger, J., Jawalekar, K., Deutsch, M. and Webster, J. Split course radiation therapy for adenocarcinoma of the pancreas. *International Journal of Radiation Oncology, Biology, Physics*, **15**, 359–364 (1988)

178. Moertel, C., Frytak, S., Hahn, R. *et al.* Therapy of locally unresectable pancreatic carcinoma: a randomized comparison of high dose (6000 rads) radiation alone, moderate dose radiation (4000 rads + 5-fluorouracil), and high dose radiation + 5-fluorouracil. *Cancer*, **48**, 1705–1710 (1981)

179. Dobelbower, R., Borgelt, B., Strubler, K. *et al.* Precision radiotherapy for cancer of the pancreas: technique and results. *International Journal of Radiation Oncology, Biology, Physics*, **6**, 1127–1133 (1980)

180. Whittington, R., Solin, L., Mohiuddin, M. *et al.* Multimodality therapy of localized unresectable pancreatic adenocarcinoma. *Cancer*, **54**, 1991–1998 (1984)

181. Gastrointestinal Tumor Study Group. Treatment of locally unresectable carcinoma of the pancreas: comparison of combined-modality therapy (chemotherapy plus radiotherapy) to chemotherapy alone. *Journal of the National Cancer Institute*, **80**, 751–755 (1988)

182. Haslam, J., Cavanaugh, P. and Stroup, S. Radiation therapy in the treatment of irresectable adenocarcinoma of the pancreas. *Cancer*, **32**, 1341–1345 (1973)

183. Kopelson, A.B., Harisiadis, L., Tretter, P. and Chang, C. The role of radiation therapy in cancer of the extra-hepatic biliary system: an analysis of thirteen patients and a review of the literature of the effectiveness of surgery, chemotherapy and radiotherapy. *International Journal of Radiation Oncology, Biology, Physics*, **2**, 881–894 (1977)

184. Buskirk, S., Gunderson, L., Adson, M. *et al.* Analysis of failure following curative irradiation of gallbladder and extrahepatic bile duct carcinoma. *International Journal of Radiation Oncology, Biology, Physics*, **10**, 2013–2023 (1984)

185. Fogel, T. and Weissberg, J. The role of radiation therapy in carcinoma of the extrahepatic bile ducts. *International Journal of Radiation Oncology, Biology, Physics*, **10**, 2251–2258 (1984)

186. Miller, T. and Fuller, L. Radiation therapy of carcinoma of the pancreas. Report on 91 cases. *American Journal of Roentgenology*, **80**, 787–791 (1958)

187. Pilepich, M. and Miller, H. Preoperative irradiation in carcinoma of the pancreas. *Cancer*, **41**, 1945–1949 (1980)

188. Dembo, A., Van Dyk, J., Japp, B. *et al.* Whole abdominal irradiation by a moving-strip technique for patients with ovarian cancer. *International Journal of Radiation Oncology, Biology, Physics*, **5**, 1933–1942 (1972)

189. Dembo, A., Bush, R., Beale, F. *et al.* A randomized clinical trial of moving strip versus open field whole abdominal irradiation in patients with invasive epithelial cancer of ovary (abstract). *Proceedings of the American Society of Clinical Oncology*, **C-571**, 146 (1983)

190. Fazekas, J. and Maier, J. Irradiation of ovarian carcinomas. A prospective comparison of the open-field and moving-strip techniques. *American Journal of Roentgenology*, **120**, 118–123 (1974)

191. van Bunningen, B., Bouma, J., Kooijman, C. *et al.* Small bowel complications after total abdominal irradiation for cancer of the ovary stage I and II (abstract). *Proceedings of the European Society of Therapeutic Radiation Oncology*, p. 309 (1988)

192. Macbeth, F., Macdonald, H. and Williams, C. (1988) Total abdominal and pelvic radiotherapy in the management of early stage ovarian carcinoma. *International Journal of Radiation Oncology, Biology, Physics*, **15**, 353–358 (1988)

193. Loeffler, J., Rosen, E., Niloff, J. *et al.* Whole abdominal irradiation for tumors of the uterine corpus. *Cancer*, **61**, 1332–1335 (1988)

194. Greer, B. and Hamburger, A. Treatment of intraperitoneal metastatic adenocarcinoma of the endometrium by the whole-abdomen moving-strip technique and pelvic boost irradiation. *Gynecologic Oncology*, **16**, 365–373 (1983)

195. Potish, R., Twiggs, L., Adcock, L. and Prem, K. Role of whole abdominal radiation therapy in the management of endometrial cancer; prognostic importance of factors indicating peritoneal metastases. *Gynecologic Oncology*, **21**, 80–86 (1985)

196. Fabian, C., Reddy, E., Jewell, W. *et al.* Phase I–II pilot of whole abdominal irradiation and concomitant 5-FU as an adjuvant in colon cancer: a Southwest Oncology Group Study. *International Journal of Radiation Oncology, Biology, Physics*, **15**, 885–892 (1988)

197. Brenner, H., Bibi, C. and Chaitchik, S. Adjuvant therapy for Dukes' C adenocarcinoma of colon. *International Journal of Radiation Oncology, Biology, Physics*, **9**, 1789–1792 (1983)

198. Hacker, N., Berek, J., Burnison, C. *et al.* Whole abdominal radiation as salvage therapy for epithelial ovarian cancer. *Obstetrics and Gynecology*, **65**, 60–66 (1985)

199. Hainsworth, J., Malcolm, A., Johnson, D. *et al.* Advanced minimal residual ovarian carcinoma: abdominopelvic irradiation following combination chemotherapy. *Obstetrics and Gynecology*, **61**, 619–623 (1983)

200. Schray, M., Martinez, A., Howes, A. *et al.* Advanced epithelial ovarian cancer: salvage whole abdominal irradiation for patients with recurrent or persistent disease after combination chemotherapy. *Journal of Clinical Oncology*, **6**, 1433–1439 (1988)

201. Fuks, Z., Rizel, S. and Biran, S. Chemotherapeutic and surgical induction of pathological complete remission and whole abdominal irradiation for consolidation does not enhance the cure of stage III ovarian carcinoma. *Journal of Clinical Oncology*, **6**, 509–516 (1988)

202. Rizel, S., Biran, S., Anteby, S. *et al.* Combined modality treatment for stage III ovarian carcinoma. *Radiotherapy and Oncology*, **3**, 237–244 (1985)

203. Steiner, M., Rubinov, R., Borovik, R. *et al.* Multi-modal approach (surgery, chemotherapy, and radiotherapy) in the treatment of advanced ovarian carcinoma. *Cancer*, **55**, 2748–2752 (1985)

204. Goldhirsch, A., Greiner, R., Dreher, E. *et al.* Treatment of advanced ovarian cancer with surgery, chemotherapy, and consolidation of response by whole-abdominal radiotherapy. *Cancer*, **62**, 40–47 (1988)

205. Potish, R., Adcock, L., Jones, T. *et al.* The morbidity and utility of periaortic radiotherapy in cervical carcinoma. *Gynecologic Oncology*, **15**, 1–9 (1983)

206. Habrand, J., Ghoul, A., Oberlin, O. *et al.* Late injuries induced by the irradiation at conventional dose in pediatric Hodgkin's disease. The influence of laparotomy and dose per fraction (abstract). *Proceedings of the European Society of Therapeutic Radiation Oncology*, p. 311 (1988)

207. Cosset, J., Henry-Amar, M., Malaise, E. *et al.* Small bowel radiation damage; the role of fractionation (abstract). *Proceedings of the European Society of Therapeutic Radiation Oncology*, p. 274 (1988)

208. Sassy, T., Breiter, N., Guttenberger, R. and Trott, K. Repair kinetics and repair capacity of the x-irradiated rat colon (abstract). *Proceedings of the European Society of Therapeutic Radiation Oncology*, p. 240 (1988)

209. Cox, J., Guse, C., Asbell, S. *et al.* Tolerance of pelvic normal tissues to hyperfractionated radiation therapy: results of protocol 83-08 of the Radiation Therapy Oncology group. *International Journal of Radiation Oncology, Biology, Physics*, **15**, 1331–1336 (1988)

210. Lipsett, J., Desai, K., Pezner, R. *et al.* Acute normal tissue tolerance to seven day per week accelerated fractionation. *International Journal of Radiation Oncology, Biology, Physics*, **10**, 1049–1052 (1984)

211. Edsmyr, F., Anderson, L., Esposti, P. *et al.* Irradiation therapy with multiple small fractions per day in urinary bladder cancer. *Radiotherapy and Oncology*, **4**, 197–203 (1985)

212. Wang, C. Altered frament of uterine cancer. *Acta Radiologica*, **56**, 289 (1961)

213. Caspers, R., Jobsen, J., Gerts, M. *et al.* Acute toxicity after radiotherapy of true pelvis (abstract). *Proceedings of the European Society of Therapeutic Radiation Oncology*, p. 103 (1988)

214. Letschert, J., Lebesque, J. and de Boer, R. Dose-volume correlation in radiation-related late small bowel complications (abstract). *Proceedings of the European Society of Therapeutic Radiation Oncology*, p. 307 (1988)

215. Vigliotti, A., Rich, T., Romsdahl, M. *et al.* Postoperative adjuvant radiotherapy for adenocarcinoma of the rectum and rectosigmoid. *International Journal of Radiation Oncology, Biology, Physics*, **13**, 999–1006 (1987)

216. Schild, S., Martenson, J., Gunderson, L. *et al.* Postoperative adjuvant therapy of rectal cancer: an analysis of disease control, survival, and prognostic

factors. *International Journal of Radiation Oncology, Biology, Physics*, **17**, 55–62 (1989)

217. Potish, R., Jones, T. and Levitt, S. Factors predisposing to radiation-related small-bowel damage. *Radiology*, **132**, 479–482 (1979)

218. van Nagell, J., Parker, J., Maruyama, Y. *et al.* The effect of pelvic inflammatory disease on enteric complications following radiation therapy for cervical cancer. *American Journal of Obstetrics and Gynecology*, **128**, 767–711 (1977)

219. Maruyama, Y., Van Nagell, J., Utley, J. *et al.* Radiation and small bowel complications in cervical carcinoma therapy. *Radiology*, **112**, 699–703 (1974)

220. Bush, S., Smith, A. and Zink, S. Pion radiotherapy at Lampf. *International Journal of Radiation Oncology, Biology, Physics*, **8**, 2181–2186 (1982)

221. Potish, R. Prediction of radiation-related small-bowel damage. *Radiology*, **135**, 219–221 (1980)

222. LoIudice, T., Baxter, D. and Balint, J. Effects of abdominal surgery on the development of radiation enteropathy. *Gastroenterology*, **73**, 1093–1097 (1977)

223. Izar, F., Bachaud, J., Delannes, M. and Daly, N. The incidence of severe chronic ileitis after abdominal and/or pelvic external irradiation with high photon beam (abstract). *Proceedings of the European Society of Therapeutic Radiation Oncology*, p. 308 (1988)

224. Phillips, T., Ross, G., Goldstein, L. *et al. In vivo* radiobiology of heavy ions. *International Journal of Radiation Oncology, Biology, Physics*, **8**, 2121–2125 (1982)

225. Ellis, F. and Weatherburn, H. RBE and clinical response in radiotherapy with neutron beams. *British Journal of Radiology*, **57**, 817–822 (1984)

226. Duncan, W., Arnott, S., Jack, W. *et al.* A report of a randomized trial of d(15) + Be neutrons compared with megavoltage X-ray therapy of bladder cancer. *International Journal of Radiation Oncology, Biology, Physics*, **11**, 2043–2049 (1985)

227. Battermann, J. Results of d + T fast neutron irradiation on advanced tumors of bladder and rectum. *International Journal of Radiation Oncology, Biology, Physics*, **8**, 2159–2164 (1982)

228. Pointon, R., Read, G. and Greene, D. A randomized comparison of photons and 15 MeV neutrons for the treatment of carcinoma of the bladder. *British Journal of Radiology*, **58**, 219–224 (1985)

229. Woodruff, K., Castro, J., Quivey, J. *et al.* Postmortem examination of 22 pancreatic carcinoma patients treated with helium ion irradiation. *Cancer*, **53**, 420–425 (1984)

230. Concannon, J., Dalbow, M., Weil, C. and Hodgson, S. Radiation and actinomycin D mortality studies: circadian variations in lethality due to independent effects of either agent. *International Journal of Radiation Biology*, **24**, 405–411 (1973)

231. Concannon, J., Summers, R., Cole, C. *et al.* Effects of X-radiation and actinomycin D on intestinal epithelium of dogs. *Radiology*, **97**, 157–164 (1970)

232. Phillips, T., Wharam, M. and Margolis, L. Modification of radiation injury to normal tissues by chemotherapeutic agents. *Cancer*, **35**, 1678 (1975)

233. Donaldson, S., Jundt, S., Ricour, C. *et al.* Radiation enteritis in children. *Cancer*, **35**, 1167–1178 (1975)

234. Rich, T., Lokich, J. and Chaffey, J. A pilot study of protracted venous infusion of 5-fluorouracil and concomitant radiation therapy. *Journal of Clinical Oncology*, **3**, 402–406 (1985)

235. Rotman, M., Macchia, R., Silverstein, M. *et al.* Treatment of advanced bladder carcinoma with irradiation and concomitant 5-fluorouracil infusion. *Cancer*, **59**, 710–714 (1987)

236. Sedlacek, S. and Pearlman, N. Locally advanced adenocarcinoma of the rectum (ACR): concurrent preoperative chemotherapy (CT) and radiation therapy (RT) (abstract). *Proceedings of the American Society of Clinical Oncology*, **6**, A363, p. 11 (1987)

237. Figueredo, A., Basrur, V. and Knight, P. Pilot study of radiation therapy (RT) and 5-fluorouracil (5FU) infusion in adenocarcinoma of rectum (ACR) (abstract). *Proceedings of the American Society of Clinical Oncology*, **6**, A356, p. 11 (1987)

238. Shehata, W., Meyer, R., Jazy, F. *et al.* Regional adjuvant irradiation for adenocarcinoma of the cecum. *International Journal of Radiation Oncology, Biology, Physics*, **13**, 843–846 (1987)

239. Danjoux, G. and Calton, G. Delayed complications in colorectal carcinoma treated by combination radiotherapy and 5-fluorouracil. ECOG pilot study. *International Journal of Radiation Oncology, Biology, Physics*, **5**, 311 (1979)

240. Gastrointestinal Tumor Study Group. Prolongation of the disease free interval in surgically treated rectal cancer. *New England Journal of Medicine*, **312**, 1465 (1985)

241. Gunderson, L., Collins, R., Earle, J. *et al.* Adjuvant treatment of rectal cancer: randomized prospective study of irradiation ± chemotherapy. *Proceedings of the 28th Annual ASTRO Meeting*, p. 169 (1986)

242. Thomas, P., Douglass, H., Stablein, D. and Schein, P. Radiation and chemotherapy for locally unresectable adenocarcinoma of the pancreas: results of a multi-institutional randomized trial. *American Journal of Clinical Oncology: Cancer Clinical Trials*, **8**, 15 (1985)

243. Wong, C., Harwood, A., Cummings, B. *et al.* Postoperative local abdominal irradiation for cancer of the colon above the peritoneal reflection. *International Journal of Radiation Oncology, Biology, Physics*, **11**, 2067–2071 (1985)

244. Fisher, B., Wolmark, N., Rockette, H. *et al.* Postoperative adjuvant chemotherapy or radiation therapy for rectal cancer: results from NSABP protocol R-01. *Journal of the National Cancer Institute*, **80**, 21–28 (1988)

245. Balslev, I., Pedersen, M., Teglbjaerg, P. *et al.* Postoperative radiotherapy in Dukes' B and C

irradiation. *American Journal of Roentgenology*, **12**, 27–46 (1924)

305. Fajardo, L. and Colby, T. Pathogenesis of veno-occlusive liver disease after radiation. *Archives of Pathology and Laboratory Medicine*, **104**, 584–588 (1980)

306. Ingold, J., Reed, G., Kaplan, H. and Bagshaw, M. Radiation hepatitis. *American Journal of Roentgenology*, **93**, 200–208 (1965)

307. White, D. (1976) The histopathologic basis for functional decrements in late radiation injury in diverse organs. *Cancer*, **37**, 1126–1143 (1976)

308. Wharton, J., Delclos, L., Gallager, S. and Smith, J. Radiation hepatitis induced by abdominal irradiation with the cobalt-60 moving strip technique. *American Journal of Roentgenology, Radium Therapy and Nuclear Medicine*, **117**, 73–80 (1973)

309. Reed, G. and Cox, A. The human liver after radiation injury. *American Journal of Pathology*, **48**, 597–611 (1966)

310. Tefft, M., Mitus, A., Das, L. *et al.* Irradiation of the liver in children: review of experience in the acute and chronic phases, and in the intact normal and partially resected. *American Journal of Roentgenology*, **108**, 365–385 (1970)

311. Johnson, P., Grossman, F. and Atkins, H. Radiation induced hepatic injury. Its detection by scintillation scanning. *American Journal of Roentgenology*, **99**, 453–462 (1967)

312. Samuels, L., Grosfeld, J. and Kartha, M. Radiation hepatitis in children. *Journal of Pediatrics*, **78**, 68–73 (1971)

313. Fellows, K., Vawter, G. and Tefft, M. Hepatic effects following abdominal irradiation in children: detection by [198]Au scan and confirmation by histologic examination. *American Journal of Roentgenol-*

*ogy, Radiation Therapy and Nuclear Medicine*, **103**, 422–454 (1968)

314. Kim, T., Panahon, A., Friedman, M. and Webster, J. Acute transient radiation hepatitis following whole abdominal irradiation. *Clinical Radiology*, **27**, 449–454 (1976)

315. Rowland, R., Peterse, A., Kimber, R. and Ward, G. Radiation veno-occlusive liver disease. *Australian and New Zealand Journal of Medicine*, **11**, 534–538 (1981)

316. Phillips, R., Karnofsky, D., Hamilton, L. and Nickson, J. Roentgen therapy of hepatic metastases. *American Journal of Roentgenology, Radium Therapy and Nuclear Medicine*, **71**, 826–834 (1954)

317. Friedman, M. Primary hepatocellular cancer – present results and future prospects. *International Journal of Radiation Oncology, Biology, Physics*, **9**, 1841–1850 (1983)

318. Shafer, A. and Selinkoff, P. Preoperative irradiation and chemotherapy for initially unresectable hepatoblastoma. *Journal of Pediatric Surgery*, **12**, 1001–1007 (1977)

319. Hansen, M., Ranek, L., Walbom, S. and Nissen, N. Fatal hepatitis following irradiation and vincristine. *Acta Medica Scandinavica*, **212**, 171–174 (1982)

320. Rotman, M., Kuruvilla, A., Choi, K. *et al.* Response of colo-rectal hepatic metastases to concomitant radiotherapy and intravenous infusion of 5-fluorouracil. *International Journal of Radiation Oncology, Biology, Physics*, **12**, 2179–2187 (1986)

321. Rosenthal, O., Stark, C., Choi, K. *et al.* Adriamycin (A) by continuous infusion (CI) and concomitant radiation therapy (RT) in hepatocellular carcinoma (abstract). *Proceedings of the American Society of Clinical Oncology*, **6**, A362 (1987)

# 19

# Gastrointestinal and hepatic morbidity of chemotherapy

**E.M. Alstead and M.J.G. Farthing**

Gastrointestinal side effects of antineoplastic chemotherapy are common but are usually self-limiting (Table 19.1). Nausea and vomiting are the most prominent and are of particular importance since they may be restricting factors in therapy. Drug-related liver damage can also limit treatment regimens and in some instances carries a high morbidity and mortality. Difficulties can arise in determining whether symptoms are due to chemotherapeutic drugs, the underlying disease or to intestinal and liver infections in the immunocompromised host. The more serious toxic effects of these drugs on the gastrointestinal tract can often be predicted from the drug dosage, route of administration, concomitant therapy and underlying disease. Hepatotoxic effects are often idiosyncratic and sporadic and therefore more difficult to predict.

## Gastrointestinal symptoms during chemotherapy

### Nausea and vomiting

The most prominent adverse effects of chemotherapy from the patients' point of view are nausea and vomiting. Inadequate control of these symptoms may lead to biochemical disturbances and psychological distress; both can result in discontinuation of therapy or poor compliance. Despite recent advances in the management of this problem, 30–40% of patients continue to experience acute vomiting with chemotherapy, despite treatment with antiemetics. Delayed and anticipatory vomiting are now recognized as increasingly important problems during cancer chemotherapy [1]. Effective management of nausea and vomiting is an important aspect of the total care of oncology patients, improving patient compliance and enhancing the therapeutic index of chemotherapy regimens, thereby resulting in a decrease in the overall morbidity and mortality of cancer chemotherapy. Antineoplastic drugs vary in their emetic potential (Table 19.2). The most important drugs in order of toxicity are intravenous cisplatin, mustine, dacarbazine, cyclophosphamide and doxorubicin. In addition there is also variation between patients in their susceptibility to vomiting induced by a particular chemotherapeutic agent. Some newer cytotoxic drugs are also less emetic than previous agents. For example, mitozantrone is less emetic than doxorubicin and carboplatin and much less than cisplatin.

Vomiting is generally caused by central, rather than by direct gastrointestinal effects, although the exact mechanisms of chemotherapy-induced emesis are still poorly understood [1]. The vomiting centre is in the medullary reticular formation [2,3], posterior to the fourth ventricle. More recent evidence has failed to demonstrate a discrete area and a theory of 'sequential activation' has been proposed [4]. This theory acknowledges the existence of a

**Table 19.1 Common gastrointestinal side effects of antineoplastic agents**

Dysphagia and odynophagia
Nausea and vomiting
    Early
    Late
    Anticipatory
Diarrhoea
Constipation and distension

**Table 19.2 Emetic potential of antineoplastic agents**

| *High* (>60%) | *Moderate* (30–60%) | *Low* (<30%) |
|---|---|---|
| Cisplatin | 5-Fluorouracil | Busulphan |
| Ifosfamide | Doxorubicin | Chlorambucil |
| Cyclophosphamide (intravenous) | Daunorubicin | 6-Thioguanine |
| Doxorubicin | L-Asparaginase | Vincristine |
| Mustine | Mitomycin C | Oestrogens |
| Dacarbazine | Bleomycin | Progestogens |
| Streptozotocin | Hydroxyurea | Corticosteroids |
| Cytarabine | Melphalan | Androgens |
| Actinomycin D | Etoposide | |
| Mithramycin | Teniposide | |
| Procarbazine | 6-Mercaptopurine | |
| Methotrexate (high-dose) | Methotrexate | |
| | Thiotepa | |
| | Vinblastine | |

threshold for the initiation of the vomiting process and may explain why some of the epiphenomena of vomiting may be activated without triggering vomiting itself [1]. Adjacent to the vomiting centre is the chemoreceptor trigger zone (CTZ) and area postrema, which are a major source of afferent impulses to the emetic centre. The emetic properties of many drugs and toxins are mediated through CTZ stimulation, although for some antineoplastic agents the mechanism by which they cause vomiting remains ill-defined. Differences in the mechanism of vomiting may explain why several classes of antiemetics are useful in its prevention. Despite the identification of several important neurotransmitters, no single antiemetic agent has been able to counteract chemotherapy-induced emesis with universal success. This suggests that complex patterns of chemoreception and neurotransmission occur within the vomiting centre axis [1]. In experimental and clinical situations there is frequently a delay between the emetic stimulus and the response. This is seen to varying degrees with different cytotoxic agents and suggests an indirect rather than a direct mechanism of action in either or both the CTZ and the medullary reticular formation. Endogenous opioids may act as intermediaries in this process.

The prevalence and severity of nausea and vomiting increases with dose, especially with antimetabolite drugs. The time of onset of vomiting after drug administration varies [5]. Vomiting is immediate with dacarbazine [6] and delayed and protracted with cyclophosphamide, doxorubicin and cisplatin [7]. When drugs are used in combination, the emetic effect appears to be additive. Clinical management of chemotherapy-induced emesis involves appropri-

ate drug treatment as well as patient support and education. In addition, it is important to exclude medical causes of nausea and vomiting such as subacute intestinal obstruction, raised intracranial pressure and other drugs and to ensure adequate hydration and correction of metabolic disturbances.

Acute vomiting responds well to antiemetic drugs. Recent studies have noted that 60–90% of patients treated with cisplatin experience significant nausea and vomiting 24–120 h after therapy. Symptoms are most prevalent at 48–72 h and, although severity directly correlates with degree of control in the first 24 h, patients with no vomiting in the first 24 h can experience delayed emesis. Effective regimens include oral metaclopramide and dexamethasone or prochlorperazine. Steroids are useful in combinations with either metoclopramide or phenothiazines. Benzodiazepines are particularly useful in the management of anticipatory nausea and vomiting. Domperidone and nabilone (a cannabinoid) have also been used. Selective 5-hydroxytryptamine-3 antagonists may also be useful in the future when they have been fully evaluated.

Anticipatory nausea and vomiting is experienced by 20–40% of patients receiving chemotherapy. Chemotherapy-induced emesis is a behaviour modifying event that serves as the stimulus for a classically conditioned Pavlovian reflex which manifests as anticipatory vomiting [1]. This manifestation stresses the importance of the input from the limbic system and higher centres [7]. Several factors have been identified which may indicate which patients are more likely to develop this symptom [1,5]. Anticipatory vomiting has been reported to be more common in patients of 50 years of age or more, although other studies have stressed its occurrence in young patients [7]. It also appears to be more common in patients with severe initial nausea and vomiting, in those with a premorbid susceptibility to motion sickness, and in those who develop the sensations of sweating or weakness after therapy.

Anticipatory nausea and vomiting are also thought to be associated with the frequency and length of treatment regimens and disease status, and are refractory to standard antiemetic therapy. Benzodiazepines, however, have been shown to reduce the symptoms, presumably due to their anxiolytic and amnesic effects [8]. Techniques aimed at behaviour modification and systemic relaxation have been used with benefit [9]. The most expedient way to deal with anticipatory nausea and vomiting is to prevent it by effective pharmacological management of nausea and vomiting from the initiation of chemotherapy. Adjuvant therapy with amnesic anxiolytics is probably also of value. An alternative approach is to attempt to enhance the endogenous antiemetic tone, possibly by the administration of low doses of an opiate analogue such as naloxone. Acupuncture techniques may also be helpful by promoting endogenous enkephalin release. At present, however, the most effective antiemetic regimens use combinations of drugs which block several of the identified stimulatory pathways [1].

## Dysphagia and odynophagia

Dysphagia and pain on swallowing are common symptoms, most usually due to opportunistic infection. Oesophageal mucosal injury is not commonly induced by chemotherapeutic agents but is associated with other drugs given concomitantly such as non-steroidal anti-inflammatory agents or antibiotics. Sudden onset, painful dysphagia in a patient receiving chemotherapy is typical of herpetic [10] or cytomegalovirus oesophagitis, but may be due to *Candida* spp.

## Diarrhoea

Despite the often extensive morphological damage to the intestinal mucosa during chemotherapy [11], many patients have only transient symptoms. Watery diarrhoea occurs with many chemotherapeutic agents including dactinomycin, doxorubicin, cisplatin, cytarabine (cytosine arabinoside), daunorubicin, floxuridine, 5-fluorouracil (5-FU), 6-mercaptopurine (6-MP), methotrexate and mithramycin. Bloody diarrhoea due to mucosal sloughing has been described after high-dose therapy with antimetabolites such as 5-FU. Steatorrhoea is also reported to occur although this is uncommon, even in patients treated with combination chemotherapy [12]. Diarrhoea is usually mild and self-limiting and symptomatic treatment only is required.

Extensive mucosal necrosis associated with bloody diarrhoea, abdominal pain and protein-losing enteropathy occurs particularly in patients receiving sequential therapy with drug regimens that include cytarabine [13]. After the first week of therapy in these patients only a single cell layer of atypical epithelial cells remained, but in patients who survived the initial injury mucosal regeneration was almost complete within 2 weeks unless infection supervened. Associated opportunistic intestinal infections due to viruses, bacteria and fungi are common and may themselves cause diarrhoea [14]. In general, diarrhoea is a self-limiting symptom which does not interrupt the course of chemotherapy.

## Constipation, distension and abdominal pain.

In patients receiving antineoplastic drugs, constipation may result from diminished oral food and fluid intake and from the use of opiates and anticholinergics for pain relief. Vinca alkaloids may cause constipation and pseudo-obstruction by direct damage to the enteric nervous system [15,16]. This syndrome is more common and severe in older patients in whom the mortality is high [15]. Simple symptomatic management is all that is usually required. Colicky abdominal pain may also occur in patients given antineoplastic chemotherapy and is thought to be due to oedema of the gut wall as part of a generalized hypersensitivity reaction [17]. These symptoms have been reported to be associated with the administration of L-asparaginase, antibiotics, busulphan and cisplatin.

# Gastrointestinal complications of chemotherapy

## Mouth

The oral cavity is subject to constant mechanical, thermal and chemical trauma and heavy bacterial colonization and thus has a high epithelial cell turnover. For this reason it is exquisitely susceptible to the cytotoxic effects of antineoplastic drugs. Patients receiving these drugs are susceptible to oral mucositis and ulceration, gingivitis, oral haemorrhage and infections. Xerostomia and neuropathies (manifesting as pain and paraesthesiae) have also been reported [18]. There is no way to predict which patients will experience stomatotoxic effects, although pre-existing dental disease may predispose to the development of oral mucositis. In one study approximately 40% of patients receiving chemotherapy for tumours other than those of the head and neck developed oral complications [18]. Patients receiving chemotherapy for haematological malignancies seem to be more susceptible than those with solid tumours.

The commonest oral complication of cancer chemotherapy is mucositis. This results from direct cytotoxicity to the stem cells in the basal layer of the epithelium leading to impaired epithelial cell turnover, epithelial thinning, desquamation and ulceration. Mucositis may also occur secondary to bone marrow suppression in which opportunistic oral infection is the primary aetiological factor in the presence of neutropenia. The drugs most commonly associated with mucositis are 5-FU, methotrexate, cyclophosphamide, hydroxyurea, cytarabine, daunorubicin, doxorubicin, mitomycin, mithramycin, actinomycin D and bleomycin sulphate. Oral haemorrhage may occur secondary to thrombocytopenia. Neurological complications present as pain and paraesthesiae and are associated with cisplatin and the vinca alkaloids.

Infection is probably the most ominous oral complication. One study reported a 33% incidence

abnormalities of liver biochemistry [74,80]. Interval treatment with methotrexate is, however, often associated with transient liver biochemical abnormalities which usually normalize before the next treatment course [81]. Ultrastructural studies show variable hepatocyte damage which includes fatty change, membrane whorls and increased numbers of autophagic vacuoles. Ito cell hyperplasia, increased residual bodies in Kupffer cells [82] and biliary epithelial changes [83] have also been reported. Hepatic fibrosis has also been described in patients taking azathioprine [74].

Interstitial fibrosis in the form of hepatoportal sclerosis and other forms of non-cirrhotic fibrosis are also induced by antineoplastic drugs. 6-MP [84] and azathioprine cause an apparently dose-dependent hepatotoxicity. The injury is primarily cholestatic, but may also be accompanied by some hepatocellular necrosis. Liver biochemistry test abnormalities are variable, but in most cases the lesion is reversible when the drug is discontinued [85].

Drug-induced vascular lesions are well recognized, notably peliosis hepatis. Peliosis has been particularly associated with oestrogens but also with 6-thioguanine [86], androgens [87–89] and azathioprine [90]. Hepatic vein thrombosis and veno-occlusive disease are also commonly reported, the latter being particularly associated with azathioprine [85]. It has been speculated that peliosis hepatis, sinusoidal dilatation, perisinusoidal fibrosis and veno-occlusive disease caused by thiopurines (thioguanine and azathioprine), may be due to toxic effects of 6-thioguanine nucleotides on the sinusoids or centrilobular veins. The risk of developing such a toxic reaction may be particularly high in subjects who accumulate high plasma concentrations of 6-thioguanine nucleotides because of a genetic deficiency in thiopurine methyltransferase activity [88]. Cytarabine has been shown in experimental animals to increase the concentration and toxicity of 6-thioguanine in the liver [90].

Veno-occlusive disease has been reported in 20% of patients with leukaemia receiving combination chemotherapy with total body irradiation in preparation for bone marrow transplantation [91] (Figure 19.2). Pre-existing liver disease is an important risk factor for veno-occlusive disease especially in patients receiving chemotherapy in combination with radiotherapy; thus drugs which cause veno-occlusive disease should be used with caution in patients who have had hepatitis.

Hepatic vein thrombosis, Budd-Chiari syndrome and occlusion of small hepatic venules have been described in association with a number of chemotherapeutic agents. Oestrogens are the most commonly implicated agent in the Budd-Chiari syndrome [92]. Veno-occlusive disease is relatively common in patients receiving chemotherapy [28],

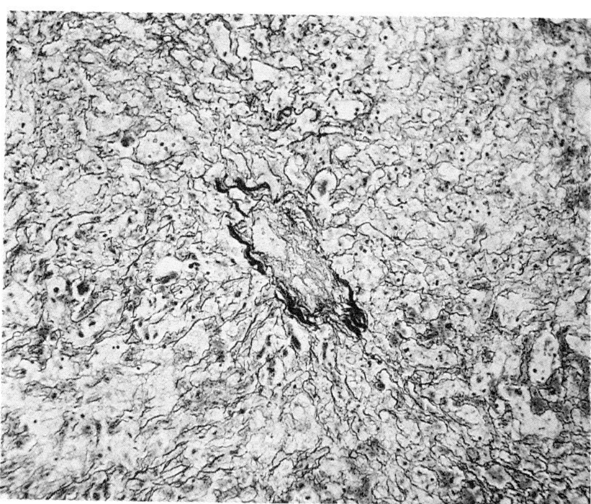

**Figure 19.2** Percutaneous liver biopsy showing veno-occlusive disease in a patient who received combination chemotherapy and irradiation prior to bone marrow transplant. Reticulin stain showing a central vein almost entirely occluded by a fine meshwork of reticulin fibres. The surrounding liver shows disruption of liver cell plates and intense congestion. Provided by Dr J. Sloane

and is frequently attributed to thioguanine, cytarabine, mithramycin C, azathioprine, dacarbazine [93] and doxorubicin. Histologically there is occlusion of terminal hepatic veins and congestion with necrosis of the perivenous area [28]. Fatal massive hepatic necrosis with widespread veno-occlusion has also been reported with the alkylating agent dacarbazine.

Hepatic tumours such as adenomas, hepatocellular carcinoma, cholangiocarcinoma and angiosarcoma have all been reported in association with antineoplastic chemotherapy [72]. Hepatic neoplasms also occur following anticancer hormonal treatment with both oestrogenic and androgenic steroids but also have been reported in association with methotrexate and chlorambucil [72,80].

## Summary and conclusions

Gastrointestinal side effects of antineoplastic chemotherapy are common, but are usually temporary and self-limiting. Apart from nausea and vomiting, which may be severe, they do not commonly influence the course of chemotherapy. Hepatic morbidity is rarer and may be due to direct toxicity, metabolic idiosyncracy or hypersensitivity to antineoplastic agents. It is possible to avoid some of the gastrointestinal side effects with careful planning of therapy, consideration of dosages and routes of administration and appropriate prophylaxis, notably for vomiting. Hepatic side effects are more likely to be idiosyncratic and therefore more difficult to avoid.

# References


1. Edwards, C.M. Chemotherapy induced emesis mechanisms and treatment: a review. *Journal of the Royal Society of Medicine*, **81**, 658–661 (1988)
2. Borison, H.L., Borison, R. and McCarthy, L.E. Role of the area postrema in vomiting and related functions. *Federation Proceedings*, **43**, 2955–2958 (1984)
3. Borison, H.L. and Wang, S.C. Physiology and pharmacology of vomiting. *Pharmacology Reviews*, **5**, 192–230 (1953)
4. Miller, A.D. and Wilson, V.J. 'Vomiting center' reanalysed: an electrical stimulation study. *Brain Research*, **270**, 154–158 (1983)
5. Craig, J.B. and Powell, B.L. Review: The management of nausea and vomiting in clinical oncology. *American Journal of Medical Sciences*, **294**, 34–45 (1987)
6. Gralla, R.J., Tyson, L.B. and Borden, L.B. A review of recent studies and a report of a random assignment trial comparing metoclopramide with delta-9-tetrahydrocannabinol. *Cancer Treatment Reports*, **68**, 163–172 (1984)
7. Moher, D., Arthur, A.Z. and Pater, J.L. Anticipatory nausea and/or vomiting. *Cancer Treatment Reviews*, **11**, 257–264 (1984)
8. Greenberg, D.B., Surman, O.S., Clarke, J. and Baer, L. Alprazolam for phobic nausea and vomiting related to cancer chemotherapy. *Cancer Treatment Reports*, **71**, 549–550 (1987)
9. Morrow, G.R. and Morrell, C. Behavioural treatment for the anticipatory nausea and vomiting induced by cancer chemotherapy. *New England Journal of Medicine*, **307**, 1476–1480 (1982)
10. Buss, D.H. and Scharv, J.M. Herpesvirus infection of oesophagus and other visceral organs in adults. Incidence and clinical significance. *American Journal of Medicine*, **66**, 457–462 (1979)
11. Smith, F.P., Kisner, K.L., Widerlite, L. and Schein, P.S. Chemotherapeutic alteration of small intestinal morphology and function: a progress report. *Journal of Clinical Gastroenterology*, **1**, 203–207 (1979)
12. Shaw, M.T., Spector, M.H. and Ladman, A.J. Effects of cancer, radiotherapy and cytotoxic drugs on intestinal structure and function. *Cancer Treatment Reviews*, **6**, 141–151 (1979)
13. Young, R.C., Goldberg, D. and Schein, P.S. Enhanced antitumour effect of cytosine arabinoside given in a schedule dictated by kinetic studies *in vivo*. *Biochemical Pharmacology*, **22**, 277–289 (1973)
14. McClelland, D.B.L. Bacterial and viral infections of the gastrointestinal tract. In *Immunology of the Gastrointestinal tract* (ed. P. Asquith), Churchill Livingstone, Edinburgh, London, New York, pp. 214–245 (1979)
15. Desai, D.V., Ezdinli, E.Z. and Stutzman, L. Vincristine therapy of lymphomas and chronic lymphocytic leukaemia. *Cancer*, **26**, 352–359 (1970)
16. Sandler, S.G., Tobin, W. and Henderson, E.S. Vincristine-induced neuropathy. *Neurology*, **19**, 367–374 (1969)
17. Weiss, R.B. Hypersensitivity reactions to cancer chemotherapy. *Seminars in Oncology*, **9**, 5–13 (1982)
18. Vuolo, S.J. Oral complications of cancer chemotherapy and dental care for the cancer patient receiving antineoplastic drug therapy: a literature review. *New York Journal of Dentistry*, **57**, 50–59 (1987)
19. Konzelman, J.L. Oral implication of radiotherapy and chemotherapy. *Journal of Oral Medicine*, **38**, 76–78 (1983)
20. Bott, S., Prakash, C. and McCalluss, R.W. Medication-induced oesophageal injury: survey of the literature. *American Journal of Gastroenterology*, **82**, 758–763 (1987)
21. Smith, B. The myenteric plexus in drug-induced neuropathy. *Journal of Neurology, Neurosurgery and Psychiatry*, **30**, 506–510 (1967)
22. Sninsky, C.A. Vincristine alters myoelectrical activity and transit of the small intestine in rats. *Gastroenterology*, **92**, 472–478 (1987)
23. McDonald, G.B., Sharma, P., Hackman, R.C. *et al.* Esophageal infections in immunosuppressed patients after bone marrow transplantation. *Gastroenterology*, **88**, 1111–1117 (1985)
24. Howiler, W. and Goldberg, H.I. Gastroesophageal involvement in herpes simplex. *Gastroenterology*, **70**, 775–778 (1976)
25. Nash, G. and Ross, J.S. Herpetic oesophagitis: a common cause of oesophageal ulceration. *Human Pathology*, **5**, 339–345 (1974)
26. McDonald, G.B., Shulman, H.M., Sullivan, K.M. and Spencer, G.D. Intestinal and hepatic complications of human bone marrow transplantation. Part I. *Gastroenterology*, **90**, 460–477 (1986)
27. Millard, P.R., Herbertson, B.M., Nagington, J. and Evans, D.B. Morphological consequence and significance of CMV infections in renal transplant patients. *Quarterly Journal of Medicine*, **42**, 585–596 (1973)
28. McDonald, G.B. and Tirumali, N. Intestinal and liver toxicity of neoplastic drugs. *Western Journal of Medicine*, **140**, 250–295 (1984)
29. Hunt, J.N., Smith, J.L., Jiang, C.L. and Kessler, M.S. Effect of synthetic prostaglandin E analog on aspirin-induced gastric bleeding and secretion. *Digestive Diseases and Sciences*, **28**, 897–902 (1983)
30. Mairligit, G.M., Faintuch, J., Levin, B. *et al.* Gastroduodenal mucosal injury during hepatic arterial infusion of chemotherapeutic agents. Lack of cytoprotection of prostaglandin $E_1$ analogue. *Gastroenterology*, **92**, 566–569 (1987)
31. Schuger, L., Peretz, T., Goldin, E. *et al.* Duodenal epithelial atypia: a specific complication of hepatic arterial infusion chemotherapy. *Cancer*, **61**, 663–666 (1988)
32. Ohnuma, T. and Holland, J.F. Nutritional consequences of cancer chemotherapy and immunotherapy. *Cancer Research*, **34**, 2395–2406 (1977)
33. Milles, S.S., Muggia, A.L. and Spiro, H.B. Colonic

# 20

# Central nervous system manifestations of radiotherapy

**W.M. Wara and D.A. Larson**

Irradiation of central nervous system structures can result in central nervous system injury. However, the actual risk of injury associated with any specific combination of clinical variables and radiation factors is poorly understood. Much of the literature on the tolerance of the central nervous system to therapeutic irradiation is incomplete or anecdotal. Nevertheless, several circumstances in which adverse reactions may occur are known and allow clinicians to assess the possibility of injury following a particular course of radiotherapy.

Adverse effects of irradiation of the human brain are usually categorized according to time of clinical manifestations:

1. Acute reactions which occur during the course of treatment;
2. Early delayed reactions which occur a few weeks to a few months following irradiation; and
3. Late delayed reactions which appear several months to years after treatment.

Adverse effects of radiation to the human spinal cord, radiation myelopathies, are usually subdivided into:

1. Transient radiation myelopathies which appear within the first year or so following treatment, and
2. Delayed radiation myelopathies, usually appearing later.

The risk for occurrence of these reactions and their severity depend both on technical factors such as radiation fraction size, total radiation dose, number of elapsed days from start to completion of radiation, volume of central nervous system tissue irradiated, and number and distribution of beam ports, as well as on clinical factors such as patient age, presence of central nervous system injury due to tumor or prior surgery, presence of infection or vascular disease, and treatment with chemotherapy in addition to radiation.

## Brain injury

### Acute reactions

Acute reactions occur during a course of radiation treatment. Patients suffering acute reactions either develop an increase in pre-existing neurological deficits or demonstrate a clinical syndrome indicative of increased intracranial pressure. In most cases reactions are mild and of little significance. They are commonly thought to be due to radiation-induced edema, although no objective evidence is available to prove the hypothesis. Computed tomographic (CT) scans obtained during the course of treatment usually do not demonstrate increased peritumoral edema [1]. The previous practice of commencing radiotherapy treatment to the brain with a few low-dose fractions to avoid edema is usually unnecessary [2], except for patients with considerably elevated intracranial pressure due to a large or critically located brain tumor, despite high-dose dexamethasone [3].

Acute reactions are seen infrequently with conventional dose fractionation schedules (180–200 cGy/day given 5 days per week to a total dose of 6000 cGy to a portion of the brain). Larger individual fractions of radiation up to 600 cGy are well tolerated acutely, provided the total dose is lowered appropriately [4,5]. However, with larger fractions (two fractions of 750 cGy each over 3 days, or 1000 cGy in a single fraction to the whole brain) up to 50% of patients develop acute complications including headache, nausea, vomiting and pyrexia, and 10% of patients may develop cerebral herniation [6,7].

Modern clinical experience indicates that constant daily radiation doses of 200 cGy are well tolerated acutely, even with large total doses. For occasional patients who develop acute reactions, and for patients with poor neurological function, concomitant corticosteroid administration usually leads to rapid resolution of signs and symptoms, even though survival is not significantly affected.

## Early delayed reactions

Early delayed reactions occur a few weeks to a few months following irradiation, but are not frequently recognized, although they are analogous to transient radiation myelopathies following spinal cord irradiation, seen more frequently (see below). Clinically, most patients demonstrating early delayed reactions develop either exacerbations of pre-existing signs and symptoms, or somnolence, seen mainly in children with acute lymphoblastic lymphoma (ALL). Other patients may occasionally develop new neurological abnormalities.

The somnolence syndrome occurs in up to 75% of children with ALL who undergo prophylactic irradiation of the central nervous system [8,9]. It is characterized by somnolence, anorexia and irritability, without accompanying focal neurological abnormalities. Symptoms develop 1–2 months following completion of radiation and resolve spontaneously within 2–5 weeks. They are more severe in children under 3 years of age. Cerebrospinal fluid pleocytosis or mild protein elevation may be present, and diffuse slowing may be seen on EEG [10]. It is not entirely clear how radiation fraction size affects the incidence of somnolence. Parker *et al.* [11] reported somnolence in 40% of children receiving 125 cGy per fraction compared with 75% of children receiving 150 cGy per fraction to the same total dose (2400 cGy). Littman *et al.* [9] observed an equal incidence (58%) and severity of somnolence in children receiving either 100 cGy or 180 cGy per fraction to the same total dose (1800 cGy). In general, relapse and survival rates in children with ALL are not adversely affected by the somnolence syndrome. Such children may have the same risk to suffer cognitive dysfunction as children with ALL who do not develop the somnolence syndrome [12]. Occasionally somnolence may develop after conventional treatment in brain tumor patients.

Early delayed reactions manifesting as new neurological deficits are uncommon. Rider [13] described two patients who developed transient reactions approximately 10 weeks after radiation therapy for extracranial lesions. Both developed nausea, vomiting, dysarthria, dysphagia, ataxia, horizontal nystagmus and a positive Romberg sign. Recovery began after 1 month and was complete within two. Boldrey and Sheline [14] described eight patients who developed transient reactions 10 weeks after radiation therapy for low grade gliomas, meningiomas and pituitary adenomas. None of the reactions could be attributed to tumor progression since the symptoms resolved within 6 weeks. Hoffman, Levin and Wilson [15] described 51 patients with malignant gliomas treated with radiation and carmustine (BCNU). Changes suggesting tumor progression were seen in 25 patients within 18 weeks after radiation therapy. However, spontaneous improvement was seen in seven of the 25 affected; therefore, therapeutic decisions resulting in changes in management should be made cautiously during this period.

Early delayed reactions are usually transient and associated with an uneventful recovery. CT scans may reveal changes consistent with demyelination during the reaction period. It is thought that early delayed reactions, whether manifesting as the somnolence syndrome or otherwise, are a result of demyelination due to a temporary inhibition of myelin synthesis [8]. The latency and recovery times of early delayed reactions correspond to the turnover time of myelin [15,16].

## Late delayed reactions

Late delayed reactions are manifest several months to years following radiotherapy and are usually progressive and irreversible, and sometimes fatal. Clinical signs and symptoms depend on the region of brain irradiated and may be related to the development of necrosis. Other late occurring clinical sequelae include pituitary-hypothalamic dysfunction, decreased intellectual ability, necrotizing leukoencephalopathy or mineralizing microangiopathy, and radiation-induced tumors. The pathogenesis of the various manifestations of late delayed reactions is not completely understood. It is probable that multiple mechanisms are involved, including effects of radiation on brain vasculature [17] or myelination [18] and their relative importance may depend on the latent interval. Vascular changes probably become more important with time [2].

### *Radiation necrosis*

The risk for the development of brain radionecrosis as distinguished from transient injury is difficult to establish for several reasons: autopsies are not commonly performed, studies frequently fail to include the number of exposed patients who have survived at least as long as the latent period, and it is difficult to compare the results of various dose fractionation schedules used. However, the data of Marks *et al.* [19] are frequently quoted. They reported 139 patients with various intracranial tumors treated with standard doses (180–200 cGy to a minimum total dose of 4500 cGy, with most patients receiving 5000–6000 cGy in 5–7 weeks) although only one of two parallel opposed fields was treated each day. Pathologically documented cerebral necrosis was seen in seven of 139 patients (5%), and two additional patients developed clinically diagnosed radionecrosis. However, only 24 of the 139 patients underwent reoperation or autopsy, so this risk estimate may represent a lower limit. However, these data, representing patients treated during 1974–1976, were recently updated and compared with results in patients treated during 1976–1981 when the dose was reduced by an average of 7% [20]. No cases of radionecrosis were seen in 198 patients in the latter series. It is concluded that the risk of radionecrosis is extremely low for patients treated to 5400 cGy in 30 fractions over 42 days, but increases rapidly as one escalates to doses above 6000 cGy.

Recently Lee *et al.* [21] reported 9606 patients treated with radiation therapy for nasopharyngeal carcinoma using unconventional, large fractions ranging from 250 to 420 cGy over 38–42 days to a total dose of 4560–6000 cGy, using techniques which included the temporal lobes in the treatment fields. Late temporal lobe radionecrosis was diagnosed by correlating clinical features and CT scans rather than by biopsy. The incidence rate in this series was only 1%, and this too may represent an underestimate.

It is recognized that comparisons of the risk for developing radionecrosis between various dose fractionation schemes are difficult. As a result several formulae have been developed to mathematically combine total dose ($D$), total number of radiation fractions ($N$) and elapsed time ($T$) from start to completion of radiotherapy to produce a single number which can be related to outcome. Examples are the Nominal Standard Dose (NSD) formula of Sheline *et al.* [2]:

$$\text{NSD (neuret)} = D \times N^{-0.44} \times T^{-0.06}, \qquad (20.1)$$

to be applied to irradiation of the brain, and the Equivalent Dose (ED) formula of Wara *et al.* [22]:

$$\text{ED (ret)} = D \times N^{-0.377} \times T^{-0.058}, \qquad (20.2)$$

usually applied to irradiation of the spinal cord. Although firm data are lacking, present evidence indicates that the threshold for brain necrosis is approximately 1000–1100 neuret, or an equivalent dose of 1250 ret.

The diagnosis of radionecrosis in patients without intracranial tumors can be inferred from findings at CT or magnetic resonance imaging (MRI). However, in patients with tumors the diagnosis is made with difficulty. At present CT or MRI cannot reliably distinguish radiation necrosis from recurrent tumor. Both may present similar, non-specific, clinical and radiological findings, and biopsy is required to confirm the diagnosis of radionecrosis if abnormalities are seen at the tumor site [16].

Surgical resection of focal areas of radiation necrosis frequently results in clinical improvement with occasional complete recovery. Resection is of little value in patients with diffuse lesions, lesions crossing midline, or lesions involving the brain stem or optic nerves. Little clinical benefit is seen following biopsy only, other than to establish the etiology. Corticosteroids frequently result in clinical improvement of neurological deficits when surgery is not possible [16]. Anticoagulant agents have been reported to lead to dramatic clinical and CT improvement [23], although confirmation of this effect in randomized trials is lacking.

## *Necrotizing leukoencephalopathy and mineralizing microangiopathy*

These reactions were first recognized as complications of treatment for childhood ALL. Necrotizing leukoencephalopathy, also called disseminating necrotizing leukoencephalopathy and subacute leukoencephalopathy, is manifest by the progressive development of personality changes, disorientation, memory loss and frank dementia. It is seen in up to 15% of children receiving cranial radiation therapy and intrathecal or high-dose intravenous methotrexate [10,24]. The risk for its occurrence appears to be low in children who receive radiation therapy treatment following methotrexate administration, as opposed to those who receive methotrexate following irradiation or concurrent irradiation [10].

Children who develop leukoencephalopathy demonstrate non-enhancing periventricular hypodensities on CT. With time, ventricular dilatation and broadening of the sulci may occur [10]. Similar abnormal CT findings have been reported in asymptomatic patients, and probably represent subclinical leukoencephalopathy. It should be noted, however, that children in remission from ALL after receiving intrathecal methotrexate and less than 2500 cGy cranial irradiation may develop cognitive impairment even though white matter changes are not seen on MRI [25].

The pathogenesis of this syndrome is thought to be demyelination of the cerebral hemispheric white matter, although other lipid membrane reactions may be involved. Histopathologically, lesions are characterized by demyelination, multifocal areas of coagulation necrosis, and gliosis.

Most children who develop this syndrome survive with some degree of permanent neurological deficit; in some the outcome is fatal, although a few may recover completely. Leukoencephalopathy has also been described in adults treated for various cancers with radiotherapy, chemotherapy, or both [26,27].

Mineralizing microangiopathy presents as headache, focal seizures, ataxia, behavior disorders, or perceptual motor disability. It is seen in approximately 25% of children who survive at least 9 months following central nervous sytem radiotherapy for ALL, and is seen more frequently in children under 10 years of age at the time of treatment [10]. CT scans may show calcification of the basal ganglia. Histopathologically, small blood vessels are seen to be occluded by calcium deposits within their walls. Brain tissues surrounding these vessels may be mineralized and necrotic [28].

## Radiological abnormalities

Late radiation injury may present radiologically as focal necrosis or as diffuse white matter injury. Both types of injury may appear together. On CT, focal necrosis produces a low density region with surrounding edema and variable mass effect, with an irregular margin of contrast enhancement. This pattern is easily interpreted when seen following irradiation of an extracranial lesion, but may be difficult to distinguish from that of tumor following irradiation of an intracranial lesion. MRI demonstrates edema, with increased signal on T2-weighted images, but does not provide appearances specific for tumor or focal necrosis. In some cases the distinction can be made by examining the blood–brain barrier and local glucose metabolism with positron emission tomography [29].

Diffuse white matter injury usually presents on CT as bilateral, diffuse low density lesions involving much of the hemispheric white matter, but is more frequently appreciated on MRI, which is extremely sensitive to white matter edema. Such lesions are usually indistinguishable from white matter changes seen in non-irradiated, otherwise normal, older people or in persons with cerebral vascular disease. Depending on criteria used for defining injury following irradiation, diffuse white matter injury may be seen in a large percentage of patients following brain irradiation [30,31]. The incidence of such injury increases with volume of brain irradiated, radiation dose, interval between irradiation and imaging, and patient age. Severe radiological changes correlate with clinical neurological findings, whereas the significance of mild and moderate radiological abnormalities is unknown [32]. Cerebral atrophy frequently accompanies diffuse white matter injury, although the clinical significance of this observation is unknown; many patients with diffuse white matter injury and cerebral atrophy have no obvious intellectual compromise, especially those under 40 years of age [27]. The radiological presentation of necrotizing leukoencephalopathy, a diffuse white matter injury, may be observed after irradiation and chemotherapy or after chemotherapy alone [26]. Diffuse white matter injury may occur at a somewhat lower dose and after a longer latent period than focal necrosis [33].

In exceptional circumstances such as with radiosurgery where radiation is delivered in a single fraction to a small intracranial target, damage to major intracranial arteries may occur, possibly resulting in brain necrosis at a site not immediately adjacent to the radiation field; arteriography may demonstrate occluded or stenosed arteries within the radiation field [34,35].

## Pituitary-hypothalamic dysfunction

Effects of brain irradiation on endocrine activity have long been recognized. Growth hormone deficiency, the most common deficiency, is noted in a large fraction of children receiving at least 2400 cGy to the hypothalamus during the whole brain cranial irradiation, and begins as early as 3 months following treatment [36]. Lustig *et al.* [37] demonstrated that such patients usually have functional pituitary somatotropes and a deficiency of endogenous hypothalamic growth hormone releasing factor (GRF), presumably reflecting the relative radioresistance of the pituitary and the relative radiosensitivity of the hypothalamic GRF secretory apparatus and higher neural centers. Other hypothalamic syndromes presenting as hypoadrenalism, hypogonadism, hypothyroidism and hyperprolactinemia following brain irradiation have been described. Mechanick, Hochberg and LaRocque [38] identified 15 patients with clinically evident hypothalamic dysfunction 2–9 years following whole brain irradiation for extrahypothalamic astrocytoma or medulloblastoma. Hypothalamic endocrine dysfunction (hyperprolactinemia) or behavioral changes (anxiety, depression, lability, belligerence, thirst and changes in sleep-wake cycle, appetite, etc.) were seen in all patients, without evidence on follow-up CT of an evident hypothalamic abnormality. Although the number of patients at risk was not precisely identified, it is likely that hypothalamic dysfunction in long-term survivors following whole brain irradiation is not rare. Younger children are at greater risk to develop hypothalamic dysfunction. The reverse syndrome has also been noted, with hypersensitive activity producing precocious puberty. Fortunately this entity is rare.

## Impaired intellectual function

Cognitive dysfunction in children is a recognized sequel of radiation therapy for brain tumors and ALL. Less information exists on the relationship between cranial irradiation and subsequent intellectual impairment in adults. In either case, causes of such dysfunction may be difficult to determine since surgery, chemotherapy, radiation therapy, psychological stress and effectiveness of rehabilitation are often thought to be contributory.

Recently Mulhern *et al.* [39] studied 40 children in continuous complete remission from ALL in order to assess memory functioning 5 years after CNS prophylaxis. Initially patients had been randomly assigned to receive CNS prophylaxis with either 1800 cGy cranial irradiation plus intrathecal methotrexate, or intrathecal methotrexate plus intravenous high-dose methotrexate. No treatment- or age-related differences were seen on 16 standardized memory measures. However, scores of the combined groups of patients were significantly lower than age-corrected norms on tests of visual-spatial memory and verbal memory.

Peckham *et al.* [40] studied 23 long-term survivors of childhood ALL who had received 2400 cGy cranial irradiation and intrathecal methotrexate and standard chemotherapeutic agents 8–10 years previously. Cognitive function had been evaluated at the time of diagnosis and periodically thereafter. Long-term assessment of levels of school achievement demonstrated that children achieved lower than expected levels in both reading and mathematics, in comparison with pretreatment and most recent IQ scores. In addition, most children experienced difficulty with attention and concentration, memory, sequencing and comprehension when performing school tasks. A small number of children performed better than expected, indicating that individual tutoring and parental support may reduce some learning deficits.

Recently Bordeaux *et al.* [41] evaluated the effect of radiotherapy and surgery on neuropsychological function in two groups of children: seven who underwent surgery and seven who underwent radiotherapy. Treatment groups were composed of children aged 56–196 months at the time of evaluation who had heterogeneous tumor diagnoses and locations. Children underwent neuropsychological testing before and after therapy. Comparisons of pretherapy findings with normative values indicated that both groups performed within the average range of most measures, although deficits at baseline were observed on test of fine-motor, psychomotor and timed-language skills, all probably attributable to tumor-related effects. Comparisons of pre- and post-therapy neuropsychological test findings demonstrated no significant interval changes for either group, possibly suggesting that surgery and radiotherapy are not associated with acute effects on neuropsychological functions. Testing in these children was performed at an average of 11 months, as opposed to testing done well beyond 1 year in many other studies. A recent study by Kramer *et al.* [25] reports a dissociation between MRI results and neurocognitive measures. He documented that in nine children with normal scans only three had average IQ scores.

Hochberg and Slotnick [42] studied 13 adult patients with high grade astrocytomas who had survived at least 1 year after being treated with the combination of surgery, external beam irradiation to 6000 cGy and lomustine (CCNU) chemotherapy. The 13 patients had failed to return to pretreatment educational or vocational levels and were therefore examined with neuropsychological tests of specific and generalized higher cortical functions. All demonstrated diffuse cortical dysfunction, including difficulty in problem solving and in coping with novel situations. Their performance was unrelated to tumor type or location and could not be explained by existing focal deficits, psychotic or depressive thought disorders, metabolic difficulties, and/or hydrocephalus.

Looper *et al.* [43] and Johnson *et al.* [44] reported survivors of small cell lung cancer who had received prophylactic or therapeutic cranial irradiation in addition to chemotherapy. Three-quarters of patients in both studies had evidence of neurological problems. In many cases this dysfunction was severe, either causing significant impairment of activity of daily living or requiring institutionalization. Onset typically occurred 2–3 years after treatment. Frequent problems included memory loss, confusion, dementia, ataxia, psychomotor retardation and optic atrophy. CT scans were available in all patients at the time of initial evaluation in Johnson's series, and were normal in 75% of patients. Of patients undergoing serial CT scans, progressive abnormalities were present in 61%.

## Radiation-induced tumors

Radiation-induced brain tumors are rare today but with improved survival in childhood malignancies their incidence may increase. Before a histologically verified tumor can be attributed to prior irradiation, it must arise within the radiation field and it should be of a different type from any prior central nervous system tumor. Liwnicz *et al.* [45] reviewed 96 such cases in the literature and found 50 meningiomas, 24 gliomas and 22 sarcomas. Most radiation-induced gliomas were found to occur in children and young adults but there was no apparent correlation between dose and latency. Such a correlation was noted with radiation-induced meningiomas, with a latency of 31.3 years following low-dose irradiation and 20.8 years following high-dose irradiation.

More recently, Ron *et al.* [46] studied over 10 000 children treated for tinea capitis with low-dose orthovoltage irradiation between 1948 and 1960, and compared them with matched general population controls and siblings who did not receive radiation treatment. The 30-year cumulative risk for the subsequent development of neural tumors in patients exposed as children was 0.8%. The estimated relative risk as compared with controls was 6.9. Increased risks were found for meningiomas, gliomas, nerve-sheath tumors and other neural tumors. A strong dose-response relationship was noted with a relative risk of approximately 20 after doses of approximately 250 cGy. Tumors occurred between 6 and 29 years after radiation (mean 17.6 years). Unfortunately, it is currently impossible to extrapolate these findings to obtain those expected in patients treated with modern high energy linear accelerators, with different resultant dose distributions and higher prescribed doses (usually 1800–6000 cGy), since cell killing probably influences radiogenic risks. The mechanism of radiation tumor induction is unknown at the present time.

### Risk factors

The incidence of late delayed reactions is increased in patients treated with methotrexate and radiotherapy for ALL. In addition, late delayed reactions are seen in long-term surviving patients with small cell carcinoma of the lung who received prophylactic cranial irradiation of 3000 cGy in ten fractions [47]. Patients with underlying vascular disease secondary to diabetes mellitus, Cushing's disease or acromegaly may be at increased risk for the development of radiation injury [48–50], as are patients with an underlying CNS infection [51] or those who have received chemotherapy [52,53]. It is generally thought that children under the age of 3 years are at increased risk of developing radiation injury since myelination in young children is not complete [2].

## Spinal cord injury
### Transient radiation myelopathy

Patients with transient radiation myelopathy describe sudden, electric-like shocks radiating down the spine to the extremities on neck flexion (Lhermitte's sign). Symptoms are usually symmetrical but are unrelated to a specific dermatome distribution, and neurological examination is otherwise normal. Carmel and Kaplan [54] reported the finding in 15% of 377 patients treated with mantle field irradiation for Hodgkin's disease, with latent periods after radiotherapy of 1–29 months (median 4 months). The average duration of symptoms was 5.3 months.

It is believed that transient radiation myelopathy results from transient demyelination in the posterior columns and/or lateral spinothalamic tracts within the radiation field. Presumably radiation inhibits the normal proliferation of myelin-producing oligodendroglial cells in the irradiated area. The latent period is consistent with temporary blockage in the synthesis of myelin. It is believed that symptoms result from stretching of the demyelinated, hypersensitive posterior fibers of the cord. In general, the clinical picture reverses spontaneously without specific therapy, although subsequent radiation myelitis has been reported occasionally, mostly in cases where commonly accepted spinal cord tolerance doses have been exceeded.

### Delayed radiation myelopathy

Patients with delayed radiation myelopathy typically present with a several month history of progressive neurological signs and symptoms, such as paresthesias and decreased pain and temperature sensation. The latent period may range from several weeks to many years. A bimodal frequency distribution of latencies has been reported, with peaks at 13 and at 26 months [55], possibly corresponding with white matter parenchymal damage and vascular damage, respectively [56]. A shorter latency period is associated with higher doses, lower age, and retreatment with radiation. Symptoms usually progress over 6 months to involve all spinal cord systems, although occasionally they develop acutely following infarction of the spinal cord as a result of radiation-induced vascular changes. Symptoms are usually irreversible, although occasional temporary remissions have been reported following treatment with corticosteroids or hyperbaric oxygen, and about 50% of patients die from secondary complications.

The diagnosis of radiation myelopathy is usually a diagnosis of exclusion, and requires that the neurological lesion lies within the radiation field and that local metastatic or primary spinal cord tumors be ruled out. Cerebrospinal fluid (CSF) pressure is usually normal. Mild elevations in CSF protein concentration may be seen. Myelography may be normal or may show an area of expansion or attenuation at the irradiated site [4,57]. In general, CT and MRI have not been useful to date in helping make this diagnosis, although midsagittal MRI images of the spine can easily demonstrate fatty replacement of marrow in vertebral bodies, thus sharply delineating the upper and lower borders of the radiation field in patients receiving commonly accepted spinal cord radiation doses [58]. Electrophysiological measurements of spinal cord nerve conduction velocities are slowed following commonly accepted doses of radiation therapy to the spinal cord [59] but it is not yet known if such measurements can be used to monitor or predict the development of myelopathy.

Pathological changes are seen in all cord elements, but particularly in white matter, and pathogenesis is usually attributed either to extensive demyelination progressing to white matter necrosis (white matter parenchymal lesion) or to intramedullary vascular damage progressing to hemorrhagic necrosis or infarct (vascular lesion) following irradiation. Histopathological studies demonstrate varying degrees of endothelial swelling in small arteries and arterioles, endothelial proliferation, collagen and hyaline deposition, intimal and medial necrosis, and vascular occlusion, together with patchy demyelination and Wallerian degeneration.

The relationship between various dose fractionation schemes and risk for radiation myelitis is incompletely understood. However, for a given total dose increased risk is associated with larger fractions, decreased number of treatments, and treatment of larger lengths of spinal cord. Larger total doses for a given daily fractionation are also associated with increased risk. Wara *et al.* [22] applied the equivalent dose formula shown in Equation 20.2 to reported cases of spinal cord injury following radiation therapy and found a threshold dose of approximately 1000 ret. In general, a dose of 4500 cGy in 25 fractions leads to myelitis in no more than 5% of patients. However, this risk may be increased by predisposing factors. Pre-existing hypertension is known to increase the likelihood of spinal cord damage in rats and may have a similar effect in humans [60]. Some chemotherapeutic agents probably increase the risk. Younger patients may be at increased risk. The thoracic cord may be more radiosensitive than the cervical cord. It is sometimes thought that risk is increased in patients whose cords have suffered previous injury from tumor and surgery, although one study found no such increased risk [61].

There is no known effective treatment of delayed radiation myelopathy, although temporary remissions have been reported following administration of steroids or hyperbaric oxygen therapy. Although long-term survival is possible, the probability of dying of radiation myelopathy is approximately 30% for thoracic cord injuries and 70% for cervical cord injuries [62].

# References


1. Deck, M.D.F. Imaging techniques in the diagnosis of radiation damage to the central nervous system. In *Radiation Damage to the Nervous System* (eds H.A. Gilbert and R.A. Kagan), Raven Press, New York, pp. 107–127 (1980)
2. Sheline, G.E., Wara, W.M. and Smith, V. Therapeutic irradiation and brain injury. *International Journal of Radiation Oncology, Biology, Physics*, **6**, 1215–1228 (1980)
3. Plowman, P.N., Fuentos, J. and Harnett, A.N. Early radiation swelling remains a problem in the management of paediatric brain tumors. *British Journal of Radiology*, **60**, 931–932 (1987)
4. Kramer, S. and Lee, K.F. Complications of radiation therapy: the central nervous system. *Seminars in Roentgenology*, **9**, 75–83 (1974)
5. Borgelt, B., Gelber, R., Kramer, S. *et al.* The palliation of brain metastases: final results of the first two studies by the Radiation Therapy Oncology Group. *International Journal of Radiation Oncology, Biology, Physics*, **6**, 1–9 (1980)
6. Young, D.F., Posner, J.B., Chu, F. and Nisce, L. Rapid-course radiation therapy of cerebral metastases: results and complications. *Cancer*, **34**, 1069–1076 (1974)
7. Hindo, W.A., DeTrana, F.A. III, Lee, M-S and Hendrickson, F.R. Large dose increment irradiation in treatment of cerebral metastases. *Cancer*, **26**, 138–141 (1970)
8. Freeman, J.E., Johnston, P.G.G. and Voke, J.M. Somnolence syndrome after prophylactic cranial irradiation in children with acute lymphoblastic leukemia. *British Medical Journal*, **iv**, 523–525 (1973)
9. Littman, P., Rosenstock, J., Gale, G. *et al.* The somnolence syndrome in leukemic children following reduced daily dose fractions of cranial radiation. *International Journal of Radiation Oncology, Biology, Physics*, **10**, 1851–1853 (1984)
10. Bleyer, W.A. and Griffin, T.W. White matter necrosis, microangiopathy and intellectual abilities in survivors of childhood leukemia, association with central nervous system irradiation and methotrexate therapy. In *Radiation Damage to the Nervous System* (eds H.A. Gilbert and A.R. Kagan), Raven Press, New York, pp. 155–174 (1980)
11. Parker, D., Malpas, J.S., Sandland, R. *et al.* Outlook following 'somnolence syndrome' after prophylactic cranial irradiation. *British Medical Journa,l* **iv**, 554 (1978)
12. Trautman, P.D., Erickson, C., Shaffer, D. *et al.* Prediction of intellectual deficits in children with acute lymphoblastic leukemia. *Journal of Developmental and Behavioral Pediatrics*, **9**, 122–128 (1988)
13. Rider, W.D. Radiation damage to the brain – a new syndrome. *Journal of the Canadian Association of Radiologists*, **14**, 67–69 (1963)
14. Boldrey, E. and Sheline, G.E. Delayed transitory clinical manifestations after radiation treatment of intracranial tumors. *Acta Radiologica*, **5**, 5–10 (1967)
15. Hoffman, W.F., Levin, V.A. and Wilson, C.B. Evaluation of malignant glioma patients during the postirradiation period. *Journal of Neurosurgery*, **50**, 624–628 (1979)
16. Edwards, M.S.B. and Wilson, C.B. Treatment of radiation necrosis. In *Radiation Damage to the Nervous System* (eds H.A. Gilbert and A.R. Kagan), Raven Press, New York, pp. 129–143 (1980)
17. Martins, A.N., Johnston, J.S., Henry, J.M. *et al.* Delayed radiation necrosis of the brain. *Journal of Neurosurgery*, **47**, 336–345 (1977)
18. Lampert, P., Tom, M.I. and Rider, W.D. Disseminated demyelination of the brain following Co$^{60}$ (gamma) radiation. *A.M.A. Archives of Pathology*, **68**, 322–330 (1959)
19. Marks, J.E., Baglan, R.J., Prassad, S.C. and Blank, W.F. Cerebral radionecrosis: incidence and risk in relation to dose, time, fractionation and volume. *International Journal of Radiation Oncology, Biology, Physics*, **7**, 243–252 (1981)

20. Marks, J.B. and Wong, J. The risk of cerebral radionecrosis in relation to dose, time and fractionation. *Progress in Experimental Tumor Research*, **29**, 210–218 (1985)

21. Lee, A.W.M., Ng, S.H., Ho, J.H.C. *et al.* Clinical diagnosis of late temporal lobe necrosis following radiation therapy for nasopharyngeal carcinoma. *Cancer*, **61**, 1535–1542 (1988)

22. Wara, W.M., Phillips, T.L., Sheline, G.E. and Schwade, J.G. Radiation tolerance of the spinal cord. *Cancer*, **35**, 1558–1562 (1975)

23. Rizzoli, H.V. and Pagnanelli, D.M. Treatment of delayed radiation necrosis of the brain. A clinical observation. *Journal of Neurosurgery*, **60**, 589–594 (1984)

24. Aur, J.A., Simons, J.V., Verzosa, M.S. *et al.* Leukoencephalopathy in children with lymphocytic leukemia receiving preventive central nervous system therapy. *Sangre (Barcelona)*, **23**, 1–12 (1978)

25. Kramer, J.H., Norman, D., Brant-Zawadzki, M. *et al.* Absence of white matter changes on magnetic resonance imaging in children treated with CNS prophylaxis therapy for leukemia. *Cancer*, **61**, 928–930 (1988)

26. Lee, Y., Nauert, C. and Glass, J.P. Treatment-related white matter changes in cancer patients. *Cancer*, **57**, 1473–1482 (1986)

27. Stylopoulos, L.A., George, A.E., de Leon, M.J. *et al.* Longitudinal CT study of parenchymal brain changes in glioma survivors. *American Journal of Neuroradiology*, **9**, 517–522 (1988)

28. Price, R.A. and Birdwell, D.A. The central nervous system in childhood leukemia III. Mineralizing microangiopathy and dystrophic calcifications. *Cancer*, **42**, 717–728 (1978)

29. Doyle, W.K., Budinger, T.F., Valk, P.E. *et al.* Differentiation of cerebral radiation necrosis from tumor recurrence by [$^{18}$F]FDG and $^{82}$Rb positron emission tomography. *Journal of Computer Assisted Tomography*, **11**, 563–570 (1987)

30. Constine, L.S., Konski, A., Ekholm, S. *et al.* Adverse effects of brain irradiation correlated with MR and CT imaging. *International Journal of Radiation Oncology, Biology, Physics*, **15**, 319–330 (1988)

31. Tsuruda, J.S., Kortman, K.E., Bradley, W.G. *et al.* Radiation effects on cerebral white matter: MRI evaluation. *American Journal of Roentgenology*, **8**, 431–437 (1987)

32. Curran, W.J., Hecht-Leavitt, C., Schut, L. *et al.* Magnetic resonance imaging of cranial radiation lesions. *International Journal of Radiation Oncology, Biology, Physics*, **13**, 1093–1098 (1987)

33. Mikhael, M.A. Radiation damage to the central nervous system: a delayed therapeutic hazard. In *Radiation Damage to the Nervous System* (eds H.A. Gilbert and A.R. Kagan), Raven Press, New York, pp. 59–91 (1980)

34. Marks, M.P., Delapaz, R.L., Fabrikant, J.I. *et al.* Intracranial vascular malformations: imaging of charged-particle radiosurgery. Part II. Complications. *Radiology*, **168**, 457–462 (1988)

35. Brant-Zawadzki, M., Anderson, M., DeArmond, S.J. *et al.* Radiation-induced large intracranial vessel occlusive vasculopathy. *American Journal of Roentgenology*, **134**, 51–55 (1980)

36. Duffner, P.K., Cohen, M.E., Voorhees, M.L. *et al.* Long-term effects of cranial irradiation on endocrine function in children with brain tumors. *Cancer*, **56**, 2189–2193 (1985)

37. Lustig, R.H., Schriock, E.A., Kaplan, S.L. and Grumbach, M.M. Effects of growth hormone-releasing factor on growth hormone release in children with radiation-induced growth hormone deficiency. *Pediatrics*, **76**, 274–279 (1985)

38. Mechanick, J.I., Hochberg, F.H. and LaRocque, A. Hypothalamic dysfunction following whole brain irradiation. *Journal of Neurosurgery*, **65**, 490–494 (1986)

39. Mulhern, R.K., Wasserman, A.L., Fairclough, D. and Ochs, J. Memory function in disease-free survivors of childhood acute lymphocytic leukemia given CNS prophylaxis with or without 1800 cGy cranial radiation. *Journal of Clinical Oncology*, **6**, 315–320 (1988)

40. Peckham, V.C., Meadows, A.T., Bartel, N. and Marrero, O. Educational late effects in long-term survivors of childhood acute lymphocytic leukemia. *Pediatrics*, **81**, 127–133 (1988)

41. Bordeaux, J.D., Dowell, R.E., Copeland, D.R. *et al.* A prospective study of neuropsychologic sequelae in children with brain tumors. *Journal of Child Neurology*, **3**, 63–68 (1988)

42. Hochberg, F.H. and Slotnick, B. Neuropsychologic impairment in astrocytoma survivors. *Neurology*, **30**, 172–177 (1980)

43. Looper, J.D., Einhorn, L.H., Garcia, A. *et al.* Severe neurologic problems following successful therapy for small cell lung cancer (SCLC). *Proceedings of the Annual Meeting of the American Society of Clinical Oncology*, **3**, 231 (1984)

44. Johnson, V.E., Becker, B., Goff, W.B. *et al.* Neurologic, neuropsychologic and computed cranial tomography scan abnormalities in 2–10 year survivors of small cell lung cancer. *Journal of Clinical Oncology*, **3**, 1659–1667 (1985)

45. Liwnicz, B.H., Berger, T.S., Liwnicz, R.G. and Aron, B.S. Radiation-associated gliomas: a report of four cases and analysis of postradiation tumors of the central nervous system. *Neurosurgery*, **17**, 436–435 (1985)

46. Ron, E., Modan, B., Boice, J.D. *et al.* Tumors of the brain and nervous system after radiotherapy. *New England Journal of Medicine*, **319**, 1033–1039 (1988)

47. Volk, S.A., Mansour, R.P., Gandara, D.R. and Redmond, J. Morbidity in long-term survivors of small cell carcinoma of the lung. *Proceedings of the American Society of Clinical Oncology*, 185 (1983)

48. Smith, B.M., McGinnis, W., Cook, J. and Latourette, H. Central nervous system changes complicating the use of radiotherapy for the treatment of a nasophary-

ngeal neoplasm in a diabetic patient. *Cancer,* **43**, 2239–2242 (1979)

49. Bloom, B. and Kramer, S. Conventional radiation therapy in the management of acromegaly. In *Secretory Tumors of the Pituitary Gland* (eds P.McL. Black, N.T. Zervas, E.C. Ridgway and J.B. Martin), Raven Press, New York, pp. 179–190 (1984)

50. Aristizabal, S.A., Boone, M.L. and Laguna, J. Endocrine factors influencing radiation injury to central nervous tissue. *International Journal of Radiation Oncology, Biology, Physics,* **5**, 349–353 (1975)

51. Cumberlin, R.L., Luk, K.H., Wara, W.M. *et al.* Medulloblastoma: treatment results and effect on normal tissues. *Cancer,* **43**, 1014–1020 (1979)

52. Burger, P.C., Mahaley, M.S. Jr., Dudka, L. and Vogel, F.S. The morphologic effects of radiation administered therapeutically for intracranial gliomas: a postmortem study of 25 cases. *Cancer,* **44**, 1256–1272 (1979)

53. Weiss, H.D., Walker, M.D. and Wiernik, P.H. Neurotoxicity of commonly used antineoplastic agents. *New England Journal of Medicine,* **291**, 127–133 (1974)

54. Carmel, R.J. and Kaplan, H.S. Mantle irradiation in Hodgkin's disease. An analysis of technique, tumor eradication and complications. *Cancer,* **37**, 2813–2825 (1976)

55. Schultheiss, T.E., Higgins, E.M. and El-Mahdi, A.M. The latent period in clinical radiation myelopathy. *International Journal of Radiation Oncology, Biology, Physics,* **10**, 1109–1115 (1984)

56. Schultheiss, T.E., Stephens, L.C. and Maor, M.H. Analysis of the histopathology of radiation myelopathy. *International Journal of Radiation Oncology,* **14**, 27–32 (1988)

57. Atkins, H.L. and Tretter, P. Time-dose considerations in radiation myelopathy. *Acta Radiologica,* **5**, 79–94 (1966)

58. Ramsey, R.G. and Zacharias, C.E. MR imaging of the spine after radiation therapy: easily recognizable effects. *American Journal of Neuroradiology,* **144**, 1131–1135 (1985)

59. Dorfman, L.J., Donaldson, S.S., Gupta, P.R. and Bosley, T.M. Electrophysiologic evidence of subclinical injury to the posterior columns of the human spinal cord after therapeutic radiation. *Cancer,* **50**, 2815–2819 (1982)

60. Asscher, A.W. and Anson, S.G. Arterial hypertension in radiation damage to the nervous system. *Lancet,* **ii**, 1343–1346 (1962)

61. Kopelson, G. Radiation tolerance of the spinal cord previously damaged by tumor and operations: long term neurological improvement and time-dose-volume relationships after irradiation of intraspinal gliomas. *International Journal of Radiation Oncology, Biology, Physics,* **8**, 925–929 (1982)

62. Schultheiss, T.E., Stephens, L.C. and Peters, L.J. Survival in radiation myelopathy. *International Journal of Radiation Oncology, Biology, Physics,* **12**, 1765–1769 (1986)

# 21

# Central nervous system morbidity secondary to chemotherapy

E.D. Kramer, B.H. Cohen and R.J. Packer

Over the past 25 years long-term disease control and survival rates have significantly improved for many forms of cancer. As more successful cancer treatments have emerged, the likelihood of nervous system (NS) morbidity caused by antineoplastic therapy has increased [1–10]. The development of new chemotherapeutic agents and the delivery of agents at higher dosages, in various combinations and by different routes have contributed to improving disease control, but also have increased the incidence of neurological sequelae. Neurotoxicity may involve either the central nervous system (CNS) or peripheral nervous system (PNS). Frequent forms of expression include acute or chronic progressive occurring encephalopathies, seizures, meningitides, cerebellar ataxia, spinal cord syndromes, parenchymal necrosis, and cranial and peripheral neuropathies. At times it is difficult to distinguish chemotherapy-induced complications from effects of prior therapy or metastatic disease.

Intrinsic factors that predispose the nervous system to treatment-related brain injury have been most intensively investigated for radiation therapy-induced sequelae and proposed mechanisms of damage have been extended to chemotherapeutic-related damage [11–16]. Because the majority of cells in the brain and spinal cord, including neurons and astrocytes, undergo little, if any, postnatal cellular division, acute effects of many chemotherapeutic agents are less prominent in the CNS than they are in other organs. Chemotherapeutic agents that cause intracellular metabolic dysfunction such as methotrexate are more likely to cause acute CNS complications [17,18]. Of all of the cells in the brain, the capillary endothelial cells are the most rapidly dividing. Their injury has been implicated as the primary reason for delayed radiation-induced CNS damage [14]. For unknown reasons, similar brain injury has not been seen after chemotherapy. On the other hand, another possible mechanism of radiation-induced damage – sublethal astrocytic and oligodendroglial cellular injury resulting in faulty myelinization and abnormal glial proliferation – has been increasingly implicated.

Another factor that limits the frequency and degree of CNS damage secondary to chemotherapeutic agents is the blood–brain barrier (BBB) [19]. Because the BBB limits the amount of ionized and water soluble drug that can reach the brain, it limits the detrimental CNS effects of these agents. However, as new means are used to overcome this barrier, including the use of higher doses of medications, the employment of intra-arterial infusions and the delivery of drugs with osmotic agents that disrupt the BBB, drugs that previously caused little CNS dysfunction are producing severe, sometimes acute, neurological damage [20,21].

## Alkylating agents

### Nitrogen mustard (mechlorethamine-HN$_2$)

Standard doses of nitrogen mustard are rarely associated with neurotoxicity. Fever, hemiplegia and coma have been reported in a patient with Hodgkin's lymphoma following two times standard, or 0.4 mg/kg of nitrogen mustard given intravenously [22]. At post-mortem examination, cortical focal gliosis and neuronal loss were found. This was considered an idiosyncratic reaction to the drug.

Increased systemic or regional doses of nitrogen mustard have been associated with a higher incidence of neurological complications [23–25]. Hearing loss, tinnitus and vestibular dysfunction occasionally occur after high-dose intracarotid therapy [23].

Intracarotid infusions have resulted in seizures, hemiplegia, coma and death [26–28]. Post-mortem examination in one patient who developed focal neurological dysfunction after intracarotid therapy revealed demyelination and gliosis ipsilateral to the infusions [26]. Lower motor neuron damage manifested by weakness and loss of reflexes occurs after high-dose intra-arterial administration of nitrogen mustard for tumors of the pelvis and limbs [29,30]. The role of nitrogen mustard in these complications has been supported by the laboratory studies of Mahaley *et al.* who demonstrated that the agent concentrated in the VIIIth central nerve of dogs [31], and of Woodhall *et al.* who showed histopathological changes in dog sciatic nerves after topical application, subepineural injection, or regional perfusion of nitrogen mustard [32].

## Cyclophosphamide (Cytoxan)

Cyclophosphamide usually causes little neurotoxicity. Rapid intravenous infusion has been associated with transient (seconds to minutes) symptoms of dizziness, facial flushing, tingling in the posterior pharynx and euphoria [33]. Visual blurring was noted in five of 29 children receiving $750 \, mg/m^2$ every other day for five doses; this was transient in three patients, but lasted 3 days and 2 weeks in the remaining two patients [34]. Single intravenous doses of $1500 \, mg/m^2$ given to nine patients and $1200 \, mg/m^2$ given to one were associated with laboratory findings of inappropriate secretion of antidiuretic hormone [35]. Abnormal laboratory findings resolved within 3 days in all patients.

## Ifosfamide

Ifosfamide is an analogue of cyclophosphamide. Although the latter rarely causes neurological toxicity, ifosfamide is associated with severe but often reversible neurotoxicity. In phase I and II studies, doses of $1600 \, mg/m^2/day$ given intravenously over 15 min for 5 days every 3–5 weeks were associated with mental status changes (ranging from irritability to confusion to coma), cerebellar dysfunction, weakness, cranial nerve dysfunction and seizures in 13 of 61 patients (21%) during 20 of 143 (14%) treatment courses [36]. Electroencephalographic (EEG) slowing of background frequencies to the delta range occurred. Spike activity was recorded from one patient who shortly thereafter had a generalized seizure. Symptoms resolved in all patients within 3 days after completion of therapy. More recently Gieron, Barak and Estrada reported severe encephalopathy characterized by coma in two children [37]. These patients with recurrent cancer experienced complications after 2 days of treatment with $1.8 \, g/m^2/day$ intravenously given over 1 hour of a planned 5 day course of treatment. EEGs were consistent with encephalopathy with slowing in the delta range, and also revealed the presence of electrographic seizures in one child. Again, all findings were reversible upon cessation of therapy.

Toxicity from this agent may be enhanced by impaired hepatic or renal function. Increased toxicity has been demonstrated in adults with poor hepatic or renal function, as indicated by low serum albumin or elevated serum creatinine [38,39]. The build-up of chloracetaldehyde, a metabolite of ifosfamide that requires liver aldehyde dehydrogenase for degradation, is believed to be in part responsible for the resulting neurological complication.

In children who had received a prior cumulative dose of $300 \, mg/m^2$ of cisplatin, a significant correlation with neurotoxicity was observed (C.B. Pratt, 1987, personal communication). The manner in which cisplatin influences ifosfamide neurotoxicity is not proven, but is believed to be primarily due to associated renal damage and poor clearance of toxic ifosfamide metabolites. Similarly, the effect of prior cranial irradiation is not clear but may intensify toxicity [40].

Although close monitoring is advised, prior therapy-induced encephalopathy does not appear to preclude further treatment with this drug [36]. One report suggests that alternate day administration decreases toxicity due to improved clearance of chloracetaldehyde.

## Thiotepa

Thiotepa has resulted in neurological toxicity when used intrathecally [41]. Two of ten patients treated in one intrathecal trial developed neurological complications. One patient experienced back pain, progressive lower extremity weakness, leg pain and areflexia after the second course of treatment with $10 \, mg/m^2$. Electromyography in this patient disclosed diffuse lower motor neuron abnormalities. The second patient developed a progressive myelopathy after the eighth intrathecal treatment and died because of resultant respiratory paralysis. Animal experiments performed in monkeys by Weiss *et al.* revealed that intracisternal doses may result in transient extensor rigidity and opisthotonus [42].

Recently there has been a rebirth of interest in thiotepa use, primarily utilizing higher intravenous dosages than previously given (often followed by bone marrow rescue). Since this drug penetrates the CNS readily with peak lumbar and ventricular drug concentrations nearly identical to simultaneous plasma concentrations, increased neurological toxicity can be expected.

# Nitrosoureas: carmustine (BCNU), lomustine (CCNU), semustine (Me-CCNU), PCNU

## Intravenous infusion at conventional dosages

Systemic administration of the nitrosoureas at conventional doses is not usually associated with neurotoxicity. In an isolated report, Ramirez *et al.* found a 9% incidence of dizziness, loss of equilibrium and ataxia in 223 patients who received 1.5 mg/kg/day intravenous carmustine (BCNU) for 5 days [43].

## Intracarotid infusion

Intracarotid infusions of BCNU have resulted in considerable complications [44–51]. In 1973, DeWys and Fowler demonstrated necrotizing arteriolitis of the ipsilateral internal carotid system in dogs after 2–4 mg/kg given intracarotidly [52]. This dose approximates to an intravenous dose of 200 mg/m$^2$ in man [53]. Matched animals receiving only the ethanol diluent did not experience this complication. In monkeys, Crafts, Levin and Nielsen determined that the intracarotid delivery of 1–20 mg/kg/week given in four weekly doses did not reproduce these findings [54]. Differences in intracranial circulation were offered as an explanation of this disparity. They suggested that doses below 115 mg/m$^2$ should be safe in human trials.

Madajewicz *et al.* treated 31 patients for intracranial metastasis with 100 mg/m$^2$ intracarotid infusions in four weekly doses of BCNU [44]. During the infusion all patients experienced ipsilateral periorbital pain, with or without occipital pain. Two patients experienced mild focal seizures during the infusion that responded to diazepam. Two others had focal seizures 6 and 24 h after treatment that resolved spontaneously. Another two experienced transient confusion and disorientation 4 and 24 h after treatment. Acute focal seizures during the infusion occurred in one of 26 (4%) patients and within the first 24 h in eight (30%) patients in another series [45]. Bremer *et al.* [48] reported periorbital/occipital pain in 23 (62%) patients and mild transient confusion and disorientation in 14 (38%) patients from a series of 37 persons treated with 100 mg/m$^2$ intracarotid BCNU. Transient cortical blindness occurred in one patient and transient hemiparesis occurred in another [48].

More serious and persisting complications caused by intracarotid BCNU are permanent visual loss, focal brain necrosis and leukoencephalopathy (Figure 21.1). Unilateral blindness due to local retinal vasculitis occurred in nine of 111 (8%) patients treated by Greenberg *et al.* using 200 mg/m$^2$ doses [55]. The effect of catheter placement on

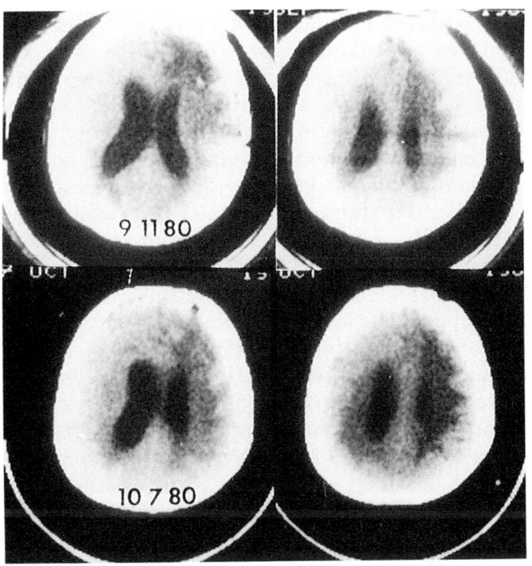

**Figure 21.1** Serial matched non-enhanced axial CT image demonstrating progressive left hemispheric white matter hypo-attenuation after intracarotid BCNU

visual toxicity was studied in 29 patients with glioma. Patients receiving infra-ophthalmic and supra-ophthalmic artery infusions of either BCNU (200 mg/m$^2$ every 2 months) or cisplatin (60 mg/m$^2$ every month) were prospectively studied [51]. Supra-ophthalmic infusions of BCNU did not cause any clinical or electrophysiological abnormality in the visual pathway, although 80% of these patients developed ipsilateral delayed cerebral necrosis (see below). All patients who received infra-ophthalmic artery BCNU infusions demonstrated ipsilateral abnormalities on electroretinography and one patient developed ipsilateral visual loss. The authors suggested that pre-treatment of patients with intravenous corticosteroids and the administration of drug over 10–15 min was a factor in the low incidence of visual loss encountered. Although intracarotid infusions of BCNU have been associated with carotid [52], ophthalmic [47] and retinal and choroidal artery [56] vasculopathy and thrombosis, they found no delayed ischemic oculopathy in their patients. A direct toxic effect of BCNU on the retina was suggested in this report [51].

Focal parenchymal necrosis has been found ipsilateral to intracarotid infusions of BCNU when supra-ophthalmic catheter positions have been used to mitigate ophthalmic side effects. One report described a 50-year-old man with a frontal glioblastoma who received three doses of 400 mg over a 3 month period [49]. Post-mortem examination revealed extensive cavitation and coagulation necrosis confined to the BCNU perfusion territory. This patient had received no prior treatment with either radiation or methotrexate. Foo *et al.* treated five patients with 11 doses of 200 mg/m$^2$ at 2 month intervals [58]. BCNU neurotoxicity, as seen by computed tomography, occurred in all four evaluable patients, including ipsilateral white matter hypodensities, non-specific gyral enhancement and delayed calcifications. One autopsy report suggested that parenchymal damage was responsible for these findings. The authors concluded that toxicity precluded treating additional patients in this manner.

It is possible that intracarotid BCNU toxicity is exacerbated by a streaming effect at the catheter tip. Streaming, during which inadequate mixing occurs between the drug with its diluent, produces non-uniform distribution of drug to different vessels [58]. At low infusion rates of 2 ml/min infusate, streaming occurred in an *in vitro* model with resultant drug concentrations five times greater than expected in various intracranial vessels. A direct toxic effect of excess ethanol diluent and drug precipitation prior to administration may contribute to focal BCNU toxicity [59,60].

Leukoencephalopathy has also been reported after intracarotid infusion of BCNU. Mahaley *et al.* reported delayed neurotoxicity in five of 16 patients treated for newly diagnosed anaplastic gliomas and in two of 26 patients with recurrent gliomas [50]. Patients had received 200 mg/m$^2$ by intracarotid infusion and neurological compromise commenced several weeks following the second or third course of treatment. Persistent confusion, hemiplegia, dysphasia, hemianopsia and hemianesthesia developed in the absence of electrolyte imbalances or tumor recurrence. Serial computed tomography revealed either no changes, new areas of hypodensity or ipsilateral gyral enhancement and punctate calcification in the middle cerebral artery territory. In the only case available for clinicopathological correlation, coagulative white matter necrosis was apparent and pathologically indistinguishable from similar necrosis induced by irradiation.

### High-dose bone marrow rescue

Systemic administration of 'high-dose' BCNU also causes neurotoxicity when given with autologous bone marrow rescue (ABMR) to circumvent the usual dose-limiting bone marrow suppression. In one study, three patients were given between 1500 and 2950 mg/m$^2$ of BCNU over a 3-day period followed by ABMR [61]. All three patients developed clinical evidence of multifocal CNS disease in the absence of recurrent tumor 4–12 weeks after treatment and died within 6 weeks of the onset of neurological compromise. Post-mortem examination revealed scattered foci of coagulative necrosis and swollen axis cylinders throughout the white matter of the CNS. Fibrinoid necrosis of small vessel

accompanied some of the lesions. Burger *et al.* found similar pathological findings and also larger symmetric areas of caseating necrosis in four patients after 1500–3450 mg/m$^2$ of BCNU [62]. Clinical symptoms included encephalopathy and seizures in one patient, encephalopathy, diplopia and quadriparesis in one, encephalopathy, diplopia and ataxia in the third patient and one was neurologically asymptomatic. Neurological deterioration occurred between 27 and 47 days after treatment. Such severe neurological sequelae have not been reported in patients receiving less than 1500 mg/m$^2$ of intravenous BCNU.

High-dose BCNU neurotoxicity may occur without prior irradiation or chemotherapy [49]. The lesions produced are pathologically indistinguishable from those ascribed to methotrexate and delayed radiation necrosis [63–66]. An unresolved issue is whether prior irradiation or chemotherapy potentiates such damage.

## Antimetabolites

### Methotrexate

Methotrexate is an inhibitor of dihydrofolate reductase, a necessary enzyme for cell growth. Inhibition of dihydrofolate reductase reduces production of tetrahydrofolate, a coenzyme needed for methylation reactions in the synthesis of purine nucleotides and thymidylate. Methotrexate also impairs other enzyme systems, including those involved in glucose transport and phosphorylation, which do not necessarily have antitumor properties and are important in the synthesis of various neurotransmitters [67].

Methotrexate is a relatively water-soluble compound and significant penetration into the CNS does not occur unless the drug is given in large intravenous dosages (as in the high-dose protocols) or is given directly into the ventricular system or lumbar sac. Although leukovorin, as a source of folinic acid to bypass the block, penetrates into the brain parenchyma, the levels achieved may not be sufficient to restore brain tetrahydrofolate levels [68,69]. There are a number of neurotoxic effects of methotrexate and although their mechanisms are not all known, the clinical spectrum is fairly well defined. These reactions may be acute, subacute or delayed, and usually occur only after high-dose intravenous or direct intrathecal or intravenous administration. The acute and subacute neurotoxicities are generally self-limiting and reversible. The chronic delayed toxicities are severe and usually irreversible [70,71].

### Acute effects following intrathecal (IT) injection

A mild to moderate aseptic meningitis (arachnoiditis) may occur after intrathecal methotrexate.

Symptoms begin as early as 2 hours after the injection, but may take 3 days to develop. Symptoms are similar to other meningitides, and include meningismus, nausea, vomiting and lethargy. The cerebrospinal fluid (CSF) opening pressure is frequently elevated and the CSF contains white blood cells, including polymorphonuclear cells. Elevated CSF protein may also be present [72–74]. A number of factors may be important in the pathogenesis of this syndrome, including dose and frequency of administration, patient age, clearance of the drug from the CSF and the solution used to dissolve the methotrexate [72]. The meningitis will usually resolve without therapy, although steroids have been used to treat severe cases [72–75]. In one report in which patients were receiving prophylactic therapy, this syndrome occurred in 29 of 73 courses (40%) [73]. Another series in which patients were being treated for meningeal leukemia, 17 of 31 patients (55%) developed aseptic meningitis; this did not seem to be related to the concurrent administration of cranial irradiation [74].

### Acute encephalopathy following high- or moderate-dose methotrexate

A reversible encephalopathy is seen in 2.3–15% of patients after high-dose or moderate-dose methotrexate treatment [76–79]. In a group of 158 patients with osteogenic sarcoma treated with high-dose methotrexate ($8$–$10\,g/m^2$ body surface area), four had the acute onset of neurological signs about 10 days after treatment. The spectrum of neurological disorder included hemiparesis, aphasia, seizures and altered sensorium. The acute phase of this syndrome lasted approximately 3 days. Two patients recovered fully and two others had residual weakness [76]. In another series of patients treated in a similar fashion for osteogenic sarcoma, nine of 60 patients (15%) developed 14 neurological events. These events occurred as early as a few hours, and as late as 20 days after infusion. The 14 neurological events included hemiparesis (5), seizures (8), alteration of sensorium (3), aphasia (3), ascending paralysis (1) and dystonia (1). One patient with hemiparesis had transient focal hypodensity on computed tomography (CT). All others who were studied had normal CTs. Seven EEGs were done, six showing focal theta and delta slowing, and one demonstrating spike and slow wave. Seven patients had lumbar punctures, and two had elevated CSF protein ($88\,mg/dl$ and $198\,mg/dl$). CSF methotrexate levels were in the normal range in those patients in whom the levels were measured. Once the patient was treated with leukovorin, no additional neurological events occurred [80]. This syndrome has also been reported in three patients receiving lower doses of $2.76\,g/m^2$. All of these patients made a full recovery [77].

The mechanism of injury is not fully determined. Since the brain is composed mainly of undividing or slowly dividing cells, impaired DNA synthesis is not a likely mechanism of acute injury. Methotrexate may impede glucose metabolism or neurotransmitter synthesis [69,80–83]. In rats, intravenous high-dose methotrexate has been shown to cause altered behavior, slowing of the EEG and reduced glucose metabolism. These effects were not apparent when rats were given adequate leukovorin [82,83].

### Subacute effects of intrathecal and intravenous infusion

An encephalopathy or myelopathy has been reported to occur in some patients days to weeks after multiple doses of intrathecal methotrexate [67,72,74,84] or after high-dose methotrexate [77]. Rarely, after intrathecal methotrexate, a spinal cord syndrome of paresis or paralysis may occur. Seizures, altered sensorium and cerebellar signs have been reported to occur after intrathecal or high-dose therapy. Delayed clearance from the blood and CSF appear to be the cause of these syndromes. Seizures and altered sensorium are usually self-limited. However, recovery from spinal cord syndromes is variable.

### Chronic toxicity after intraventricular instillation

Prolonged exposure of methotrexate to the CNS will result in severe and permanent injury. This is most likely to occur after intraventricular instillation of the drug in the setting of obstructive hydrocephalus. This syndrome was first reported in three children with obstructive hydrocephalus due to posterior fossa brain tumors. Patients developed coagulative brain necrosis after multiple doses of methotrexate given through an Ommaya reservoir. Patients without obstructive hydrocephalus treated in the same fashion did not develop coagulation necrosis [85]. In another report, two patients developed encephalopathy (aphasia, hemiparesis and altered sensorium) after methotrexate was instilled into the brain parenchyma via a misplaced catheter tip [86]. One child improved after systemic steroids and the other did not recover.

### Chronic leukoencephalopathy

The most significant toxicity of methotrexate is leukoencephalopathy (Figure 21.2) occurring months to years after methotrexate therapy. The severity is variable and the course may be static or progressive [69–74,87,88]. This syndrome generally occurs in four clinical settings:

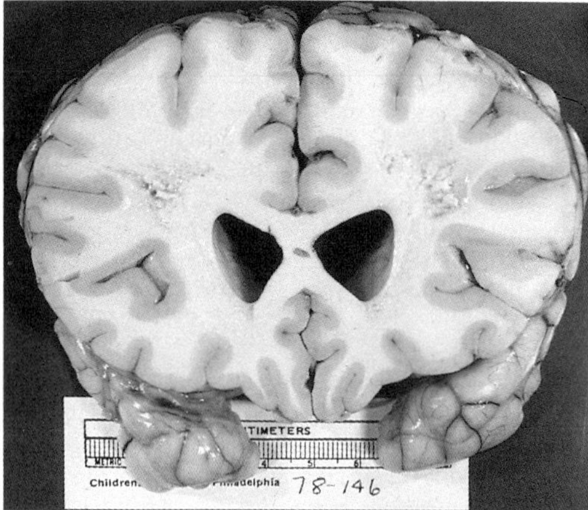

**Figure 21.2** Poorly demarcated, symmetrical foci of necrosis in deep white matter of child treated with methotrexate and radiation for central nervous system leukemia

1. Children with acute lymphocytic leukemia who received presymptomatic intrathecal methotrexate (with or without cranial irradiation).
2. Patients with brain tumors and leukemia treated with cranial irradiation and either intrathecal or high-dose intravenous methotrexate.
3. Patients with meningeal tumor treated with intrathecal methotrexate (with or without irradiation).
4. Patients with osteogenic sarcoma treated with high-dose intravenous methotrexate.

Signs and symptoms include dementia, memory disturbances, pseudobulbar palsy, ataxia, spasticity and seizures. In severe cases patients progress into vegetative states, coma and death. Computed tomography reveals cortical atrophy and white matter hypodensity [88]. The most distressing aspect of methotrexate leukoencephalopathy is that it occurs in many patients apparently cured of their malignancy.

This syndrome may occur in patients who had received methotrexate without cranial irradiation, but the effects of methotrexate are exacerbated by prior irradiation [85]. Methotrexate is believed to interfere with myelin production and maintenance, and may be the primary factor in causing leukoencephalopathy. Irradiation is believed to damage the endothelial cells, and in patients who received prior irradiation additional methotrexate may leak into the brain parenchyma, resulting in synergistic damage.

The pathological changes in the brains of patients with this syndrome are limited to the white matter.

Regions of scattered foci of necrosis without an inflammatory response are present (Figure 21.3). There are varying amounts of mineralization, reactive astrocytosis and necrotizing microangiopathy. In severe cases the individual foci become confluent, leaving large regions of necrosis [88–90]–(Figure 21.4).

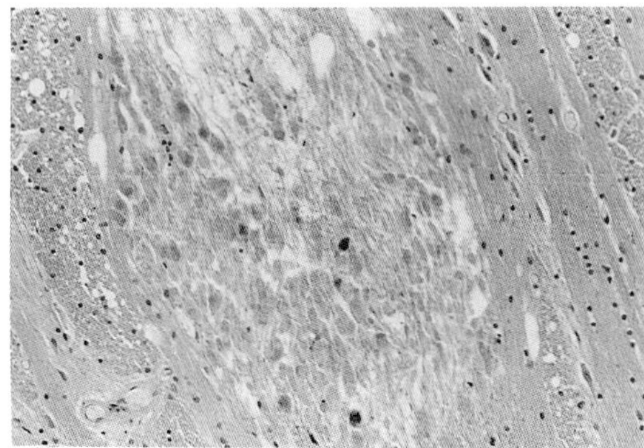

**Figure 21.3** Necrosis of pontine fiber tracts displaying typical damage secondary to therapy with methotrexate and radiation. Note rounded swelling of damage fibers and lack of cellular response. Stain, haematoxylin and eosin; × 250

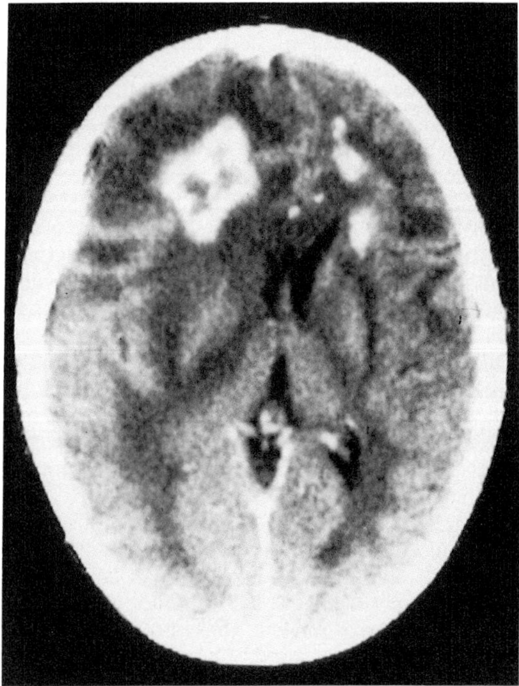

**Figure 21.4** Contrast enhanced axial CT image demonstrating widespread white matter hypo-attenuation with areas of focal calcification after intrathecal methotrexate

## 5-Fluorouracil (5-FU)

A reversible cerebellar syndrome characterized by varying degrees of truncal or appendicular ataxia, dysmetria, hypotonia, coarse nystagmus and slurred speech occurs in a dose-related fashion with this agent [71,91–94]. With doses of 7.5–15 mg/kg/week, fewer than 1% and with doses of 20 mg/kg/week, 7% of patients experience such side effects [93,95]. Symptoms begin within hours to days after administration of drug and resolve 1–6 weeks after the drug is stopped or the dose is lowered [71,92,96]. Peak plasma levels rather than total cumulative dose appear to correlate with neurological compromise [71,92].

High-dose 5-FU therapy $(0.8–1.9\,g/m^2$ given every 2 weeks) has also been associated with encephalopathy. Confusion, memory impairment and dementia were seen in 50% of patients in one report [97]. Higher doses $(3.4\,g/m^2/\text{one dose})$ caused lethargy and coma with concordant EEG slowing in 40% of patients without cerebellar signs in another report [98]. These cortical symptoms resolved by 2 months of drug discontinuation. Extrapyramidal movement disorders [99], blurred vision [100], diplopia and extraocular movement disorders [101] have also infrequently occurred. These rare deficits have uniformly resolved upon discontinuation of 5-FU.

Neuropathological examinations of patients who have experienced neurotoxicity from 5-FU have revealed a loss of neurons and a glial reaction in the dentate and inferior olivary nuclei and in the cerebellar granular and Purkinje cell layers [91,102]. Similar findings have been noted in patients who had no clinical neurotoxicity [91] and, conversely, no abnormal histopathological changes have been found in some patients who have experienced neurological side effects [101].

The mechanism of neurotoxicity is not known. It is believed to be related to the accumulation of degradation products of 5-FU [102,103]. Fluorocitrate and fluoroacetate have been shown to concentrate in the cerebella of mice treated with 5-FU and to produce similar histopathological changes in the cerebella of cats.

## Cytosine arabinoside (Ara-C, arabinosyl cytosine, cytarabine)

Only one report, describing two patients with 'stocking glove paresthesias' suggests that conventional intravenous doses of Ara-C (cytarabine) $(100–200\,mg/m^2)$ are neurotoxic [104]. However, larger intravenous dosages have resulted in greater neurotoxicity. When given at a dose of $3\,mg/m^2$ every 12 h for a minimum of six doses there is a 16–47% incidence of neurological complications [105–107].

A generally reversible cerebellar syndrome consisting of dysarthria, ataxia and disdiadochokinesia was initially defined by Lazarus *et al.* [105]. Two subsequent reports demonstrated that cumulative intravenous doses of $18\,g/m^2$ or greater carry an age-related risk of severe irreversible cerebellar toxicity. Herzig *et al.* showed that this effect was significantly increased in patients over 50 years of age [108]. Gottlieb *et al.* recommended that no patient over the age of 55 should receive high-dose intravenous Ara-C and that high-dose use of this drug should be discontinued in any patient at the first appearance of cerebellar symptoms [109].

Post-mortem findings in severely affected patients consistently reveal diminished cellularity and gliosis in the Purkinje cell layer of the cerebellum [105]. The cause of these findings is not clear. As the deaminases needed for the catabolism of Ara-C are not present in CSF, high levels of the uracil metabolite and its possible potentiating effect on the parent drug may be responsible [110,111]. It has also been postulated that Ara-C exerts its effect by interference with the Purkinje cell DNA, with resulting damage to intracellular homeostasis and structural integrity [112].

Intrathecally administered Ara-C $(30–70\,mg/m^2)$ does not cause cerebellar disease [113,114]. Use of this agent in this manner has been associated with an aseptic meningitis similar to that caused by methotrexate, and both transient [115] and permanent [116] paraparesis. Additionally, disseminated necrotizing leukoencephalopathy, seizures and central and peripheral myelinopathies have been reported in association with intrathecal Ara-C [113,117–119]. However, a direct causative relationship between Ara-C and these latter neurological sequelae has not been established.

One isolated report described a case of acute demyelinating polyneuropathy (Guillain-Barré syndrome) after $36\,mg/m^2$ of Ara-C [119].

# Other agents

## Vincristine

Peripheral neuropathy is the dose-limiting side effect of vincristine [120]. A symmetrical peripheral neuropathy occurs in virtually all patients who receive repeated doses of this drug [120,121]. Cranial and autonomic neuropathies also occur and may be severe. The effects are cumulative and generally reversible when the drug is discontinued. Post-adolescent patients and those with hepatic dysfunction may be at higher risk for developing earlier and more severe complications [72,120,122].

Asymptomatic loss of the Achilles tendon reflex may occur after only one or two doses of vincristine. Further treatment causes the loss of more proximal deep tendon reflexes [116,120]. Maximum reflex loss occurs approximately 17 days after a single dose and resolution may be complete at 1–3 months [120].

Muscle weakness may follow reflex loss and also begins distally [116,120,123]. In adults 23–36% are affected. Weakness of the ankle and toe dorsiflexors and foot evertors may result in 'foot drop'. If therapy is continued a gait disorder and eventual quadriparesis may ensue. Accompanying muscle wasting is uncommon [120,123]. Complete resolution usually takes months [124]. Cramps in the thighs and calves may occur during the recovery phase of the illness. These can be quite bothersome but tend to respond to dantrolene or other muscle relaxants.

Sensory symptoms are relatively common. Though objective sensory loss has been hard to document, distal painful paresthesias are reported in approximately 50% of patients [120,121,123]. Jaw pain, reported in 6–8% of patients, occurs after the first or second dose, starts within hours and may last days [116]. This complication does not usually recur on repeated doses [116].

Cranial neuropathies, similar to other vincristine neuropathies, are most often bilateral. Any of the cranial nerves may be affected. One report cited the incidence of bilateral ptosis, abducens nerve palsy and facial palsy as 10%, 6% and 4%, respectively [120]. Trigeminal nerve toxicity has been suggested as the mechanism of jaw pain [125]. Dysphonia from vocal cord paralysis [116,122], dysphagia [122] and optic neuropathy [125–127] have been attributed to vinca toxicity.

Autonomic neuropathies may be the earliest symptoms of toxicity [116,121]. Colicky abdominal pain and constipation occur in one-third to one-half of patients and often precede reflex changes. Adynamic ileus occurred in 12% of patients from one series [120]. Bladder atony [120,124], impotence [116,128] and orthostatic hypotension [120,129–131] are less frequent but have been cited in patients with relatively mild peripheral neuropathy.

The syndrome of inappropriate antidiuretic hormone secretion has been described in both adults and children treated with vincristine [131,132]. Seizures, believed secondary to hyponatremia, have occurred in this setting. Two series have reported seizure rates of 1% [133] and 4% [134] not associated with metabolic abnormality. Although vincristine was implicated in these seizures, all patients received further therapy without recurrence.

Unusual reports of severe toxicity can be found. Patients progressing to complete paraplegia after one and two doses may represent idiosyncratic reactions. A patient with a Charcot-Marie-Tooth variant experienced such a reaction and the authors warned against use of vincristine in patients with pre-existing neuropathies [135]. Patients with diabetic neuropathy, however, did not show increased toxicity in one series [135]. One recent report suggested that concurrent Guillian-Barré syndrome caused such symptoms in their patient [137]. Encephalopathy and seizures occurred in an 8-year-old girl after receiving her second dose of drug and a brain biopsy showed a pattern of microtubule dissociation thought to be due to vincristine [138]. Accidental intrathecal administration of vincristine has resulted in death despite attempts at CSF washout [139–141].

The pathogenesis of vincristine neurotoxicity may be related to the drug's effect on microtubule formation. These structures are important in axoplasmic transport and are constantly being synthesized in the cell body. Abnormal density and length of microtubules are noted in axons exposed to the drug *in vitro*. Histological observations indicate that the process is a primary axonal degeneration rather than a myelinopathy [142].

## L-Asparaginase

Acute and delayed encephalopathy are caused by this agent. Acute encephalopathy can occur during the first days of treatment [143]. A 21–60% incidence of encephalopathy has been associated with various intravenous doses [144–147], although in general this complication has been related to higher drug dosages or repeated drug infusion [72]. Symptoms range from lethargy and confusion to stupor and coma. Reports of seizures are rare [147]. Neurological examination usually reveals no focal deficits. The L-asparaginase-induced encephalopathy is reversible in almost all patients.

The delayed L-asparaginase encephalopathy begins about a week after therapy [148]. Symptoms are similar to the earlier onset form. Resolution of this complication, however, may take weeks and the mechanism is probably different. Electroencephalographic findings of diffuse slowing parallel the clinical encephalopathies in both cases [72,145,147].

L-Asparaginase neurotoxicity is believed to be caused by the systemic metabolic abnormalities produced by this drug, since the drug itself does not cross the BBB [149,150]. The activity of L-asparaginase releases large quantities of L-aspartic and L-glutamic acids as well as ammonia compounds. These compounds readily cross the BBB and may interfere with the entry of other essential amino acids into the CNS. CNS levels of asparagine have been shown to be depleted in patients who have developed delayed toxicity [150]. Infusions of L-asparagine in three patients resulted in neurological improvement in two, and probable improvement in the remaining patient treated [148]. Additionally, the related hepatic dysfunction of L-asparaginase may limit the metabolism of ammonia and increase the likelihood of encephalopathy [150]. Encephalopathy has occurred with various preparations of drug making it unlikely that impurities and carrying agents are causative factors.

L-Asparaginase may also induce coagulopathy after only one or two doses with resulting CNS involvement [152–154]. Cerebrovascular thrombotic or hemorrhagic complications have been reported to occur in 0.9–2.8% of patients who receive 6000 units/m$^2$ intravenously 3 times weekly [153–156]. Higher doses appear to be related to a greater frequency of complications. Intensive protocols (25 000 units/m$^2$ intravenously/week) have resulted in a 2.8% rate of intracranial vascular complications [157]. Thrombosis most often occurs in the sagittal sinus or surface cortical veins [158] (Figures 21.5 and 21.6). Clinical manifestations include headache,

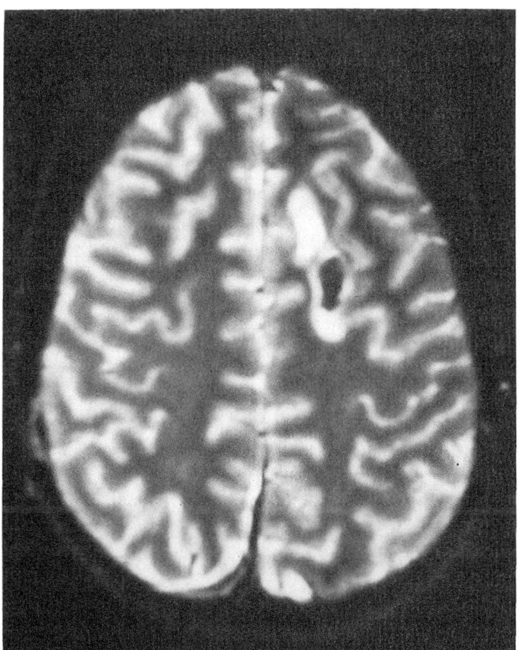

**Figure 21.6** T$_2$ weighted axial magnetic resonance image in the same patient demonstrating a venous infarct in the left parietal region

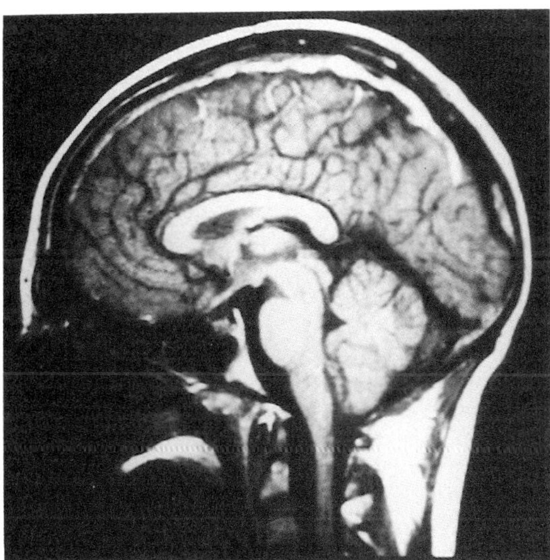

**Figure 21.5** Sagittal T$_1$ weighted magnetic resonance image revealing clot in the superior sagittal sinus. The patient received L-asparaginase prior to developing severe headaches and seizures

focal seizures, hemiparesis and encephalopathy. When L-asparaginase is used three times weekly for 3 weeks thrombotic events usually occur within 10 days of the 7–9th dose of medication. Pre-treatment with fresh frozen plasma has been recommended prior to further treatment with this agent, and recurrence of symptoms has not been reported [156,158,159].

The pathogenesis of cerebral thrombosis is believed to be related to L-asparaginase-induced coagulative abnormalities. Increased clotting times, especially the partial thromboplastin time, are common. Decreased levels of fibrinogen [156,160],

factors IX [161] and XI [161], plasminogen [156,160,162] and antithrombin III [156,160,162] have been reported. Fibrinolysis is also affected. Reduced inhibition in the fibrinolytic activities of plasmin, urokinase and human tissue plasminogen activator have been demonstrated [163]. There is a rebound effect after stopping therapy and the rebound state has been implicated as causing a secondary hypercoagulable state and thrombosis [162].

## Cisplatin (*cis*-platinum)

Cisplatin until recently was given exclusively by the intravenous route; however, intracarotid infusions are now being employed. The major neurotoxic effects of intravenous cisplatin are hearing loss and peripheral neuropathies.

Ototoxicity caused from cisplatin is well described and is related to the cumulative dose; deafness is infrequent [164–167]. Tinnitus occurs in 9%, symptomatic hearing loss in 6%, and high frequency hearing loss by audiometric examination in 24% of patients treated with up to 60 mg/m$^2$. The high frequencies are vulnerable at lower cumulative dosages, but frequencies in the speech range can be involved if the patient continues to be treated with the drug. In one childhood study, patients were treated with 90 mg/m$^2$ every 3 weeks. One-half of the patients developed significant hearing loss at 8000 Hz when a cumulative dose of 270 mg/m$^2$ was reached. Significant loss in the speech frequencies (2000 Hz) occurred in 30% of children at a cumulative dose of 540 mg/m$^2$ and in 50% at 810 mg/m$^2$. Patients were followed for 15 months and hearing function did not improve after cessation of treatment [167]. A study of the ototoxic effects of cisplatin in children with brain tumors showed similar results. Hearing in the 250–2000 Hz range remained stable up to a cumulative dose of 474 mg/m$^2$ [168]. Patients in this study did not receive further cisplatin if greater than a 20 dB loss occurred at or below 2000 Hz.

In some reports irradiation involving the cochlea has been reported to enhance the ototoxicity of cisplatin [168,169]. In a study of chinchillas, prior cochlear irradiation enhanced the degree of cisplatin-induced ototoxicity. The mechanism of the synergy between cisplatin and irradiation is unknown [169]. However, it may be related to radiation-induced increased permeability of the striae vascularis allowing for increased cisplatin drug levels. Cisplatin hearing loss is most likely secondary to cochlear rather than auditory nerve damage. The hair cells have been implicated as the most likely site of damage [170,171]. Because the ototoxic effect can be anticipated, patients receiving cisplatin should be tested with audiograms prior to each administration.

The appearance of a predominantly sensory peripheral neuropathy is also dose-related and well characterized [172–175]. In an adult study where patients were treated with cisplatin and doxorubicin (Adriamycin), 92% developed varying degrees of neuropathy [174]. Complaints of numbness and tingling precede the loss of reflexes, and depression of vibratory sensation. Marked sensory ataxia may occur in severe cases. Joint position, light touch and pin sensation are less frequently involved. Motor strength is not usually impaired. Patients do not develop symptoms until cumulative dosages of about 200 mg/m$^2$ are reached. Complete resolution of symptoms may be demonstrated over months to years [175]. The mechanism of injury is not known, although other heavy metals can produce peripheral neuropathies. Pathological findings in nerves disclose a decrease in large diameter myelinated fibers, segmental demyelination and axonal degeneration. Recent information suggests that WR2721 may protect against cisplatin neurotoxicity [175].

Other less well described neurotoxic effects of cisplatin have been reported including cerebral herniation [176], reversible increased intracranial pressure and papilledema [177], transient and permanent retrobulbar neuritis [177] and seizures [178]. In addition to direct neurotoxicity, cisplatin alters renal function resulting in wasting of sodium and magnesium which may result in tetany and seizures [179].

When given via the carotid artery, with or without mannitol to open the BBB, severe encephalopathy may result. Intra-arterial cisplatin can cause focal intraparenchymal necrosis in the vascular distribution of arterial supply, indistinguishable from that caused by intra-arterial carmustine (BCNU). The incidence of this complication is unknown but was reported in nine of 37 patients in one series [22].

## Procarbazine

Procarbazine may cause fully reversible encephalopathy and peripheral neuropathy [72]. When used orally at doses of 100–300 mg/day, neurological complications are uncommon. One series cited the development of CNS involvement, ranging from mild drowsiness to profound stupor, in 16 of 51 (31%) of patients treated with 200–1000 mg/day orally [180]. Other reports have described a lower rate of confusion and lethargy in patients receiving doses ranging from 150 to 400 mg/day orally [181]. EEG tracings in six patients who became stuporous during such treatment have revealed diffuse slow wave activity consistent with encephalopathy. More uncommonly, transient delirium has been reported during oral therapy with this drug [182]. Consistent with animal experiments, mild CNS symptoms may resolve in spite of continued therapy.

Distal symmetric paresthesias occur in 10–17% of patients [180,183]. Proximal myalgias which remit during continued therapy and ataxia have also been associated with procarbazine [72]. Again, these side effects are reversible upon stopping therapy.

Other less common side effects may occur. Orthostatic hypotension was found in 8% of patients in one series [183]. Hypertension may occur in patients taking sympathomimetic agents, tricyclic antidepressants or tyramine-containing foods [184]. These complications are believed to be caused by inhibition of the monoamine oxidase system. Delayed hepatic drug detoxification of concomitantly administered antiemetic phenothiazines, barbiturates and narcotics may contribute to the CNS effects [72,185]. A disulfuram-like 'flush syndrome' has followed alcohol ingestion in patients treated with this agent [186,187].

The cause of procarbazine toxicity is not well established. The agent readily crosses the BBB [188]; however, a specific direct effect is not known. As a hydrazine derivative, procarbazine is capable of depleting plasma pyridoxal phosphate (vitamin B$_6$) and this mechanism has been implicated in the development of peripheral neuropathy [189]. Administration of exogenous pyroxidine has not been effective in avoiding or reversing neurological complications [180,190].

Intravenous procarbazine continues to be used in experimental clinical trials. The development of

**Table 21.1 Additional chemotherapeutic agents causing infrequent neurotoxicity**

| Class/agent | Dose/route | Neurotoxicity | Frequency |
|---|---|---|---|
| Alkylating agents: | | | |
| Spirohydantoin | 6 mg/m$^2$ 3×/wk i.v. | Encephalopathy, ataxia [193] | Common |
| Chlorambucil | 1.5 mg/kg orally | Encephalopathy, ataxia [194], myoclonus | Single report |
| | 5 mg/kg orally | Encephalopathy [195], seizures, ataxia | Single report |
| Nitrosoureas: | | | |
| PCNU | 40–60 mg/m$^2$ intracarotid | Headache, blindness [196], agitation | Common |
| Triazines: | | | |
| DTIC | 1000–3000 mg/m$^2$ i.v. over 5 days | Facial paresthesias [197] | Rare |
| | 500 mg × 5 days i.v. × 2 cycles | Dementia, seizures [198] | Rare |
| | 625 mg/m$^2$ i.v. day 1 and 4 × 3 cycles | Cerebral hemorrhage [199], seizures | Common |
| Antimetabolites: | | | |
| 5-Azacytidine | 200–250 mg/m$^2$/day × 5 days | Encephalopathy [200], weakness, muscle tenderness and pain | Frequent |
| Vinca alkaloids: | | | |
| Vinblastine | 5–6 mg/m$^2$ over 1–2 weeks or 0.4 mg/kg i.v. | Similar to vincristine [119,120], often not seen due to dose-limiting hematological effects | Rare |
| Vindesine | 1–7 mg/m$^2$ i.v. over 24 h or 0.5–7 mg/m$^2$ i.v. bolus | Similar to vincristine [201–204] | Frequent |
| Podophyllotoxins: | | | |
| VP-16 | 300–400 mg/m$^2$/day × 5 days | Peripheral neuropathy [205,206] | Possible |
| | 800 mg/m$^2$ × 3 days i.v. (high-dose) | Exacerbation of [207] pre-existing neurological deficits including hemiparesis and seizures, encephalopathy | Common |
| Doxorubicin | Intravenous | Radiation recall [208] | Rare |
| Actinomycin D | Intravenous | Radiation recall [209] | Rare |
| Bleomycin | 10 mg/kg i.v. with vinblastine 0.2 mg/kg i.v. | Raynaud's phenomenon [210] | Common |
| Others: | | | |
| Hexamethylmelamine | 300–320 mg/m$^2$/day or 8 mg/kg/day orally × 21 days | Encephalopathy [211] Headache, extrapyramidal movement disorders, ataxia, seizures, neuropathy | Common |
| Corticosteroids | Varying doses | Dysphoric states, insomnia | Common |

serious persistent CNS symptoms including somnolence and psychosis has occurred at various dosage schedules and has limited its usefulness via this route [191].

For additional chemotherapeutic agents and their neurotoxicities, and for an overview of the common causative agents of neurological complications, see Tables 21.1 and 21.2.

## Antiemetics

Antiemetics are necessary medications for patients receiving chemotherapy. Phenothiazines (promethazine, prochlorperazine, chlorpromazine) and other drugs exert antiemetic effects because they are dopamine antagonists, acting at the medullary chemoreceptor trigger zone. The most common side effect of these drugs is sedation. The most problematic side effect with any of these medications is the acute onset of extrapyramidal reactions usually after intravenous injection, but rarely after oral administration. These reactions consist of involuntary movements causing torticollis, oculogyric crisis, forced protrusion of the tongue, facial grimacing and akathisias (involuntary restlessness). These effects are transient and not serious, but may cause considerable distress.

Metoclopromide is an extremely effective antiemetic that appears to have a relatively high incidence of reactions. In one series, at dosages equal to or above 2 mg/kg, 15% of patients developed extrapyramidal reactions and 33% developed akathisia [192]. The extrapyramidal effects may be easily reversed with intravenous diphenhydramine (1 mg/kg) and the incidence of severity may be reduced if diphenhydramine is given concurrently with the antiemetic.

**Table 21.2 Neurological side effects and frequently associated agents**

| CNS | |
| --- | --- |
| Acute encephalopathy: | Myelopathy: |
|   Methotrexate IT HD [73,74,76,78] |   Methotrexate IT HD [84] |
|   L-asparaginase [145,148] |   Ara-C IT [84,115] |
|   Hexamethylmelamine [211] |   Thiotepa IT [84] |
|   5-Fluorouracil [98] | |
|   Procarbazine [185] | |
|   BCNU IC [44,45] | |
|   Cisplatin IC [178] | |
|   Ara-C HD [105,107] | |
| Chronic encephalopathy: | Acute cerebellar reactions: |
|   Methotrexate IT [72,73] |   5-Fluorouracil [92] |
|   Ara-C IT [89] |   Ara-C HD [105–107] |
|   BCNU IC [48,49] |   Hexamethylmelamine [211] |
| **PNS** | |
| Cranial nerve dysfunction: | Other: |
|   Vincas [116,120] |   Vincas [116,120] |
|   Cisplatin [165] | |
|   5-Fluorouracil [92] | |
| Neuropathy: | Antidiuretic hormone secretion: |
| Sensory: |   Cyclophosphamide [35] |
|   Vincas [124] |   Vincas [124] |
|   Cisplatin [174] | |
|   Procarbazine [182] | |
| Sensorimotor: | |
|   Vincas [116,120] | |
|   Hexamethylmelamine [211] | |
|   5-Azacytidine [200] | |

IT, intrathecal; HD, high-dose; IC, intracarotid

## References


1. Dawson, D.M., Rosenthal, D.S. and Moloney, W.C. Neurological complications of acute leukemia in adults: changing rate. *Annals of Internal Medicine*, **79**, 541–544 (1973)
2. Hansen, H.H. Should initial treatment of small cell carcinoma include systemic chemotherapy and brain irradiation? *Cancer Chemotherapy Reports*, **4**(Suppl.), 239–241 (1973)
3. Meadows, A.T. and Evans, A.T. Effects of chemotherapy on the central nervous system. *Cancer*, **37**, 1079–1985 (1976)
4. McIntosh, S., Lathskin, E.H., O'Brien, R.T. *et al.* Chronic neurologic disturbance in childhood leukemia. *Cancer*, **37**, 853–857 (1976)
5. Moss, H.A., Nannis, E.D. and Poplack, D.G. The effects of prophylactic treatment of the central nervous system on the intellectual functioning of children with acute lymphocytic leukemia. *American Journal of Medicine*, **71**, 47–52 (1981)
6. Eise, C. Intellectual abilities among survivors of childhood leukemia as a function of CNS irradiation. *Archives of Disease in Childhood*, **53**, 391–395 (1978)
7. Meadows, A.T., Massari, D.J. Fergusson, J. *et al.* Declines in IQ scores and cognitive dysfunctions in children with acute lymphocytic leukemia treated with irradiation. *Lancet*, **ii**, 1015–1018 (1981)
8. Raimondi, A.J. and Tomita, T. Advantages of 'total' resection of medulloblastoma and disadvantages of full head post-operative radiation therapy. *Child Brain*, **5**, 550–551 (1979)
9. Hirsch, J.F., Reiner, D., Czerichow, P. *et al.* Medulloblastoma in childhood: survival and functional results. *Acta Neurochirurgica*, **48**, 1–15 (1979)
10. Duffner, P.K., Cohen, M.E. and Thomas, P.R.M. Late effects of treatment on the intelligence of children with posterior fossa tumors. *Cancer*, **51**, 233–237 (1983)
11. Price, R.A. and Jamieson, P.A. The central nervous system in childhood leukemia. II. Subacute leukencephalopathy. *Cancer*, **35**, 306–318 (1975)
12. Price, R.A. and Birdwell, D.A. The central nervous system in childhood leukemia. III. Mineralizing micrangiopathy and dystrophic calcification. *Cancer*, **42**, 717–728 (1978)
13. Crosley, C.J., Rorke, L.B., Evans, A.E. and Nigro, M. Central nervous system lesions in childhood leukemia. *Neurology*, **28**, 678–685 (1978)
14. Rottenberg, D.A., Chernik, N.L., Deck, M.D.F. *et*

*al.* Cerebral necrosis following radiotherapy of extracranial neoplasms. *Annals of Neurology*, **1**, 339–357 (1977)

15. Wright, T.L. and Bresnan, M.J. Radiation-induced cerebrovascular disease in childhood. *Neurology*, **26**, 540–543 (1976)

16. Sheline, G.E. Irradiation injury of the human brain: a review of clinical experience. In *Radiation Damage to the Nervous System* (eds M.A. Gilbert and A.R. Kagan), Raven Press, New York, pp. 39–58 (1980)

17. Allen, J.C., Rosen, G. and Mehta, B.M. Leukoencephalopathy following high-dose IV methotrexate with leucovorin rescue. *Cancer Treatment Reports*, **64**, 1261–1273 (1980)

18. Packer, P.J., Grossman, R.I. and Belasco, J.B. High-dose systemic methotrexate associated acute neurologic dysfunction. *Medical and Pediatric Oncology*, **11**, 159–161 (1983)

19. Chabner, B.A., Myers, C.E., Coleman, C.N. and Johns, D.G. The clinical pharmacology of antineoplastic agents (first of two parts). *New England Journal of Medicine*, **292**, 1107–1113 (1975)

20. Neuwelt, E.A., Glasberg, M., Frenkel, E. and Barnett, P. Neurotoxicity of chemotherapeutic agents after blood-brain-barrier modification: neuropathologic studies. *Annals of Neurology*, **14**, 316–324 (1983)

21. Martinez-Prieto, J.N., Yung, A., Feun, L. and Lee, Y. Toxicity of intracarotid chemotherapy for patients with malignant brain tumors. *Cancer Bulletin*, **38**, 49–53 (1986)

22. Bethlenfalvay, N.C. and Bergin, J.J. Severe cerebral toxicity after intravenous nitrogen mustard therapy. *Cancer*, **29**, 366–369 (1972)

23. Lawrence, W. Jr, Kuehn, P., Masle, E.T. *et al.* An abdominal tourniquet for regional chemotherapy. *Journal of Surgical Research*, **1**, 142–151 (1961)

24. Clifford, P., Beecher, J.L., Harries, J.R. *et al.* Nitrogen mustard therapy with aortic occlusion in nasopharyngeal carcinoma. *British Medical Journal*, **ii**, 1256–1260 (1973)

25. Conrad, M.E. Jr and Crosby, W.H. Massive nitrogen mustard therapy in Hodgkin's disease with protection of bone marrow by tourniquets. *Blood*, **16**, 1089–1103 (1960)

26. French, J.D., West, P.M., van Amerongen, F.K. and Magoun, H.W. Effects of intracarotid administration of nitrogen mustard on normal brain and brain tumors. *Journal of Neurosurgery*, **9**, 378–389 (1952)

27. Ariel, I.M. Intra-arterial chemotherapy for metastatic cancer to the brain. *American Journal of Surgery*, **102**, 647–650 (1961)

28. Owens, G. Chemotherapy of primary gliomas of the brain. *New York State Journal of Medicine*, **64**, 1933–1937 (1964)

29. Brunschweig, A. and Brochkuner, A. Postoperative rupture of major vessels after radical pelvic operation. *American Journal of Obstetrics and Gynecology*, **80**, 481–484 (1960)

30. Creech, O., Ryan, R.F. and Krementz, E.T. Regional chemotherapy of isolated perfusions in the treatment of melanoma of the extremities. *Plastic and Reconstructive Surgery*, **28**, 333–346 (1961)

31. Mahaley, M.S. Jr, Huneycutt, H., Boone, H. *et al.* Localization of methylbis(2-chloroethyl-1,2-C$^{14}$) amine hydrochloride in nervous tissue after intravenous injection or regional cerebral perfusion in dogs. *Cancer Chemotherapy Reports*, **11**, 29–32 (1961)

32. Woodhall, B., Mahaley, S. Jr, Boone, S. *et al.* The effect of chemotherapeutic agents upon peripheral nerves. *Journal of Surgical Research*, **2**, 373–381 (1962)

33. Tashima, C.K. Immediate cerebral symptoms during rapid intravenous administration of cyclophosphamide. *Cancer Chemotherapy Reports*, **59**, 441–442 (1975)

34. Kende, G., Sirkin, S.R., Thomas, P.R.M. *et al.* Blurring of vision. A previously undescribed complication of cyclophosphamide therapy. *Cancer*, **44**, 69–71 (1979)

35. Steele, S.T., Serpick, A.A. and Block, J.B. Antidiuretic response to cyclophosphamide in man. *Journal of Pharmacology and Experimental Therapeutics*, **185**, 35–39 (1973)

36. Pratt, C.B., Horowitz, M.E., Meyer, W.H. *et al.* Phase II trial of ifosfamide in children with malignant solid tumors. *Cancer Treatment Reports*, **71**, 131–135 (1987)

37. Gieron, M.A., Barak, L.S. and Estrada, J. Severe encephalopathy associated with ifosfamide administration in two children with metastatic tumors. *Journal of Neuro-Oncology*, **6**, 29–30 (1988)

38. Meanwell, C.A., Kelly, K.A. and Blackledge, G. Avoiding ifosfamide/mesna encephalopathy. *Lancet*, **ii**, 406 (1986)

39. Perren, T.J., Turner, R.C. and Smith, I.E. Encephalopathy with rapid infusion ifosfamide/mesna. *Lancet*, **i**, 390–391 (1987)

40. Nicoll, J.J. Radiation reaction enhanced by ifosfamide. *British Journal of Radiology*, **59**, 1039–1041 (1986)

41. Gutin, P.H., Levi, J.A., Wiernik, P.H. and Walker, M.D. Treatment of malignant meningeal disease with intrathecal thiotepa: a phase II study. *Cancer Treatment Reports*, **61**, 885–887 (1977)

42. Weiss, H.D., Walker, M.D., Wiernik, P.H. and Dallgard, D. Preclinical and phase I clinical studies of intrathecal *N,N',N''*-triethylenephosphoramide (thiotepa-NSC 6396). *Proceedings of the American Association for Cancer Research*, **15**, 65 (1974)

43. Ramirez, G., Wilson, W., Grage, T. *et al.* Phase II evaluation of 1,3-bis(2-chlorethyl)-1-nitrosourea (BCNU; NSC-409962) in patients with solid tumors. *Cancer Chemotherapy Reports*, **56**, 787–790 (1972)

44. Madajewicz, S., West, C.R., Park, H.C. *et al.* Phase II study – intra-arterial BCNU therapy for metastatic brain tumors. *Cancer*, **47**, 653–657 (1981)

45. West, C.R., Avellanosa, A.M., Barua, N.R. *et al.*

dose cytosine arabinoside: clinical response to therapy in acute leukaemia. *Medical Pediatrics and Oncology*, **10**, 239–250 (1982)

108. Herzig, R.H., Herzig, G.P., Wolff, S.N. *et al.* Central nervous system effects of high-dose cytosine arabinoside. *Seminars in Oncology*, **14**, 21–24 (1987)

109. Gottlieb, D., Bradstock, K., Koutts, J. *et al.* The neurotoxicity of high-dose cytosine arabinoside is age related. *Cancer*, **60**, 1439–1441 (1987)

110. Hande, K.R., Stein, R.S., McDonough, D.A. *et al.* Effects of high-dose cytarabine. *Clinical Pharmacology and Therapeutics*, **31**, 669–674f (1982)

111. Lopez, J.A. and Agarwal, R.P. Acute cerebellar toxicity after high-dose cytarabine associated with CNS accumulation of its metabolite, uracil arabinoside. *Cancer Treatment Reports*, **68**, 1309–1310 (1984)

112. Winkelman, M.D. and Hines, J.D. Cerebellar degeneratiaon caused by high-dose systemic cytosine arabinoside. *Annals of Neurology*, **12**, 77 (1982)

113. Benger, A., Browman, G.P., Walker, I.R. *et al.* Clinical evidence of a cumulative effect of high-dose cytarabine on the cerebellum in patients with acute leukemia: a leukemia intergroup report. *Cancer Treatment Reports*, **69**, 240–241 (1985)

114. Young, D.F. and Posner, J.B. Nervous system toxicity of chemotherapeutic agents. In *Handbook of Clinical Neurology, Part II. Neurologic Manifestations of Systemic Diseases* (eds P.J. Vinken and G.W. Bruyn), North-Holland, New York, pp. 91–131 (1980)

115. Breuer, A.C., Pitman, S.W., Dawson, D.M. and Schoene, W.C. Paraparesis following intrathecal cytosine arabinoside: a case report with neuropathologic findings. *Cancer*, **40**, 2817–2822 (1977)

116. Holland, J.F., Schorland, C., Gailani, S. *et al.* Vincristine treatment of advanced cancer: a cooperative study of 392 cases. *Cancer Research*, **33**, 1258–1264 (1973)

117. Mena, H., Garcia, J.H. and Velandia, F. Central and peripheral myelinopathy associated with systemic neoplasia and chemotherapy. *Cancer*, **48**, 1724–1737 (1981)

118. Eden, O.B., Goldie, W., Wood, T. *et al.* Seizures following intrathecal cytosine arabinoside in young children with acute lymphoblastic leukemia. *Cancer*, **42**, 53–58 (1978)

119. Johnson, N.T., Crawford, S.W. and Sargur, M. Acute acquired demyelinating polyneuropathy with respiratory failure following high-dose systemic cytosine arabinoside and marrow transplantation. *Bone Marrow Transplantation*, **2**, 203–207 (1987)

120. Sandler, S.G., Tobin, W. and Henderson, E.S. Vincristine-induced neuropathy: a clinical study of 50 leukemic patients. *Neurology*, **19**, 367–374 (1969)

121. Hildebrand, J. *Lesions of the Nervous System in Cancer Patients*, Raven Press, New York, pp. 49–70 (1978)

122. Bohannon, K.A., Miller, D.G. and Diamond, H.D. Vincristine in the treatment of lymphoma and leukemias. *Cancer Research*, **23**, 613–621 (1963)

123. Bradley, W.G., Lassman, L., Pearce, G.W. *et al.* The neuromyopathy of vincristine in man: clinical, electrophysiological and pathological studies. *Journal of Neurological Sciences*, **10**, 107–131 (1970)

124. Gottlieb, R.J. and Cuttner, J. Vincristine-induced bladder atomy. *Cancer*, **28**, 674–675 (1971)

125. Norton, S.W. and Stockman, J.A. Unilateral optic neuropathy following vincristine chemotherapy. *Journal of Pediatric Ophthalmology and Strabismus*, **16**, 190–193 (1979)

126. Sanderson, P.A., Kuwabara, T. and Cogan, D.G. Optic neuropathy presumably caused by vincristine therapy. *American Journal of Ophthalmology*, **81**, 146–150 (1976)

127. Awidi, A.W. Blindness and vincristine. *Annals of Internal Medicine*, **93**, 781 (1980)

128. Weiss, H.D. The physiology of human penile erection. *Annals of Internal Medicine*, **76**, 793–799 (1972)

129. Carmichael, S.M., Eagleton, L., Ayers, C.R. *et al.* Orthostatic hypotension during vincristine therapy. *Archives of Internal Medicine*, **126**, 290–292 (1970)

130. DiBella, N.J. Vincristine-induced orthostatic hypotension: a prospective clinical study. *Cancer Treatment Reports*, **64**, 359–360 (1980)

131. Whittaker, J.A., Parry, D.H., Bunch, C. and Weatherall, D.J. Coma associated with vincristine therapy. *British Medical Journal*, **iv**, 335–357 (1973)

132. Stuart, M.J., Cuaso, C., Miller, M. and Oski, F.A. Syndrome of recurrent increased secretion of antidiuretic hormone following multiple doses of vincristine. *Blood*, **45**, 315–320 (1975)

133. Johnson, F.L., Bernstein, I.D., Hartmann, J.R. *et al.* Seizures associated with vincristine sulfate therapy. *Journal of Pediatrics*, **82**, 699–702 (1973)

134. Hardisty, R.M., McElwain, T.J. and Darby, C.W. Vincristine and prednisone for the induction of remission in acute childhood leukaemia. *British Medical Journal*, **ii**, 662–665 (1969)

135. Weiden, P.L. and Wright, S.E. Vincristine neurotoxicity. *New England Journal of Medicine*, **286**, 1369–1370 (1972)

136. Casey, E.B., Jellife, A.M., LeQuesne, M. *et al.* Vincristine neuropathy: clinical and electrophysiological observations. *Brain*, **96**, 69–86 (1973)

137. Norman, M., Elinder, G. and Finkel, Y. Vincristine neuropathy and a Guillain-Barré syndrome: a case with acute lymphatic leukaemia and quadraparesis. *European Journal of Haematology*, **39**, 75–76 (1987)

138. Hurwitz, R.L., Mahoney, D.H., Armstrong, D.L. and Browder, T.M. Reversible encephalopathy and seizures as a result of conventional vincristine administration. *Medical and Pediatric Oncology*, **16**, 216–219 (1988)

139. Schochet, S., Lampert, P.W. and Earle, K.M. Neuronal changes induced by intrathecal vincristine sulfate. *Journal of Neuropathology and Experimental Neurology*, **27**, 645–658 (1968)

140. Shepherd, D.A., Steuber, C.P., Starling, K.A. and Fernbach, D.J. Accidental intrathecal administration of vincristine. *Medical and Pediatric Oncology*, **5**, 85–88 (1978)

141. Slyter, H., Liwnicz, B., Herrick, M.K. and Mason, R. Fatal myeloencephalopathy caused by intrathecal vincristine. *Neurology*, **30**, 867–871 (1980)

142. Sahenk, Z., Brady, S.T. and Mendell, J.R. Studies on the pathogenesis of vincristine-induced neuropathy. *Muscle and Nerve*, **10**, 80–84 (1987)

143. Pratt, C.B., Choi, S.I. and Holton, C.P. Low-dosage asparaginase treatment of childhood acute lymphocytic leukemia. *American Journal of Diseases of Children*, **121**, 406–409 (1971)

144. Oettgen, H.F., Stephenson, P.A., Schwartz, M.K. *et al.* Toxicity of *E. coli* L-asparaginase in man. *Cancer*, **25**, 253–278 (1970)

145. Moure, J.M.B., Whitecar, J.P. and Bodey, G.P. Electroencephalogram changes secondary to asparaginase. *Archives of Neurology*, **23**, 365–368 (1970)

146. Ohnuma, T., Holland, J.F., Freeman, A. *et al.* Biochemical and pharmacological studies with asparaginase in man. *Cancer Research*, **30**, 2297–2305 (1970)

147. Land, V.J., Sutow, W.W., Fernbach, D.J. *et al.* Toxicity of L-asparaginase in children with advanced leukemia. *Cancer*, **30**, 339–347 (1972)

148. Ohnuma, T., Holland, J.F., Freeman, A. *et al.* Biochemical and pharmacological studies with asparaginase in man. *Cancer Research*, **30**, 2297–2305 (1970)

149. Schwartz, M.K., Lash, E.D., Oettgen, H.F. and Tomao, F.A. L-Asparaginase activity in plasma and other biological fluids. *Cancer*, **25**, 244–252 (1970)

150. Riccardi, R., Holcenberg, J., Glaubiger, D. and Poplack, D. L-Asparaginase pharmacokinetics and L-asparaginase in the cerebrospinal fluid. *Proceedings of the American Association of Cancer Research*, **21**, 336 (1980)

151. Wriston, J.C. and Yellin, T.O. L-Asparaginase: a review. *Advances in Enzymology*, **39**, 185–248 (1973)

152. Cairo, M.S., Lazarus, K., Gilmore, R.L. and Baehner, R.L. Intracranial hemorrhage and focal seizures secondary to use of L-asparaginase during induction therapy of acute lymphocytic leukemia. *Journal of Pediatrics*, **97**, 829–833 (1980)

153. Priest, J.R., Ramsay, N.K., Latchaw, R.E. *et al.* Thrombotic and hemorrhagic strokes complicating early therapy for childhood acute lymphoblastic leukemia. *Cancer*, **46**, 1548–1554 (1980)

154. Priest, J.R., Ramsay, N.K.C., Steinherz, P.G. *et al.* A syndrome of thrombosis and hemorrhage complicating L-asparaginase therapy for childhood acute lymphoblastic leukemia. *Pediatrics*, **100**, 984–989 (1982)

155. Weimann, M.C. and Calabresi, P. Pharmacology of antineoplastic agents. In *Medical Oncology* (eds P. Calabresi, P.S. Schein and S.A. Rosenberg), Macmillan, New York, pp. 342–344 (1985)

156. Priest, J.R. Ramsay, N.K.C., Bennett, A.J. *et al.* The effect of L-asparaginase on antithrombin, plasminogen, and plasma coagulation during therapy for acute lymphoblastic leukemia. *Journal of Pediatrics*, **100**, 990–995 (1982)

157. Clavell, L.A., Gelber, R.D., Cohen, H.J. *et al.* Four-agent induction and intensive asparaginase therapy for treatment of childhood acute lymphoblastic leukemia. *New England Journal of Medicine*, **315**, 657–663 (1986)

158. Feinberg, W.M. and Swenson, M.R. Cerebrovascular complications of L-asparaginase therapy. *Neurology*, **38**, 127–133 (1988)

159. Packer, R.J., Rorke, L.B., Lange, B.J. *et al.* Cerebrovascular accidents in children with cancer. *Pediatrics*, **76**, 194–201 (1985)

160. Pui, C.H., Jackson, C.W., Chesney, C. *et al.* Sequential changes in platelet function and coagulation in leukemic children treated with L-asparaginase, prednisone and vincristine. *Journal of Clinical Oncology*, **1**, 380–385 (1983)

161. Bezeaud, A., Drouet, L., Leverger, G. *et al.* Effect of L-asparaginase therapy for acute lymphoblastic leukemia on plasma vitamin K-dependent coagulation factors and inhibitors. *Journal of Pediatrics*, **108**, 698–701 (1986)

162. Buchanan, G.R. and Holtkamp, C.A. Reduced antithrombin III levels during L-asparaginase therapy. *Medical and Pediatric Oncology*, **8**, 7–14 (1980)

163. Vellenga, E., Kluft, C., Mulder, N.H. *et al.* The influence of L-asparaginase therapy on the fibrinolytic system. *British Journal of Haematology*, **57**, 247–254 (1984)

164. VonHoff, D.D., Schilsky, R., Reichert, C.M. *et al.* Toxic effects of *cis*-dichlorodiammineplatinum (II) in man. *Cancer Treatment Reports*, **63**, 1527–1531 (1979)

165. Piel, I.J., Meyer, D., Perlia, C.P. and Wolfe, V.I. Effects of *cis*-dichlorodiammineplatinum (NSC-119875) on hearing function in man. *Cancer Chemotherapy Reports*, **58**, 871–875 (1974)

166. Panatierre, F.J. Cisplatinum toxicity. An analysis based on three SWOG studies. *Proceedings of the American Association for Cancer Research*, **22**, 157 (1981)

167. McHaney, V.A., Thibadeau, G., Hayes, F.A. and Green, A. Auditory function of children receiving cisplatinum chemotherapy. *Proceedings of the American Association for Cancer Research*, **22**, 401 (1981)

168. Granowetter, L., Rosenstock, J.G. and Packer, R.J. Enhanced cisplatinum neurotoxicity in pediatric patients with brain tumors. *Journal of Neuro-Oncology*, **1**, 293–297 (1983)

169. Baranak, C.C., Wetmore, R.F. and Packer, R.J. Cisplatinum ototoxicity after radiation treatment: an animal model. *Journal of Neuro-Oncology*, **6**, 266–267 (1988)

170. Stadnicki, S.W., Fleischman, R.W., Schaeppi, U. and Meriam, P. *Cis*-dichlorodiammine platinum II

(NSC-119875): hearing loss and other toxic effects in Rhesus monkeys. *Cancer Chemotherapy Reports*, **59**, 467–480 (1975)

171. Fleischman, R.W., Stadnicki, S.W., Ethier, M.F. *et al.* Ototoxicity of *cis*-dichlorodiammine platinum II in the guinea pig. *Toxicology and Applied Pharmacology*, **33**, 320–332 (1975)

172. Aschraf, M., Scotchel, P.L., Krall, J.M. and Fink, E.B. Cisplatinum-induced hypomagnesemia and peripheral neuropathy. *Gynecological Oncology*, **16**, 309–318 (1983)

173. Thompson, S.W., Davis, L.E., Kornfeld, M. *et al.* Cisplatin neuropathy. *Cancer*, **54**, 1269–1275 (1984)

174. Roelofs, R.I., Hrushesky, W., Rogin, J. and Rosenberg, L. Peripheral sensory neuropathy and cisplatin chemotherapy. *Neurology*, **34**, 934–938 (1984)

175. Mollman, J.E., Glover, D.J., Hogan, M. and Furman, R. Cisplatin neuropathy: risk factors, prognosis and protection by WR-2721. *Cancer*, **61**, 2192–2195 (1988)

176. Walker, R.W., Cairncross, J.G. and Posner, J.B. Cerebral herniation in patients receiving cisplatin. *Journal of Neuro-Oncology*, **6**, 61–65 (1988)

177. Ostrow, S., Hahn, D., Wiernik, P.H. and Richards, R.D. Ophthalmologic toxicity after *cis*-dichlorodiammineplatinum (II) therapy. *Cancer Treatment Reports*, **62**, 1591–1594 (1978)

178. Berman, I.J. and Mann, M.P. Seizures and transient cortical blindness associated with cisplatinum (II) diamminechloride (PDD) therapy in a 30-year-old man. *Cancer*, **45**, 764–766 (1980)

179. Stuart-Harris, R., Ponder, B.A.J. and Wrigley, P.F.M. Tetany associated with cisplatin. *Lancet*, **ii**, 1303 (1980)

180. Brunner, K.W. and Young, C.W. A methylhydrazine derivative in Hodgkin's disease and other malignant neoplasms: therapeutic and toxic effects studied in 51 patients. *Annals of Internal Medicine*, **63**, 69–86 (1965)

181. Stolinsky, D.C., Solomon, J., Pugh, R.P. *et al.* Clinical experience with procarbazine in Hodgkin's disease, reticulum cell sarcoma, and lymphosarcoma. *Cancer*, **26**, 984–990 (1970)

182. Mann, A.M. and Hutchinson, J.L. Manic reaction associated with procarbazine hydrochloride therapy of Hodgkin's disease. *Canadian Medical Association Journal*, **97**, 1350–1353 (1967)

183. Samuels, M.L., Leary, W.B., Alexanian, R. *et al.* Clinical trials with *N*-isopropyl-a-(2-methylhydrazino)-*p*-toluamide hydrochloride in malignant lymphoma and other disseminated neoplasia. *Cancer*, **20**, 1187–1194 (1967)

184. DeVita, V.T., Hahn, M.A. and Oliverio, V.T. Monoamine oxidase inhibition by a new carcinostatic agent, *N*-isopropyl-1-(2-methylhydrazino)-*p*-toluamide (MIH). *Proceedings of the Society for Experimental Biology and Medicine*, **120**, 561–565 (1965)

185. Lee, I.P. and Lucier, G.W. The potentiation of barbiturate-induced necrosis by procarbazine. *Journal of Pharmacology and Experimental Therapeutics*, **196**, 586–593 (1976)

186. Brule, G., Schlumberger, J.R. and Griscelli, C. *N*-isopropyl-a-(2-methylhydrazino)-*p*-toluamide hydrochloride (NSC-77213) in the treatment of solid tumors. *Cancer Chemotherapy Reports*, **44**, 31–38 (1965)

187. Mathe, G., Schweisguth, O., Schneider, M. *et al.* Methylhydrazine in treatment of Hodgkin's disease and various forms of haematosarcoma and leukaemia. *Lancet*, **ii**, 1077–1080 (1963)

188. Oliverio, V.T., Denham, C., DeVita, V.T. and Kelley, M.G. Some pharmacolaogic properties of a new antitumor agent, *N*-isopropyl-a-(2-methylhydrazino)-*p*-toluamide hydrochloride (NSC-77213). *Cancer Chemotherapy Reports*, **42**, 1–7 (1964)

189. Chabner, B.A., DeVita, V.T., Considine, N. *et al.* Plasma pyridoxal phosphate depletion by the carcinostatic procarbazine. *Proceedings of the Society for Experimental Biology and Medicine*, **132**, 1119–1122 (1969)

190. Billmeier, G.J. and Holton, C.P. Procarbazine hydrochloride in childhood cancer. *Journal of Pediatrics*, **75**, 892–895 (1969)

191. DeVita, V.T., Serpick, A. and Carbone, P.P. Preliminary clinical studies with ibenzmethyzine. *Clinical Pharmacology and Therapeutics*, **7**, 542–546 (1966)

192. Allen, J.C., Gralla, R., Reilly, L. *et al.* Metaclopramide: dose-related toxicity and preliminary antiemetic studies in children receiving cancer chemotherapy. *Journal of Clinical Oncology*, **8**, 1136–1141 (1985)

193. Heideman, R., Packer, R.J., Reaman, G. *et al.* Spiromustine (NSC 172112) (SHM): results of a phase I clinical trial and pharmacokinetics in pediatric patients (abstract). *Proceedings of the American Society for Clinical Oncology*, **6**, A153 (1987)

194. Gren, A.A. and Naiman, J.L. Chlorambucil poisoning. *American Journal of Diseases of Children*, **116**, 190–191 (1968)

195. Wolfson, S. and Olney, M.B. Accidental ingestion of a toxic dose of chlorambucil: report of a case in a child. *Journal of the American Medical Association*, **165**, 239–240 (1957)

196. Stewart, D.J., Grahovac, Z., Russel, N.L. *et al.* Phase I study of intracarotid PCNU. *Journal of Neuro-Oncology*, **5**, 245–250 (1987)

197. Moertel, C.G., Rettemeier, R.G. *et al.* Study of 5-(3,3-dimethyl-1-1-triazeno) imidazole-4-carboxamide (NSC 45388) in patients with gastrointestinal carcinoma. *Cancer Chemotherapy Reports*, **54**, 471–473 (1970)

198. Patterson, A.H.G. and McPherson, T.A. A possible neurologic complication of DTIC. *Cancer Treatment Reports*, **61**, 106 (1977)

199. Gams, R.A. and Carpenter, J.T. Central nervous system complications after combination treatment with adriamycin (NSC 123127) and 5-(3,3-dimethyl-

1-triazeno) imidazole-4-carboxamide (NSC 45388). *Cancer Chemotherapy Reports*, **58**, 753–754 (1974)

200. Levi, J.A. and Wiernik, P.H. A comparative clinical trial of 5-azacytidine and guanazide in previously treated adults with acute nonlymphocytic leukemia. *Cancer*, **38**, 36–41 (1976)

201. Obrist, R., Paravicini, U., Hartmann, D. *et al.* Vindesine. A clinical trial with special reference to neurological side effects. *Cancer Chemotherapy and Pharmacology*, **2**, 223–237 (1979)

202. Gralla, R.J., Tan, C.T. and Young, C.W. Vindesine: a review of phase II trials. *Cancer Chemotherapy and Pharmacology*, **2**, 271–274 (1979)

203. Carroll, D.S., Gralla, R.J. and Kemeny, N.E. Phase II evaluation of vindesine in patients with advanced colorectal carcinoma. *Cancer Treatment Reports*, **63**, 2097–2098 (1979)

204. Ohnuma, T., Greenspan, E.M. and Holland, J.F. Initial clinical study with vindesine: tolerance to weekly IV bolus and 24-hour infusion. *Cancer Treatment Reports*, **64**, 25–30 (1980)

205. Falkson, G., van Dyke, J.J., van Eden, E.B. *et al.* A clinical trial of the oral form of 4′-dimethyl-epipodophyllotoxin-B-D ethylidine glucoside (NSC 141540) VP 16-213. *Cancer*, **35**, 1141–1144 (1975)

206. Littlewood, T.J., Bentley, D.P. and McQueen, I.N. High-dose etoposide does not cause peripheral neuropathy. *Cancer Chemotherapy and Pharmacology*, **19**, 180–181 (1987)

207. Leff, R.S., Thompson, J.M., Daly, M.B. *et al.* Acute neurologic dysfunction after high-dose etoposide therapy for malignant glioma. *Cancer*, **62**, 32–35 (1988)

208. Mayer, E.G., Paulter, C. and Aristzapal, S. Complications of irradiation related to apparent drug potentiation by Adriamycin. *International Journal of Radiation Oncology, Biology, Physics*, **1**, 1179–1188 (1976)

209. D'Angio, G.J. Clinical and biological studies of actinomycin-D and roentgen irradiation. *American Journal of Roentgenology*, **87**, 106–109 (1962)

210. Teutsch, C., Lipton, A. and Harvey, H.A. Raynaud's phenomenon as a side effect of chemotherapy with vinblastine and bleomycin for testicular carcinoma. *Cancer Treatment Reports*, **61**, 925–926 (1977)

211. Legha, S.S., Slavik, M. and Carter, S.K. Hexamethylmyelamine: an evaluation of its role in the therapy of cancer. *Cancer*, **38**, 27–35 (1976)

# 22

# Neuropsychological sequelae of radiotherapy

A.S. Gamis, J.P. Neglia and L.L. Robison

Among the myriad of late effects that have been found in long-term survivors of childhood cancer, neuropsychological sequelae have increasingly been recognized in patients with the two most common pediatric cancers, acute lymphoblastic leukemia (ALL) and brain tumors. The application of central nervous system (CNS) therapy is unique to the treatment programs of these two neoplasms. It is this therapy, which combines cranial irradiation with or without intrathecal or systemic chemotherapy, that has been implicated in the etiology of the neurocognitive deficits in these patients. It has been argued that cranial irradiation is a significant risk factor for the development of this impairment.

Radiotherapy has played an important role in the treatment of childhood ALL and brain tumors [1]. With long-term disease-free survival among all childhood cancers now exceeding 60%, it is increasingly appropriate that attention be directed to the quality of life which follows curative therapy. In this chapter, studies of the neuropsychological sequelae in these two particular cancers will be examined, with particular emphasis on the effects of cranial irradiation. The clinical implications of these findings, as they relate to treatment, in addition to the very important need for ongoing neuropsychological evaluation and educational intervention in these children and young adults is also discussed.

## Acute lymphoblastic leukemia (ALL) of childhood

Craniospinal irradiation was introduced into the treatment regimens of childhood ALL in the late 1960s and early 1970s. Prior to effective presymptomatic CNS therapy, CNS relapse rates were reported to be as high as 75%. With the use of 2400 cGy of craniospinal irradiation, CNS relapse rates declined to less than 10%. Further studies revealed that similar efficacy could be achieved by reducing the field of irradiation to only the cranium while adding intrathecal methotrexate. This prophylactic regimen remains the gold standard with which newer methods are compared.

More recent research has been directed toward the identification of patient subgroups that require more (or less) intensive therapy. Among those patients considered to be at high risk (high initial leukocyte count, T cell disease, lymphomatous characteristics, age at diagnosis of <2 or >8 years and thrombocytopenia [1]), cranial irradiation continues to be important for the prevention of CNS relapse. Approximately 2–3% of children with ALL have CNS involvement at the time of initial diagnosis. For these children and those who relapse in the CNS, current treatment therapy for CNS leukemia usually includes 2400 cGy to the entire craniospinal axis in addition to intrathecal methotrexate.

More recent CNS prophylactic regimens have employed a variety of combinations of radiation and chemotherapy including craniospinal irradiation alone, cranial irradiation with intrathecal chemotherapy (most often methotrexate), intrathecal methotrexate alone or in combination with intrathecal cytosine arabinoside (cytarabine) and hydrocortisone ('triple' therapy), a combination of systemic and intrathecal methotrexate or, most recently, high-dose intravenous methotrexate alone with leukovorin (folinic acid) rescue. The initially accepted dose of CNS irradiation was 2400 cGy, although subsequent studies have indicated equal efficacy with the use of 1800 cGy. In addition, use of intrathecal therapy alone for CNS prophylaxis has been found to be effective in patients with low or moderate risk ALL [2]. Current studies are reporting successful prevention of CNS relapse in >90–95% of childhood ALL patients receiving these prophylactic regimens.

Results from over 40 studies examining neuropsychological sequelae in children with ALL have now been reported with a wide variety of findings. While many investigations have found that neuropsychological sequelae are secondary to cranial irradiation, several have not found this association. Moreover, in those studies that suggest a causal relationship between neuropsychological complications and cranial irradiation, the specific patient groups at risk and the specific nature of the neuropsychological sequelae vary. Several reasons have been suggested for this discordance [3,4]. Methodologic limits of the studies include variability in ages of patients tested, small sample sizes, biased selection criteria, inappropriate control groups or failure to include control groups, and lack of consistent testing measures. This has made the overall interpretation of these studies difficult and may have produced biased results. Thus, for the pediatric oncologist who must design and prescribe the treatment protocol for each patient, and the pediatrician and/or specialist who will care for the long-term survivors, the results of neuropsychological studies in populations of ALL patients must be carefully examined and interpreted with caution.

The majority of studies to date have utilized the Wechsler Intelligence scales (WPPSI, WISC, WISC-R, WAIS) and the Wide Range Achievement Test (WRAT) [5] to identify and define the scope of neuropsychological dysfunction. Twelve subtests make up the WISC-R (the test most often used for this age group) from which performance, verbal, and full scale IQ scores are derived (Table 22.1) [6]. Verbal IQ is derived from subtests which measure experience, education, environment, culture, social judgement, ability to concentrate, attention span, rote memory and verbal expression. Performance IQ measures visual perception, motor coordination, visual alertness, visual memory, speed and accuracy of learning, comprehension of a total situation and analysis of abstract design. Scores of subtests are scaled to a mean value of 10, and IQ scores are based upon a mean of 100. The WRAT measures

academic achievement in three subcategories: reading, spelling and arithmetic. Other tests, or portions of tests, utilized in evaluating neuropsychological dysfunction have included the Halstead–Reitan Neuropsychological Battery, the Beery Developmental Test of Visual-Motor Integration, the McCarthy Scales of Children's Abilities, the Burt Reading test, the British Abilities scale, the Stanford–Binet Intelligence scale, the Bender–Gestalt test of perceptual motor function, the Peabody Individual Achievement test, and interviews and questionnaires with parents and teachers.

Early studies of neuropsychological function failed to identify significant deficiencies in patients who had received CNS prophylaxis [7,8]. In the first published study of neuropsychological dysfunction and CNS prophylaxis no statistical differences were found between patients who had received CNS prophylaxis (consisting of cranial irradiation with or without intrathecal methotrexate) and ALL or Wilms' tumor patients who had not received any CNS therapy [7]. However, slightly lower scores were seen in the children receiving CNS prophylaxis. Obetz *et al.* [8], evaluating 33 ALL patients 6–96 months after diagnosis, found no significant neuropsychological deficits; however, they did find that in those patients tested more than 2 years after CNS prophylaxis, 48–50% had abnormal test results. Thus, while they concluded that no significant deficits occurred, there was a trend indicating that measurable sequelae may not arise or become apparent until several years after CNS therapy.

Studies have shown that few neurocognitive deficits exist at the time of the initial diagnosis of childhood ALL [4,7,9,10]. However, neuropsychological studies of long-term survivors of childhood ALL have revealed a significantly higher frequency of deficits when compared with classmates [11], with solid tumor patients who had not received CNS therapy [12], and with siblings [13]. Cognitive performance of ALL patients has also been found to be consistently lower than classmates who were matched for age, sex and social class [11]. Neither behavioral nor school attendance differences could be found to account for these findings. Prospective neuropsychological evaluations found significant declines in those patients who had received cranial irradiation (median score 88) when compared with children in two control groups consisting of ALL (intrathecal methotrexate only) and Wilms' tumor who had median IQs of 109 and 114, respectively [12]. Compared with IQ at dignosis, 61% (11/18) had greater than a 10-point decline in their full-scale IQ scores. While these findings have been questioned [3], the significant disparity seen in IQ function between the groups and the extent of neuropsychological dysfunction observed in each irradiated patient is unlikely to be fully attributed to methodologic issues.

**Table 22.1 WISC-R subtests**

| Performance IQ | Verbal IQ |
| --- | --- |
| Picture completion | General information |
| Picture arrangement | General comprehension |
| Block design | Arithmetic |
| Object assembly | Similarities |
| Coding | Vocabulary |
| Mazes | Digit span |

The findings of Whitt *et al.* [14] and Mulhern *et al.* [15] suggest that all ALL patients exhibit neuropsychological declines regardless of the type of CNS prophylaxis, thus implicating the intensive chemotherapeutic regimens. While these studies did not find CNS prophylaxis to be the causative factor, many other investigations do point to the prophylactic CNS treatment as the reason for neuropsychological dysfunction. Several studies in which solid tumor patients were used as controls have found relative deficits in cognitive and academic abilities of ALL patients who received CNS prophylaxis [9,10,12,16–19]. As both groups received chemotherapy, were chronically ill and had experienced life-threatening illnesses, the use of CNS prophylaxis was implicated. Only two studies have found no difference between ALL patients and other cancer patients [7,20]. In these studies results demonstrated that there was a trend to lower function in the ALL patients, and those who received higher dosages of radiation (2400 cGy) tended to score lower on intelligence tests. To investigate the effect of CNS therapy upon neuropsychological function, Moss, Nannis and Poplack [13] matched 24 irradiated ALL children (2400 cGy concurrent with intrathecal methotrexate or cytosine arabinoside (cytarabine)) and 13 ALL patients who had received no CNS prophylactic therapy to siblings. When compared with siblings, only the CNS irradiated group performed significantly lower, with deficits observed in full-scale, performance and verbal IQ. Of interest was the finding that the irradiated group continued as a whole to function in the average range. However, by using the sibling controls as a means of determining the patient's IQ prior to irradiation, there was a decline from the 79th percentile to the 47th percentile.

Some studies have directly examined the question of whether cranial irradiation is the reason for neuropsychological sequelae by comparing two groups of ALL; those who received CNS radiation plus intrathecal chemotherapy and those receiving only intrathecal chemotherapy (Table 22.2 and 22.3). The majority have found significant differences among the irradiated and non-irradiated groups [9,12,21–25], although several have seen no difference [8,15,26,27]. Interestingly, in one study neuropsychological sequelae were lacking in patients in whom CNS irradiation was delayed until 6 months after induction therapy, while in those patients irradiated during the induction/consolidation phase of therapy significant deficits in neuropsychological function were found [21]. In addition to IQ deficits in studies comparing irradiated and non-irradiated ALL patients, cranial irradiation has also been associated with computed tomography (CT) abnormalities of the brain and an increased frequency of difficulties in school [22,28].

Several studies have directly or indirectly examined the question of dose of CNS radiation and neuropsychological function in groups of children receiving 1800 or 2400 cGy of cranial irradiation (Table 22.4). Two studies comparing these dosages have found no significant difference in cognitive function between the two groups [25,27]. Tamaroff *et al.* [25] found both groups to have significant deficits compared with normal values. Williams *et al.* [27], in contrast, found no evidence of neuropsychological dysfunction in either group; however, this study was severely limited by a short period of follow-up. Recent reports have examined the effects of 1800 cGy with intrathecal therapy versus intrathecal and intravenous methotrexate therapy. Ochs, Parvey and Mulhern [26] and Mulhern *et al.* [15]

**Table 22.2 A summary of studies comparing children with ALL who received 2400 cGy of prophylactic cranial irradiation with control groups who received no CNS irradiation**

| Author [ref.] | Diagnosis to test interval (years) | WISC-R | | | WRAT | | |
| --- | --- | --- | --- | --- | --- | --- | --- |
| | | FSIQ | PIQ | VIQ | Spelling | Reading | Arithmetic |
| Eiser [21] | 5.0 | ↓ | ↓ | ↔ | NA | ↔[a] | NA |
| Obetz [8] | 2.9 | ↔ | ↔ | ↔ | NA | NA | NA |
| Meadows [29] | 3.0 | ↓[a] | NA | NA | NA | NA | NA |
| Pavlovsky [22] | 5.0 | ↓[a] | ↓[a] | NA | NA | NA | NA |
| Pfefferbaum [23] | 8.0 | ↓ | ↔ | ↓ | ↔ | ↔[a] | ↓ |
| Rowland [24] | 4.7 | ↓ | ↓ | ↓ | ↓ | ↔ | ↓ |
| Copeland [9] | 7.8 | ↓ | ↓ | ↓ | ↓ | NA | ↓ |
| Whitt [14] | 4.5 | ↔ | ↔ | ↔ | ↔ | ↔ | ↑ |
| Tamaroff [25] | 6.2 | ↓ | ↓ | ↔ | NA | NA | NA |
| Williams [27] | 1.6 | ↔ | ↔ | ↔ | ↔ | ↔ | ↓ |

↓, irradiated group scored significantly lower than control group; ↑, irradiated group scored significantly higher than control group; ↔, no significant difference found between irradiated and control groups; NA, not available or tested; [a], utilized evaluations other than WISC-R or WRAT

**Table 22.3 A summary of studies comparing children with ALL who received 1800 cGy of prophylactic cranial irradiation with control groups who received no CNS irradiation**

| Author [ref.] | Diagnosis to test interval (years) | WISC-R | | | WRAT | | |
|---|---|---|---|---|---|---|---|
| | | FSIQ | PIQ | VIQ | Spelling | Reading | Arithmetic |
| Tamaroff [25] | 3.2 | ↓ | ↓ | ↔ | NA | NA | NA |
| Ochs [26] | 4.0 | ↔ | NA | NA | NA | NA | NA |
| Williams [27] | 0.5 | ↔ | ↔ | ↔ | ↔ | ↔ | ↓ |
| Mulhern [15] | 5.7 | ↔ | NA | NA | NA | NA | NA |

↓, irradiated group scored significantly lower than control group; ↑, irradiated group scored significantly higher than control group; ↔, no significant difference found between irradiated and control groups; NA, not available or tested; [a]utilized evaluations other than WISC-R or WRAT

**Table 22.4 A summary of studies which compared children with ALL who received either 1800 cGy or 2400 cGy of prophylactic cranial irradiation**

| Author [ref.] | Diagnosis to test interval (years) | WISC-R | | | WRAT | | |
|---|---|---|---|---|---|---|---|
| | | FSIQ | PIQ | VIQ | Spelling | Reading | Arithmetic |
| Meadows [29] | 1.0 | ↔ | ↓ | NA | NA | NA | NA |
| Harten[a] [20] | 5.8 | ↔[c] | ↓[c] | NA | NA | NA | NA |
| Robison[b] [31] | 7.0 | ↓ | ↓ | NA | NA | NA | NA |
| Tamaroff [25] | 6.2 | ↔ | ↔ | ↔ | NA | NA | NA |
| Williams [27] | 1.6 | ↔ | ↔ | ↔ | ↔ | ↔ | ↔ |
| Trautman[a] [30] | 4.0 | ↔ | ↔ | ↔ | ↔[c] | ↔[c] | ↔[c] |

↓, 2400 cGy group scored significantly lower than 1800 cGy group; ↔, no significant difference found between irradiated and control groups; NA, not available or tested; [a], scores were lower but did not reach statistical significance; [b], actual dose of radiation ranged from 2000 to 2700 cGy, therefore values listed represent the effect of the higher doses of CNS irradiation; [c], utilized evaluations other than WISC-R or WRAT

both found no significant neuropsychological sequelae in those patients irradiated with 1800 cGy (Table 22.3). Mulhern speculated that this dose of irradiation may be safer than 2400 cGy. Meadows, Massari and Obringer [29], however, in early follow-up studies, found impairment of visual motor skills among patients who had received 1800 cGy. Both Trautman *et al.* [30] and Harten *et al.* [20] suggested that neuropsychological test scores may be lower with increasing radiation dosage (1800–2400 cGy); however, neither study found statistically significant differences. Robison *et al.* [31] found that in males older than 5 years of age a higher dose of radiation (range: 2000–2700 cGy) resulted in lower performance IQs and full-scale IQs. Clearly, further study is needed to better clarify the differences in neuropsychological effect between 1800 and 2400 cGy of cranial irradiation.

In ALL patients who have received more than 2400 cGy of cranial irradiation, significant declines in neuropsychological sequelae have been seen [32]. In a study of 29 children who received two courses of cranial irradiation for isolated CNS relapse (total maximum dose of 4800 cGy), neuropsychological test scores were compared with 50 long-term survivors of childhood ALL who had received CNS prophylactic irradiation and had remained in remission [32]. Wechsler intelligence test scores of the study group showed significant deficits compared with normative values and with the comparison group. Achievement test scores (WRAT) were even more severely affected by the additional cranial irradiation; 20% were functioning in the mentally retarded range with eight having full-scale IQs (WISC-R) less than 70. Not only were these deficits severe in nature, investigators found that an increasing interval between diagnosis of ALL and IQ testing correlated positively with lower IQ scores. A younger age at diagnosis also was associated with poorer neuropsychological function in these patients. Other correlates with poor neuropsychological outcome included abnormalities on CT and seizures, both of which independently were associated with 10–15 IQ point decrements. Thus, doses of CNS irradiation in excess of 2400 cGy clearly appear to be associated with marked neurocognitive dysfunction.

That CNS radiation can cause neuropsychological sequelae is no longer questionable. What needs consideration is what agent or combination of agents is also implicated and which subgroups of patients are most susceptible. When addressing these questions it is important to consider the possibility that an interactive effect may exist between treatment modalities as well as with patient characteristics such as age and sex. Investigators have raised the question whether neuropsychological dysfunction may be the result of synergistic actions of cranial irradiation and methotrexate administered intrathecally or intravenously. The number of therapeutic modalities used has been reported to be directly related to the degree of CNS toxicity [1]. Early studies have implicated the combination of radiation and methotrexate as synergistically toxic to the CNS [33,34]. McIntosh *et al.* [34] found that the occurrence of significant neuropsychological dysfunction in irradiated patients coincided with the escalation of systemic methotrexate. While not directly implicating this combination, other data support this synergism [7]. This trend was recently examined by Fallovollita *et al.* [35] in 70 patients who had received 2400 cGy of cranial irradiation either alone or with intrathecal methotrexate. Significantly lower scores were seen in those patients receiving the intrathecal methotrexate. In patients under 5 years of age at diagnosis, the addition of methotrexate decreased IQ scores by an average of 10–11 points. The timing and/or sequence of administration of the intrathecal methotrexate in relation to cranial irradiation may influence neuropsychological toxicity. The Children's Cancer Study Group has presented data suggesting a significant protective effect when intrathecal methotrexate is administered prior to CNS irradiation [36]. Animal data have demonstrated this protective effect on neuronal tissue by the preradiation injection of intrathecal methotrexate. This may explain the finding by Eiser [21] of IQ deficits only in those patients receiving cranial irradiation early (without prior intrathecal methotrexate) and not in patients who received cranial irradiation 6 months post-diagnosis (after intrathecal methotrexate had been administered).

Other chemotherapeutic agents, including cytosine arabinoside (cytarabine), hydrocortisone and dexamethasone have been administered intrathecally, but to date have not been implicated in neuropsychological sequelae when administered without irradiation. Two studies which included these variables in their analysis did not find neuropsychological dysfunction to correlate with the particular intrathecal agent, methotrexate or cytosine arabinoside, when administered with irradiation [13,28]. Interestingly, Tamaroff *et al.* [37] examined neuropsychological function in patients who had received intrathecal methotrexate without CNS irradiation and compared it with solid tumor patients. No neuropsychological deficits were found in either of these two unirradiated groups.

Most investigations have included analyses designed to ascertain possible risk factors for neuropsychological sequelae in ALL patients. These analyses are based on the clinical observation that a proportion of patients receiving CNS prophylaxis have no evidence of neurological or neuropsychological dysfunction, while others clearly show significant sequelae. This was clearly observed in the evaluation of neuropsychological sequelae in ALL patients who had CNS relapses and had received 2400–4800 cGy of cranial irradiation with intrathecal medications [32]. Despite the severe neuropsychological sequelae noted in many of these patients, one-third exhibited no significant such dysfunction.

Among the many risk factors examined (Table 22.5), age of the patient at the time of diagnosis and

**Table 22.5 Risk factors for neuropsychological sequelae in children with ALL**

Cranial irradiation (≥2400 cGy, ?1800 cGy)
Concurrent use of intrathecal methotrexate
Concurrent use of high-dose intravenous methotrexate
Age ≤6–8 years at time of CNS irradiation
CT scan abnormalities (intracerebral calcifications)
? Intensive systemic chemotherapy
? Female gender
? Somnolence syndrome
? Socioeconomic status
? Parental education

irradiation has been most studied. Eiser and Lansdown [11] were the first to find that age was a significant risk factor. Their data indicated that only in those patients receiving CNS prophylaxis before the age of 5 years did neuropsychological sequelae result. Those aged over 5 years, even though they received the same CNS prophylaxis, exhibited no sequelae. Most studies have replicated these findings [9,12,13,16,18,22,23,31,32,35,38,39]. A few have not found significant differences in age groups [8,14,15,27,30], while others have reported that older age correlated with neuropsychological sequelae [20]. Jannoun [38] analysed three age groups (under 3 years, 3–6 years and over 6 years) and found neuropsychological dysfunction to be greatest in those under 3 years of age at diagnosis, but also significant in the 3–6-year-old group compared with their siblings. This age association has also been documented by Carli *et al.* [40] who found that CT abnormalities were age-related. Among their 12 patients with intracerebral calcifications, 11 were under 5 years of age when irradiated. Pavlovsky *et al.* [22] has also found young age, neuropsychological dysfunction and CT abnormalities to correlate. In general, patients under 4–5 years of age at diagnosis appear to be at greatest risk for radiation-associated neuropsychological dysfunction.

Other risk factors have been examined to assess their contribution to neuropsychological sequelae. In some studies female gender, especially when associated with young age, has placed the patient at greater risk for sequelae [18,31,35]. Others have found no significant differences between males and females [12,14,39]. An early study indicated that the somnolence syndrome, which occurs in a significant proportion of cranially irradiated patients, may predispose patients to increased risk for neuropsychological sequelae [41]. Jannoun and Chessells [39] also found a trend of increased learning disabilities in patients who had somnolence syndrome. This, however, has not been seen in other studies [30,42]. The patient's socioeconomic status and parental education have also been suggested to correlate with neuropsychological dysfunction in ALL patients [14,30,43].

As was first recognized by Obetz *et al.* [8] and confirmed by others [12,38], neuropsychological dysfunction does not often become manifest until 2–3 years after cranial irradiation is administered. It has been suggested that many impairments may not actually manifest themselves until many years later when such skills are required for specific tasks performed later in life [42]. In a prospective, longitudinal study, Jannoun and Chessells [39] noted a decline in neuropsychological function which occurred at 2–3 years post-diagnosis. However, following the cessation of all chemotherapy a modest improvement was noted. Other investigators have also argued that the decline in neuropsychological function may be transient [20]. Peckham *et al.* [43], in their evaluation of academic achievement, found no further progression in neuropsychological dysfunction after the first 5 years. These plateaus or reversals of intellectual decline may actually reflect educational intervention and/or adaptation on the part of the patient. Twaddle *et al.* [19] attributed the finding of a progressive decline in their ALL patients to a slower developmental rate. They reasoned that the children treated with cranial irradiation learned at a slower rate and thus fell farther and farther behind their peers. This, they argued, exhibited itself as a progressive decline, and suggested it could be transient if educational efforts were directed towards improving their learning ability and rate of development and thus narrowing the gap with their peers.

Examination of an association between neuropsychological dysfunction and CNS abnormalities detected on CT scans has been the subject of several studies in irradiated patients. Three abnormalities including subacute leukoencephalopathy (which is seen as areas of white matter hypodensity), mineralizing microangiopathy (characterized by intracerebral calcifications), and cerebral atrophy (which appears as ventricular and subarachnoid space dilatation) have been studied [44]. These findings have not been seen in patients treated with intrathecal chemotherapy alone [45]. Brouwers *et al.* [46] sought to determine what neurological damage was causing the neuropsychological deficits. Utilizing a test evaluating simple reaction time to an auditory stimulus, they examined 23 children with ALL who were off therapy and had received 2400 cGy of CNS irradiation and intrathecal methotrexate or cytosine arabinoside (cytarabine). Based upon concurrent CT scans, patients were divided into three groups: (1) those with no abnormalities; (2) those with cerebral atrophy; and (3) those who had intracerebral calcifications. Mean ages at diagnosis for these groups were 8.1 years, 9.6 years and 4.5 years, respectively. Significant delays in reaction time were found in the two groups with CT scan abnormalities. A significantly greater delay was seen in those patients with intracerebral calcifications in comparison with those with cerebral atrophy. Calcifications were primarily located in the basal ganglia which has been found to be the primary site of development of calcifications following CNS irradiation [44]. Findings indicated the delays in reaction time to be secondary to attention deficits rather than motor difficulties [46]. A CT scan finding of calcifications accurately predicted 100% of their patients with significant neuropsychological dysfunction. In addition to attention deficits, this study also found significant deficits in memory and verbal fluency correlating with CT scan abnormalities. The group with the intracerebral calcifications also had a significantly lower mean age than the other two groups. Intracranial calcifications have also been seen more often in children who have had higher doses of CNS irradiation for relapses in the CNS and were a risk factor which independently accounted for an average 10–15 IQ point decline [32]. Of further interest is the finding by Riccardi *et al.* [47] that CT scan changes may take years to develop. They found that while periventricular hypodensities decreased with time, intracerebral calcifications took years to become apparent.

Other means of correlating radiation-associated neuropsychological dysfunction with organic damage have been investigated. Evaluations of hearing and vision abilities in children with ALL receiving CNS irradiation have not found any deficits which could account for neuropsychological dysfunction or academic disabilities [48,49]. Recent work has shown significant correlation between evoked potentials and neuropsychological dysfunction in children who were long-term survivors of ALL [50]. These investigators found that the patients who exhibited neuropsychological disabilities also had significant delays in cognitive processing time as measured by the latency of the P3 wave of auditory event-related EEG potentials. This test may offer an objective value to evaluate neuropsychological dysfunction, although more studies are needed.

Clearly, children with ALL who have received CNS therapy including radiation are at risk for neuropsychological dysfunction. By and large it would appear that cranial irradiation plays a prominent role in the development of these sequelae. These sequelae, along with those involving dysfunction in growth, endocrine and neurological function have led to the investigation of alternatives to cranial irradiation for CNS prophylaxis in children with ALL.

## Pediatric brain tumors

Brain tumors, the second most common pediatric neoplasm, comprise 20% of all childhood cancers and are the most common of the solid tumors. As with ALL, survival for pediatric patients with brain tumors has risen over the years, with long-term survival (>5 years) now approaching 50% [51]. Brain tumors are, however, a heterogeneous group of neoplasms with a variety of histological types and sites of origin with survival and therapy dependent upon these variables. Traditionally, the therapeutic modalities available have included surgery and/or radiotherapy. Only recently has chemotherapy begun to play a role in brain tumor treatment. Recent SEER data indicate that CNS irradiation is administered to approximately 70% of children with brain tumors [51]. Dosage and volume will vary in the treatment of brain tumors compared with ALL in which radiation is more standardized. Local (less than whole brain) irradiation is restricted to those CNS neoplasms which are unlikely to spread, while cranial (whole brain) irradiation is utilized when a tumor has the potential for extensive CNS involvement. Craniospinal (whole CNS, neuraxis) irradiation is administered in those types of tumors with a propensity to metastasize along the neuraxis [52]. When cranial or craniospinal irradiation is used, boosts (increased total dose) are given to the local tumor bed. The typical dose is influenced by the tolerance of normal brain, the total volume to be irradiated, and the age of the patient. Total doses used typically range from 4500 cGy for the whole brain to 5400 cGy for locally irradiated brain tumors and local boosts. Doses are often reduced in those children under 3 years of age. Currently it is felt that reduction below 4000 cGy increases the likelihood of tumor relapse [53].

With long-term disease-free survival becoming more likely for these patients, evaluation of their quality of survival becomes more relevant. Initially this evaluation was limited to observations of functional abilities [54]. In a study of 22 children with medulloblastoma surviving 5–17 years after diagnosis, 18 (82%) were noted to be leading active lives (Bloom's categories I or II), while only two were totally disabled. This interpretation seemed to confirm previous reports in which a significant majority of survivors were leading active lives [55]. However, it is important to point out that in Bloom's definition of category I, which described patients with 'no disability', were those patients 'who are said to be slow at learning, but who, on general examination, are bright and appear intelligent'. Thus many of these patients with 'no disability' actually may have had some degree of intellectual dysfunction. Hirsch *et al.* [56] have more recently shown that this classification may not be an accurate indicator of true disability in childhood survivors of brain tumors. Physician assessment in this study found that 73% of the long-term survivors were in categories I or II, thus indicating little or no disability, yet only 11% of these patients scored in the average or above-average range (IQ >90) when tested. Others have also found that evaluations which were dependent upon a physician's global assessment of function underestimated both the severity and range of neurocognitive deficits [57]. Thus, these global test results must be cautiously interpreted.

In contrast to the optimistic report of Bloom, Wallace and Henk [54], several other early reports indicated that many patients were experiencing cognitive and functional disabilities following therapy for their brain tumors [53,58]. Li, Winston and Gimbrere [59] more recently found that 24% of brain tumor patients (compared with only 4% of other childhood cancer patients) were partially or severely disabled and could be classified in Bloom's categories III or IV, respectively.

Modern testing has made possible more detailed examination of these late effects. However, as in ALL, studies have not used uniform testing procedures, not consistently eliminated selection bias, and have often included patients with various brain tumors in various locations. This lack of control, combined with the neurocognitive variables inherent to brain tumors by virtue of their primary location, makes interpretation and comparison of these studies difficult. However, the majority of data accumulated so far strongly implicates CNS irradiation as a significant contributor to neuropsychological dysfunction.

Bamford *et al.* [60] using selected subtests of the Revised Stanford–Binet Scale and the patient's education record, evaluated 30 patients randomly selected from 64 long-term survivors of childhood brain tumors; 17 were noted to be below average in intelligence and academic achievement, four remained in normal classes but required special help, 11 were placed in special education classes and two were severely retarded. Among the etiological factors speculated upon, cranial irradiation was suspected to be a significant cause of the intellectual dysfunction seen in these patients. Hirsch *et al.* [56] sought to determine whether cranial irradiation (in addition to site of origin and presence of hydrocephalus at diagnosis) was a significant etiological factor by comparing medulloblastoma patients who received radiotherapy and cerebellar astrocytoma patients who were treated with surgery only. Of 28 medulloblastoma patients who received neuropsychological testing, only 11% achieved a full-scale IQ >90 compared with 62% of the astrocytoma patients who scored within the normal range. Of the irradiated patients 58% were found to have IQs between 70 and 90, and an additional 31% were profoundly affected with IQs <70. Academic achievement was also found to be severely affected, as only four of 16 school-age medulloblastoma children were keeping pace with their peers. In comparison, of 22 astrocytoma patients (no irradiation), 16 were maintaining reasonable academic levels of achievement. This study further suggested that while the surgical resection and location of the tumor (those with brainstem involvement were more severely affected) influenced the patients' cognitive abilities, irradiation played the primary role. Unfortunately, confounding the association of irradiation and IQ was the use of chemotherapy in a significant proportion of the medulloblastoma patients. Among the agents used, intrathecal methotrexate was administered to many of the patients. As noted previously, this agent has been implicated to potentiate the neurotoxic effect of CNS irradiation [1]. Notably, these patients did perform considerably worse than those in other studies who received radiation only.

Both Eiser [61] and Spunberg *et al.* [62] in their evaluations of neuropsychological sequelae of children with various brain tumors found significant proportions (30–78%) of the patients to have below average IQs. While neither study could discern an obvious etiological agent, Spunberg *et al.* did find that patients with poor prognosis tumors, who therefore received higher doses of irradiation, performed worse on neuropsychological tests. Of nine patients evaluated, four who received <4000 cGy of cranial irradiation had an IQ >70. Both patients who were irradiated with >5000 cGy had IQs below 55. However, due to the small size of the study, no significance could confidently be placed in these findings. Li, Winston and Gimbrere [59] did find a slight trend toward decreased function in irradiated patients. In that study, 13/30 (43%) irradiated brain tumor children were classified in Bloom's functional

categories (modified) III and IV, while only 11/72 (15%) unirradiated brain tumor patients had similar functional disabilities. Educational achievement was also found to be slightly worse among the irradiated brain tumor patients than among those treated with surgery alone.

Silverman *et al.* [63] were the first to employ a case-control approach in neuropsychological testing of pediatric brain tumor patients after cranial irradiation, using the patient's siblings as the control. Patients having had posterior fossa medulloblastomas were studied if they had no evidence of supratentorial disease, no supratentorial surgery, no chemotherapy and had received craniospinal irradiation. These strict inclusion criteria were employed to eliminate the variables which might have potentially confounded the neuropsychological effects of cranial irradiation. Nine of 13 long-term survivors were studied. All had received craniospinal irradiation (3500–4080 cGy) and posterior fossa boosts (total dosage: 4510–5460 cGy). Their ages ranged from 2.5 to 25 years (median: 7 years) at the time of irradiation with testing occurring 3–7.5 years later. Results of the testing (Wechsler, WRAT) showed that the patient group scored within the low-average to average range, while the sibling control group tested in the average to high-average range. Even more significant were the direct differences between each patient and his sibling. Patients had significant neuropsychological deficits in both mean full scale IQ ($-16.4$; $P<0.001$) and mean performance IQ ($-21.4$; $P<0.001$), as well as lower scores in mean verbal IQ ($-9.1$). Academic achievement (WRAT) was also lower in the patients, though significant deficits were seen only in the arithmetic subtest (mean deficit, 15.7). Cranial irradiation was implicated as the principle source of the neuropsychological sequelae in these patients. Interestingly, further evaluation revealed that these deficits were most pronounced in the younger patients (Figure 22.1). No dose effect could

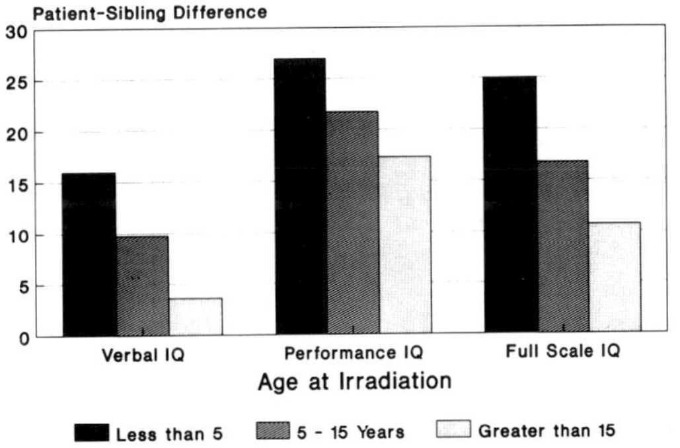


**Figure 22.1** Mean IQ differences between brain tumor patients and their siblings based upon age at time of irradiation

be discerned though the narrow range of dose and the small size of the study population did not allow for adequate assessment of this variable. Among the patients studied was an 18-year-old whose sibling was an identical twin. Although this patient was older at the time of treatment, deficits (none statistically significant) were found in both the Wechsler (PIQ, FSIQ) and the WRAT (arithmetic, reading, spelling) compared with the twin sibling.

A recent prospective study [64] examined newly diagnosed primary brain tumor patients at the following set intervals: (1) diagnosis (or within 1 month); (2) post-irradiation (3 months after the first test and 4 months after diagnosis); and (3) serial follow-ups every 6 months after the second test until 4 years after diagnosis. Forty-three patients were evaluated at least twice. They ranged in age at diagnosis from 10 months to 14 years 7 months (mean, 7.5 years). For the entire group ($n = 43$), mean IQ scores were 91 at diagnosis, 98 at the 4-month date, 91 1 year after diagnosis, and 90 at 2–4 years after diagnosis. Irradiation was either administered to the whole brain (2500–5760 cGy; median 4500) with 1000 cGy boosts to the tumor bed, or locally (4680–5580 cGy; median 5500), or not at all. Mean IQ changes from the first (at diagnosis) to the second (after irradiation) evaluation showed significant improvement in the patients receiving whole brain (88.5–93.4) and local irradiation (98.4–105.4), and an upward trend in those not irradiated (92.0–94.8). At the 4-month point, there was no significant IQ difference between the three different groups. However, subsequent testing revealed highly significant declines in IQ ($-12.7$) only in those receiving whole brain irradiation. Delayed drops in IQ have also been seen in several previous retrospective studies [60,63]. No decline in cognitive function was evident in the locally irradiated group or in the patients not irradiated. From this study it appears that whole brain irradiation is a significant contributor to neuropsychological dysfunction. Danoff *et al.* [65] also examined the effect of treatment volume (local versus whole brain versus whole CNS) on neurocognitive function. They found that among the 36 patients evaluated, mental retardation (IQ <69) occurred in six patients (17%), all of whom had received only local irradiation. Five of these six mentally retarded patients had cerebral astrocytomas. Several other studies have noted that patients with supratentorial tumors had worse prognoses for neuropsychological function than those with infratentorial tumors, supporting the importance of primary tumor site and treatment area in these long-term effects [59,66].

As noted above, the evaluation of neuropsychological function in survivors of childhood brain tumors is confounded by multiple potential etiological variables (Table 22.6). Ellenberg and associates [64] attempted to discern through multivariate analysis

**Table 22.6 Risk factors for neuropsychological sequelae in children with brain tumors**

Cranial or craniospinal irradiation
Increasing radiation dosage
Supratentorial location of primary tumor
Concurrent use of intrathecal methotrexate
Age ≤8 years at time of CNS irradiation
? Secondary hydrocephalus

the relative contribution of these different variables. Age, especially as it interacts with cranial irradiation, appears to be a principle prognostic factor for future neuropsychological function. When patients were grouped by age, only those younger than 7.5 years at the time of cranial irradiation experienced a significant decline in intellectual function [64]. Those receiving local irradiation or no irradiation had no change, and those older than 7.5 years who had received cranial irradiation had slight but statistically non-significant declines in IQ. Overall there was a highly age-dependent effect in those patients receiving craniospinal irradiation. Those patients aged under 5 years exhibited >20 point IQ declines, those between 6 and 8 years of age averaged 10 point IQ drops, while those older than 8 years had no evidence of intellectual deterioration. Bloom, Wallace and Henk [54] had earlier recognized this age-dependent effect and recommended a 10–20% reduction in radiation dosage for those under 3 years of age. Eiser [61] also found age differences when children were grouped into those under 5 years, those between 5 and 10 years, and those over 10 years. With each increasing age group, neuropsychological sequelae diminished in incidence and severity. This age-dependent variable has been seen in most other studies evaluating brain tumor patients [59,60,63,65,67].

The use of chemotherapy in conjunction with irradiation for brain tumors is a relatively new method of multimodality therapy. Therefore few studies have yet examined whether the patients receiving both modalities are at a greater risk for neuropsychological sequelae as seems to occur in ALL patients. The implications of the study by Hirsch *et al.* [56] indicating severe neuropsychological sequelae associated with cranial irradiation has been questioned as the cohort of patients studied included several who had received adjuvant chemotherapy. That study did report sequelae of a greater degree and in a higher percentage of patients (81% scored below an IQ of 90, and 31% were below 70) than have other similar studies which excluded patients treated with chemotherapy. Duffner, Cohen and Thomas [68] noted significant intellectual dysfunction in those patients who had received both modalities. Unfortunately, control patients receiving radiotherapy alone were not included in the study thus making it difficult to determine the effect of the chemotherapy. In both of these studies several subjects received methotrexate intravenously and/or intrathecally. Ellenberg *et al.* [64] examined 12 patients who received chemotherapy-containing regimens which did not include methotrexate or intrathecal drugs, and found no significant synergistic neuropsychological toxicity with cranial irradiation. The administration of chemotherapy alone, as previously noted, does not appear to have neuropsychological consequences in ALL patients [37]. In infants with medulloblastomas, a regimen of MOPP (nitrogen mustard, vincristine, procarbazine, prednisone) without cranial irradiation has not been found to contribute to neuropsychological deficits [69]. Other variables such as hydrocephalus, incomplete tumor resection and secondary complications have not been found to be significant factors associated with the development of these sequelae. It would thus appear that cranial irradiation contributes significantly to neuropsychological sequelae, and that this adverse effect may be amplified with the use of methotrexate.

As in ALL patients, significant proportions of long-term survivors appear to have cognitive deficits secondary to their curative therapy, more so than can be attributed to the primary neoplasm or its secondary effects. With the improving survival of children diagnosed with brain tumors, future therapeutic regimens must take these findings into consideration in order to minimize these late effects, while continuing to improve the probability of that patient's relapse-free survival.

# Areas of impairment and recommendations for educational intervention

For the physician, health care worker or teacher who will care for these long-term survivors of childhood ALL or brain tumors, it is critical that these problems be recognized and appropriate intervention be implemented. While deficits have been found in every cognitive area, impairment has most frequently been found in the non-verbal skills in both ALL [4] and brain tumor patients [63]

**Table 22.7 Areas of neuropsychological impairment in children after CNS irradiation**

Attention and concentration
Visual perception and integration
Non-verbal (spatial) memory
Mathematical skills
Abstract reasoning
Sequencing tasks
Perceptual organization
Quantitative skills
Verbal associative skills

(Table 22.7). As noted earlier, these skills have been evaluated in most studies with the performance subtests of the WISC-R, and by arithmetic academic achievement in the WRAT. In addition, memory tasks appear to be more significantly impaired if they are based upon visual-spatial abilities rather than verbal skills [9]. This impairment of visual-spatial skills has also been implicated as the etiology of difficulties in arithmetic achievement.

Tasks requiring freedom from distractibility are particularly difficult for the child surviving ALL or brain tumor therapy [70]. Peckham *et al.* [43] found that 83% of a group of children with ALL who were irradiated (2400 cGy) exhibited difficulties in attention and concentration which interfered with acquisition of skills and information. The selective deficits found in patients may thus be due to the preponderance of timed tests comprising the performance IQ as well as the arithmetic (a timed test) [4,46] and the information [4] subtests which, in part, make up the verbal IQ score. Poplack and Brouwers [71] noted that the apparent deficits in memory so often noted by investigators were also most likely secondary to attentional deficits. Attention deficit or distractibility has been correlated with CT scan abnormalities, specifically intracranial calcifications within the basal ganglia [46]. Before this association was known, Eiser [21] interestingly had found that this specificity of cognitive impairment (i.e. non-verbal) was consistent with a brain injury, rather than the psychosocial stresses of chronic illness which would be more global.

As these children return to the mainstream, it is clear that more must be done to ensure that they receive appropriate educational opportunities. A survey completed by teachers who had long-term survivors of ALL in their classrooms indicated that most (70%) needed more information regarding the child's illness, prognosis and late neurocognitive effects [72]. They were unsure of how much to expect of the children and indicated that they were more lenient with these children. Bamford *et al.* [60] noted earlier in brain tumor patients that without better understanding of the child's disease and/or immediate prognosis the teacher would be unwilling to 'insist upon reasonable academic effort, with unfortunate consequences for the child's career'. Not only do teachers require better education regarding the child's potential and level of tolerance [61], but so do the parents who may be overly protective of the child who survived cancer [60]. Not surprisingly, it has been found that those children who received active encouragement from their parents did much better in their academic performance [57].

Combined with these fears of encouraging appropriate effort among the ALL survivors is the fact that neuropsychological tests in schools have often underestimated the severity and true extent of the cognitive deficits. Meadows *et al.* [12] found that among 13 children who scored one standard deviation below normal in more than two WISC-R subtest scores, six had normal IQ scores. Similar insensitivity of screening procedures was seen in an earlier study of ALL survivors [73] where four of five children judged to be 'normal' were found to have abnormal neuropsychological function. Thus, as seen in other reports [57], despite significant focal deficits, screening tests looking for global IQ deficits or casual observations by parents and school teachers would have missed these children. As a result one finds a child who has a greater than expected learning disorder receiving little of the needed encouragement and education.

Early educational intervention is of great importance in these children. It is this type of child in which deficits of a small, but significant degree are found who can most benefit from early intervention. While it is always the wish of those involved to 'mainstream' the children, it has been argued that this may create a cycle of failure, frustration, depression and regression [57]. Programs aimed at the attainment of learning skills would be most helpful in this population. Teaching of these basic learning skills such as sequencing and organization of ideas [43] along with multimodal presentations of subjects (auditory, visual, kinesthetic) may also be of great benefit. Special training to attain attentional and concentrational skills [43] and better methods to overcome memory deficits are also of significant importance.

The ideal educational setting would provide learning aids to overcome the areas of deficit specific to each child. Areas of strength should be exploited to encourage academic achievement [57] and minimize the academic failures and subsequent frustrations that these children may experience while trying to overcome their cognitive problems. To date, no studies have reported the efficacy of such interventional programs for pediatric cancer survivors. Attempts to provide these children with programs designed to teach such skills are now under way in a few centers. In the meantime, detailed neuropsychological evaluation of these long-term survivors is greatly needed in order to identify focal cognitive deficits so that educational intervention may be focused to their needs. The ultimate goal is to provide a complete therapeutic program that includes both cure of the child's cancer and reattainment of their original quality of life.

## References


1. Bleyer, W.A. Central nervous system leukemia. In *The Leukemias* (ed. D.G. Poplack), *Pediatric Clinics of North America*, **35**, 789–814, W.B. Saunders, Philadelphia (1988)
2. Tubergen, D.G., Gilchrist, G.S., Sather, H.N. *et al.* Intrathecal methotrexate provides adequate central nervous system therapy in acute lymphoblastic leukemia patients with intermediate risk factors and an age less than ten years. *Proceedings of the American Society of Clinical Oncology*, **7**, 688 (1988)
3. Williams, J.M. and Davis, K.S. Central nervous system prophylactic treatment for childhood leukemia: neuropsychological outcome studies. *Cancer Treatment Reviews*, **13**, 113–127 (1986)
4. Fletcher, J.M. and Copeland, D.R. Neurobehavioral effects of central nervous system prophylactic treatment of cancer in children. *Journal of Clinical and Experimental Neuropsychology*, **10**, 455–538 (1988)
5. Jastak, J.F. and Jastak, S. *Wide Range Achievement Test*, revised edn, Jastak Assoc. Inc., Wilmington, Delaware (1978)
6. Wechsler, D. *Manual for the Wechsler Intelligence Scale for Children – Revised*, Psychological Corporation, New York (1974)
7. Soni, S.S., Marten, G.W., Pitner, S.E. *et al.* Effects of central nervous system irradiation on neuropsychologic functioning of children with acute lymphocytic leukemia. *New England Journal of Medicine*, **293**, 113–118 (1975)
8. Obetz, S.W., Smithson, W.A., Groover, R.V. *et al.* Neuropsychologic follow-up study of children with acute lymphocytic leukemia. *American Journal of Pediatric Hematology/Oncology*, **1**, 207–213 (1979)
9. Copeland, D.R., Fletcher, J.M., Pfefferbaum-Levine, B. *et al.* Neuropsychological sequelae of childhood cancer in long-term survivors. *Pediatrics*, **75**, 745–753 (1985)
10. Stehbens, J.A., Kolier, C.T. and Wilson, B.K. Achievement and intelligence test-retest performance in pediatric cancer patients at diagnosis and one year later. *Journal of Pediatric Psychology*, **8**, 47–56 (1983)
11. Eiser, C. and Lansdown, R. Retrospective study of intellectual development in children treated for acute lymphoblastic leukaemia. *Archives of Disease in Childhood*, **52**, 525–529 (1977)
12. Meadows, A.T., Gordon, J., Massari, D.J. *et al.* Declines in IQ score and cognitive dysfunctions in children with acute lymphocytic leukaemia treated with cranial irradiation. *Lancet*, **ii**, 1015–1018 (1981)
13. Moss, H.A., Nannis, E.D. and Poplack, D.G. The effects of prophylactic treatment of the central nervous system on the intellectual functioning of children with acute lymphocytic leukemia. *American Journal of Medicine*, **71**, 47–52 (1981)
14. Whitt, J.K., Wells, R.J., Lauria, M.M. *et al.* Cranial radiation in childhood acute lymphocytic leukemia. *American Journal of Diseases of Children*, **138**, 730–736 (1984)
15. Mulhern, R.K., Wasserman, A.L., Fairclough, D. and Ochs, J. Memory function in disease-free survivors of childhood acute lymphocytic leukemia given CNS prophylaxis with or without 1800 cGy cranial irradiation. *Journal of Clinical Oncology*, **6**, 315–320 (1988)
16. Eiser, C. Effects of chronic illness on intellectual

development – a comparison of normal children with those treated for childhood leukaemia and solid tumours. *Archives of Disease in Childhood*, **55**, 766–770 (1980)

17. Lansky, S.B., Cairns, G.F., Cairns, N.U. *et al.* Central nervous system prophylaxis: studies showing impairment in verbal skills and academic achievement. *American Journal of Pediatric Hematology/Oncology*, **6**, 183–190 (1984)

18. Stehbens, J.A. and Kisker, C.T. Intelligence and achievement testing in childhood cancer: three years post diagnosis. *Journal of Developmental and Behavioral Pediatrics*, **5**, 184–188 (1984)

19. Twaddle, V., Britton, P.G., Craft, A.C. *et al.* Intellectual function after treatment for leukaemia or solid tumours. *Archives of Disease in Childhood*, **58**, 949–952 (1983)

20. Harten, G., Stephani, U., Henze, G. *et al.* Slight impairment of psychomotor skills in children after treatment of acute lymphoblastic leukemia. *European Journal of Pediatrics*, **146**, 189–197 (1984)

21. Eiser, C. Intellectual abilities among survivors of childhood leukaemia as a function of CNS irradiation. *Archives of Disease in Childhood*, **53**, 391–395 (1978)

22. Pavlovsky, S., Castano, J., Leiguardo, R. *et al.* Neuropsychological study in patients with ALL. *American Journal of Pediatric Hematology/Oncology*, **5**, 79–86 (1983)

23. Pfefferbaum-Levine, B., Copeland, D.R., Fletcher, J.M. *et al.* Neuropsychological assessment of long-term survivors of childhood leukemia. *American Journal of Pediatric Hematology/Oncology*, **6**, 123–128 (1984)

24. Rowland, J.H., Glidewell, O.J., Sibley, R.F. *et al.* Effects of different forms of central nervous system prophylaxis on neuropsychologic function in childhood leukemia. *Journal of Clinical Oncology*, **2**, 1327–1335 (1984)

25. Tamaroff, M., Salwen, R., Miller, D.R. *et al.* Neuropsychologic sequelae in irradiated (1800 Rads (r) and 2400 r) and non-irradiated children with acute lymphoblastic leukemia (ALL). *Proceedings of American Society of Clinical Oncology*, **4**, 165 (1985)

26. Ochs, J., Parvey, L.S. and Mulhern, R. Prospective study of central nervous system changes in children with acute lymphoblastic leukemia receiving two different methods of central nervous system prophylaxis. *Neurotoxicology*, **7**, 217–226 (1986)

27. Williams, J.M., Ochs, J., Davis, K.S. *et al.* The subacute effects of CNS prophylaxis for acute lymphoblastic leukemia on neuropsychological performance: a comparison of four protocols. *Archives of Clinical Neuropsychology*, **1**, 183–192 (1986)

28. Brouwers, P., Riccardi, R., Fedio, P. and Poplack, D.G. Long-term neuropsychologic sequelae of childhood leukemia: correlation with CT brain scan abnormalities. *Journal of Pediatrics*, **106**, 723–728 (1985)

29. Meadows, A.T., Massari, D. and Obringer, A. Cognitive function in children after 1800 rad cranial irradiation (CRT) or periodic intrathecal methotrexate (IT MTX): a preliminary report. *Proceedings of the American Society of Clinical Oncology*, **3**, 71 (1984)

30. Trautman, P.D., Erickson, C., Shaffer, D. *et al.* Prediction of intellectual deficits in children with acute lymphoblastic leukemia. *Developmental and Behavioral Pediatrics*, **9**, 122–128 (1988)

31. Robison, L.L., Nesbit, Jr., M.E., Sather, H.N. *et al.* Factors associated with IQ scores in long-term survivors of childhood acute lymphoblastic leukemia. *American Journal of Pediatric Hematology/Oncology*, **6**, 115–120 (1984)

32. Mulhern, R.K., Ochs, J., Fairclough, D. *et al.* Intellectual and academic achievement status after CNS relapse: a retrospective analysis of 40 children treated for acute lymphoblastic leukemia. *Journal of Clinical Oncology*, **5**, 933–940 (1987)

33. Price, R.A. and Jamieson, P.A. The central nervous system in childhood leukemia. II. Subacute leukoencephalopathy. *Cancer*, **35**, 306–318 (1975)

34. McIntosh, S., Klatskin, E.H., O'Brien, R.T. *et al.* Chronic neurologic disturbance in childhood leukemia. *Cancer*, **37**, 853–857 (1976)

35. Fallovollita, J., Bleyer, A., Robison, L. *et al.* Intellectual dysfunction after cranial irradiation (CrRT) in young children with acute lymphoblastic leukemia (ALL): concurrent intrathecal methotrexate (IT MTX) is a contributing factor. *Proceedings of American Society of Clinical Oncology*, **6**, 257 (1987)

36. Balsom, B., Bleyer, A., Robison, L. *et al.* Cranial irradiation (CrRT) in young children: can intellectual deficits be prevented with pretreatment methotrexate (MTX)? *Proceedings of the American Society of Clinical Oncology*, **6**, 155 (1987)

37. Tamaroff, M., Miller, D.R., Murphy, M.L. *et al.* Immediate and long-term post therapy neuropsychological performance in children with acute lymphoblastic leukemia treated without central nervous system radiation. *Journal of Pediatrics*, **101**, 524–529 (1982)

38. Jannoun, L. (1983) Are cognitive and educational development affected by age at which prophylactic therapy is given in acute lymphoblastic leukaemia? *Archives of Disease in Childhood*, **58**, 953–958 (1983)

39. Jannoun, L. and Chessells, J.M. (1987) Long-term psychological effects of childhood leukemia and its treatment. *Pediatric Hematology and Oncology*, **4**, 293–308 (1987)

40. Carli, M., Perilongo, G., Laverda, A.M. *et al.* Risk factors in long-term sequelae of central nervous system prophylaxis in successfully treated children with acute lymphocytic leukemia. *Medical and Pediatric Oncology*, **13**, 334–340 (1985)

41. Ch'ien, L.T., Aur, R.J., Stanger, S. *et al.* Long-term neurological implications of somnolence syndrome in children with acute lymphocytic leukemia. *Annals of Neurology*, **8**, 273–277 (1980)

42. Berg, R.A., Ch'ien, L.R., Lancaster, W. *et al.* Neuropsychological sequelae of postradiation somno-

lence syndrome. *Journal of Developmental and Behavioral Pediatrics*, **4**, 103–107 (1983)

43. Peckham, V., Meadows, A.T., Bartel, N. and Marrero, O. Educational late effects in long-term survivors of childhood acute lymphocytic leukemia. *Pediatrics*, **81**, 127–133 (1988)

44. Bleyer, W.A. and Griffin, T.W. White matter necrosis, mineralizing microangiopathy, and intellectual abilities in survivors of childhood leukemia: associations with central nervous system irradiation and methotrexate therapy. In *Radiation Damage to the Nervous System* (eds H.A. Gilbert and A.R. Kagan), Raven Press, New York, p. 155 (1980)

45. Bleyer, W.A. Neurologic sequelae of methotrexate and ionizing radiation: a new classification. *Cancer Treatment Reports*, **65** (Suppl. 1), 89–98 (1981)

46. Brouwers, P., Riccardi, R., Poplack, D. and Fedio, P. Attentional deficits in long-term survivors of childhood acute lymphoblastic leukemia (ALL). *Journal of Clinical Neuropsychology*, **6**, 325–336 (1984)

47. Riccardi, R., Brouwers, P., Di Chiro, D. and Poplack, D. Abnormal computed tomography brain scans in children with acute lymphoblastic leukemia: serial long-term follow-up. *Journal of Clinical Oncology*, **3**, 12–18 (1985)

48. Hoover, D.L., Smith, L.E., Turner, S.J. *et al.* Ophthalmic evaluation of survivors of acute lymphoblastic leukemia. *Ophthalmology*, **95**, 151–155 (1988)

49. Thibadoux, G.M., Pereira, W.V., Hodges, J.M. and Aur, R.J. Effects of cranial radiation on hearing in children with acute lymphocytic leukemia. *Journal of Pediatrics*, **96**, 403–406 (1980)

50. Heukrodt, C., Powazek, M., Brown, W.S. *et al.* Electrophysiological signs of neurocognitive deficits in long-term leukemia survivors. *Journal of Pediatric Psychology*, **13**, 223–236 (1988)

51. Duffner, P.K., Cohen, M.E., Myers, M.H. and Heise, H.W. Survival of children with brain tumors: SEER program, 1973–1980. *Neurology*, **36**, 597–601 (1986)

52. Heideman, R.L., Packer, R.J., Albright, L.A. *et al.* Tumors of the central nervous system. In *Principles and Practice of Pediatric Oncology* (eds P.A. Pizzo and D.G. Poplack), J.B. Lippincott, Philadelphia, pp. 505–554 (1989)

53. Deutsch, M. Radiotherapy for primary brain tumors in very young children. *Cancer*, **50**, 2785–2789 (1982)

54. Bloom, H.J., Wallace, E.N. and Henk, J.M. The treatment and prognosis of medulloblastoma in children. *AJR*, **105**, 43–62 (1969)

55. Bouchard, J. and Peirce, C.B. Radiation therapy in management of neoplasms of central nervous system, with special note in regard to children: twenty years experience, 1939–1958. *American Journal of Roentgenology, Radiation Therapy and Nuclear Medicine*, **84**, 610–628 (1960)

56. Hirsch, J.F., Renier, D., Czernichow, P. *et al.* Medulloblastoma in childhood. Survival and functional results. *Acta Neurochirurgica*, **48**, 1–15 (1979)

57. LeBaron, S., Zeltzer, P.M., Zeltzer, L.K. *et al.* Assessment of quality of survival in children with medulloblastoma and cerebellar astrocytoma. *Cancer*, **62**, 1215–1222 (1988)

58. Smith, R.A., Lampe, I. and Kahn, P.A. The prognosis of medulloblastoma in children. *Journal of Neurosurgery*, **18**, 91–97 (1961)

59. Li, F.P., Winston, K.R. and Gimbrere, K. Follow-up of children with brain tumors. *Cancer*, **54**, 135–138 (1984)

60. Bamford, F.N., Jones, P.M., Pearson, D. *et al.* Residual disabilities in children treated for intracranial space-occupying lesions. *Cancer*, **37**, 1149–1151 (1976)

61. Eiser, C. Psychological sequelae of brain tumours in childhood: a retrospective study. *British Journal of Clinical Psychology*, **20**, 35–38 (1981)

62. Spunberg, J.J., Chang, C.H., Goldman, M. *et al.* Quality of long-term survival following irradiation for intracranial tumors in children under the age of two. *International Journal of Radiation Oncology, Biology, Physics*, **7**, 727–736 (1981)

63. Silverman, C.L., Palkes, H., Talent, B. *et al.* Late effects of radiotherapy on patients with cerebellar medulloblastoma. *Cancer*, **54**, 825–829 (1984)

64. Ellenberg, L., McComb, J.G., Siegel, S.E. and Stowe, S. Factors affecting intellectual outcome in pediatric brain tumor patients. *Neurosurgery*, **21**, 638–644 (1987)

65. Danoff, B.F., Cowchock, S., Marquette, C. *et al.* Assessment of the long-term effects of primary radiation therapy for brain tumors in children. *Cancer*, **49**, 1580–1586 (1982)

66. Kun, L.E., Mulhern, R.K. and Crisco, J.J. Quality of life in children treated for brain tumors – intellectual, emotional, and academic function. *Journal of Neurosurgery*, **58**, 1–6 (1983)

67. Mulhern, R.K. and Kun, L.E. Neuropsychologic function in children with brain tumors: III. Interval changes in the six months following treatment. *Medical and Pediatric Oncology*, **13**, 318–324 (1985)

68. Duffner, P.K., Cohen, M.E. and Thomas, P. Late effects of treatment on the intelligence of children with posterior fossa tumors. *Cancer*, **51**, 233–237 (1983)

69. Baram, T.Z., van Eys, J., Dowell, R.E. *et al.* Survival and neurologic outcome of infants with medulloblastoma treated with surgery and MOPP chemotherapy. *Cancer*, **60**, 173–177 (1987)

70. Goff, J., Anderson, H. and Cooper, P. Distractibility and memory deficits in long-term survivors of acute lymphoblastic leukemia. *Developmental and Behavioral Pediatrics*, **1**, 158–163 (1980)

71. Poplack, D.G. and Brouwers, P. Adverse sequelae of central nervous system therapy. In *Late Effects in Successfully Treated Children with Cancer* (ed. M.E. Nesbit Jr.), *Clinics in Oncology*, **4**, 263–283, W.B. Saunders, London (1985)

72. Eiser, C. How leukaemia affects a child's schooling. *British Journal of Social and Clinical Psychology*, **19**, 365–368 (1980)

73. Meadows, A.T. and Evans, A.E. Effects of chemotherapy on the central nervous system. *Cancer*, **37**, 1079–1085 (1976)

# 23

# Ocular morbidity in radiotherapy

**A.N. Harnett and J.L. Hungerford**

The eye and orbit are relatively uncommon sites for malignant tumours but these are by no means rare. Surgery and radiotherapy are the two most important forms of treatment for primary neoplasms in and around the eye and radiotherapy is usually the treatment of choice for secondary ocular and adnexal tumours.

The two commonest primary neoplasms of the eye are uveal malignant melanoma and retinoblastoma. Ocular melanomas usually arise in the choroid. Although these tumours were formerly treated exclusively by enucleation of the eye, smaller melanomas are now frequently excised locally from the choroid or treated by brachytherapy using radioactive scleral plaques. In this way the eye may often be preserved with useful vision. Larger melanomas may be treated by charged particle irradiation with protons or helium ions, though frequently with less satisfactory visual results. External beam radiotherapy is now the treatment of choice for preservation of the eye and of vision in the majority of retinoblastomas and the sight-preserving capabilities of radiotherapy are particularly important in one-third of cases in which the disease affects both eyes. In combination with chemotherapy, radiotherapy has virtually eliminated the need for surgical exenteration in orbital rhabdomyosarcoma and has allowed vision to be preserved in most cases. Orbital lymphomas are often of low grade and may be treated successfully and with minimum morbidity by radiotherapy alone.

The choroid is the most frequent site for secondary tumours in the orbital region, with carcinoma of the breast being far the commonest primary source. The posterior pole of the eye is a site of election for metastatic carcinoma and both eyes are often involved, with a serious threat to vision. These tumours are usually radiosensitive and vision can often be preserved by radiotherapy for the rest of the patient's life. Similarly good responses can be obtained from palliative radiotherapy of metastatic orbital deposits. Radiation therapy has been used successfully in the management of benign conjunctival conditions and of orbital disorders such as dysthyroid exophthalmos and indeterminate lesions referred to as pseudolymphoma or pseudotumour. It may have a role to play in the treatment of benign but sight-threatening haemangiomas of the choroid and retina.

The overall ocular morbidity of radiotherapy and chemotherapy depends on the combined sensitivities of the various anatomical constituents of the globe to radiation and chemical damage, on the dose of therapy required to destroy tumours of different histological types, on the size and number of tumours present, and on the location within the eye of intraocular tumours. The eye is composed of substructures with widely varying sensitivity, ranging from highly radiosensitive tissues such as the lens through structures of medium sensitivity such as the retina and choroid to highly radioresistant tissues like the cornea and sclera. Tumours vary in their radiosensitivity from highly sensitive neoplasms, e.g. retinoblastoma and lymphoma, to relatively radioresistant lesions such as melanoma. Intraocular tumours may present when only a few millimetres in diameter so that focal treatments are possible. Some, like retinoblastoma, may be multiple or they may be too close to the optic disc or macula or too large for safe focal therapy. In each instance a whole retina approach may offer both better local tumour control and a better visual result. The most appropriate treatment method is now chosen from the wide choice of whole orbit, eye or retina techniques or focal approaches available after appraisal of all the tumour characteristics outlined above. The eye and

**Table 23.1 Malignancies in which radiotherapy may be employed and where ocular morbidity may result**

| | |
|---|---|
| Acute leukaemia<br>  Cranial irradiation<br>  Total body irradiation | Paranasal sinuses<br>  Ethmoid<br>  Maxillary antrum<br>  Frontal |
| Skin<br>  Facial } e.g. basal cell and<br>  Scalp } squamous cell<br>         carcinomas |   Sphenoid<br><br>Nasopharynx<br><br>Nasal cavity and palate |
| CNS tumours<br>  Particularly frontal<br>  (astrocytomas,<br>  oligodendrogliomas) | Parotid<br><br>Middle ear |
| Pituitary and craniopharyngiomas | |

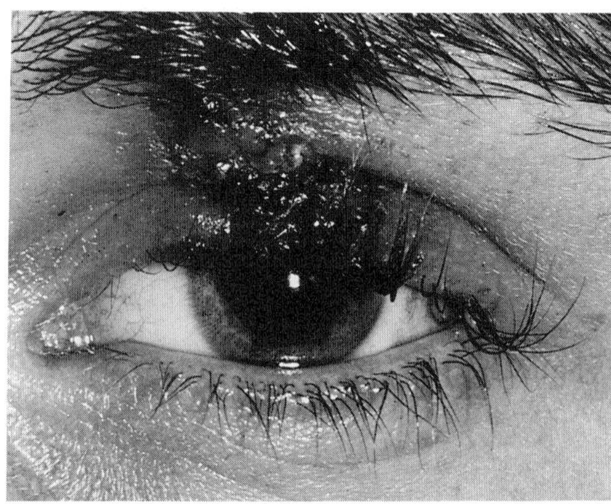

**Figure 23.1** Circumscribed erythema of the eyelid following proton beam radiotherapy for a choroidal melanoma

orbit may be included in the treatment volume when non-ocular malignancies are treated definitively or prophylactically. Significant ocular morbidity may stem from the treatment by radiotherapy of carcinomas of the nasopharynx and paranasal sinuses and from the treatment of common malignancies such as leukaemia. Table 23.1 lists the sites of malignant disease where radiotherapy may be employed with potential hazard to the eye.

# Acute effects of therapeutic irradiation

The complications which may arise as a result of ocular radiotherapy may be divided into acute and late effects. Acute effects occur early and are usually reversible, limiting long-term morbidity. Erythema of the skin initially appears after about 8 days from commencing treatment, depending on the field size, fractionation, and type of radiation (see Figure 23.1). This may be reduced or restricted by using megavoltage radiotherapy with its skin sparing effect due to build-up, although sometimes full skin dose is required. Obvious erythema is seen in the third week of a conventionally fractionated course of radiotherapy, and may progress to dry desquamation followed by moist desquamation. The skin changes settle within a few weeks of completion of treatment. Specific instructions to the patient undergoing radiation or the patient's parent are important in order to minimize skin reactions, and include avoidance of washing, scratching, trauma, friction from clothes, heat and sunlight, irritating drugs and placement of adhesive tapes. Depilation of the eyelashes, eyebrow and even scalp hair at the exit portal of the radiation beam (Figure 23.2) may be seen. When radiation therapy is given for basal cell

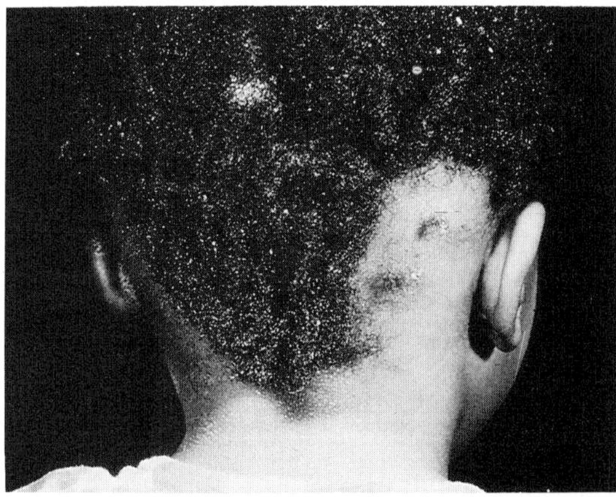

**Figure 23.2** Alopecia due to exit portal following external beam radiotherapy for retinoblastoma using an anterior field

carcinomas of the eyelid, or when the eye is included in the treatment volume for maxillary antrum, loss of eyelashes is usually permanent. Loss of eyebrow hair has even been recorded when a radioactive cobalt eye plaque has been used for the treatment of choroidal melanoma, and is usually associated with the more serious complication of lacrimal gland damage [1].

The acute conjunctival reaction includes hyperaemia, chemosis and an associated exudative watery discharge. There is an increased tendency for infection to occur, and when these symptoms

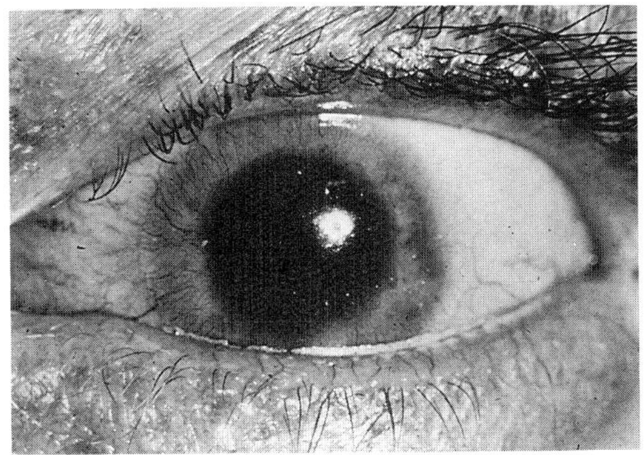

**Figure 23.3** Radiation-induced punctate epithelial keratitis

develop prophylaxis with antibiotics is recommended. Again, the reaction usually resolves quickly. Acute corneal toxicity presents with epithelial oedema leading to punctate epithelial keratopathy (Figure 23.3). Symptomatic relief of discomfort may be obtained from artificial tear drops. Perilimbal injection may be seen in association with mild kerato-uveitis which may be helped by topical steroids. As with the skin and conjunctival changes, the acute corneal toxicity quickly settles. No further acute effects are expressed in the remaining ocular tissues but they are not exempt from later morbidity.

Chronic effects are more serious and usually irreversible; they are responsible for visual complications. This category is discussed with respect to functional damage on the external eye and orbit, followed by an analysis on the direct effect on the eye itself. The emphasis is placed on why patients lose vision and how visual loss may be limited, rather than on a comprehensive list of the late effects of radiation therapy on each ocular tissue, which may already be found in the literature [1–6].

# Late effects of therapeutic irradiation

## The external eye and orbit

Thinning, atrophy, telangiectasis and pigmentary changes in the skin are late complications of radiotherapy which are well recognized and reported. However, it is loss of lid substance causing lid shrinkage and lagophthalmos, or lid deformity which may lead to serious morbidity. This may be combined with or compounded by deficiency in any of the tear film components, leading to loss of the film's stability with dry spots appearing on the corneal and conjunctival epithelium. Consideration should be given to:

1. Minimizing eyelid shrinkage.
2. Reducing keratinization of the lids.
3. Preserving the tear film.

### Eyelid

Following radiotherapy lid deformities may occur, especially if pre-existing lid abnormalities such as ectropion exist. If the tarsus is included in the radiation field, contraction can lead to a characteristic colobomatous lid deformity (Figure 23.4). Occasionally late lid necrosis may occur; this is usually

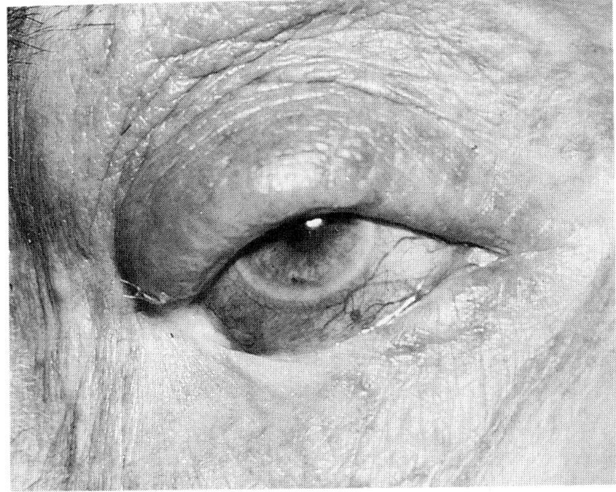

**Figure 23.4** Colobomatous lower eyelid defect following poorly fractionated radiotherapy for a basal cell carcinoma

related to extensive tumours involving the entire lid, sites of atrophic skin, previous injury or surgical treatment, or to large dose per fraction radiotherapy prescriptions. These problems may be lessened by the following recommendations:

1. Avoiding treating the whole eyelid when possible, and increasing fractionation when this is not possible.
2. Avoiding irradiating the more sensitive upper eyelid; otherwise increasing fractionation from 1–2 weeks treatment to 3–5 weeks treatment when this cannot be avoided.
3. Restricting direct exposure to the sun after recent radiation therapy.
4. Always increasing fractionation for basal/squamous cell carcinomas around the eye, compared with other facial sites.

Ideally there should be close collaboration with the ophthalmologist and radiation oncologist so that the most appropriate treatment may be instituted.

## Lacrimal apparatus

### Lacrimal glands

The maintenance of the tear film is dependent on both a normal production of tears and blinking, which will be affected by eyelid problems. Blinking prevents dry spots occurring, and maintains a continuous tear film on the ocular surface. This improves the optical properties of the cornea by smoothing surface irregularities. The tear film protects the epithelial cells and has an antimicrobial action. Most of the basal tear production is from the accessory or minor lacrimal glands which are mainly situated in the superior conjunctival fornix and upper lid. The major lacrimal duct can supplement this basal tear production, but is also responsible for reflex tear production. Doses of 30–40 Gy to the entire eye do not usually affect tear production, but when the dose to lacrimal tissue exceeds 50 Gy many patients develop dry eye syndrome and the prospects of maintaining vision are poor [5]. MacFaul and Bedford [1] reported damage to the lacrimal gland and ducts from cobalt plaque irradiation when placed anterior to the equator on the temporal side of the globe. This is due to radiation from the posterior surface of the plaque, which cannot be shielded as it emits high energy gamma rays. This problem of plaque therapy can be avoided by using shielded iodine-125 or ruthenium-106 plaques. When using external beam radiotherapy, efforts should be made to shield the major lacrimal gland, although this may preserve only the reflex tear production. However, it is often possible slightly to extend the shielding to include the lateral part of the upper eyelid and thus preserve function of the most significant area of accessory lacrimal tissue.

### Tear composition

The tear film is composed of three layers and a deficiency of any of the three tear film components may result in rapid break-up of the film, leading to a dry eye.

1. The deep layer consists of glycoprotein mucin which is provided by goblet cells of the conjunctiva. More recently the lacrimal gland has been shown to contribute to mucin production [7]. Mucin coats the relatively hydrophobic epithelial cell membranes and therefore allows spreading of the aqueous tears.
2. The middle aqueous layer emanates from the accessory and major lacrimal glands.

3. The superficial lipid layer is derived from meibomian glands, which are situated in the eyelids and are more numerous in the upper lid. This layer retards evaporation of the aqueous layer.

The importance of reducing the portal size or increasing shielding to protect the major lacrimal gland and part of the upper eyelid is apparent. Karp, Streeter and Cogan [8] have demonstrated histologically post-irradiation involutional atrophy of the meibomian glands of the eyelids in eight patients who underwent exenteration. Seven of the eight patients were reported to have received a dose between 45 and 69 Gy; no details of fractionation were given. Roth *et al.* [9] reported meibomian gland destruction with the resultant loss of the oily layer of the tear film when fast neutrons were employed. Of 93 eyes, 22 had permanent loss of meibomian gland function. However, Bessell *et al.* [10] supported the findings of Parson *et al.* [5] that patients receiving less than 30 Gy to the orbit did not develop disordered ocular lubrication. In this group of patients treated for ocular lymphoma, the incidence of disordered ocular lubrication was only 4.5% when 30–39 Gy was received.

### Dry eye syndrome and its management

When the entire eye and lacrimal tissues have been irradiated symptoms will vary depending on the dose received. Mild symptoms of discomfort, burning and foreign body sensation contrast with the severe dry eye syndrome of a red, painful, scratchy eye, which is photophobic secondary to corneal epithelial defects and sensitive to the drying effects of the wind. Over a period of months, vision may be lost due to corneal desiccation with scarring and opacification (Figure 23.5). The incidence of corneal ulceration may be greatly reduced by using

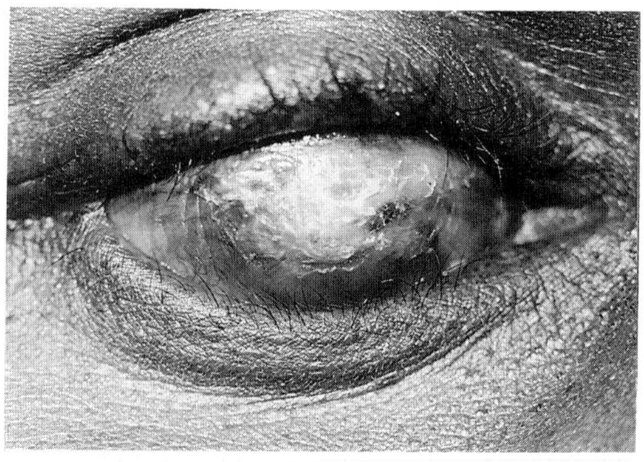

**Figure 23.5** Advanced corneal changes due to dryness and lid shrinkage following poorly fractionated radiotherapy for retinoblastoma

increased fractionated radiotherapy, and by employing central corneal shielding when possible. Should anterior segment complications develop, early and aggressive management is advised. Administration of artificial tears through the day and lubricating ointment such as liquid paraffin (Lacri-Lube) at night is very beneficial and is often sufficient to control mild or moderate dry eye symptoms. These measures will also reduce infection. Lateral tarsorrhaphy is seldom performed and rarely helpful; it should be considered when other management has failed. Similarly, protective spectacles are unhelpful. Enucleation or evisceration may be required for a painful, non-seeing eye.

### Lacrimal drainage system

MacFaul and Bedford [1] observed that occlusion of the canaliculus, sac and nasolacrimal duct commonly occurred when radiation was used for treatment of tumours situated near the inner canthus and the lacrimal sac. However, this was probably the result of poorly fractionated radiotherapy and less sophisticated techniques. Bessell *et al.* [6] record no such problems when using up to 50 Gy in 20 fractions over 4 weeks. In the series of Parsons *et al.* [5], high-dose irradiation only rarely led to nasolacrimal duct occlusion, unless it had been disrupted by tumour or prior surgery. Only one patient was recognized to develop epiphora secondary to obstruction of a previously normal nasolacrimal duct in the presence of normal puncta and canaliculi. Stenosis of the lacrimal puncta or canaliculi is more common following high-dose irradiation. Syringing of the lacrimal passages, insertion of a plastic tube to maintain patency and surgical treatment do not appear to be effective in prevention or treatment.

In summary, these complications are only seen after high-dose irradiation. Tumour involvement or previous surgery to the nasolacrimal drainage system increases the risk of occlusion. For tumours located near these structures, even when the tumours are very small such as a basal cell carcinoma at the inner canthus, employing increasingly fractionated radiotherapy is likely to prevent or minimize this complication.

### Conjunctiva and cornea

The importance of eyelid deformities and tear production including conjunctival secretions has already been discussed; a dry eye will cause corneal and conjunctival epithelial damage and consequent visual loss. The other serious late effects on these tissues are limited to high doses. Over 50 Gy, keratin plaques tend to form in damaged conjunctiva and, particularly when these arise on the tarsal

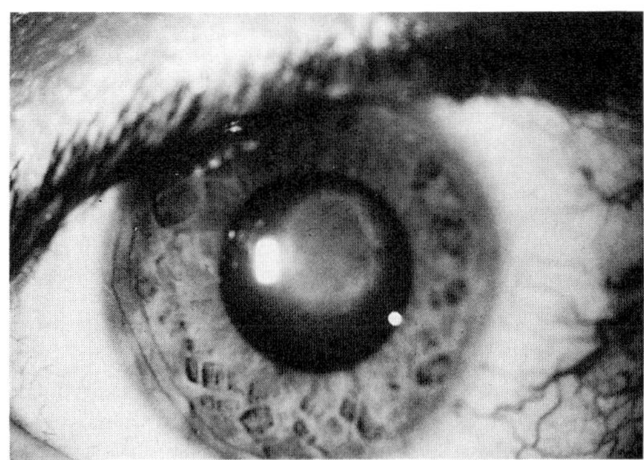

**Figure 23.6** Radiation-induced conjunctival telangiectasia in an eye which has also developed a radiation cataract

surface of the upper eyelid, they abrade the corneal epithelium and cause repeated ulceration. Conjunctival telangiectasia is more frequently seen, occurring at lower doses, and does not lead to problems apart from occasional bleeding (Figure 23.6). Similarly high doses affect the cornea causing epithelial keratitis and corneal hypoaesthesia. These problems are often exacerbated by lid deformities, reduced lacrimation, trichiasis, chemosis and conjunctival keratinization. Progressive corneal epithelial desquamation and ulceration may result. Such complications are difficult to manage, partly because they are often inter-related. It is therefore helpful to consider how they may be minimized at the initial treatment. As already outlined, corneal ulceration is greatly reduced by increasing fractionation, using corneal shielding, and prescribing artificial tears and lubricating ointment. Thinning of the sclera may follow the use of radioactive eye plaques but perforation never occurs and no treatment is required (Figure 23.7).

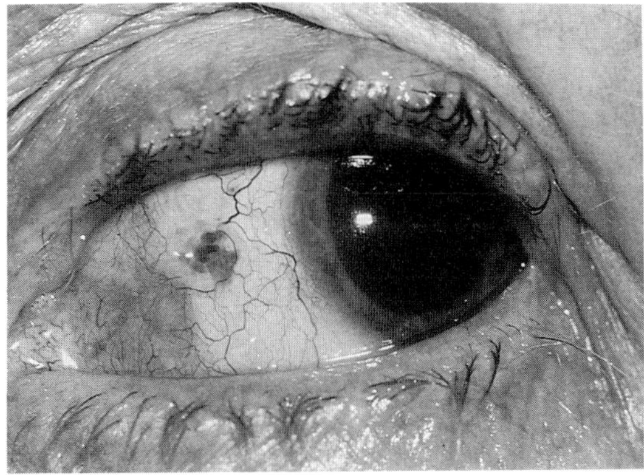

**Figure 23.7** Scleral thinning following cobalt-60 scleral plaque therapy for a ciliary body melanoma

## Orbit

Orbital radiotherapy in infancy may damage ossification centres. Retardation of the orbital bone growth is most marked in the very young. Infants treated for retinoblastoma are generally more seriously affected by this side effect than older children receiving radiotherapy for rhabdomyosarcoma. The characteristic reduction in middle facial

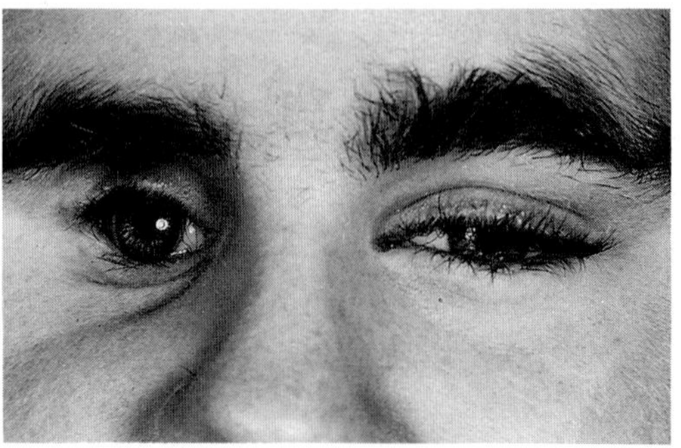

(a)

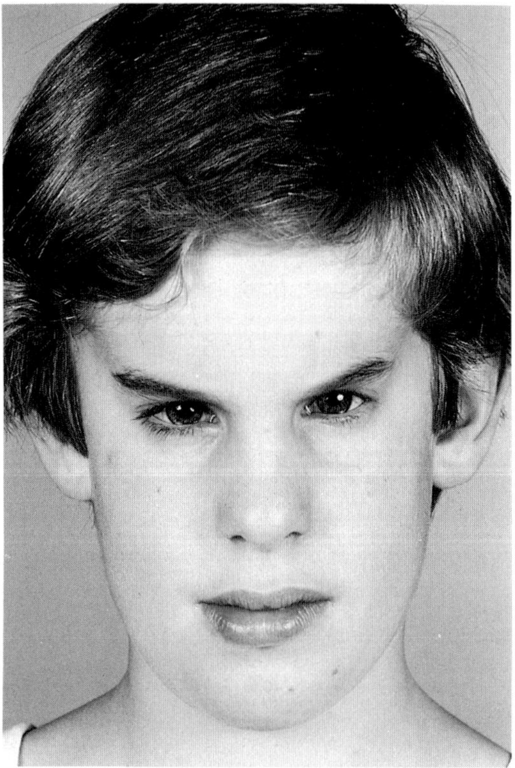

(b)

**Figure 23.8 a** Facial asymmetry following unilateral orbital radiotherapy for retinoblastoma in infancy; **b** symmetrical middle facial deformity following bilateral orbital radiotherapy for retinoblastoma in infancy

growth is more noticeable when treatment is unilateral (Figure 23.8a) than when it is bilateral as in many cases of retinoblastoma (Figure 23.8b). This effect may be reduced by employing megavoltage treatment with a linear accelerator, which has the advantages of the lack of differential absorption in bone compared with orthovoltage therapy, and the sharper beam profile with less penumbra being obtained with this machine. Lower doses and highly accurate small fields for retinoblastoma can be employed which will also reduce the severity of this complication [11].

## The globe

The previous section has laid particular emphasis on the serious complications to anterior ocular structures (including the eyelids, conjunctiva, cornea and nasolacrimal apparatus) which are often overlooked and yet responsible for visual loss. The vision-threatening direct effects on the eye itself will now be discussed. Cataracts, vitreous haemorrhage, retinal damage and optic atrophy are the most widely recognized causes of visual loss.

## Lens

The lens is the most radiation-sensitive ocular structure and cataract is the best known ocular complication of radiotherapy (Figure 23.6). However, the significance of cataract has been overstated compared with morbidity at other sites in the eye for the following reasons:

1. Initial estimates of the dose of radiation required to cause a cataract were too low.
2. Many lens opacities are not clinically significant and vision is not affected.
3. Cataracts affecting vision are eminently treatable by surgical extraction. However, there may be little point in performing cataract surgery if there is marked morbidity of the cornea and retina.

In their classic dosimetric studies Merriam and Focht [12] explored the relationship between radiation cataract and dose. Using a phantom, they analysed the results of radiotherapy in 173 patients treated for various clinical conditions. They found that the minimum cataractogenic dose for a single fraction was 2 Gy while for fractionated treatment of 3 weeks to 3 months a total of 4 Gy was necessary to produce a cataract. For doses over 11.5 Gy all patients developed cataracts irrespective of the fractionation employed. It was noted that the lower the lens dose, the longer was the time to the development of a cataract and the greater chance of it being stationary rather than progressive.

By contrast, Schipper, Tan and Van Peperzeel

[13] found that, in a fractionated course of radiotherapy for the treatment of retinoblastoma, the minimum cataractogenic dose was 8 Gy. This was twice as high as the 4 Gy reported by Merriam and Focht. There would appear to be considerable evidence for this higher figure. Merriam and Focht used an ionization chamber which had a greater diameter than the total thickness of the lens and performed their studies retrospectively, whereas Schipper's treatments were all performed prospectively on children with retinoblastoma who were being treated with a direct lateral field. In addition, after cranial irradiation, where the anterior margin of the field is close to the lens even under ideal conditions of patient immobilization and positioning, many cases of radiation cataract should have been seen and reported if the minimum cataractogenic dose is 4 Gy. This would be particularly so when using the older dose for cranial irradiation of 24 Gy rather than 18 Gy. However, most clinicians have been unable definitely to attribute the few lens opacities that are seen after cranial irradiation to the radiotherapy [14,15]. Harnett, Hirst and Plowman [16] achieved full documentation of dose through the eye, taking measurements at 0.5 mm intervals using thermoluminescent dosimeters. They concluded that doses to the lens appeared much higher than were originally appreciated and that a minimum cataractogenic dose of 4 Gy for a fractionated treatment must be an underestimate.

With the development and increasing use of total body irradiation, valuable information has been provided concerning cataract induction. Even with single doses of 10 Gy, a radiation cataract does not invariably occur. In this treatment, of course, no eye shielding can be used. In Seattle, 40% of patients developed cataracts at 2 years and 75% within 5 years [17]. A reduction in this complication can be achieved. Barrett, Nichols and Gibson [18] used the same dose (10 Gy), but the dose rate was much lower (0.02 Gy/min as opposed to 0.05–0.08 Gy/min in the Seattle series). They have seen a 20% incidence of cataract between 3 and 6 years after treatment. Similarly a sparing effect was achieved with a 20% incidence when total body irradiation was fractionated [19]. Bessell *et al.* [6] performed an ophthalmological review of a large series of patients receiving radiotherapy to the orbit for lymphoma. The mean lens dose was 15 Gy. A corneal shield was used with the anterior field in all patients unless there was evidence of tumour in the intraconal space immediately behind the globe which would have been underdosed if a corneal shield was used [10]. In some cases the lens received a much higher dose up to 45 Gy. Only 11 of 73 patients developed typical posterior subcapsular lens opacities, of which eight interfered with vision. None have been reported to have required cataract surgery.

The radiation-sensitive cells are found in the germinative zone in the pre-equational region of the anterior lens epithelium [20–22]. This is the only area of the lens that is undergoing significant mitotic activity. After a variable and considerable latent period, the degenerate or fragmented cells migrate or are pushed by remaining viable epithelial cells to the posterior part of the lens where a cataract may be formed. It may be stationary or progressive, and in the latter case diffuse cloudiness and eventual opacity of the entire irradiated region of the lens may occur. MacFaul and Bedford [1] were the first to categorize into four groups the clinical appearance of radiation-induced cataract and their relationship to the type of radiation therapy used.

## Radioactive eye plaques and cataract induction

Cataract induction is a recognized complication of cobalt-60 eye plaque radiotherapy [1]. It is more commonly seen in patients with relatively large melanomas involving the peripheral choroid or ciliary body [1,23]. Other types of radioactive eye plaques have been developed in an attempt to reduce complications. Foerster *et al.* [24] found no cataract formation in patients treated for choroidal melanoma with ruthenium-106/rhodium-106 beta ray plaques. After a mean scleral contact dose of 443 Gy, 10.8% of patients with a ciliary body melanoma developed a cataract because of the more anterior position of their tumour, the interval from radiation to cataract formation varying from 0.65 to 50 months in this group. Radiation cataract may occur many years after radiotherapy. It is interesting to note, therefore, that with a follow-up of up to 16 years, the long-term incidence of radiation cataract is no higher [25]. When iodine 125 plaques have been used radiation cataract has occurred more frequently than following ruthenium therapy [26].

## Management of radiation-induced cataracts

The management of radiation-induced cataract reducing vision may seem straightforward, as surgical extraction is the definitive treatment. However this is rather a simplistic approach, as even in surgically uncomplicated cases the late effects of radiation on other parts of the eye may prevent a good immediate visual result or lead to subsequent deterioration in vision. When planning radiotherapy, consideration should be given to ways of reducing lens dose [5,6,16,27–29]. Reducing the dose to the front of the eye will also pay dividends in minimizing complications to the anterior ocular tissues including the conjunctiva and cornea which would otherwise compound lens morbidity and make surgery more difficult and less likely to be successful. Corneal opacities may contraindicate lens extraction, particularly when the contralateral eye has normal vision. When choroidal melanoma is treated by radioactive eye plaques, there may be concern in operating on an eye which may contain viable tumour and operation should be postponed until no further shrinkage of the tumour can be detected. If lens opacity precludes an ophthalmoscopic view, follow-up should be by ultrasound.

Cataract surgery appears particularly unsuccessful after cobalt-60 plaque irradiation. Augsburger and Shields [30] found 13 of 287 treated eyes developed mature radiation cataracts, of which seven underwent cataract extraction. The visual acuity initially improved in six eyes, but this was not maintained and deterioration occurred several months later in every case. The investigators felt the results signified that the effects of cobalt-60 plaque therapy on the whole eye, particularly on the retina, are likely to be pronounced if the effects on the lens are sufficient to produce a mature radiation cataract. The use of other types of plaque (ruthenium-106 and iodine-125) may appear to reduce this morbidity but follow-up intervals have been shorter and late retinal effects may have been underestimated. Furthermore the older series included patients treated with large cobalt-60 plaques which are no longer recommended.

Correction of aphakia may be by spectacles, contact lenses or by an intraocular lens prosthesis. When only one eye has been treated and aphakia is unilateral, the optics of spectacles do not allow restoration of binocular vision. Binocularity may be re-established using contact lenses but many eyes are too dry after radiotherapy to tolerate this form of optical correction. As a result, many eyes which would otherwise see well are functionally useless. There are grounds for cautious use of intraocular lenses. Some eyes are subject to episodes of uveitis following radiotherapy and the risks of intraocular lens insertion are slightly greater than in otherwise healthy eyes. Nevertheless the functional benefit more than justifies their use in those who are unilaterally aphakic following radiotherapy.

### Retina, choroid and optic nerve

These structures are relatively radioresistant. Radiation retinopathy has not been documented in patients treated with doses up to 24 Gy for acute leukaemia [15]. Similarly, when ocular lymphoma has been treated by radiation therapy with doses up to 37.5 Gy [31] and up to 45 Gy [6], no radiation-induced retinopathy has been observed. Ten patients who had received a radiation dose of 25–30 Gy were investigated by fundus fluorescein angiography and no retinovascular changes were demonstrated [6]. With the trend to use more highly fractionated and lower doses of radiation in retinoblastoma, even although the ocular tissues in the very young are more sensitive, it appears that

chorioretinopathy will rarely be seen. Doses of 50–60 Gy for retinoblastoma often produced diffuse retinal changes but only one of 22 eyes had decreased vision due to radiation retinopathy [2]; two eyes of one patient developed apparent optic nerve ischaemia and one of those eyes received two courses of radiation. The investigators conclude that gratifying long-term visual results may be obtained even for many very large tumours. In a later report, Egbert *et al.* [32] performed a histopathological study of posterior ocular abnormalities after irradiation for retinoblastoma. Again, a high dose of 60 Gy external beam radiotherapy and slightly larger fractions than would now be recommended (2–2.5 Gy) were used. They observed frequent abnormalities of the retinal vessels, significant changes in the ciliary arteries and, less commonly, lesions in the central retinal artery. These changes could lead to visual loss due to central retinal artery occlusion, anterior ischaemic optic neuropathy or choroidal ischaemia.

Parsons *et al.* [5] described severe radiation retinopathy in 12 of 13 patients receiving 50–70 Gy over 5–9 weeks. Chronic radiation damage to these tissues is usually the result of disruptions in their vascular supply and is primarily a form of micro-occlusive vascular disease. After irradiation, vascular lumens are narrowed or obliterated and abnormal vascular permeability occurs. Nerve fibre layer infarcts, exudates and haemorrhages may occur. Macular exudates and oedema due to abnormal vascular permeability will result in decreased visual acuity. This form of retinopathy is now seen mainly in patients who have received radiotherapy for nasopharyngeal carcinomas (Figure 23.9). Elmassri

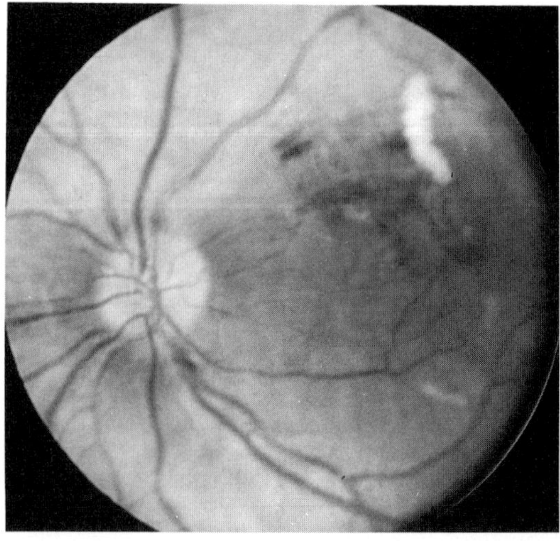

**Figure 23.9** Radiation retinopathy following treatment of a nasopharyngeal carcinoma

[33] emphasized the role of the choroid in radiation retinopathy and pointed out that some pale areas seen after plaque therapy for retinoblastoma are, in fact, infarcts of the choroidal lobule and not exudates. He endorsed the term radiation chorioretinopathy. Hayreh [34] demonstrated fluorescein leakage from telangiectatic vessels after treatment of choroidal melanoma by cobalt-60 plaques after very high scleral doses.

After doses of over 50 Gy, retinal pigment epithelial changes are seen which may extend to large areas of pigmentary mottling and extensive pigment epithelial atrophy. At ophthalmoscopic examination the sclera may be clearly visualized when there are large areas of chorioretinal thinning.

Anterior ischaemic optic neuropathy and posterior vascular occlusions in the optic nerve and chiasm lead to visual loss but are rarely seen at doses under 60 Gy. When radioactive eye plaques are positioned adjacent to the disc the high local doses employed cause vascular changes in the choroid and retina and associated retinal neuro-epithelial degeneration, resulting in optic atrophy (Figure 23.10). Augsburger and Shields [30] stressed that when cobalt-60 eye plaques produced mature radiation cataract, then associated retinal damage resulting in visual loss would be present. When ruthenium-106/rhodium-106 eye plaques were used, Foerster *et al.* [24] found a 10% incidence of radiation retinopathy to the retina outside the tumour site with an average of 700 Gy delivered to the scleral base of the tumour; with the doses employed all plaques produce local radiation retinopathy. Lommatzsch [35], however, reported that only 25.8% achieved good visual acuity after ruthenium plaque treatment, and 73 of 132 cases develo

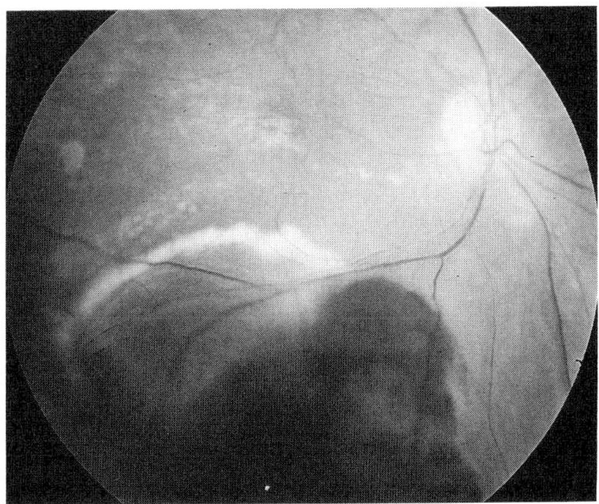

**Figure 23.11** Radiation maculopathy following iodine-125 plaque therapy for a paramacular choroidal melanoma

ped serious complications including macula degeneration, partial and/or complete atrophy of the optic nerve. The difference in this complication rate may be due to reduction in the scleral dose, or may be the result of the longer follow-up in the Lommatzsch series. Radiation retinopathy following plaque therapy is also dependent on the position within the eye of the treated tumour and the dose employed. Foerster *et al.* [24] found radiation retinopathy to be more frequent in tumours at the posterior pole (Figure 23.11). The more posterior the tumour and the higher the dose, the greater is the likelihood of retinopathy affecting the macula or of optic neuropathy. With a melanoma dose of up to 100 Gy to the tumour apex there will be a greater possibility of radiation damage to vision for a tumour in a given position than with a retinoblastoma dose of 40 Gy.

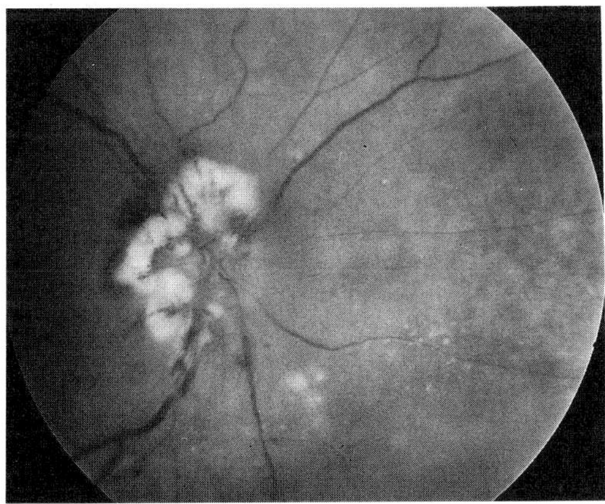

**Figure 23.10** Ischaemic optic neuropathy following ruthenium-106/rhodium-106 plaque therapy for a juxtapapillary choroidal melanoma

## Management of radiation choroidoretinopathy and optic neuropathy

The visual outcome in untreated radiation choroidoretinopathy is variable. The prognosis for vision depends on the location and extent of the areas of retinal capillary closure characteristic of this condition. When the degree of capillary closure is small, spontaneous improvement may occur with resolution of the microvascular abnormalities and of the leakage seen at diagnosis. This effect has been attributed to retinal vascular remodelling [36]. When capillary closure is extensive in the macular area, vision may be lost as a result of exudation from microvascular abnormalities or from ischaemic macular oedema. The former is amenable to treatment by laser photocoagulation [37,38], but treatment of the latter is not very effective in preserving visual function. When peripheral vascular closure is predominant, central vision may be threatened by neovascularization leading to vitreous haemorrhage. The aetiology of this process is probably identical with that leading to diabetic retinopathy in which hypoxic retina produces a vasoproliferative factor. Just as it does in diabetic retinal disease, rendering the hypoxic areas anoxic by panretinal photocoagulation frequently brings about regression of the new vessels and removes the threat of intraocular haemorrhage [39]. Radiation damage to the retinal pigment epithelium (RPE) may result in untreatable impairment of the function of the overlying photoreceptors. A further, though uncommon, side effect of extensive damage to this layer is impairment of bulk fluid transport across the retina leading to intractable serous retinal detachment. Acetazolamide has been shown to be effective in this situation following non-radiation-induced RPE damage but has yet to be assessed in radiation choroidoretinopathy.

Loss of vision following radiation damage to the optic nerve or chiasm results directly from ischaemic atrophy of nerve fibres rather than as an indirect consequence of exudation or neovascularization as in radiation choroidoretinopathy. Consequently, this side effect is not amenable to laser photocoagulation. Its incidence can be minimized by maintaining fraction sizes administered to the optic nerve or chiasm at or below 2 Gy. Attempts have been made to treat early ischaemic optic neuropathy by hyperbaric oxygen.

### Vitreous haemorrhage

Vitreous haemorrhage is a manifestation of retinal damage. Bleeding can result from fragile vasculature and neovascular tufts, leading to a haemorrhagic retinitis or a vitreous haemorrhage. An organized vitreous haemorrhage may produce a traction retinal detachment. Minimal bleeding will present as vitreous floaters; however, when vitreous haemorrhage occurs following radiotherapy, it is usually more severe and vision may be reduced to light perception only. Egbert *et al.* [2] examined visual results and ocular complications following radiotherapy for retinoblastoma. Vitreous haemorrhage occurred in seven eyes and only one eye was enucleated. The haemorrhages typically cleared spontaneously, and only one of the saved eyes had decreased vision due to remaining vitreous blood. It is of note that most children received a high dose of 50–60 Gy, so this complication is not unexpected.

Harnett [11] analysed a series of 193 eyes treated for retinoblastoma at St Bartholomew's and Moorfields Hospitals. The results obtained using different fractionation schedules were examined and a lower total dose was employed. Enucleation was performed for three eyes in the reduced fraction group (nine or ten fractions) due to vitreous haemorrhage, whereas no eyes were enucleated for treatment related complications in the 20-fraction group. Control by conservative treatment with the regime of 40 Gy in 20 fractions over 28 days achieved results equal in terms of local tumour control and vision to those reported by other centres using higher doses. Now 40–50 Gy conventionally fractionated radiotherapy is widely used for the management of retinoblastoma.

## Second primary tumours

The incidence of a new primary malignancy occurring after treatment with radiation, chemotherapy or with both for an ocular tumour is very small. It occurs many years after primary management, except in patients treated for retinoblastoma where the incidence is appreciably greater than would normally be expected. It is confined almost exclusively to the genetic form of the disease, which presents as bilateral involvement in about 85% of cases. One or more tumours other than retinoblastoma may occur in the orbit, head and neck or distant sites; even patients who have been treated surgically by enucleation, photocoagulation, cryosurgery and who have not received radiotherapy or chemotherapy are not exempt from developing second tumours.

Abramson, Ellsworth and Zimmerman [40] followed a large series of patients treated for bilateral retinoblastoma between 1922 and 1972 and found that 10% of 742 patients developed second non-ocular primary tumours, of which about 70% were osteogenic sarcomas (Figure 23.12). A later report [41] stated that there was a 15–20% chance of developing a second non-ocular neoplasm with an interval of 1–42 years after treatment of the ocular tumour, although data were not provided to support these figures. Francois *et al.* [42] added credibility to these statements, finding that approximately 15% of bilateral retinoblastoma cases developed osteosarcoma. It is of note that it was exceptional to see this second tumour in unilateral cases. Kitchin and Ellsworth [43] found 45 of 506 (nearly 9%) of retinoblastoma cases developed a second tumour within or outside the irradiated region after a latency period of 13 years on average. Only one of these second tumours was observed in a unilateral retinoblastoma and 23 of the tumours were osteogenic sarcomas. Osteosarcoma arising at a distance in the femur has been calculated to be 500 times more frequent than expected in retinoblastoma patients [40]. In a series of 22 patients with bilateral

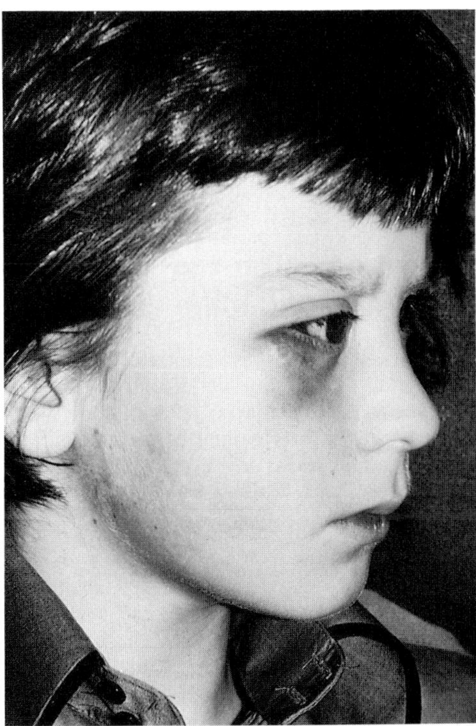

**Figure 23.12** Osteogenic sarcoma following orbital radiotherapy for retinoblastoma

retinoblastoma who did not receive any radiotherapy, three cases of second primary non ocular tumours have been documented [44]. When this is considered together with the significant increase in malignancy at sites which are distant from the irradiation, it is clear that hereditary retinoblastoma on its own merits and independent of treatment is associated with an increased incidence of malignancy. Further evidence has been provided by reports of an increased incidence of malignant tumours in members of families with genetically determined retinoblastoma, but who have not themselves expressed the gene by developing an ocular tumour [42,45].

It would be unreasonable to close the discussion at this point without considering whether radiation induction is an important aetiological factor in the development of second primary tumours. There are many reports of second tumours occurring within the radiation field and orbit or in adjacent tissues. Alberti *et al.* [46] reported ten patients developing tumours within the radiation field among 500 patients treated in Essen from 1960 to 1983. Most were soft tissue sarcomas. An even larger series by Draper, Sanders and Kingston [47] found 21 of 882

retinoblastoma survivors developing osteosarcomas, of which eight were sited within the field of radiation. There were also six cases of soft tissue sarcoma, two of which could possibly be attributed to radiation. Osteogenic sarcoma is a rare malignancy most frequently arising from the femur, tibia or humerus; fewer than 1% develop at the level of the cranium and less than 1% of cranial sarcomas develop in the orbit. It therefore cannot be a chance finding that osteosarcoma of the orbit is 1000 times greater in retinoblastoma survivors. Meadows *et al.* [48] reviewed 102 children treated in ten paediatric oncology centres and found 17 developed a second primary neoplasm, 11 of which occurred in a previously irradiated area.

Two papers have documented a total of four cases of orbital leiomyosarcoma, a rare ocular neoplasm occurring after radiotherapy for retinoblastoma [49,50]. Squamous cell carcinomas of the eyelids have been reported by Forrest [51] and Albert *et al.* [52] occurring 29 years and 62 years respectively after radiotherapy, although it is difficult to be dogmatic about the pathogenesis in this situation. Other eyelid tumours such as sebaceous cancer may occur many years after radiotherapy [51,53,54]. In the case described by Lemos, Santa Cruz and Baba [54], the patient was treated in 1958 with orthovoltage radiation.

There are several reports of malignancies arising in other adjacent tissues. Most tumours are sarcomas. Ferlito, Recher and Tamozzoli [55] report a fibrosarcoma of the mandible occurring after radiotherapy, but the case is complicated by the fact that the child received two courses of radiotherapy to the right eye in addition to chemotherapy which included an alkylating agent. Similarly, a patient who developed an orbital malignant fibrous histiocytoma was treated with two courses of radiotherapy and cyclophosphamide [56]. Nishizawa *et al.* [57] document a malignant fibrous histiocytoma of the maxilla that developed in a 20-year-old man who 19 years earlier had received irradiation.

It is now recognized that patients who carry the retinoblastoma gene, located within the *q*14 segment of the long arm of chromosome 13, are particularly sensitive to radiation and are more susceptible to develop a further malignancy within the irradiated tissue [58]. Weichselbaum and Little [59] pointed to the close proximity of the retinoblastoma gene to the gene controlling repair after radiation damage as offering explanation for the increased incidence of new tumours following radiation. However, it should be remembered that some series show the percentage of second primary tumours in retinoblastoma survivors to be the same, whether they have had radiotherapy or not [44].

Radiotherapy is the commonest conservative management for the treatment of retinoblastoma, and yet may be implicated in the development of second primary tumours. The issue has been complicated by many reports of post-radiation malignancies where treatment was given with unsophisticated and crude radiotherapy. In addition radiotherapy has been combined with chemotherapy using alkylating agents which are recognized as being particularly carcinogenic. Recently Meadows [60] clearly showed the important relationship between alkylating agents and the incidence of second malignant neoplasms in patients treated for a first malignancy during childhood. Examples have been given of patients receiving two or more courses of radiation who later developed second malignancies or who were treated with orthovoltage radiation. Indeed, in the case of orbital leiomyosarcoma described by Font, Jurco and Brechner [50], a dose of 160 Gy had been administered. When very large doses of X-ray radiation were used between 1930 and 1945, one-third of the retinoblastoma patients developed a second malignant tumour within the irradiated area [61]. Sagerman *et al.* [62] showed that the incidence of these tumours was directly linked with the dose administered, being greatly decreased when the total radiation dose was reduced from 80 to less than 45 Gy. A dose of 40 Gy conventionally fractionated at 2 Gy per day over 4 weeks is now recommended using a 4 or 6 MV linear accelerator. In patients who have limited disease at presentation, small fields measuring 3.2 cm × 2.8 cm at the isocentre can be used to treat the back of the eye and avoid the anterior chamber and spare the lens [29]. This will result in a lower integral dose and sharply defined field borders will reduce penumbra and thus the radiation dose to the surrounding tissues.

It is relevant that there are so few cases documented of second tumours occurring in unilateral retinoblastoma cases. Abramson, Ellsworth and Zimmerman [40] reported three cases, two with distant tumours and one who had a rhabdomyosarcoma of the temple. As 15% of the inherited form of retinoblastoma is unilateral, these cases could presumably be hereditary cases with germinal mutations. Some cases reported and referred to in the literature as second primary tumours [42,63] may now be recognized as ectopic intracranial retinoblastoma (or trilateral retinoblastoma).

### Recommendations

Taking into account the development of second primary tumours which occur in:

1. non-irradiated patients;
2. at distant sites;
3. in bilateral retinoblastoma; and
4. in unaffected family members of retinoblastoma patients;

and allowing for improved radiotherapy techniques and the elimination of alkylating agents when

possible, it seems likely that radiation will rarely be directly responsible for carcinogenesis. This adds support to the observation of Abramson, Ronner and Ellsworth [44] that whether receiving radiotherapy or not, the percentage of retinoblastoma survivors having a second primary tumour is the same.

# Complications after the management of benign disease

Occasionally radiotherapy is employed in the management of non-malignant conditions of the eye such as pterygia, dysthyroid exophthalmos and sight-threatening haemangiomas of the choroid and retina. The complications arising from the treatment of pterygia are not well recognized and clear recommendations on management are not available in the literature.

### Pterygium

Pterygium is a triangular fold of tissue which extends from the conjunctiva over the cornea. Although it is not a malignancy, radiotherapy may be employed in its management. It is fleshy and usually occurs on the nasal side. It most commonly affects people who spend most of their time outdoors, particularly farmers in sunny, dusty and windblown areas, and is thought to be an irritative phenomenon due to ultraviolet light. The pterygium may enlarge and encroach on the pupillary area and require surgical excision. Recurrence often follows with rates of over 60% being reported. If treatment is supplemented by local β-ray treatment, recurrence is reduced virtually to nil [64,65]. Beta-ray treatment using a strontium applicator has been used; there has been great variation in the doses employed, up to a total dose of 52 Gy [66]. Four patients in this series developed deep scleral ulceration and *Pseudonomas* endophthalmitis. These authors felt the sclera could not be considered to be resistant to radiation necrosis even after modest doses of β-irradiation [67]. Persistent bare sclera following pterygium treatment may require surgical intervention to prevent subsequent scleral ulceration and the risk of infection [68]. Sectorial lens opacities were seen in 19 eyes, and radiation-induced cataracts impairing vision in three eyes. However, β-irradiation-induced cataract is rarely seen with β of less than 30 Gy [69]. However, even with lower doses a thinned vascular area of conjunctiva surrounded by telangiectatic vessels may commonly be seen. Thus a more cautious attitude has been suggested. Tarr and Constable [66] recommended the use of lower doses of radiation so that complications would be reduced, even though this might be less effective in preventing recurrence. They inferred using a dose of less than 24 Gy. However, Talbot [65] reduced the dose to 10 Gy and over a maximum follow-up of 5 years there was no increase in recurrence rate and no serious complications.

We make the following recommendations:

1. Each fraction should be <8 Gy.
2. A total dose of 20 Gy should not be exceeded.

Persistent bare sclera should not be left but dealt with surgically.

# Ocular morbidity after treatment of malignancy at other sites

Ocular complications may occur as the result of radiotherapy for central nervous system (CNS) tumours, head and neck tumours and from the treatment of leukaemia. The malignancies which may be implicated are listed in Table 23.1. The acute and late effects of therapeutic irradiation arising from the treatment of skin tumours adjacent to the eye have already been discussed. Local lead masks or lead cut-outs may occasionally be needed to protect the eye when using superficial X-rays (usually <150 kV X-rays). Treatment of tumours arising in the parotid, middle ear, palate, nasal cavity and sinuses may lead to ocular problems unless careful attention is paid to immobilization and planning, using a combination of fields which both encompass the tumour volume and minimize radiation dose to the eye. Unless these tumours are locally very extensive at these sites, they may not lie immediately adjacent to the eye. Use of a single high energy electron field is simple and may avoid the possibility of ocular complications following the use of paired wedged megavoltage fields. When the latter treatment is employed, thermoluminescent dosimetry (TLD) measurements should be made over the eye to estimate the dose received and enforce changes in the prescription when necessary.

Three groups are particularly important with respect to ocular morbidity and will be discussed in greater detail:

1. Acute leukaemia is a common malignancy; many patients have been treated with cranial irradiation and increasingly total body irradiation is being used.
2. Nasopharynx and paranasal sinus tumours, although not common tumours in Caucasians, cause the most marked complications due to their close proximity to the eye and the high dose required to achieve cure.
3. CNS and pituitary tumours may be in close proximity to the eye and optic tract.

## Acute leukaemia

Cranial prophylactic irradiation is established as having an important part to play in reducing the incidence of leukaemic relapse. In addition to encompassing the cranial meninges, the posterior pole of the eye together with proximal optic nerve and its dural sheath are included in the radiotherapy treatment volume [27,70], and this may reduce the incidence of ocular relapse [71]. Solitary anterior chamber relapse is very rare [72]. Dose estimates in the lens [27] and dosimetric analysis through the eye in cranial irradiation [16] have been performed; the lens may receive approaching 40% of the prescribed dose with unsophisticated techniques. However, even using doses up to 24 Gy (18 Gy is now most frequently used), Weaver *et al.* [15] could not definitely attribute any ocular abnormalities to radiation and all patients had normal visual acuity; similar observations were reported by Elliott, Oakhill and Goodman [14].

Cataracts may occur after chemoradiotherapy and bone marrow transplantation; 40% of patients treated in Seattle developed cataracts after single fraction 10 Gy total body irradiation within 2 years of treatment, and 75% within 5 years [17]. The incidence is reduced to 20% when a fractionated regime is used [19]. Barrett, Nicholls and Gibson [18] reported a similar incidence (six of 30 children) using low dose rate single fraction treatment; only one child required surgery because of visual impairment.

## Nasopharynx and paranasal sinus tumours

The problems relating to ocular morbidity when treating tumours at these sites are due to their close proximity to the eye and the high doses employed in treatment. Not infrequently it is necessary to include one eye in the treatment volume. For example, when a maxillary antrum tumour has eroded through the orbital floor, the clinician is obliged to treat the eye within the radiation portals and it is difficult to shield any part of the eye. In the situation where the tumour is not so extensive, the eye may be protected by using a lead block. It is also important to consider the dose that the contralateral eye receives. Shukovsky and Fletcher [73] examined the retinal and optic nerve complications in patients with tumours of the ethmoid sinus and nasal cavity treated with irradiation. High doses of megavoltage irradiation were delivered to the retina and optic nerve. They documented macular and retinal degeneration, optic nerve atrophy, central artery thrombosis and blindness, and concluded that doses in excess of 6800 cGy in 6 weeks would result in the loss of sight in the treated eye within 2–5 years following radiotherapy. These patients were treated in the 1960s and with more sophisticated techniques and equipment, and with slightly lower doses now used (attempting not to exceed 60 Gy) these complications are reduced.

Later, in 1976, Chan and Shukovsky [74] reported the visual results of patients receiving approximately 60 Gy in 30 fractions in 6 weeks to the entire eye during radiotherapy for tumours of the nasal cavity and paranasal sinuses. Two-thirds of those treated had no clinical difficulty with eyesight or eye complications. Similarly patients receiving radiotherapy for nasopharyngeal tumours need careful attention in an effort to reduce and minimize ocular morbidity. The posterior aspect of the eye is often included in the treatment volume and radiation retinopathy will often be seen (Figure 23.9). Again, it is helpful to limit the dose to the eye to 60 Gy maximum, given in 2 Gy fraction sizes.

## CNS and pituitary tumours (including craniopharyngiomas)

The majority of patients who receive radiotherapy for CNS tumours have anaplastic astrocytomas or glioblastoma multiforme. Due to the latent interval for the expression of late effects, many patients do not survive long enough for their malignant glioma to enter the period of risk. However, with the high doses employed, doses to the ocular tissues and pathways must be considered and limited whenever possible. Full immobilization head shells should be used, and eye shielding using lead blocks may be required in the situation of frontal lobe neoplasms. Fraction sizes of under 2 Gy should be given. The late responses of the optic pathways are of particular importance in the radiotherapy of pituitary adenomas and craniopharyngiomas, both tumours which are compatible with prolonged survival or cure after treatment. Radiation damage to the optic chiasma may be one cause of visual loss which can lead to blindness. Both total dosage and fractionation are important where visual pathway damage is concerned. Harris and Levene [75] reported visual loss in five patients in a series of 55 treated for pituitary adenomas or craniopharyngiomas and found that, within their dosage range, no patient who received fractions of less than 2.5 Gy per day showed such visual loss. Similarly, Aristizabal, Caldwell and Arilla [76] found that radiation damage to the optic pathways occurred at doses above 46 Gy conventionally fractionated in only five of 122 patients. The usual radiation prescription recommended for pituitary tumours now is 45 Gy in 25 fractions in 35 days.

## Chemotherapy

There is only limited documentation of ocular morbidity due to chemotherapy. This may be attributed to the facts that:

1. Chemotherapy is used systemically and rarely locally, apart from steroids, in contrast to radiation therapy.
2. Other side effects and complications tend to be more severe and possibly life-threatening, thus distracting from ocular problems.
3. When ocular complications occur both chemotherapy and radiotherapy may have been employed, and it is then difficult to discern which has been the causative agent.

Many of the commonly used chemotherapeutic drugs may be found in the tears and cause symptoms. As more intensive regimes are employed, with marrow ablative chemotherapy regimens and total body irradiation, there may be an increase in ocular problems. Awareness and prompt management including routine review of such patients by an ophthalmologist will minimize complications. In general, however, chemotherapy rarely causes ocular morbidity.

## Accidental damage from chemotherapy

Most chemotherapeutic agents cause severe inflammation and pain if introduced into the eye. In the preparation and dispensing of these drugs, eye protection with plastic goggles should always be worn. When a cytotoxic drug is accidentally sprayed in the eye, it may cause a punctate keratitis. The anthracyclines (particularly doxorubicin) and vincristine are especially irritant. The eye should be washed immediately and thoroughly with water, topical chloramphenicol prescribed, and an eye patch worn until healing has occurred. Topical use of 5-fluorouracil for skin malignancies around the eye may also lead to ocular problems. Inflammation of the eyelids, circumorbital oedema, conjunctival irritation and corneal erosions may occur.

## Systemic chemotherapy

Chemotherapeutic programmes are likely to cause myelosuppression and, infrequently, this may be reflected in the eye. Thrombocytopenia may lead to vitreous haemorrhage (Figure 23.13) with sudden deterioration of vision and blindness. Rarely, neutropenia may lead to bacterial conjunctivitis or even endophthalmitis, a risk which is increased by local irradiation. However, many drugs when given systemically may cause a chemical conjunctivitis. This is most frequently recognized with methotrexate, even when used at low doses so that folinic acid rescue is not required. The symptom is relieved by prescribing folinic acid eye drops, commencing 24 h after administration of the methotrexate and continuing 6-hourly for up to 3 days. 5-Fluorouracil, particularly when given by infusion with the high doses employed, may cause increased lacrimation

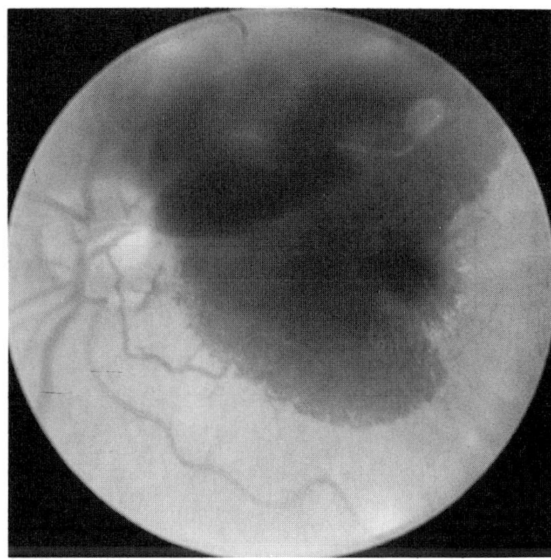

**Figure 23.13** Vitreous haemorrhage following
chemotherapy for leukaemia.

and conjunctivitis. Effectively, it produces lacrimal
gland irritation, leading to excessive lacrimation and
the appearance of the drug in the tears. Treatment
should be given with artificial eye drops and topical
steroids. Cessation or reduction in the chemotherapeutic drug may be required. The low grade
conjunctival irritation may be irreversible and lead
to further complications, including ectropion. Other
drugs that have been found in lacrimal secretions
include bleomycin and the anthracyclines, particularly epirubicin. The conjunctivitis which they produce is often associated with an oral mucositis. It is
important to exclude and treat fungal or viral
infection which may be present and exacerbate the
situation; otherwise, if the symptom is particularly
severe, a dose reduction will have to be made.

The vinca alkaloids (particularly vincristine) have
been reported to cause ptosis, cranial nerve palsies,
nystagmus, corneal hypoaesthesia, optic neuropathy
and transient cortical blindness. The eye complications have sometimes been the first manifestation of
vincristine neurotoxicity. Cisplatin is associated with
papilloedema, optic and retrobulbar neuritis and
cortical blindness. When these serious complications
occur, treatment with the drug has to be stopped.
Cyclophosphamide has been reported to cause
transient blurred vision. It is well established that
busulfan is associated with posterior subcapsular
cataracts. Chan and Shukovsky [74] reported a
series of patients with malignant tumours of the
nasal cavity and paranasal sinuses in whom the
entire eye was included in the treated tumour dose
volume. Ocular complications were much more
frequent in patients treated with 5-fluorouracil (5-

FU) in conjunction with high-dose radiotherapy
compared with those receiving identical megavoltage radiotherapy alone, whereas the survival for
the two groups was not improved by the combined
modality treatment. The radiotherapy and 5-FU
group had a 40% incidence of complete loss of
vision in the treated eye at 3 years, compared with
10% in the radiotherapy alone group. A clinically
significant cataract developed in 50% of those
receiving radiotherapy and 5-FU compared with
10% in the radiotherapy group. All patients receiving 5-FU developed a corneal lesion, compared with
under 20% for those receiving radiotherapy alone.
Just under 80% of patients receiving 5-FU had
chronic conjunctivitis compared with nearly 30% of
patients receiving radiotherapy alone. Although
visual, lens, corneal and conjunctival morbidity
were all increased with chemotherapy, there were
only 40 patients in the analysis and so the results
should be interpreted with some caution. However,
other clinicians have also noticed an increased risk
of injury following radiation in patients simultaneously receiving chemotherapy [5,77]. In Parsons'
analysis, only one severe radiation injury was
sustained below 50 Gy, and this occurred in a patient
who was also receiving chemotherapy.

Cataracts may occur after treatment with corticosteroids. Elliott, Oakhill and Goodman [14] examined 37 children who had completed treatment for
acute lymphoblastic leukaemia and found 12 had
posterior subcapsular lens opacities, none of which
were optically significant. Treatment had included
corticosteroids and cranial irradiation, but no dose
relationship with steroids was evident. Similarly, in
18 long-term survivors of acute leukaemia who had
not been irradiated, there was no dose relationship
shown when the total number of weeks of steroid
treatment varied from 4 to 106; all had normal eye
examination and no lens changes were observed
[15].

Treatment with steroids for periods of longer than
1 year and with a daily dose greater than 10 mg of
prednisolone are risk factors which have been shown
to be significant for the development of posterior
subcapsular cataracts [78]. This study was carried
out in patients with non-malignant disease; patients
with cancer rarely receive steroids for such long
periods. Increased intraocular pressure and
glaucoma may follow the topical administration of
corticosteroids.

## High-dose chemoradiotherapy

Frequent and serious ocular complications have
been documented following high-dose chemoradiotherapy and marrow transplantation [79].
Forty of 90 cases developed dry eye syndrome and
considerable relief was achieved with tear substi-
tutes, lubricants, occasional use of steroids, and

moisture chambers. Four patients contracted herpes zoster ophthalmitis and five herpes simplex keratitis, both responding to antiviral treatment. Trophic corneal ulcers were also observed, particularly in severe dry eye syndrome or severe systemic graft-versus-host disease (GVHD). Patients with fulminating GVHD complained of intense eye pain, photophobia and blurred vision. Examination revealed massive subconjunctival haemorrhages, sterile mucopurulent exudates, pseudomembrane formation and massive geographic denudement of the corneal epithelium, together with secondary herpes simplex infections of the lid and cornea. The dry eye syndrome invariably became severe and chronic in these patients. Patients who receive bone marrow transplants and total body irradiation have a high incidence of dry eye syndrome, viral keratitis and trophic disturbances of the cornea, and so should be reviewed by an ophthalmologist.

## Second tumours

It has been emphasized that retinoblastoma patients have a significantly increased incidence of developing second primary tumours and that chemotherapy, and particularly alkylating agents, increases the risk still further [60]. The most recent survival figure for retinoblastoma in Great Britain is 88% at 3 years [80]. Only 48 of the 431 children received chemotherapy and in this series it appears to have little influence on survival. Chemotherapy is recommended for high-risk patients including those with optic nerve involvement beyond the lamina cribrosa, particularly if the resected end is involved and if there is heavy choroidal involvement and in those with extrascleral extension, orbital recurrence, trilateral disease and metastatic involvement. In most centres alkylating agents are avoided, especially when chemotherapy is used as an adjuvant treatment.

## Hormonal therapy

Finally, hormonal treatment has been implicated in ocular morbidity. Optic neuritis has been described following treatment with the most commonly used hormonal medication, the anti-oestrogen tamoxifen. A reduction in visual acuity, retinopathy and corneal opacities have also been reported [81]. However, these complications are rarely seen and appear to be confined to patients treated with high doses (mean dose 240 mg/day) for a period exceeding 12–18 months [82]. It is exceptional to see any ocular complications in patients treated with up to 40 mg tamoxifen daily; this is the standard dose that has been used in many breast cancer patients, both as an adjuvant treatment and also for metastatic and locally advanced disease.

## Acknowledgements

We thank Miss L. MacMillan for typing the manuscript.

## References

1. MacFaul, P.A. and Bedford, M.A. Ocular complications after therapeutic irradiation. *British Journal of Ophthalmology*, **54**, 237–247 (1970)

2. Egbert, P.R., Donaldson, S.S., Moazed, K. and Rosenthal, A.R. Visual results and ocular complications following radiotherapy for retinoblastoma. *Archives of Ophthalmology*, **96**, 1826–1830 (1978)

3. Haik, B.G., Jereb, B., Abramson, D.H. and Ellsworth, R.M. Ophthalmic radiotherapy. In *Complications in Ophthalmic Surgery* (ed. N.T. Iliff), Churchill Livingstone, pp. 449–485 (1988)

4. Nakissa, N., Rubin, P., Strohl, R. and Keys, H. Ocular and orbital complications following radiation therapy of paranasal sinus malignancies and review of literature. *Cancer*, **51**, 980–986 (1983)

5. Parsons, J.T., Fitzgerald, C.R., Hood, C.I. *et al.* The effects of irradiation on the eye and optic nerve. *International Journal of Radiation Oncology, Biology, Physics*, **9**, 609–622 (1983)

6. Bessell, E.M., Henk, J.M., Whitelocke, R.A.F. and Wright, J.E. Ocular morbidity after radiotherapy of orbital and conjunctival lymphoma. *Eye*, **1**, 90–96 (1987)

7. Vaughan, D. and Asbury, T. Tears. In *General Ophthalmology*, Lange Medical Publications, Los Altos, California, pp. 53–57 (1977)

8. Karp, L.A., Streeter, B.W. and Cogan, D.G. Radiation-induced atrophy of the meibomian glands. *Archives of Ophthalmology*, **97**, 303–305 (1979)

9. Roth, J., Brown, N., Catterall, M. and Beal, A. Effects of fast neutrons on the eye. *British Journal of Ophthalmology*, **60**, 236–244 (1976)

10. Bessell, E.M., Henk, J.M., Wright, J.E. and Whitelocke, R.A.F. Orbital and conjunctival lymphoma treatment and prognosis. *Radiotherapy and Oncology*, **13**, 237–244 (1988)

11. Harnett, A.N. Ocular radiotherapy: a review of current management. *British Journal of Radiology*, **22**(Suppl.), 122–132 (1988)

12. Merriam, G.R. and Focht, E.F. A clinical study of radiation cataracts and the relationship to dose. *American Journal of Roentgenology*, **77**, 759–785 (1957)

13. Schipper, J., Tan, K.E.W.P. and Van Peperzeel, H.A. Treatment of retinoblastoma by precision megavoltage radiation therapy. *Radiotherapy and Oncology*, **3**, 117–132 (1985)

14. Elliott, A.J., Oakhill, A. and Goodman, S. Cataracts in childhood leukaemia. *British Journal of Ophthalmology*, **69**, 459–461 (1985)

15. Weaver, R.G., Chauvenet, A.R., Smith, T.J. and

Schwartz, A.C. Ophthalmic evaluation of long-term survivors of childhood – acute lymphoblastic leukaemia. *Cancer*, **58**, 963–968 (1986)

16. Harnett, A.N., Hirst, A. and Plowman, P.N. The eye in acute leukaemia. 1. Dosimetric analysis in cranial radiation prophylaxis. *Radiotherapy and Oncology*, **10**, 195–202 (1987)

17. Applebaum, F.R. and Thomas, E.D. Treatment of acute leukaemia in adults with chemoradiotherapy and bone marrow transplantation. *Cancer*, **55**, 2201–2209 (1987)

18. Barrett, A., Nicholls, J. and Gibson, B. Late effects of total body irradiation. *Radiotherapy and Oncology*, **9**, 131–135 (1987)

19. Deeg, H.J., Flournoy, N., Sullivan, K.M. *et al.* Cataracts after total body irradiation and marrow transplantation: a sparing effect of dose fractionation. *International Journal of Radiation Oncology, Biology, Physics*, **10**, 957–964 (1984)

20. Ham, W.T. Jr. Radiation cataract. *Archives of Ophthalmology*, **50**, 618–643 (1953)

21. Rubin, P. and Casarett, G.W. Organs of special sense: the eye and the ear. In *Clinical Radiation Pathology*, W.B. Saunders, Philadelphia, pp. 674–695 (1968)

22. International Commission of Radiological Protection. Non-stochastic effects of ionizing radiation. In *ICRP Publication 41*, **14**, 17–19, Pergamon Press, Oxford (1984)

23. Bedford, M.A. The use and abuse of cobalt plaques in the treatment of choroidal malignant melanomata. *Transactions of the Ophthalmology Society of the UK*, **93**, 139–143 (1973)

24. Foerster, M.H., Bornfeld, N., Schulz, U. *et al.* Complications of local beta irradiation of uveal melanomas. *Graefe's Archive for Clinical and Experimental Ophthalmology*, **224**, 336–340 (1986)

25. Lommatzsch, P.K. Beta-irradiation of choroidal melanoma with 106-Ru/106-Rh applicators: 16 years' experience. *Archives of Ophthalmology*, **101**, 713–717 (1983)

26. Rotman, M., Packer, S., Long, R. *et al.* Ophthalmic plaque irradiation of choroidal melanoma. In *Intraocular Tumours* (eds P.K. Lommatzsch and F.C. Blodi), Springer-Verlag, Berlin, pp. 341–346 (1983)

27. Kline, R.W., Gillin, M.T. and Kun, L.E. Cranial irradiation in acute leukaemia: dose estimate in the lens. *International Journal of Radiation Oncology, Biology, Physics*, **5**, 117–121 (1979)

28. Hancock, S.L. Anterior eye protection with orbital neoplasia. *International Journal of Radiation Oncology, Biology, Physics*, **12**, 123–130 (1986)

29. Harnett, A.N., Hungerford, J.L., Lambert, G.D. *et al.* Improved external beam radiotherapy for the treatment of retinoblastoma. *British Journal of Radiology*, **60**, 753–760 (1987)

30. Augsburger, J.J. and Shields, J.A. Cataract surgery following cobalt-60 plaque radiotherapy for posterior uveal malignant melanoma. *Ophthalmology*, **92**, 815–822 (1985)

31. Jereb, B., Lee, H., Jakobiec, F.A. and Kutchev, J. Radiation therapy of conjunctival and orbital lymphoid tumours. *International Journal of Radiation Oncology, Biology, Physics*, **10**, 1013–1019 (1984)

32. Egbert, P.R., Fajardo, L.F., Donaldson, S.S. and Moazed, K. Posterior ocular abnormalities after irradiation for retinoblastoma: a histopathological study. *British Journal of Ophthalmology*, **64**, 660–665 (1980)

33. Elmassri, A. Radiation chorioretinopathy. *British Journal of Ophthalmology*, **70**, 326–329 (1986)

34. Hayreh, S.S. Post-radiation retinopathy. A fluorescence fundus angiographic study. *British Journal of Ophthalmology*, **54**, 705–714 (1970)

35. Lommatzsch, P.K. Beta irradiation with Ru-106/Rh-106. Applicators of choroidal melanomas: sixteen years' experience. In *Intraocular Tumours* (eds P.K. Lommatzsch and F.C. Blodi), Springer-Verlag, Berlin, pp. 355–363 (1983)

36. Noble, K.G. and Kupersmith, M.J. Retinal vascular remodelling in radiation retinopathy. *British Journal of Ophthalmology*, **68**, 475–478 (1984)

37. Chee, P.H.Y. Radiation retinopathy. *American Journal of Ophthalmology*, **66**, 860–865 (1968)

38. Gass, J.D.M. A fluorescein angiographic study of macular dysfunction secondary to retinal vascular disease. *Archives of Ophthalmology*, **80**, 606–617 (1968)

39. Ray Chaudhuri, P., Austin, D.J. and Rosenthal, A.R. Treatment of radiation retinopathy. *British Journal of Ophthalmology*, **65**, 623–625 (1981)

40. Abramson, D.H., Ellsworth, R.M. and Zimmerman, L.E. Non-ocular cancer in retinoblastoma survivors. *Ophthalmology Transactions*, **81**, 454–457 (1976)

41. Abramson, D.H., Ellsworth, R.M. and Kitchin, F.D. Osteogenic sarcoma of the humerus after cobalt plaque treatment for retinoblastoma. *American Journal of Ophthalmology*, **90**, 374–376 (1980)

42. Francois, J., De Sutter, E., Coppieters, R. and De Bie, S. Late extraocular tumours in retinoblastoma survivors. *Ophthalmologica*, **181**, 93–99 (1980)

43. Kitchin, D. and Ellsworth, R.M. Pleiotrophic effects of the gene for retinoblastoma. *Journal of Medical Genetics*, **11**, 244–246 (1974)

44. Abramson, D.H., Ronner, H.J. and Ellsworth, R.M. Second tumours in non-irradiated bilateral retinoblastoma. *American Journal of Ophthalmology*, **87**, 624–627 (1979)

45. Gordon, H. Family studies in retinoblastoma. In *Medical Genetics Today* (ed. D. Bergsma), John Hopkins Press, Baltimore, pp. 185–190 (1974)

46. Alberti, W., Hopping, W., Havers, W. *et al.* Non-ocular malignancies in retinoblastoma: analysis of 500 patients (abstract). *Proceedings of the 3rd Annual Meeting of the European Society for Therapeutic Radiology and Oncology*, p. 252 (1984)

47. Draper, G.J., Sanders, B.M. and Kingston, J.E. Second primary neoplasms in patients with retinoblastoma. *British Journal of Cancer*, **53**, 661–671 (1986)

48. Meadows, A.T., D'Angio, G.J., Mike, V. *et al.*

Patterns of second malignant neoplasms in children. *Cancer*, **40**, 1903–1911 (1977)

49. Folberg, R., Cleasby, G., Flanagan, J.A. *et al.* Orbital leiomyosarcoma after radiation therapy for bilateral retinoblastoma. *Archives of Ophthalmology*, **101**, 1562–1565 (1983)

50. Font, R.L., Jurco, S. and Brechner, R.J. Post-radiation leiomyosarcoma of the orbit complicating bilateral retinoblastoma. *Archives of Ophthalmology*, **101**, 1557–1561 (1983)

51. Forrest, A.N. Tumours following radiation about the eye. *Transactions of the American Academy of Ophthalmology and Otolaryngology*, **65**, 694–717 (1960)

52. Albert, D.M., Charles, N.J., McGhee, C.N. *et al.* Development of additional primary tumours after 62 years in the first patient with retinoblastoma cured by radiation therapy. *American Journal of Ophthalmology*, **97**, 189–196 (1984)

53. Boniuk, M. and Zimmerman, L.E. Sebaceous carcinoma of the eyelid, eyebrow, caruncle and orbit. *Transactions of the American Academy of Ophthalmology and Otolaryngology*, **72**, 619–642 (1968)

54. Lemos, L.B., Santa Cruz, D.J. and Baba, N. Sebaceous carcinoma of the eyelid following radiation therapy. *American Journal of Surgical Pathology*, **2**, 305–311 (1978)

55. Ferlito, A., Recher, G. and Tamazzoli, L. Radiation-induced fibrosarcoma of the mandible following treatment for bilateral retinoblastoma. *Journal of Laryngology and Otology*, **93**, 1015–1020 (1979)

56. Tewfik, H.H., Tewfik, F.A. and Latourette, H.B. Post-irradiation malignant fibrous histiocytoma. *Journal of Surgical Oncology*, **16**, 199–202 (1981)

57. Nishizawa, S., Hayashida, T., Horiguchi, S. *et al.* Malignant fibrous histiocytoma of maxilla following radiotherapy for bilateral retinoblastoma. *Journal of Laryngology and Otology*, **99**, 501–504 (1985)

58. Coia, L.R., Frazekas, J.T. and Kramer, S. Post-irradiation sarcoma of the head and neck. *Cancer*, **46**, 1982–1985 (1980)

59. Weichselbaum, R.R. and Little, J.B. Familial retinoblastoma and ataxia telangiectasia. *Cancer*, **45**, 775–779 (1980)

60. Meadows, A.T. Risk factors for second malignant neoplasms: report from the late effects study group. *Bulletin of Cancer*, **75**, 125–130 (1988)

61. Editorial. The changing pattern of retinoblastoma. *Lancet*, **ii**, 1016–1017 (1971)

62. Sagerman, R.H., Cassidy, J.R., Tretter, P. and Ellsworth, R.M. Radiation-induced neoplasia following external beam therapy for children with retinoblastoma. *American Journal of Roentgenology, Radium Therapy and Nuclear Medicine*, **105**, 529–535 (1968)

63. Jakobiec, F.A., Tso, M.O.M., Zimmerman, L.E. and Danis, P. Retinoblastoma and intracranial malignancy. *Cancer*, **39**, 2048–2058 (1977)

64. Ozarda, A.T. Evaluation of post-excisional strontium-90 beta ray therapy for pterygium. *Southern Medical Journal*, **70**, 1304 (1977)

65. Talbot, A.N. Complications of beta ray treatment of pterygium. *Transactions of the Ophthalmological Society of New Zealand*, **31**, 62–63 (1979)

66. Tarr, K.H. and Constable, I.J. Late complications of pterygium treatment. *British Journal of Ophthalmology*, **64**, 496–505 (1980)

67. Tarr, K.H. and Constable, I.J. *Pseudomonas* endophthalmitis associated with scleral necrosis. *British Journal of Ophthalmology*, **64**, 676–679 (1980)

68. Tarr, K.H. and Constable, I.J. Radiation damage after pterygium treatment. *Australian Journal of Ophthalmology*, **9**, 97–101 (1981)

69. Hilgers, J.H.C. Strontium-90 β-irradiation cataractogenicity and pterygium recurrence. *Archives of Ophthalmology*, **76**, 329–333 (1966)

70. Bremner, M.H. and Wright, J. Ocular leukaemia in acute lymphoblastic leukaemia of childhood. *Australian Journal of Ophthalmology*, **10**, 255–262 (1982)

71. Ridgway, E.W., Jaffe, N. and Walton, D.S. Leukaemic ophthalmopathy in children. *Cancer*, **38**, 1744–1749 (1976)

72. Harnett, A.N. and Plowman, P.N. The eye in leukaemia. 2. The management of solitary anterior chamber relapse. *Radiotherapy and Oncology*, **10**, 203–207 (1987)

73. Shukovsky, L. and Fletcher, G.H. Retinal and optic nerve complications in a high dose irradiation technique of ethmoid sinus and nasal cavity. *Radiology*, **104**, 629–634 (1972)

74. Chan, R.C. and Shukovsky, L.J. Effects of irradiation on the eye. *Radiology*, **120**, 673–675 (1976)

75. Harris, J.R. and Levene, M.B. Visual complications following irradiation for pituitary adenomas and craniopharyngiomas. *Radiology*, **120**, 167–171 (1976)

76. Aristizabal, S., Caldwell, N.L. and Arilla, J. The relationship of time-dose fractionation factors to complications in the treatment of pituitary tumours by irradiation. *International Journal of Radiation Oncology, Biology, Physics*, **2**, 667–673 (1977)

77. Griffin, J.D. and Garnick, M.B. Eye toxicity of cancer chemotherapy: a review of the literature. *Cancer*, **48**, 1539–1549 (1981)

78. Spaeth, G.L. and Von Sallmann, L. Corticosteroids and cataracts. *International Ophthalmology*, **6**, 915 (1966)

79. Jack, M.K. and Hicks, J.D. Ocular complications in high-dose chemoradiotherapy and marrow transplantation. *Annals of Ophthalmology*, **13**, 709–711 (1981)

80. Sanders, B.M., Draper, G.J. and Kingston, J.E. Retinoblastoma in Great Britain 1969–80: incidence, treatment and survival. *British Journal of Ophthalmology*, **72**, 576–583 (1988)

81. Fraunfelder, F.T. *Drug Induced Ocular Side Effects and Drug Interactions*, 3rd edn, Lea and Febiger, Philadelphia and London, pp. 384–408 (1989)

82. Kaiser-Kupfer, M.I. and Lippman, M.E. Tamoxifen retinopathy. *Cancer Treatment Reports*, **62**, 315 (1978)

# 24

# Bone marrow morbidity of chemotherapy

**A.L. Jones and J.L. Millar**

Cytotoxic drugs are not tumour-specific and therefore exert different toxicities related to their effects on normal cells. However cancer cells are proliferative cells, like normal self-renewing cells and therefore are sensitive to antiproliferative drugs. There needs to be a therapeutic ratio between tumour and normal tissue cytotoxicity which can be exploited in treatment. Rapidly dividing cells, especially those of the bone marrow and gastrointestinal tract, are commonly affected by chemotherapy and bone marrow suppression is the dose-limiting factor for many drugs [1]. Tumour cells frequently develop resistance to cytotoxic drugs during treatment but normal haemopoietic cells in the bone marrow do not become resistant, therefore bone marrow toxicity can persist throughout treatment. Cumulative marrow morbidity results in more severe and prolonged toxicity with successive cycles of chemotherapy. Although acute myelosuppression usually resolves within a few weeks, some drugs cause a more delayed pattern of toxicity. These differences are important in drug scheduling to avoid irreversible myelosuppression which could prove fatal. Some drugs cause latent damage to the bone marrow but this may not become apparent clinically until months or years later.

To understand the effects of drugs on haemopoiesis it is necessary to examine the structure of the bone marrow and the hierarchy of cell development within it. A scheme of haemopoiesis is shown in Figure 24.1. The most ancestral haemopoietic cells are the stem cells which comprise less than 1% of total nucleated marrow cells. Most cytotoxic drugs affect stem cells through a variety of mechanisms and the resultant morbidity depends on the characteristics of damage to the stem cell population. Stem cells are not morphologically recognizable in man, but animal data suggest they resemble small lym-

phocytes [2]. Stem cells are unique because of their capacity for self-renewal [3] thereby maintaining the stem cell population throughout life. The stem cell population is heterogeneous and more mature stem cells have a lower capacity for self-renewal [4,5], but these cells are pluripotent and differentiate to the committed precursor cells of all haemopoietic lineages. Other cells found in bone marrow such as osteoclasts [6] and mast cells [7] are also derived from haemopoietic stem cells.

In mice the presence of stem cells can be demonstrated *in vivo*. After total body irradiation (TBI) mice become pancytopenic due to marrow failure. Haemopoietic stem cells, present in donor mouse marrow, will form discrete colonies in the spleens of irradiated recipients 7–13 days after intravenous injection of the marrow [8]. These are called colony forming units of the spleen (CFUs) and each is derived from a single stem cell. Although containing haemopoietic cells of mainly one lineage, each spleen colony is capable of forming colonies composed of haemopoietic cells of all lineages. These colonies can restore haemopoiesis in the irradiated mice. There is no equivalent assay for human stem cells. Self-renewal of stem cells in mice can be demonstrated by serial transplantation of CFUs into irradiated recipients. However, there is a decline in colony forming ability of bone marrow cells subjected to serial transplantation [9]. This demonstrates that the capacity for self-renewal is not infinite. Damage to the stem cell pool may not only exhaust its capacity to produce haematological progeny, but may also render it unsuitable for transplantation by reducing its repopulating ability.

Committed haemopoietic precursor cells undergo proliferation within the bone marrow to expand their number and provide a pool of cells which

circulating leucocytes and infection in patients with acute leukaemia. *Annals of Internal Medicine*, **64**, 328–340 (1966)

73. Brown, A.E. Neutropenia, fever and infection. *American Journal of Medicine*, **76**, 421–428 (1984)

74. Cho, S.Y. and Choi, H.Y. Opportunistic fungal infection among cancer patients. *American Journal of Clinical Pathology*, **72**, 617–621 (1979)

75. Gerson, S.L., Talbot, G.H., Hurwitz, S. *et al.* Prolonged granulocytopenia: the major risk factor for invasive pulmonary aspergillosis in patients with acute leukemia. *Annals of Internal Medicine*, **100**, 345–351 (1984)

76. Winston, D.J., Ho, W.G. and Gale, R.P. Therapeutic granulocyte transfusions for documented infections. *Annals of Internal Medicine*, **97**, 509–515 (1982)

77. Pickering, L.K., Anderson, D.C., Choi, S. *et al.* Leukocyte function in children with malignancy. *Cancer*, **35**, 1365–1371 (1975)

78. McCormack, R.T., Nelson, R.D., Bloomfield, C.D. *et al.* Neutrophilic function in lymphoreticular malignancy. *Cancer*, **44**, 920–926 (1979)

79. Pizzo, P.A. Granulocytopenia and cancer therapy. Past problems, current solutions, future challenges. *Cancer*, **54**, 2649–2661 (1984)

80. Cline, M.J. Drugs and phagocytosis. *New England Journal of Medicine*, **291**, 1187–1188 (1974)

81. Gaydos, L.S., Freireich, E.J. and Mantel, N. The quantitative relation between platelet count and hemorrhage in patients with acute leukemia. *New England Journal of Medicine*, **266**, 905–909 (1962)

82. Harker, L.A. and Slichter, S.J. The bleeding time as a screening test for evaluation of platelet function. *New England Journal of Medicine*, **287**, 155–159 (1972)

83. Higby, E.J., Cohen, E., Holland, J.F. *et al.* The prophylactic treatment of thrombocytopenic leukemic patients with platelets. A double blind study. *Transfusion*, **14**, 440–446 (1974)

84. Hoak, J.C. and Koepke, J.A. Blood transfusion and blood products. In *Clinics in Haematology* (ed. J.D. Cash), W.B. Saunders, Philadelphia, pp. 69–79 (1976)

85. Brand, A., van Leeuwen, A., Eernisse, J.G. *et al.* Platelet transfusion therapy: Optimal donor selection with a combination of the lymphocytoxicity and platelet immunofluorescence test. *Blood*, **51**, 781–788 (1978)

86. Greenblatt, D.J., Abernethy, D.R. and Shader, R.I. Pharmacokinetic aspects of drug therapy in the elderly. *The Drug Monitoring*, **8**, 249–255 (1986)

87. Dewys, W.D., Begg, C., Lavin, P.T. *et al.* Prognostic effect of weight loss prior to chemotherapy in cancer patients. *American Journal of Medicine*, **69**, 491–497 (1980)

88. Ascione, F.J. Allopurinol with mercaptopurine. *Drug Therapeutics*, **7**, 69–74 (1977)

89. Frei, E. and Canellos, G.P. Dose: a critical factor in cancer chemotherapy. *American Journal of Medicine*, **69**, 583–594 (1980)

90. Hryniuk, W. and Bush, H. The importance of dose intensity in chemotherapy of metastatic breast cancer. *Journal of Clinical Oncology*, **2**, 1281–1288 (1984)

91. Hryniuk, W. The importance of dose intensity in outcome of chemotherapy. In *Advances in Oncology*, (eds S. Hellman, V.T. De Vita and S. Rosenberg), J.B. Lippincott, Philadelphia, pp. 121–141 (1988)

92. Tannock, I.F., Boyd, N.F., De Boer, G. *et al.* A randomised trial of two dose levels of cyclophosphamide, methotrexate, and fluorouracil chemotherapy for patients with metastatic breast cancer. *Journal of Clinical Oncology*, **6**, 1377–1387 (1988)

93. Valeriote, F. and Toler, S. Extensive proliferative capacity of haemopoietic stem cells. *Cell and Tissue Kinetics*, **16**, 1–6 (1983)

94. Lohrmann, H.P. and Schreml, W. Cytotoxic drugs and the granulopoietic system. *Recent Results in Cancer Research*, **81**, 1–222 (1982)

95. Hellman, S. and Botnick, L.E. Stem cell depletion: an explanation of the late effects of cytotoxins. *International Journal of Radiation Oncology, Biology, Physics*, **2**, 181–184 (1977)

96. Braunschweiger, P.G., Schenken, L.L. and Schiffer, L.M. Adriamycin-induced delayed erythropoietic injury expressed following anemia stress. *Cancer Research*, **40**, 2257–2262 (1980)

97. Castro-Malaspina, H., Gay, R.E., Jhanwar, S.C. *et al.* Characteristics of bone marrow fibroblasts colony-forming cells (CFU-F) and their progeny in patients with myeloproliferative disorders. *Blood*, **59**, 1046–1054 (1982)

98. Ben-Ishay, Z., Prindull, G., Sharon, S. and Borenstein, A. Effects of chemotherapy on bone marrow stroma in mice with acute myelogenous leukaemia. Correlation with CFU-C and CFU-D. *Leukaemia Research*, **9**, 1059–1067 (1985)

99. Molineux, G., Xu, C., Hendry, J. and Testa, N.G. A cellular analysis of long-term haematopoietic damage after repeated treatment with cyclophosphamide. *Cancer Chemotherapy and Pharmacology*, **18**, 11–16 (1986)

100. Hays, E.F., Hale, L., Villarreal, B. and Fitchen, J.H. Stromal and haemopoietic stem cell abnormalities in long term marrow cultures of marrow from busulphan treated mice. *Experimental Hematology*, **10**, 383–392 (1982)

101. Przepiorka, D., Torok-Storb, B. and Simmons, P.J. The origin of bone marrow stroma after transplantation. Implications for graft failure. In *Hematopoiesis: Long-Term Effects of Chemotherapy and Radiation* (eds N.G. Testa and R.P. Gale), Marcel Dekker, New York and Basel, pp. 279–287 (1988)

102. Kovacs, C.J., Evans, M.J., Hooker, J.H. and Abernathy, R.S. A permanent defect in T-cell function resulting from adriamycin. *Experimental Hematology*, **14**, 505 (1986)

103. Morley, A. and Blake, J. An animal model of chronic aplastic marrow failure. I. Late marrow failure after busulfan. *Blood*, **44**, 49–59 (1974)

104. Trainor, K.J., Seshadri, R.S. and Morley, A.A. Residual marrow injury following cytotoxic drugs. *Leukaemia Research*, **3**, 205–210 (1979)

105. Trainor, K.J. and Morley, A.A. Screening of cytotoxic drugs for residual bone marrow damage. *Journal of the National Cancer Institute*, **57**, 1237–1239 (1976)

106. Botnick, L.E., Hannon, E.C. and Hellman, S. Multisystem stem cell failure from alkylating agents. *Cancer Research*, **38**, 1942–1947 (1978)

107. De Jong, J.P., Nikkels, P.G., Brockbank, K.G.M. *et al.* Comparative *in vitro* effects of cyclophosphamide derivatives on murine bone marrow derived stromal and hemopoietic progenitor cell classes. *Cancer Research*, **48**, 4001–4005 (1985)

108. Hodgson, G.S. and Bradley, T.R. Effects of endotoxin and extracts of pregnant mouse uterus on the recovery of haemopoiesis after 5-fluorouracil. *Cancer Treatment Reports*, **63**, 1761–1769 (1979)

109. Xu, C.X., Molineux, G., Testa, N.G. and Hendry, J.H. Long-term damage to haemopoietic cell populations after repeated treatment with BCNU or cyclophosphamide. *British Journal of Cancer*, **54**, 174–176 (1986)

110. Schreml, W. and Lohrmann, H.P. Hematotoxicity of adjuvant therapy. In *Adjuvant Therapy of Cancer* (eds S.E. Jones and S.E. Salmon), Grune and Stratton, New York, pp. 63–70 (1979)

111. Osband, M., Cohen, H., Cassady, J.R. and Faffe, N. Severe and protracted bone marrow dysfunction following long-term therapy with methyl-CCNU. *Proceedings of the American Association of Cancer Research*, **18**, 303 (1979)

112. Lohrmann, H.P., Lepp, K. and Schreml, W. 5-Fluorouracil, 1,3-bis (chloroethyl)-1-nitrosourea, and 1-(chloroethyl)-3-(4-methylcyclohexyl)-1-nitrosourea: effect on the human granulopoietic system. *Journal of the National Cancer Institute*, **68**, 541–547 (1982)

113. Lohrmann, H.P., Schreml, W., Lang, M. *et al.* Changes of granulopoiesis during and after adjuvant chemotherapy of breast cancer. *British Journal of Haematology*, **40**, 369–381 (1978)

114. Keating, M., Cork, A., Broach, Y. *et al.* Towards a clinically relevant cytogenetic classification of acute myelogenous leukaemia. *Leukaemia Research*, **11**, 119–133 (1987)

115. Michaels, S., McKenna, R., Arthur, D. *et al.* Therapy-related acute myeloid and myelodysplastic syndrome: a clinical and morphological study of 65 cases. *Blood*, **65**, 1364–1372 (1985)

116. Koeffler, P. and Rowley, J. Therapy related acute non-lymphocytic leukaemia. In *Neoplastic Diseases of the Blood* (eds G. Canellos, R. Kyle and C. Schiffer), Churchill Livingstone, New York, pp. 357–384 (1985)

117. Bergsagel, D.E., Bailey, A.J., Langley, G.R. *et al.* The chemotherapy of plasma-cell myeloma and the incidence of acute leukaemia. *New England Journal of Medicine*, **301**, 743–748 (1979)

118. De Vita, V.T. The consequences of the chemotherapy of Hodgkin's disease: the tenth David A. Karnofsky memorial lecture. *Cancer*, **47**, 1–13 (1981)

119. Reimer, R.R., Hoover, R., Fraumeni, J.F. and Young, R.C. Acute leukemia after alkylating-agent therapy of ovarian cancer. *New England Journal of Medicine*, **297**, 177–180 (1977)

120. Stott, H., Fox, W., Girling, D.J. *et al.* Acute leukaemia after busulphan. *British Medical Journal*, **ii**, 1513–1517 (1977)

121. Rosner, F., Carey, R.W. and Zarrabi, M.H. Breast cancer and acute leukemia: report of 24 cases and review of the literature. *American Journal of Hematology*, **4**, 151–172 (1978)

122. Einhorn, N. Acute leukemia after chemotherapy (melphalan). *Cancer*, **41**, 444–447 (1978)

123. Grunwald, H.W. and Rosner, F. Acute leukemia and immunosuppressive drug use: a review of patients undergoing immunosuppressive therapy for non-neoplastic diseases. *Archives of Internal Medicine*, **139**, 461–466 (1979)

124. Moorehead, P.S., Nowell, P.C., Mellman, W.J. *et al.* Chromosome preparations of leukocytes cultured from human peripheral blood. *Experimental Cell Research*, **20**, 613–616 (1960)

125. Rowley, J. Chromosome changes in leukemia cells as indicators of mutagenic exposure. In *Chromosomes and Cancer: From Molecules to Man* (eds J.D. Rowley and J.E. Ultmann), Academic Press, New York, pp. 139–159 (1983)

126. Sherr, C., Rettenmier, C., Diaz, M. *et al.* The c-fms proto-oncogene product is related to the receptor for the mononuclear phagocyte growth factor, CSF-1. *Cell*, **41**, 665–676 (1985)

127. Le Beau, M., Westbrook, C., Diaz, M. *et al.* Evidence for the involvement of GM-CSF and *fms* in the deletion (5q) in myeloid disorders. *Science*, **231**, 984–987 (1986)

128. Schreml, W., Lohrmann, H.P. and Anger, B. Stem cell defects after cytoreductive therapy in man. *Experimental Hematology*, **13**(Suppl. 16), 31–42 (1985)

129. Bonadonna, G. and Valagussa, P. Dose response effect of adjuvant chemotherapy in breast cancer. *New England Journal of Medicine*, **304**, 10–15 (1981)

130. Souhami, R.L., Harper, P.G., Linch, D. *et al.* High-dose cyclophosphamide with autologous marrow rescue for small cell carcinoma of the bronchus. *Cancer Chemotherapy and Pharmacology*, **10**, 205–207 (1983)

131. Smith, I., Evans, B.D., Harland, S.J. *et al.* High dose cyclophosphamide with autologous bone marrow rescue after conventional chemotherapy in the treatment of small cell lung cancer. *Cancer Chemotherapy and Pharmacology*, **14**, 120–124 (1985)

132. McElwain, T.J., Hedley, D.W., Burton, G. *et al.* Marrow autotransplantation accelerates haematological recovery in patients with malignant melanoma treated with high-dose melphalan. *British Journal of Cancer*, **40**, 72–80 (1979)

133. Spitzer, G., Verma, D.S., Fisher, R. *et al.* The myeloid progenitor cell – its value in predicting hematopoietic recovery after autologous bone marrow transplantation. *Blood*, **55**, 317–323 (1980)

134. Gorin, N.C. Collection, manipulation and freezing of haemopoietic stem cells. *Clinics in Haematology*, **15**, 9–45 (1986)

135. Eder, J.P., Bast, R.C., Peters, W.P. *et al.* Prediction of the optimal timing of bone marrow reinfusion after high dose chemotherapy. *Cancer Research*, **46**, 4496–4499 (1986)

136. Millar, J.L. and Smith, I.E. The viability of marrow stored at 4°C. In *Autologous Bone Marrow Transplantation* (eds J.G. McVie, O. Dalesio and I.E. Smith), Raven Press, New York, pp. 9–12 (1984)

137. Weiner, R.S., Tobias, J.S. and Yankee, R.A. The processing of human bone marrow for cryopreservation and reinfusion. *Biomedicine*, **24**, 226–231 (1976)

138. Dicke, K.A., Spitzer, G. and Zander, A.R. Autologous bone marrow transplantation. *Proceedings of the First International Symposium*, Texas, USA (1985)

139. Souhami, R. and Peters, W. High-dose chemotherapy in solid tumours in adults. *Clinics in Haematology*, **15**, 219–234 (1986)

140. Lakhani, S., Selby, P., Bliss, J. *et al.* Chemotherapy for malignant melanoma: combinations and high doses produce more responses without survival benefit. *British Journal of Cancer*, **61**, 330–334 (1990)

141. Peters, W.P., Eder, J.P., Henner, W.D. *et al.* High dose combination alkylating agent with autologous bone marrow transplantation: a phase I trial. *Journal of Clinical Oncology*, **4**, 646–654 (1986)

142. Von Fliedner, V., Higby, D.G. and Kim, U. Graft versus host reaction following blood product transfusion. *American Journal of Medicine*, **72**, 951–961 (1982)

143. McCarthy, D.H. and Goldman, J.M. Transfusion of circulating stem cells. *CRC Critical Reviews in Clinical and Laboratory Science*, **20**, 1–24 (1984)

144. Abrams, R.A., McCormack, K., Bowles, C. and Deissroth, A.B. Cyclophosphamide treatment expands the circulating stem cell pool in dogs. *Journal of Clinical Investigation*, **67**, 1392–1399 (1981)

145. Richman, C.M., Weiner, C.S. and Yankee, R.A. Increase in circulating stem cells following chemotherapy in man. *Blood*, **47**, 1031–1039 (1976)

146. Abrams, R.A., Johnston-Early, A., Kramer, C. *et al.* Amplification of granulocyte-monocyte stem cell numbers following chemotherapy in patients with extensive small cell carcinoma of the lung. *Cancer Research*, **41**, 35–41 (1981)

147. Reiffers, J., Bernard, Ph., Marit, G. *et al.* Collection of blood-derived haemopoietic stem cells and applications for autologous transplantation. *Bone Marrow Transplantation*, **1**, 371–372 (1986)

148. Socinski, M.A., Elias, A., Schnipper, L. *et al.* Granulocyte-macrophage colony stimulating factor expands the circulating haemopoietic progenitor compartment in man. *Lancet*, **ii**, 1194–1198 (1988)

149. Juttner, C., To, L.B., Haylock, D.N. *et al.* Circulating autologous stem cells collected in very early remission from acute non-lymphoblastic leukaemia produce prompt but incomplete reconstitution after high-dose melphalan or supralethal irradiation. *British Journal of Haematology*, **61**, 739–745 (1985)

150. Bell, A.J., Figes, A., Oscier, D.G. and Hamblin, T.J. Peripheral blood stem cell autografts in the treatment of lymphoid malignancy. *British Journal of Haematology*, **66**, 63–68 (1987)

151. Goldin, A., Venditti, J.M., Kline, L. *et al.* Eradication of leukemic cells (L1210) by methotrexate and methotrexate plus citovorum factor. *Nature*, **212**, 1540–1550 (1966)

152. Chabner, B.A. and Young, R.C. Threshold methotrexate concentration for *in vivo* inhibition of DNA synthesis in normal and tumourous target tissue. *Journal of Clinical Investigation*, **52**, 1804–1811 (1973)

153. Jaffe, N. Recent advances in the chemotherapy of metastatic osteogenic sarcoma. *Cancer*, **30**, 1627–1631 (1972)

154. Stoller, R.G., Hande, K.R., Jacobs, S.A. *et al.* Use of plasma pharmacokinetics to predict and prevent methotrexate toxicity. *New England Journal of Medicine*, **297**, 630–634 (1977)

155. Millar, J.L. and McElwain, T.J. Combinations of cytotoxic agents that have less than expected toxicity on normal tissues in mice. *Antibiotics and Chemotherapy*, **23**, 271–282 (1978)

156. Millar, J.L., Clutterbuck, R.D. and Smith, I.E. Improving the therapeutic index of two alkylating agents. *British Journal of Cancer*, **42**, 485–487 (1980)

157. Gore, M.E., Hills, C.A., Siddik, Z.H. *et al.* Priming reduces the bone marrow toxicity of carboplatin. *European Journal of Clinical Oncology*, **23**, 75–80 (1987)

158. Hedley, D.W., Millar, J.L., McElwain, T.J. and Gordon, M.Y. Acceleration of bone-marrow recovery by pretreatment with cyclophosphamide in patients receiving high-dose melphalan. *Lancet*, **ii**, 966–967 (1978)

159. Harland, S., Perez, D., Millar, J. and Smith, I. A randomised trial of cyclophosphamide pretreatment ('priming') before short-duration chemotherapy for small cell carcinoma. *European Journal of Cancer and Clinical Oncology*, **21**, 61–64 (1985)

160. Gentile, P. and Epremian, B.E. Approaches to ablating the myelotoxicity of chemotherapy. *CRC Critical Reviews in Oncology/Hematology*, **7**, 71–87 (1987)

161. Wils, J., Borst, A. and Schieder, H. Myeloprotective

effects of high dose medroxyprogesterone acetate. *Journal of Steroid Biochemistry*, **19**, 85 (1983)

162. Gallichio, V.S. Lithium and hematopoietic toxicity. I. Recovery *in vivo* of murine hematopoietic stem cells (CFU-S and CFU-Mix) after single-dose administration of cyclophosphamide. *Experimental Hematology*, **14**, 395–400 (1986)

163. Yuhas, J.M. Active versus passive absorption kinetics for selective protection of normal tissues by S-2-(3-aminopropylamino)-ethyl-phosphorothioic acid. *Cancer Research*, **40**, 1519–1524 (1980)

164. Glover, D., Glide, J.H., Weller, C. *et al.* WR-2721 protects against hematological toxicity of cyclophosphamide; a controlled Phase 1 trial. *Journal of Clinical Oncology*, **4**, 584–588 (1986)

165. Lee, Y-T.M. The rationale for intraarterial chemotherapy. *European Journal of Cancer and Clinical Oncology*, **9**, 1265–1268 (1987)

166. Papahadajopoulos, D., Poste, G., Vail, W.J. *et al.* Use of lipid vesicles as carriers to introduce actinomycin D into resistant tumour cells. *Cancer Research*, **36**, 2988–3012 (1976)

167. Donahue, R.E., Wang, E.A., Stone, D.K. *et al.* Stimulation of hematopoiesis in primates by continuous infusion of recombinant human GM-CSF. *Nature*, **321**, 872–875 (1986)

168. Mayer, P., Lam, C., Obenaus, H. *et al.* Recombinant human GM-CSF induces leukocytosis and activates peripheral blood polymorphonuclear neutrophils in nonhuman primates. *Blood*, **70**, 206–213 (1987)

169. Nienhuis, A.W., Donahue, R.E., Karlsson, S. *et al.* Recombinant human granulocyte-macrophage colony-stimulating factor (GM-CSF) shortens the period of neutropenia after autologous bone marrow transplantation in a primate model. *Journal of Clinical Investigation*, **80**, 573–577 (1987)

170. Welte, K., Bonilla, M.A., Gillio, A.P. *et al.* Recombinant human granulocyte colony stimulating factor. Effects on hematopoiesis in normal and cyclophosphamide-treated primates. *Journal of Experimental Medicine*, **165**, 941–948 (1987)

171. Bronchud, M.H., Scarffe, J.H., Thatcher, N. *et al.* Phase I/II study of recombinant human granulocyte colony-stimulating factor in patients receiving intensive chemotherapy for small cell lung cancer. *British Journal of Cancer*, **56**, 809–813 (1987)

172. Brandt, S.J., Peters, W.P., Attwater, S.K. *et al.* Effect of recombinant human granulocyte-macrophage colony-stimulating factor on hematopoietic reconstitution after high-dose chemotherapy and autologous bone marrow transplantation. *New England Journal of Medicine*, **318**, 869–876 (1988)

173. Morstyn, G., Souza, L.M., Keech, J. *et al.* Effect of granulocyte colony stimulating factor on neutropenia induced by cytotoxic chemotherapy. *Lancet*, **i**, 667–671 (1988)

174. Fabian, I., Bleiberg, I., Riklis, I. and Kletter, Y. Enhanced reconstitution of hematopoietic organs in irradiated mice, following their transplantation with bone marrow cells pretreated with recombinant interleukin 3. *Experimental Hematology*, **15**, 1140–1144 (1987)

175. Moore, M.A.S. and Warren, D.J. Synergy of interleukin 1 and granulocyte colony-stimulating factor: *in vivo* stimulation of stem-cell recovery and hematopoietic regeneration following 5-fluorouracil treatment of mice. *Proceedings of the National Academy of Sciences USA*, **84**, 7134–7138 (1987)

176. Leahy, A.G., Ikebuchi, Hirai, Y. *et al.* Synergism between interleukin-6 and interleukin-3 in supporting proliferation of human hemopoietic stem cells: comparison with interleukin-1 alpha. *Blood*, **6**, 1759–1763 (1988)

177. Paquette, R.L., Zhou, J.Y., Yang, Y.C. *et al.* Recombinant gibbon interleukin-3 acts synergistically with recombinant G-CSF and GM-CSF *in vitro*. *Blood*, **71**, 1596–1600 (1988)

178. Donahue, R.E., Seehra, J., Metzger, M. *et al.* Hematopoiesis in primates. *Science*, **241**, 1820–1823 (1986)

179. Bergsagel, D.E. An assessment of massive-dose chemotherapy. *Canadian Medical Association Journal*, **104**, 31–36 (1971)

180. Door, R.T. and Fritz, W.L. *Cancer Chemotherapy Handbook*, Elsevier/North Holland, New York (1980)

181. Vadhan-Raj, S., Keating, M., le Maistre, A. *et al.* Effects of recombinant human granulocyte-macrophage colony-stimulating factors in patients with myelodysplastic syndromes. *New England Journal of Medicine*, **317**, 1545–1552 (1987)

182. De Vita, V.T., Carbone, P.P., Owens, A.H. *et al.* Clinical trials with 1,3-bis(2-chloroethyl)-1-nitrosourea NSC-909962. *Cancer Research*, **25**, 1876–1881 (1985)

183. Sponzo, E.W., Arseneau, J.C. and Canellos, G.P. Procarbazine induced oxidative haemolysis: relationship in vivo red cell survival. *British Journal of Haematology*, **27**, 587–595 (1974)

184. Groopman, J.E., Mitsuipsu, R.T., Deleo, M.J. *et al.* Effect of recombinant human granulocyte-macrophage colony-stimulating factor on myelopoeiani in the acquired immunodeficiency syndrome. *New England Journal of Medicine*, **317**, 593–598 (1987)

# 25

# Bone marrow morbidity of radiotherapy

**Hans-Jochem Kolb**

Effects of ionizing irradiation on haemopoietic tissues, i.e. bone marrow, blood and lymphatic tissue, had already been observed early this century [1]. In the following decades several careful studies of haemopoietic effects of radiation were reported. Extensive systematic research was initiated in conjunction with the development of nuclear energy as well as nuclear weapons. Studies of radiation protection in animals showed that shielding of some haemopoietic tissue as well as injection of bone marrow prevented mortality from the bone marrow syndrome following total body irradiation [2,3]. In the 1950s radioactive labelling enabled the study of the cell cycle, proliferation and renewal of haemopoietic cells [4]. The formation of colonies in the spleen of irradiated mice [5] and the development of culture methods [6,7] greatly enhanced investigations of the physiology of haempoietic stem cells and their radiosensitivity. In the last decade methods for long-term cultures of haemopoietic stem cells [8] and *in vitro* cloning techniques [9] have been developed which have allowed the study of the haemopoietic microenvironment. More recently recombinant haemopoietic growth factors [10–14] have become available as tools for research in stem cell physiology and as possible remedies for radiation-induced cytopenias. However, there are still many open questions with respect to the effects of ionizing radiation on haemopoietic tissue despite intensive research during the last eight decades.

## Anatomy of the haemopoietic organ

In the evaluation of haemopoietic morbidity of radiotherapy the particularities of bone marrow as the haemopoietic organ have to be considered. Restoration of haemopoiesis rests on the survival of haemopoietic stem cells. The pluripotent haemopoietic stem cell and its 'niche' of stroma [15] represent the functional unit from which all cell lines of myelopoiesis and lymphopoiesis are reconstituted. Even Langerhans' cells in the skin [16], Kupffer's cells of the liver [17] and osteoclasts [18,19] are derived from haemopoietic stem cells. After birth these haemopoietic units are located in the bone marrow and dispersed in many bones of the skeleton. In the adult the major functional sites are the vertebrae, pelvis, ribs, sternum, skull, scapulae and the proximal parts of the humerus and femur (Figure 25.1). In children active haemopoiesis is also contained in greater parts of the long bones. Due to the high capacity of self-renewal of haemopoietic stem cells, destruction of the marrow in one part of the skeleton is easily compensated by increased activity of haemopoiesis in other parts. Therefore the volume of the bone marrow irradiated is of greatest importance for suppression of haemopoiesis. In Hodgkin's disease total nodal irradiation includes 60–70% of the total bone marrow, mantle field and para-aortic nodes about 40–50% and a segmental field of about 20–25% [20]. Craniospinal irradiation involves 25% of the bone marrow in children and in adolescents about 30–40% [20]. Haemopoietic stem cells cannot be recognized morphologically. Presumably they are present in red marrow of various parts of the body in equal concentrations. However the relative mass of haemopoietic marrow decreases with age and haemopoietic marrow is replaced by fat. In the adult most active haemopoiesis is found in the spine, the pelvis, the ribs and the sternum. In case of need, fatty marrow can be reversibly replaced by red marrow and haemopoiesis can spread peripherally

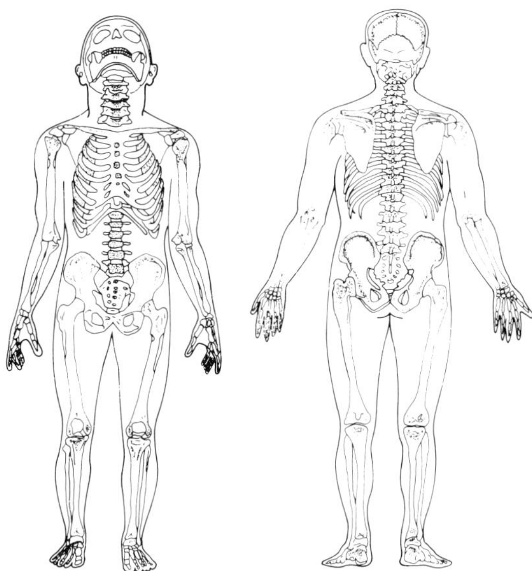

**Figure 25.1** Distribution of bone marrow in the adult

in the extremities. In myeloproliferative diseases the enlarged spleen contains extramedullary haemopoiesis. Irradiation of the spleen can reduce splenomegaly, but haemopoietic suppression may be severe if splenomegaly is associated with myelofibrosis.

In the microarchitecture of bone marrow haemopoietic stem cells may not be distributed equally [21]. In mice proliferating stem cells were found more closely to the interior surface of the bone, whereas resting stem cells were more frequent in the center of the marrow space. These findings may have implications for long-term damage caused by bone seeking isotopes or external irradiation of different quality, since resting stem cells are endowed with a high capacity of self-renewal.

Haemopoietic stem cells are circulating in the peripheral blood at low concentrations [22]. Blood stem cells have been collected by repeated leukaphereses for autologous transplantation in dogs and man. In dogs about 50 times as many mononuclear blood cells as marrow cells are needed for reconstitution of haemopoiesis following total body irradiation [23]. Higher concentrations of haemopoietic progenitor cells including more primitive progenitor cells are found in the blood of patients with chronic myelogenous leukaemia [24]. There have been doubts about the capacity of blood stem cells for self-renewal [25], but Koerbling *et al.* [26] have shown persistent allogeneic engraftment of purified blood stem cells in dogs. The significance of haemopoietic stem cells present in the peripheral

blood is not fully understood. These cells may migrate physiologically from densely populated areas to a less densely populated area thus providing optimal 'space' for haemopoiesis. Alternatively, circulating stem cells may have been spilled from the marrow in case of increased production or derangement of the barrier between marrow and sinusoidal blood.

The bone marrow is not only the site of the production of myeloid cells, but also a part of the immune system. Lymphocytes are derived from haemopoietic stem cells and together with macrophages and dendritic accessory cells they are the major cellular component of the immune system. Primary lymphoid organs are the thymus for the commitment of T lymphocytes and the bone marrow for that of B lymphocytes. In these organs lymphocytes mature from incompetent precursor cells to T and B lymphocytes. Major steps in the maturation process of T lymphocytes are acquisition of structures for antigen recognition, restriction to major histocompatibility complex (MHC) antigens necessary for cellular cooperation [27], and differentiation to helper cells, suppressor cells and cells with cytolytic functions; for B lymphocytes the maturation process includes immunoglobulin gene rearrangement and receptors for MHC antigens [28]. Secondary lymphoid organs include lymph nodes, spleen and gut-associated lymphatic tissue where the cooperation of lymphocytes and accessory cells is optimized. In their task of immune surveillance T lymphocytes recirculate in blood, tissue and lymphatic vessels. B lymphocytes are also found circulating in the blood. Extracorporeal irradiation of blood has been used for immunosuppression in organ transplantation with variable success [29]. Total lymphoid irradiation (TLI) is an effective treatment of Hodgkin's disease [30]. It includes most of the lymphoid tissue above the diaphragm in a mantle field and below the diaphragm in an inverted Y-field with only the epitrochlear, popliteal and some of the mesenteric lymph nodes remaining outside the radiation field.

# Physiology of haemopoiesis

## Haemopoietic stem cells

Haemopoietic stem cells are characterized by their high potential of self-renewal and differentiation into myeloid and lymphoid cell lines. Their morphology is that of bone marrow lymphocytes from which they cannot be distinguished. Therefore functional assays are necessary for measuring haemopoietic stem cells. In the mouse the spleen colony assays (CFU-S) allow the measurement of pluripotent haemopoietic stem cells [5]. A limited number of marrow cells is injected into lethally irradiated mice and the number of nodules is counted 7 or 12 days later. As shown by chromosomal markers, all cells of the nodule are the progeny of a single cell [31]. The colonies may consist of one cell lineage (erythropoietic, granulopoietic or megakaryocytic) or several lineages. They also contain pluripotent haemopoietic stem cells capable of producing more colonies in the spleen of secondary hosts [32].

CFU-S represent less than 1% of all haemopoietic cells and their proliferative rate is low. Only about 10% of CFU-S are in proliferation cycle. However CFU-S are heterogeneous in their capacity of self-renewal. The highest capacity of self-renewal is confined to a subset of CFU-S with a very low proliferative rate. The frequency of haemopoietic stem cells capable of permanent restitution of haemopoiesis may be as low as one in 50 000 marrow cells [33]. It has been shown by radiation-induced chromosomal markers [34] and more recently by retroviral-mediated transfer of genes [35] that the entire haemopoietic system of an irradiated mouse can be reconstituted by a single pluripotent stem cell.

Obviously the most primitive stem cells are endowed with an enormous proliferative capacity which does not decline with age [36]. The reserve capacity of the CFU-S population is probably enough to provide haemopoiesis for at least five normal life spans [21]. However in serial transfers the transferred CFU-S population failed to protect the irradiated recipient after four or five transfers [37]. This loss of regenerative capacity was not changed by allowing longer intervals between transfers or giving constant numbers of CFU-S [36]. A similar loss of regenerative capacity and a retardation of the recovery of CFU-S was observed following repeated total body irradiations with sublethal doses [38,39]. The renewal capacity of CFU-S can be measured by measuring the number of CFU-S in a femur per number of CFU-S injected 14 days previously. This renewal capacity was permanently decreased in the shielded limbs of repeatedly irradiated mice [40].

At present it is generally accepted that not all CFU-S are stem cells with a high renewal capacity and that the most immature stem cells with a high proliferative capacity are quiescent, i.e. out of cycle. Theoretically the abundant haemopoietic reserve may be due either to an abundant self-renewal capacity of stem cells or to a sufficiently large number of pluripotent stem cells without self-renewal capacity, but with an extensive proliferative capacity and expansion of their progeny. The maintenance of the entire haemopoietic system by as few as a single clone indicates an enormous proliferative capacity of the progeny of a single stem cell [34,35]. Another observation supports the theory that haemopoietic stem cells are recruited to

sustain haemopoiesis and die. Mice heterozygous for the X-linked enzyme phosphoglycerokinase showed great fluctuations in the proportion of both red cell populations instead of a stable mosaicism [41].

The regulation of the recruitment, proliferation and differentiation of pluripotent stem cells at the clonal level is still obscure. There is ample evidence from the 'homing' of transferred cells, recovery from partial body irradiation and long-term bone marrow cultures that growth of haemopoietic stem cells is locally regulated by inhibitory and stimulatory factors [42,43]. Microenvironmental regulation can be studied in long-term bone marrow cultures where an adherent layer of macrophages, adipocytes, endothelial cells and fibroblastoid reticulum cells is necessary for supporting the growth of stem cells [8]. Stromal cells have been cloned [9] and tested for production of stimulatory and inhibitory factors [44]. Interleukin 3 and interleukin 1 are humoral factors produced by stimulated T lymphocytes and macrophages respectively which are now available in pure recombinant form [13,45]. Both interleukins have a stimulatory effect on pluripotent stem cells. The combination of both acts synergistically in the stimulation of the growth of progenitors [46]. However, they may not increase the number of pluripotent stem cells *in vivo*. In mice interleukin 3 mobilizes and stimulates proliferation of CFU-S without increasing their total number [47].

In species other than mice the measurement of haemopoietic progenitor cells relies on *in vitro* cultures. Haemopoietic progenitor cells with the potential of mixed differentiation and a more limited self-renewal can be grown *in vitro* in semi-solid medium [48]. These cells produce mixed colonies in culture (CFU-GEMM for colony forming unit – granulocytic, erythrocytic, monocytic and megakaryocytic) and resemble the more differentiated subset of CFU-S [49]. In autologous bone marrow transplantation a correlation of the number of mixed colonies infused per kg body weight to the velocity of haemopoietic recovery could not be demonstrated [50]. However there is suggestive evidence that haemopoietic stem cells of man survive in culture, since such bone marrow cells have been used successfully for autologous transplantation [51]. Human haemopoietic stem cells are contained in a population of marrow cells positive for the CD34 antigen. CD34 positive marrow cells were capable of reconstituting haemopoiesis in man and baboons and CD34 negative cells failed to reconstitute baboons [52].

## Haemopoietic progenitor cells

The progeny of pluripotent stem cells becomes committed to a differentiation pathway by the influence of various growth factors which may be

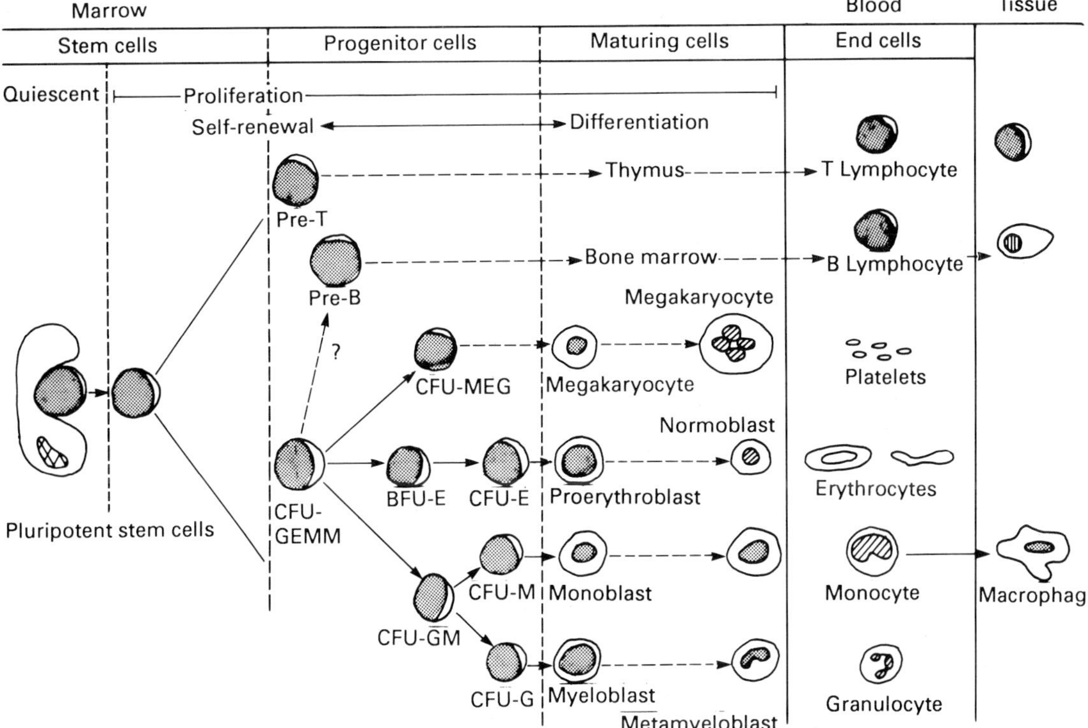



**Figure 25.2** Hierarchy of haemopoietic cells

produced locally and systemically (Figure 25.2). Progenitor cells are also morphologically undefined and have a limited potential of self-renewal. Among the growth factors only erythropoietin acts like a classical hormone with its main production in the kidney stimulated by hypoxia [53]. Growth factors for granulomonocytopoiesis (GM-CSF), granulo-poiesis (G-CSF) and monocytopoiesis (M-CSF) are produced in many tissues [54]. Presumably they act locally and, if produced in sufficient quantity, systemically. Several growth factors have become available in a pure recombinant form and their activities *in vivo* are under study.

## Maturing compartment

Maturing cells of the bone marrow are morphologically recognized as belonging to a differentiated cell line. Generally there are four divisions in each cell line from the earliest recognizable cell to the mature cell, but in granulopoiesis 12 and more divisions can occur if needed [55].

## End cells

At the completion of the maturation process cells of the myeloid series are post-mitotic and therefore less radiosensitive. In contrast cells of the lymphoid series transform and proliferate when encountering foreign antigen. Moreover recirculation as a part of their physiological function may be altered by radiation.

## Radiosensitivity of the components of the haemopoietic system

The radiosensitivity of haemopoietic progenitor cells has been determined in the mouse using the spleen colony assay and in many species including man using the colony formation *in vitro* [5,56–61]. In the mouse the dose required to reduce the CFU-S growth to 37% $(D_0)$ was between 0.7 and 1.4 Gy and the extrapolation number between 0.8 and 2.4, indicating little repair of potentially lethal damage

[5] (for review see ref. [62]). The inactivation of haemopoietic progenitor cells cultured *in vitro* was characterized by a $D_0$ between 0.6 and 1.6 Gy and an extrapolation number of between 0.8 and 1.6 [58,60,61,63]. As could be expected from the small shoulder of the survival curve the effect of dose rate on survival of CFU-S and progenitor cells was small (for review see ref. [62]). The therapeutic ratio for total body irradiation as conditioning treatment for bone marrow transplantation can be defined by non-haemopoietic toxicity in relation to haemopoietic toxicity. In mice this ratio improved at dose rates below 5 cGy/min [64]. In dogs we could not find an influence of dose rate on the inactivation of CFU-GM *in vitro* nor on the recovery of CFU-GM in the bone marrow following total body irradiation [59]. However nadirs of blood counts for leucocytes, platelets and lymphocytes were lower in dogs that were treated with the higher dose rate [65].

Controversial results have been reported about the effect of fractionation of total body irradiation on haemopoiesis. Chaffey and Hellman [66] evaluated endogenous spleen colonies in mice given fractionated total body irradiation. The number of colonies did not decrease with fractions of 200 cGy given up to 1400 cGy indicating that the number of stem cells destroyed by 200 cGy is recovered within one day. These results were not obtained with exogenous colonies produced by transferred cells. Total body irradiation in six fractions instead of one increased the $D_0$ from 0.75 Gy to 1.09 Gy [67]. In our own study of histoincompatible marrow transplantation in dogs we have seen recovery of the recipient's haemopoiesis following TBI with 13.5 Gy, if TBI was given hyperfractionated rather than in few fractions of higher doses [68]. In conclusion, damage to haemopoietic stem cells is not changed by alteration of dose rate, but by fractionation. This discrepancy can be explained by the low capacity of haemopoietic stem cells for repair of potentially lethal damage and their high capacity for regeneration.

The haemopoietic microenvironment can be seen as the 'soil' on which the 'seed' of stem cells can grow. Transplanted bones retained their stroma and lost their haemopoietic cells which were replaced by the recipient's haemopoiesis [69]. Repopulation of the marrow space of the transplanted bone by the host's haemopoietic cells was retarded by prior irradiation with 9.5 Gy. The retardation was abrogated in total body irradiated recipients. The radiosensitivity of stromal cells has been investigated *in vitro* by the formation of fibroblastoid colonies [57] or their support of haemopoiesis in long-term marrow cultures [70]. Growth of stromal cells *in vitro* as fibroblastoid colonies [57,71] was sensitive to irradiation with a $D_0$ of between 2.2 and 4 Gy, that of permanent stromal cell lines [72] with a $D_0$ of between 0.94 and 1.45 Gy. The response was influenced by the dose rate. In contrast to survival the stromal function of supporting haemopoiesis appears less radiosensitive and less dependent on the dose rate [73]. The haemopoietic stroma of human patients who had received 10–12 Gy total body irradiation and an HLA-identical marrow graft was of host type in any case [74]. However, in mice that had been locally irradiated at high doses, cultured stromal cells engrafted following intravenous injection [75].

The cellularity of bone marrow recovers faster from sublethal doses of total body irradiation than pluripotent stem cells [76]. However a slight hypocellularity may remain for a prolonged period of time. Erythropoiesis is generally more sensitive than granulopoiesis. The mitotic index falls within hours of irradiation, a minor part of the erythroblasts show abnormalities of their nucleus and mitotic abnormalities can be seen for several days. However, these changes do not correlate well with the radiation dose given [4]. The blood counts change characteristically [4]. Lymphocyte counts drop within hours of irradiation in a dose-dependent fashion, granulocyte counts show a delay of 3–4 days until they fall. Within 24–48 h an increase of granulocyte counts can be observed. Platelet counts decrease even later, after more than 5 days. Platelet and white blood counts may be influenced by several factors apart from the dose of irradiation including infection and consumption. The most reliable parameter may be the reticulocyte count which drops within 24 h in a dose-dependent way [77].

Heinz bodies are a denaturation product of haemoglobin in red cells treated with phenylhydrazine. Red cells carrying Heinz bodies are more frequent in persons professionally exposed to irradiation and in patients treated with radiotherapy [78]. Haemolysis has been the limiting toxicity of extracorporeal irradiation occurring after cumulative doses of about 100 000 cGy to the flowing blood through an arteriovenous shunt [79]. The life span of platelets was not changed up to a dose of 75 000 cGy. Extracorporeal irradiation of the blood produced prompt lymphopenia which was reversible following discontinuation [80]. Lymphopenia was associated with a prolonged transplant survival, but not with a suppressed antibody response [80].

Lymphocytes are among the most radiosensitive mammalian cells. In contrast to other cells that do not die until they undergo mitosis, most lymphocytes are killed without entering the mitotic cycle ('interphase death'). B lymphocytes are even more radiosensitive than T lymphocytes [81]. In general, T suppressor cells are more radiosensitive than T helper cells. Moreover, dose-survival analysis of *in vitro* irradiated lymphocytes reveals at least two subsets of both T cells and B cells with different radiosensitivity, a majority of 60–80% very sensitive and a minority of less sensitive lymphocytes [82].

The response of lymphocytes to radiation depends on the functional status of the cells and the method of study. Primed T helper cells are radioresistant as compared with unprimed cells. This radioresistance is seen *in vitro*, but it is not seen when tested by adoptive transfer. Irradiation may alter the pattern of recirculation of T cells [83].

Immunosuppression by irradiation is greatest when given prior to exposure to antigen [84]. Irradiation after antigen exposure can even enhance antibody production [85], presumably by preferential inactivation of suppressor cells. Total body irradiation has been used for immunosuppression prior to organ transplantation, but the doses required were quite high. At doses of greater than 3 Gy an increasing proportion of patients died of marrow aplasia [86]. In man the $LD_{50}$ of the bone marrow syndrome is probably around 4.5 Gy [87]. More experience in immunosuppression by total body irradiation has been acquired in bone marrow transplantation. In dogs a dose of about 6 Gy was required to ensure engraftment of marrow identical for antigens of the major histocompatibility complex (MHC) [88]. Marrow of sibling donors identical for one MHC-haplotype engrafted permanently in recipients irradiated with 13.5 Gy [68]. Engraftment of allogeneic marrow was enhanced by total body irradiation at higher dose rates [89,90]. Dose fractionation allowed total body irradiation with higher doses, but a hyperfractionated regimen was less immunosuppressive than a less fractionated regimen [68]. A delay of marrow infusion from 24 to 72 h following total body irradiation enhanced repopulation of thymus, spleen and marrow and improved survival [91].

# Morbidity from radiotherapy

## Total body irradiation

### Low-dose fractionated total body irradiation

Total body irradiation (TBI) in a sublethal dose range has been used for the treatment of chronic lymphocytic leukaemia and low-grade malignant lymphoma [92–98]. Total doses of 1.5–3 Gy were given in 2–5 fractions of 5–15 cGy each per week. A single dose of 3 Gy as adjuvant total body irradiation was added to local irradiation for Ewing's sarcoma [99]. Higher doses of TBI were given as a sequential and segmental irradiation in children with disseminated neuroblastoma [100] or as subtotal body irradiation excluding skull and extremities in patients with lymphoma, seminoma and other widespread tumours [96]. In all series of low-dose fractionated TBI and other large field irradiations the major side effect was myelosuppression. About 30% of the lymphoma patients developed prolonged pancytopenia and 40% thrombocytopenia. It is worth noting that myelosuppression was not different whether TBI was given in fractions of 5, 10 or 15 cGy. Occasionally, myelosuppression was improved by splenectomy [101] or even chemotherapy [97]. In some patients with hypogammaglobulinaemia the immunoglobulin levels increased following completion of TBI [101]. The beneficial effect of TBI in these low doses cannot be explained easily. Possibly inactivation of suppressor cells enhances immune reactivity and surveillance.

## Total body irradiation with bone marrow rescue

Total body irradiation with a variety of dosages and regimens is widely used as a preparative treatment for bone marrow transplantation. There is an acute suppression of the patient's haemopoiesis by the preparative regimen with severe neutropenia and thrombocytopenia within 1 week of TBI which lasts for about 2 weeks until the graft takes over haemopoiesis. Thereafter most of the haemopoiesis is produced by the grafted marrow. However there are exceptions: the stroma supporting haemopoiesis of the graft remains host type following HLA-identical transplantation [74]; in blood group-incompatible transplants isoagglutinins of the host can persist for weeks and months after transplantation indicating that the host's B lymphocytes can survive lethal doses of irradiation [102]; in a minority of patients a mixture of donor and host type haemopoiesis appears transiently or persists [103–105]. In patients given marrow from which contaminating T cells have been depleted, a mixture of donor and host type haemopoiesis or even a rejection of the graft is observed more frequently [106]. Obviously alterations of haemopoiesis cannot only be related to the preparative regimen or TBI for preparation and an effect of the haemopoietic graft on the microenvironment has to be considered. Marrow biopsies from transplanted patients are frequently slightly hypocellular for various times after transplantation while blood counts are normal. A number of investigators found a decreased content of haemopoietic progenitor cells in marrow and blood of transplanted patients [50,107,108]. Others described a proliferative defect of haemopoietic progenitors of transplanted patients in culture [109]. Even after normalization of blood counts a large proportion of haemopoietic progenitors remain in cycle [50]. The higher growth fraction indicates a marginal marrow reserve and an increased susceptibility to chemotherapy. In most patients with graft-versus-host disease the depression of haemopoietic progenitor growth could be abrogated by blocking immune T cells [110]. The recovery of the immune system of marrow transplanted patients is similar during the first 4 months for patients with syngeneic, autologous and allogeneic grafts [111]. Immune reconstitution is complete in most patients by 1–2 years unless chronic graft-versus-host disease impairs it [112].

## Local and partial body irradiation

The local effects of irradiation on the bone marrow have been studied systematically by Knospe, Blom and Crosby [113] in rats. Between 24 and 48 h after irradiation with 20–100 Gy the marrow sinusoids disintegrated and the marrow became aplastic within 4 days. Repair of sinusoids was apparent already on day 4 and the marrow was repopulated on day 14. A second phase of aplasia with concurrent loss of sinusoids ensued 1–3 months after irradiation. Regeneration of sinusoids and haemopoiesis occurred 6–12 months after a dose of 40 Gy and increasing fibrosis was seen after doses of more than 60 Gy. Local haemopoietic recovery failed in mice following single doses above 50 Gy, but fractionated exposures did not preclude recovery up to doses of 60 Gy except for megakaryocytes [114]. In man, permanent marrow aplasia was reported by Sykes *et al.* [115] in patients with breast cancer and by Slanina *et al.* [116] in patients with Hodgkin's disease after irradiation with doses above 30 Gy. Both investigators evaluated bone marrow aspirates from the sternum. In contrast Knospe *et al.* [117] used $^{59}$Fe and $^{52}$Fe and Rubin *et al.* [118] used $^{99m}$Tc-S colloid for the study of bone marrow regeneration in patients with Hodgkin's disease treated with total nodal irradiation. Both investigators found in the majority of patients commencement of regeneration between 6 months and 2 years and increasing regeneration until 5 years after irradiation.

The volume of the irradiated marrow contributes to local regeneration in the irradiated field. Morardet, Parmentier and Flamant [119] and Sacks *et al.* [120] compared regeneration in patients irradiated on a segmental field with that of patients receiving total nodal irradiation using bone scanning techniques. In the irradiated field they found very little regeneration in patients given mantle field irradiation, but definite regeneration in patients given total nodal irradiation. Autopsy findings confirmed the pattern of regeneration [30,121]. Younger age and male sex enhanced regeneration [122]. Splenectomy did not seem to influence regeneration [118].

Compensatory stimulation of unirradiated marrow does not occur if the radiation field involves less than 10–15% of the total bone marrow volume. Generalized stimulation of unirradiated bone marrow is seen after irradiation of large fields with 25–

50% bone marrow exposed. In these patients the exposed bone marrow fails to regenerate after doses above 30–40 Gy and the stimulated activity of unirradiated haemopoiesis persists for many years. In total nodal irradiation, where 50–75% of the bone marrow is exposed, several compensatory mechanisms become active. First, proliferative activity increases in the protected areas. As a second mechanism extension of haemopoiesis into the femur and humerus shafts occurs at about 1 year after irradiation and ceases after 5 years. Third, regeneration in the radiation field starts after 1 year and increases gradually until 5 years after irradiation.

Another possible mechanism for haemopoietic regeneration is migration of haemopoietic stem cells from unirradiated to irradiated parts. As first shown by Jacobson *et al.* [2], mice survived TBI in an otherwise lethal dose if the spleen was protected from the radiation by a lead shield. Haemopoietic stem cells migrated from the shielded spleen and repopulated the irradiated areas. Mobilization and migration occurred early after irradiation, since splenectomy 1–6 h after irradiation allowed survival. In irradiated, leg-shielded mice Croizat, Frindel and Tubiana [123] investigated the effects of irradiation on CFU-S in the protected hind limb. Early after irradiation the content of CFU-S in the shielded leg decreased and the extent of this fall correlated with the dose given to the irradiated bone marrow. However, the decreased content is more likely to be due to recruitment and differentiation of CFU-S to haemopoietic progenitors than migration, since migration did not increase with the radiation dose [124]. The concept of stem cell migration has been extensively discussed, but the role in larger mammals and humans remains debatable.

During the course of radiotherapy a fall in blood counts can be observed, if the radiation field is sufficiently large [118,125]. Depression of the white blood count to less than 2.5 g/l was observed in 63% of the patients treated with total nodal irradiation; depression of the platelet counts to less than 50 g/l was found in 41% of the patients [118]. Lymphocytes are the most sensitive cells and monocytes the least sensitive. However the counts of neutrophils and platelets are most critical for acute bone marrow morbidity with respect to haemorrhage and infections. The most sensitive parameter of acute bone marrow function and regeneration is probably the reticulocyte count [77]. Recovery of blood counts occurred in a period of 1 or 2 months after completion of radiotherapy [118].

However the blood count is not a good indicator of bone marrow damage. In dogs, bone marrow for autologous transplantation was obtained 4 months after TBI at sublethal doses, when blood counts were normal. Haemopoietic recovery was delayed as compared with that of dogs given untreated marrow. Additional information may be gained from the measurement of haemopoietic progenitor cells. Nothdurft *et al.* [126] found low levels of CFU-GM in the blood of partial body irradiated dogs for a prolonged period of time in the absence of neutropenia. Colony-stimulating activity of the serum reflected the neutrophil count rather than the CFU-GM concentration. In some patients with malignant lymphoma treated with radiotherapy, levels of CFU-GM were subnormal despite normal granulocyte values [127]. However there is a great variability of CFU-GM concentrations at different puncture sites of marrow and between normal individuals.

Previous cytotoxic chemotherapy influences the haemopoietic radiotolerance to a variable degree. Some drugs such as busulphan, dimethyl busulphan, nitrosourea, chlorambucil, mitomycin C and melphalan at high doses have a pronounced effect on pluripotent haemopoietic stem cells [128] and decrease the radiotolerance of haemopoiesis for prolonged periods of time. It is well known that irradiation of the spleen in patients with chronic myelogenous leukaemia who had been treated with busulphan can result in severe myelosuppression [129]. These drugs act also on resting cells and thus damage the more immature, pluripotent stem cells. Myelosuppression by other drugs, particularly anti-metabolites, is mediated by their antimitotic activity against more mature compartments of haemopoiesis and therefore of shorter duration. These drugs may aggravate myelosuppression if given shortly before or after irradiation. In particular, 5-fluorouracil increased the radiosensitivity of haemopoietic stem cells in mice [130]. Some drugs such as methotrexate and cyclophosphamide may even increase the radiotolerance of haemopoiesis if given 1–3 days prior to irradiation [131]. Therefore time as well as dose should be taken into consideration when planning combined chemoradiotherapy regimens.

Long-term effects of radiation on the immune system have been a matter of discussion for a long time, because suppression of immune surveillance may diminish the benefit from irradiation. In patients irradiated locally for the treatment of cancer of the breast, the lung, the head and neck or uterine cervix a decrease in lymphocyte counts, several *in vitro* tests of lymphocyte functions (responsiveness to mitogens and purified protein derivative, production of immunoglobulins) and skin tests are depressed immediately after irradiation; most tests become normal after several months [132,133]. Immunosuppression after radiotherapy did not depend on the irradiation of particular areas, but was rather influenced by the volume of bone marrow and blood involved [132]. Depression of lymphocyte functions after irradiation were found to be caused by monocytes producing prostaglandins [134]. However, T lymphocytes (in particular T

helper cells) remain reduced in number for more than 10 years. The alteration of T lymphocyte numbers has not correlated with the clinical outcome of the tumor. Patients treated with total nodal irradiation showed a marked impairment of their cell-mediated immune response [135]. The immuno-suppressive effect of total nodal irradiation was probably due to the generation of suppressor cells [136]. It was subsequently used for the treatment of autoimmune diseases [137] and for organ transplantation. In mice total lymphoid irradiation suppressed skin graft rejection most effectively [138], but permanent transplantation tolerance in larger mammals was only established by including the whole abdomen in the radiation field [139]. From these data it can be concluded that the volume of lymphoid tissue and/or bone marrow irradiated is important for immunosuppression. In bone marrow transplantation total lymphoid irradiation was successfully combined with cyclophosphamide in order to prevent rejection of the marrow in patients with severe aplastic anaemia [140].

The thymus is regarded as a radiosensitive organ in infancy, most of the radiosensitivity being related to the death of lymphocytes [141]. The thymic stroma and thymic epithelium appear less radiosensitive [142]. In infant mice reversible suppression of cell-mediated immune responses were observed [142]. Irradiation of the thymus was formerly used in infants and young children with an enlarged thymus gland for the treatment of the status thymicolymphaticus which was thought to be a cause of sudden death of infants [143]. In retrospective evaluations an increased incidence of leukaemia and thyroid cancer was described [144], but several studies showed disparate results [145,146].

The possible occurrence of secondary malignancies, in particular acute myeloid leukaemia, is the most serious late effect of radiotherapy. Secondary leukaemias most frequently evolve from myelodysplastic syndromes and carry abnormalities of chromosome 5, 7 or other chromosomes [147]. However the risk of secondary leukaemia, preleukaemia or acute myeloproliferative syndrome was lower in radiotherapy patients than in chemotherapy patients and highest in patients treated by combined modalities [148,149].

## Prevention and treatment of bone marrow morbidity

Severe pancytopenia due to myelosuppression from radiotherapy may last for several weeks and the life of the patient may be endangered by serious infections and haemorrhage. Therefore the dose and, if possible, the field of radiotherapy should be adjusted to prevent severe myelosuppression in patients of older age and in patients with extensive previous chemotherapy, in particular with drugs that damage the pluripotent stem cell such as busulphan, dimethyl busulphan, nitrosourea or melphalan in high-dose schedules. Myelosuppression is best controlled by blood counts including neutrophil counts, platelet counts and reticulocyte counts. Cultures of haemopoietic progenitors may reveal a persistent defect of haemopoiesis, but their variability and the time of 7–14 days required for evaluation restricts their usefulness as a guide for therapy.

In cases of severe neutropenia patients should be nursed in private rooms with simple measures of reverse isolation. Doctors, nurses and visitors should wear face masks and disinfect their hands. The patient should receive prophylactically oral mycostatics and non-absorbable antibiotics. Platelet transfusions should be given prophylactically if the platelet count drops below 20 g/l. The platelets should be obtained from single donors in order to minimize immunization and infection. They should be irradiated prior to transfusion for prevention of graft-versus-host reactions. Similarly red cell concentrates should be filtered for removal of leukocytes.

More recently GM-CSF and G-CSF have become available in a recombinant form. Studies in patients after chemotherapy [150] and in victims of a radiation accident [151] have shown increased granulocyte levels during the time of infusion. This form of therapy can prevent infection most effectively.

In cases of lymphoma of high malignancy with large tumour masses or poorly responding Hodgkin's disease, bone marrow may be obtained after chemotherapy for autologous transplantation. The bone marrow can be cryopreserved and used for rescue of haemopoiesis after total body irradiation or intensive chemotherapy including total nodal irradiation.

Acute and late sequelae of ionizing irradiation on haemopoietic tissues are now well recognized. They should be taken into consideration when planning further chemotherapy or radiotherapy. However, despite extensive use of radiotherapy and intensive research in radiobiology and physiology of haemopoiesis during three-quarters of the century, many questions are still open and many answers are still awaited.

## References


1. Heineke, H. Experimentelle Untersuchungen über die Einwirkung der Roentgenstrahlen auf das Knochenmark, nebst einigen Bemerkungen über die Roentgentherapie der Leukaemie und Pseudoleukaemie und des Sarkoms. *Deutsche Zeitschrift für Chirurgie* **78**, 196–230 (1905).
2. Jacobson, L.O., Marks, E.K., Robson, M.J. *et al.* The effect of spleen protection on mortality following X-irradiation. *Journal of Laboratory and Clinical Medicine*, **34**, 1538–1543 (1949)
3. Lorenz, E., Uphoff, D., Reid, T.R. and Shelton, E. Modification of irradiation injury in mice and guinea pigs by bone marrow injection. *Journal of the National Cancer Institute*, **12**, 197–201 (1951)
4. Bond, V.P., Fliedner, T.M. and Archambeau, J.L. *Mammalian Radiation Lethality*, Academic Press, New York (1965)
5. Till, J.E. and McCulloch, E.A. A direct measurement of the radiation sensitivity of normal mouse bone marrow cells. *Radiation Research*, **14**, 213–222 (1961)
6. Pluznik, D.H. and Sachs, L. The cloning of normal mast cells in tissue culture. *Journal of Cell Physiology*, **66**, 319–324 (1965)
7. Bradley, T.R. and Metcalf, D. *Australian Journal of Experimental Medical Science*, **44**, 287–300 (1966)
8. Dexter, T.M. and Testa, N.G. Differentiation and proliferation of haemopoietic cells in culture. In *Methods in Cell Biology*, (ed. D.M. Prescott), Academic Press, New York, pp. 387–405 (1976)
9. Haas, M. and Meshorer, A. Reticulum cell neoplasms induced in C57BL/6 mice by cultured virus grown in stromal hematopoietic cell lines. *Journal of the National Cancer Institute*, **63**, 427–436 (1979)
10. Wong, G.G., Witek, J., Temple, P.A. *et al.* Human GM-CSF: molecular cloning of the complementary DNA and purification of the natural and recombinant proteins. *Science*, **228**, 810–815 (1985)
11. Souza, L.M., Boone, T.C., Gabrilove, J. *et al.* Recombinant human granulocyte stimulating factor: effects on normal and leukemic myeloid cells. *Science*, **232**, 61–65 (1985)
12. Kawasaki, E.S., Ladner, M.B., Wang, A.M. *et al.* Molecular cloning of complementary DNA encoding human macrophage-specific colony-stimulating factor (CSF-1). *Science*, **230**, 291–296 (1985)
13. Yang, Y.C., Ciarletta, A.B., Temple, P.A. *et al.* Human IL3 (multi-CSF): identification by expression cloning of a novel haematopoietic growth factor related to muric IL3. *Cell*, **47**, 3–10 (1986)
14. Wong, G.G., Temple, P.A., Leary, A.C. *et al.* Human CSF-1: molecular cloning and expression of 4 Rb cDNA encoding the human urinary protein. *Science*, **235**, 1504–1508 (1987)
15. Schofield, R. The relationship between the spleen colony-forming cell and the haemopoietic stem cell. *Blood Cells*, **4**, 7–25 (1978)
16. Katz, S.I., Tamaki, K. and Sachs, D.H. Epidermal Langerhans cells are derived from cells originating in bone marrow. *Nature (London)*, **282**, 324–325 (1979)
17. Gale, R.P., Sparkes, R.S. and Golde, D.W. Bone marrow origins of hepatic macrophages (Kupffer cells) in humans. *Science*, **201**, 937–938 (1978)
18. Ash, P., Loutit, J.F. and Townsend, K.M.F. Osteoclasts derived from haemopoietic stem cells. *Nature (London)*, **283**, 669–670 (1980)
19. Marks, S.C. and Walker, D.G. The hematogenous

origin of osteoclasts: experimental evidence from osteopetrotic (microphthalmic) mice treated with spleen cells from beige mouse donors. *American Journal of Anatomy*, **161**, 1–10 (1981)

20. Rubin, P. and Scarantino, C.W. The bone marrow organ: the critical structure in radiation-drug interaction. *International Journal of Radiation Oncology, Biology and Physics*, **4**, 3–23 (1978)
21. Lord, B.I. and Testa, N.G. The hemopoietic system – structure and regulation. In *Hematopoiesis – Long-Term Effects of Chemotherapy and Radiation* (ed. N.G. Testa and R.P. Gale), Marcel Dekker, New York, pp. 1–26 (1988)
22. Goodman, J.W. and Hodgson, B.S. Evidence for stem cells in the peripheral blood of mice. *Blood*, **19**, 702 (1962)
23. Bodenberger, U., Kolb, H.J., Rieder, I. *et al.* Fractionated total body irradiation and autologous marrow transplantation – recovery after various marrow cell doses. *Experimental Hematology*, **8**, 384–394 (1980)
24. Goldman, J.M., Shiota, F., Th'ng, K.H. and Orchard, K.H. Circulating granulocytic and erythroid progenitor cells in chronic granulocytic leukaemia. *British Journal of Haematology*, **46**, 7–13 (1980)
25. Micklem, H.S., Anderson, N. and Ross, E. Limited potential of circulating haemopoietic stem cells. *Nature*, **256**, 41–43 (1975)
26. Koerbling, M., Fliedner, T.M., Calvo, H. *et al.* Albumin density gradient purification of canine hemopoietic blood stem cells (HBSC): long-term allogeneic engraftment without GVH-reaction. *Experimental Hematology*, **7**, 277–288 (1977)
27. Zinkernagel, R.M. Thymus and lymphohemopoietic cells: their role in T cell maturation, in selection of T cells, H-2 restriction specificity and H-2 linked Ir gene control. *Immunological Reviews*, **42**, 224–270 (1978)
28. Cooper, M.D. B-lymphocytes: normal development and function. *New England Journal of Medicine*, **317**, 1452–1456 (1987)
29. Chanana, A.D., Brecher, G., Cronkite, E.P. *et al.* The influence of extracorporeal irradiation of the blood and lymph on skin homograft rejection. *Radiation Research*, **27**, 330–346 (1966)
30. Kaplan, H.S. Radiotherapy. In *Hodgkin's Disease* (ed. H.S. Kaplan), Harvard University Press, Cambridge, Massachusetts, pp. 366–441 (1980)
31. Becker, A.J., McCulloch, E.A. and Till, J.E. Cytological demonstration of the clonal nature of spleen colonies derived from transplanted mouse marrow cells. *Nature*, **197**, 452–454 (1963)
32. Siminovitch, L., McCulloch, E.A. and Till, J.E. The distribution of colony-forming cells among spleen colonies. *Journal of Cellular and Comparative Physiology*, **62**, 327–336 (1963)
33. Micklem, H.S., Lennon, J.E., Ansell, J.D. and Gray, R.A. Numbers and dispersion of repopulating hemopoietic cell clones in radiation chimeras as function of injected cell dose. *Experimental Hematology*, **15**, 251 (1987)
34. Wu, A.M., Till, J.E., Siminovitch, L. and McCulloch, E.A. Cytological evidence for a relationship between normal hematopoietic colony-forming cells and cells of the lymphoid system. *Journal of Experimental Medicine*, **127**, 455–463 (1968)
35. Lemischka, I.R., Raulet, D.H. and Mulligen, R.C. Developmental potential and dynamic behavior of hematopoietic stem cells. *Cell*, **45**, 917 (1986)
36. Lajtha, L.G. and Schofield, R. Regulation of stem cell renewal and differentiation: possible significance in ageing. In *Advances in Gerontological Research* (ed. B.L. Strehler). Academic Press, New York, pp. 131–146 (1971)
37. Siminovitch, L., Till, J.E. and McCulloch, E.A. Decline in colony-forming ability of marrow cells subjected to serial transplantation into irradiated mice. *Journal of Cellular and Comparative Physiology*, **64**, 23–31 (1964)
38. Hendry, J.H. and Lajtha, L.G. The response of haematopoietic colony-forming units to repeated doses of X-rays. *Radiation Research*, **52**, 309–315 (1972)
39. Vos, O. Stem cell renewal in spleen and bone marrow of mice after repeated total-body irradiations. *International Journal of Radiation Biology*, **22**, 41–50 (1972)
40. Mauch, P., Rosenblatt, M. and Hellman, S. Permanent loss in stem cell renewal capacity following stress to the marrow. *Blood*, **72**, 1193–1196 (1988)
41. Burton, D.I., Ansell, J.D., Gray, R.A. and Micklem, H.S. A stem cell for stem cells in murine haematopoiesis. *Nature*, **298**, 562–563 (1982)
42. Lord, B.I., Mori, K.J., Wright, E.G. and Lajtha, L.G. An inhibitor of stem cell proliferation in normal bone marrow. *British Journal of Haematology*, **34**, 441–445 (1976)
43. Frindel, E., Croizart, H. and Vassort, F. Stimulating factors liberated by treated bone marrow: *in vitro* effect of CFU kinetics. *Experimental Hematology*, **4**, 56–61 (1976)
44. Zipori, D. Hemopoietic microenvironments. In *Hematopoiesis: Long-term Effects of Chemotherapy and Radiation* (eds N.G. Testa and R.P. Gale), Marcel Dekker Inc., New York, pp. 27–62 (1988)
45. Epstein, C.L. Interleukin 1 in hemopoiesis (abstract). *Experimental Hematology*, **16**, 415 (1988)
46. Moore, M.A.S. and Warren, D. Combination biotherapy *in vivo* and *in vitro* with IL-1, IL-3, IL-5, G-CSF, and GM-CSF (abstract). *Experimental Hematology*, **16**, 413 (1988)
47. Lord, B.I., Molineux, G., Testa, N.G. *et al.* The kinetic response of haematopoietic precursor cells *in vivo* to highly purified recombinant interleukin-3. *Lymphokine Research*, **5**, 97–104 (1986)
48. Johnson, G.R. and Metcalf, D. Pure and mixed erythroid colony formation *in vitro*, stimulated by

spleen conditioned medium with no detectable erythropoietin. *Proceedings of the National Academy of Sciences, USA*, **74**, 3879–3882 (1977)

49. Johnson, G.R. Haemopoietic multipotential stem cells in culture. In *Cell Culture Techniques* (ed. E.A. McCulloch), *Clinics in Haematology*, **13**, 309–327, W.B. Saunders, London (1979)

50. Messner, H.A., Curtis, J.E., Minden, M.D. *et al.* Clonogenic hemopoietic precursors in bone marrow transplantation. *Blood*, **70**, 1425–1432 (1987)

51. Chang, J., Coutinho, L., Morgenstern, G. *et al.* Reconstitution of haematopoietic system with autologous marrow taken during relapse of acute myeloblastic leukemia and grown in long-term culture. *Lancet*, **i**, 294–295 (1986)

52. Berenson, R.J., Andrews, R.G., Bensinger, W.I. *et al.* Autologous marrow transplantation in baboons and man using CD34+ stem cells (abstract). *Experimental Hematology*, **16**, 522 (1988)

53. Adamson, J.W. and Brown, J.E. Aspects of erythroid differentiation and proliferation. In *Molecular Control of Proliferation and Differentiation* (eds J. Papaconstantinou and W.J. Rutta), Academic Press, London, pp. 161–179 (1978)

54. Metcalf, D. *The Hemopoietic Colony Stimulating Factors*, Elsevier, New York (1984)

55. Bessis, M. *Reinterpretation des Frottis Sanguins*, Springer, Berlin (1976)

56. Senn, J.S. and McCulloch, E.A. Radiation sensitivity of human bone marrow cells measured by a cell culture method. *Blood*, **35**, 56–60 (1970)

57. Wilson, F.D., Stitzerl, K.A., Klein, A.K. *et al.* Quantitative response of bone marrow colony-forming units (CFU-C and PFU-C) in weanling beagles exposed to acute whole-body irradiation. *Radiation Research*, **74**, 289–297 (1978)

58. Nakeff, A., McLellan, W.L., Bryan, J. and Valeriote, F.A. Response of the megakaryocyte, erythroid, and granulocyte-macrophage progenitor cells in mouse bone marrow to gamma-irradiation and cyclophosphamide. In *Experimental Hematology Today* (eds S.J. Baum and G.D. Ledney), Springer, Berlin, pp. 99–104 (1979)

59. Kolb, H.J., Bodenberger, U., Geyer, S. *et al.* Total body irradiation regimens before bone marrow transplantation in dogs. In *Bone Marrow Transplantation in Europe* (eds J.L. Touraine, E. Gluckman and C. Griscelli), Excerpta Medica, Amsterdam, pp. 38–41 (1981)

60. Neumann, H.A., Loehr, G.W. and Fauser, A.A. Radiation sensitivity of pluripotent hemopoietic progenitors (CFU-GEMM) derived from human bone marrow. *Experimental Hematology*, **9**, 742–744 (1981)

61. Nothdurft, W., Steinbach, K.H. and Fliedner, T.M. *In vitro* studies on the sensitivity of canine granulopoietic progenitor cells (GM-CFC) to ionizing irradiation: Differentiation between steady state GM-CFC from blood and bone marrow. *International Journal of Radiation Oncology, Biology, Physics*, **43**, 133–140 (1983)

62. Glasgow, G.P., Beetham, K.L. and Mill, W.B. Dose rate effects on the survival of normal hematopoietic stem cells of BALB/c mice. *International Journal of Radiation Oncology, Biology, Physics*, **9**, 557–563 (1983)

63. Testa, N.G., Hendry, J.H. and Lajthy, L.G. The response of mouse hemopoietic colony formers to acute or continuous gamma radiation. *Biomedicine*, **19**, 183–186 (1973)

64. Trávis, E.L., Peters, L.J., McNeill, J. *et al.* Effect of dose rate on total body irradiation: Lethality and pathologic findings. *Radiotherapy and Oncology*, **4**, 341–351 (1985)

65. Kolb, H.J., Rieder, I., Bodenberger, U. *et al.* Dose rate and dose fractionation studies in total body irradiation of dogs. *Pathologie Biologie*, **27**, 370–372 (1979)

66. Chaffey, J.T. and Hellman, S. Radiation fractionation as applied to murine colony-forming cells in differing proliferative states. *Radiology*, **93**, 1167–1172 (1969)

67. Evans, R.G., Wheatley, C.L. and Nielsen, J.R. Modification of radiation-induced damage to bone marrow stem cells by dose rate, dose fractionation, and prior exposure to cytoxan as judged by the survival of CFU-S: Application to bone marrow transplantation (BMT). *International Journal of Radiation Oncology, Biology, Physics*, **14**, 491–495 (1988)

68. Loesslein, L.K., Kolb, H.J., Porzsolt, S. *et al.* Hyperfractionation of total body irradiation and engraftment of marrow from DLA-haploidentical littermates. *Transplantation Proceedings*, **19**, 2707–2708 (1987)

69. Chamberlin, W., Barone, J., Kedo, A. and Fried, W. Lack of recovery of murine hematopoietic stromal cells after irradiation-induced damage. *Blood*, **44**, 385–392 (1974)

70. Greenberger, J.S., Eckner, R.J., Otten, J.A. and Tennant, R.W. *In vitro* quantitation of lethal and physiologic effects of total body irradiation on stromal and hematopoietic stem cells in continuous bone marrow cultures from Rf mice. *International Journal of Radiation Oncology, Biology, Physics*, **8**, 1155–1165 (1982)

71. Friedenstein, A.J., Gorskaja, U.F. and Kulagina, N.N. Fibroblast precursors in normal and irradiated mouse hematopoietic organs. *Experimental Hematology*, **4**, 267–274 (1976)

72. Fitzgerald, T.J., Santucci, M.A., Harigaya, K. *et al.* Radiosensitivity of permanent human bone marrow stromal cell lines: effect of dose rate. *International Journal of Radiation Oncology, Biology, Physics*, **15**, 1153–1159 (1988)

73. Greenberger, J.S., Fitzgerald, T.J., Klassen, V. *et al.* Alteration in hematopoietic stem cell seeding and proliferation by both high and low dose rate irradia-

tion of bone marrow stromal cells *in vitro*. *International Journal of Radiation Oncology, Biology, Physics*, **14**, 85–94 (1988)

74. Simmons, P.J., Przepiorka, D., Thomas, E.D. and Torok-Storb, B. Host origin of marrow stromal cells following allogeneic bone marrow transplantation. *Nature*, **328**, 429–432 (1987)

75. Anklesaria, P., Kase, K., Glowacki, J. *et al.* Engraftment of a clonal bone marrow stromal cell line *in vivo* stimulates hematopoietic recovery from total body irradiation. *Proceedings of the National Academy of Sciences, USA*, **84**, 7681–7685 (1987)

76. Guzman, E. and Lajtha, L.G. Some comparisons of kinetic properties of femoral and splenic hemopoietic stem cells. *Cell and Tissue Kinetics*, **3**, 91–98 (1970)

77. Chaudhuri, J.P., Metzger, E. and Messerschmidt, O. Peripheral reticulocyte count as biological dosimetry of ionizing irradiation. *Acta Radiologica Oncology*, **18**, 155–169 (1979)

78. Gerhardt, P. Untersuchungen über den Enfluss ionisierender Strahlen auf die Erythrozyten. Teil II: Untersuchungsergebnisse. *Strahlentherapie*, **137**, 478–492 (1969)

79. Chanana, A.D., Cronkite, E.P. and Rai, K.R. The role of extracorporeal irradiation of blood in treatment of leukemia. *International Journal of Radiation Oncology, Biology, Physics*, **1**, 539–548 (1976)

80. Storb, R., Ragde, H. and Thomas, E.D. Extracorporeal irradiation of the blood in baboons. *Radiation Research*, **38**, 43–54 (1969)

81. Anderson, R.E. and Warner, N.L. Ionizing radiation and the immune response. In *Advances in Immunology* (eds F.J. Dixon and A.G. Kunkel), Vol. 26, Academic Press, New York, pp. 216–320 (1976)

82. Mello, R.S., Kwan, D. and Norman, A. Chromosome aberrations and T cell survival in human lymphocytes. *Radiation Research*, **60**, 482–488 (1974)

83. Campbell, P.A. and Cooper, H.R. Irradiation-resistant primed T cell function. *Cellular Immunology*, **17**, 74–82 (1975)

84. Taliaferro, W.H., Taliaferro, L.G. and Janssen, E.F. The localization of X-ray injury to the initial phases of antibody response. *Journal of Infectious Diseases*, **91**, 105–124 (1952)

85. Dixon, F.J. and McConahey, P.J. Enhancement of antibody formation by whole body irradiation. *Journal of Experimental Medicine*, **117**, 833–847 (1963)

86. Tubiana, M., Frindel, E., Croizat, H. and Parmentier, C. Effects of radiation on bone marrow. *Pathologie Biologie*, **27**, 326–334 (1979)

87. Mole, R.H. The $LD_{50/30}$ for uniform low LET irradiation of man. *British Journal of Radiology*, **57**, 355–369 (1984)

88. Storb, R., Raff, R.F., Appelbaum, F.R. *et al.* What radiation dose for DLA-identical canine marrow grafts? *Blood*, **72**, 1300–1304 (1988)

89. Courtenay, D.V. Studies on the protective effect of allogeneic marrow grafts in the rat following whole-body irradiation at different dose rates. *British Journal of Radiology*, **36**, 440–447 (1963)

90. Gengozian, N., Carlson, D.E. and Allen, E.M. Transplantation of allogeneic and xenogeneic (rat) marrow in irradiated mice as affected by radiation exposure rate. *Transplantation*, **7**, 259–273 (1969)

91. Lichter, A.S., Tracy, D., Lam, W.C. and Order, S. Total body irradiation in bone marrow transplantation: the influence of fractionation and delay of marrow infusion. *International Journal of Radiation Oncology, Biology, Physics*, **6**, 301–309 (1980)

92. Johnson, R.E. and Ruehl, U. Treatment of chronic lymphocytic leukemia with emphasis on total body irradiation. *International Journal of Radiation Oncology, Biology, Physics*, **1**, 387–397 (1976)

93. Chaffey, J.T., Rosenthal, D.S., Moloney, W.C. and Hellman, S. Total body irradiation as treatment for lymphosarcoma. *International Journal of Radiation Oncology, Biology, Physics*, **1**, 399–405 (1976)

94. Choi, N.C., Timothy, A.R., Kaufman, S.D. *et al.* Low dose fractionated whole body irradiation in the treatment of advanced non-Hodgkin's lymphoma. *Cancer*, **43**, 1636–1642 (1979)

95. Hoppe, R.T., Kushlan, P., Kaplan, H.S. *et al.* The treatment of advanced stage favorable histology on non-Hodgkin's lymphoma: a preliminary report of a randomized trial comparing single agent chemotherapy, combination chemotherapy, and whole body irradiation. *Blood*, **58**, 592–598 (1981)

96. Loeffler, R.K. Therapeutic use of fractionated total body and subtotal body irradiation. *Cancer*, **47**, 2253–2258 (1981)

97. Labetzki, L., Schmidt. R.E., Hartlapp, J.H. *et al.* Ganzköperbestrahlung bei malignen Lymphomen niedriger Malignität. *Strahlentherapie*, **158**, 195–201 (1982)

98. Lybeert, M.L.M., Meerwaldt, J.H. and Deneve, W. Long-term results of low dose total body irradiation for advanced non-Hodgkin lymphoma. *International Journal of Radiation Oncology, Biology, Physics*, **13**, 1167–1172 (1987)

99. Jenkin, R.D.T., Rider, W.D. and Sonley, M.J. Ewing's sarcoma – adjuvant total body irradiation, cyclophosphamide and vincristine. *International Journal of Radiation Oncology, Biology, Physics*, **1**, 407–413 (1976)

100. Green, A.A., Hustu, H.O., Palmer, R. and Pinkel, D. Total-body sequential segmental irradiation and combination chemotherapy for children with disseminated neuroblastoma. *Cancer*, **38**, 2250–2257 (1976)

101. Johnson, R.E. Role of radiation therapy in management of adult leukemia. *Cancer*, **39**, 852–855 (1977)

102. Buckner, C.D., Clift, R.A., Sanders, J.E. *et al.* ABO incompatible marrow transplants. *Transplantation*, **26**, 233–238 (1978)

103. Branch, D.R., Gallagher, M.T., Forman, S.J. *et al.* Endogenous stem cell repopulation resulting in

mixed hematopoietic chimerism following total body irradiation and marrow transplantation for acute leukemia. *Transplantation*, **34**, 226–228 (1982)

104. Carbonell, F., Ganser, A., Fliedner, T.M. *et al*. The fate of cells with chromosome aberrations after total body irradiation and bone marrow transplantation. *Radiation Research*, **93**, 453–460 (1983)

105. Baker, M.C., Lawler, S.D., Harris, H. *et al*. Radiation damage in patients treated by total-body irradiation, bone marrow grafting, and cyclosporin. *Radiation Research*, **105**, 413–424 (1986)

106. Butturini, A. and Gale, R.P. T cell depletion in bone marrow transplantation for leukemia: current results and future directions. *Bone Marrow Transplantation*, **3**, 185–192 (1988)

107. Li, S., Champlin, R., Fitchen, J.H. and Gale, R.P. Abnormalities of myeloid progenitor cells after 'successful' bone marrow transplantation. *Journal of Clinical Investigation*, **75**, 234–241 (1985)

108. Arnold, R., Schmeiser, T., Heit, W. *et al*. Hemopoietic reconstitution after bone marrow transplantation. *Experimental Hematology*, **14**, 271–277 (1986)

109. Barrett, A.J. and Adams, J.A. A proliferative defect of human bone marrow after transplantation. *British Journal of Haematology*, **49**, 159–164 (1981)

110. Raghavachar, A., Frickhofen, N., Arnold, R. *et al*. Hematopoietic colony formation after allogeneic bone marrow transplantation: enhancement by cyclosporin A and anti-T-(immune) interferon antiserum *in vitro*. *Experimental Hematology*, **14**, 621–625 (1986)

111. Witherspoon, R.P., Lum, L.G., Storb, R. and Thomas, E.D. *In vitro* regulation of immunoglobulin synthesis after human marrow transplantation. II. Deficient T and non-T lymphocyte function within 3–4 months of allogeneic, syngeneic or autologous marrow grafting for hematologic malignancy. *Blood*, **59**, 844–850 (1982)

112. Lum, L.G. The kinetics of immune reconstitution after human marrow transplantation. *Blood*, **69**, 369–380 (1987)

113. Knospe, W.H., Blom, J. and Crosby, W.H. Regeneration of locally irradiated bone marrow I. Dose dependent, long-term changes in the rat, with particular emphasis upon vascular and stromal reaction. *Blood*, **28**, 398–415 (1966)

114. El-Naggar, A.M., Hanna, R.A., Chanana, A.D. *et al*. Bone marrow changes after localized acute and fractionated X irradiation. *Radiation Research*, **84**, 46–52 (1980)

115. Sykes, M.P., Chu, F., Gee, T.S. and McKenzie, S. Follow-up on the long-term effects of therapeutic irradiation on bone marrow. *Radiology*, **113**, 179–180 (1974)

116. Slanina, J., Musshoff, K., Rahner, T.H. and Stiasny, R. Long-term side effects in irradiated patients with Hodgkin's disease. *International Journal of Radiation Oncology, Biology, Physics*, **2**, 1–19 (1977)

117. Knospe, W.H., Rayudu, V.M.S., Cardello, M. *et al*. Bone marrow scanning with $^{52}$iron ($^{52}$Fe). Regeneration and extension of marrow after ablative doses of radiotherapy. *Cancer*, **37**, 1432–1442 (1976)

118. Rubin, P., Landman, S., Mayer, E. *et al*. Bone marrow regeneration and extension after extended field irradiation in Hodgkin's disease. *Cancer*, **32**, 699–711 (1973)

119. Morardet, N., Parmentier, C. and Flamant, R. Etude par le fer 59 des effets de la radiothérapie étendue des hématosarcomes sur l'érythropoïèse. *Biomedicine*, **18**, 228–234 (1973)

120. Sacks, E.L., Goris, M.L., Glatstein, E. *et al*. Bone marrow regeneration following large field radiation. Influence of volume, dose and time. *Cancer*, **42**, 1057–1065 (1978)

121. Parmentier, C., Morardet, N. and Tubiana, M. Late effects on human bone marrow after extended field radiotherapy. *International Journal of Radiation Oncology, Biology, Physics*, **9**, 1303–1311 (1983)

122. Steere, H.A., Lillicrap, S., Clink, H.M. and Peckham, M.J. The recovery of iron uptake in erythropoietic bone marrow following large field radiotherapy. *British Journal of Radiology*, **52**, 61–66 (1979)

123. Croizat, H., Frindel, E. and Tubiana, M. Abscopal effect of irradiation on hematopoietic stem cells of shielded bone marrow. Role of migration. *International Journal of Radiation Biology*, **30**, 347–358 (1976)

124. Croizat, H., Frindel, E. and Tubiana, M. The effect of partial body irradiation on haemopoietic stem cells. *Cell and Tissue Kinetics*, **2**, 39–49 (1980)

125. Plowman, P.N. The effects of conventionally fractionated, extended portal field radiotherapy on the human peripheral blood count. *International Journal of Radiation Oncology, Biology, Physics*, **9**, 829–839 (1983)

126. Nothdurft, W., Calvo, W., Klinnert, V. *et al*. Acute and long-term alterations in the granulocyte/macrophage progenitor cell (GM-CFC) compartment of dogs after partial-body irradiation: irradiation of the upper body with a single myeloablative dose. *International Journal of Radiation Oncology, Biology, Physics*, **12**, 949–957 (1986)

127. Morardet, N., Parmentier, C., Hayat, M. and Charbord, P. Effects of radiotherapy on the bone marrow granulocyte progenitor cells (CFU-C) of patients with malignant lymphomas. II. Long-term effects. *International Journal of Radiation Oncology, Biology, Physics*, **4**, 853–857 (1978)

128. Trainor, K.J. and Morley, A.A. Screening of cytotoxic drugs for residual bone marrow damage. *Journal of the National Cancer Institute*, **57**, 1237–1239 (1976)

129. Wilson, J.F. and Johnson, R.E. Splenic irradiation following chemotherapy in chronic myelogenous leukemia. *Radiology*, **101**, 657–661 (1971)

130. De Ruiter, J., Cramer, S.J. and van Putten, L.M. Effects of local tumor treatment with surgery or irradiation followed by adjuvant chemotherapy in mice. I. Survival of marrow stem cells. *International*

*Journal of Radiation Oncology, Biology, Physics*, **5**, 1429–1432 (1979)

131. Millar, J.L., Blackett, N.M. and Hudspith, B.N. Enhanced post-irradiation recovery of the haemopoietic system in animals pretreated with a variety of cytotoxic agents. *Cell and Tissue Kinetics*, **11**, 543–553 (1978)

132. Dubois, J.B. and Serrou, B. Effects of ionizing radiation on cell-mediated immunity in cancer patients. In *Immunopharmacologic Effects of Radiation Therapy* (eds J.B. Dubois and C. Rosenfeld), Raven Press, New York, pp. 275–298 (1981)

133. Blomgren, H., Baral, E., Jarstrand, C. *et al.* Effect of external radiation therapy on the peripheral lymphocyte population. In *Immunopharmacologic Effect of Radiation Therapy* (eds J.B. Dubois and C. Rosenfeld), Raven Press, New York, pp. 299–319 (1981)

134. Blomgren, H., Wasserman, J., Rotstein, S. *et al.* Possible role of prostaglandin producing monocytes in the depression of mitogen responses of blood lymphocytes following radiation therapy. *Radiotherapy and Oncology*, **1**, 255–261 (1984)

135. Fuks, Z., Strober, S., Bobrove, A.M. *et al.* Long-term effects of radiation on T and B lymphocytes in the peripheral blood of patients with Hodgkin's disease. *Journal of Clinical Investigation*, **58**, 803–814 (1976)

136. Slavin, S., Weiss, L., Morecki, S. *et al.* Immunosuppression and induction of transplantation tolerance by fractionated total lymphoid irradiation. In *Tolerance in Bone Marrow and Organ Transplantation* (ed. S. Slavin), Elsevier, Amsterdam, pp. 105–153 (1984)

137. Kotzin, B.L., Strober, S., Engelman, E.G. *et al.* Treatment of intractable rheumatoid arthritis with total lymphoid irradiation. *New England Journal of Medicine*, **305**, 969–976 (1981)

138. Slavin, S., Strober, S., Fuks, Z. and Kaplan, H.S. Long-term survival of skin allografts in mice treated with fractionated total lymphoid irradiation. *Science*, **193**, 1252–1254 (1976)

139. Myburgh, J.A., Smit, J.A. and Browde, S. Total lymphoid irradiation in vascularized organ allotransplantation in primates. In *Tolerance in Bone Marrow and Organ Transplantation* (ed. S. Slavin), Elsevier, Amsterdam, pp. 153–166 (1984)

140. Ramsay, N.K.C., Kim, T., Nesbit, M.E. *et al.* Total lymphoid irradiation and cyclophosphamide as preparation for bone marrow transplantation in severe aplastic anemia. *Blood*, **55**, 344–346 (1980)

141. Trowell, O.A. Radiosensitivity of the cortical and medullary lymphocytes in the thymus. *International Journal of Radiation Biology*, **4**, 163–173 (1961)

142. Sharp, J.G. and Watkins, E.B. Cellular and immunological consequences of thymic irradiation. In *Immunopharmacologic Effects of Radiation Therapy* (eds J.B. Dubois, B. Serrou and C. Rosenfeld), Raven Press, New York, pp. 137–179 (1981)

143. Friedlander, A. Status lymphaticus and enlargement of the thymus with a report of a case successfully treated by the X-ray. *Archives in Pediatrics*, **24**, 490–501 (1907)

144. Simpson, C.L. and Hempelmann, L.H. The association of tumors and roentgen ray treatment of the thorax in infancy. *Cancer*, **10**, 42–56 (1957)

145. Conti, E.A., Patton, G.C., Conti, J.E. and Hempelmann, L.H. Present health of children given X-ray treatment to the anterior mediastinum in infancy. *Radiology*, **74**, 386–391 (1960)

146. Hempelmann, L.H. and Grossman, J. The association of illnesses with abnormal immunologic features with irradiation of the thymic gland in infancy: a preliminary report. *Radiation Research*, **58**, 122–127 (1974)

147. The Fourth Workshop on Chromosomes in Leukemia 1982. *Cancer Genetics and Cytogenetics*, **11**, 249–360 (1984)

148. Curtis, R.E., Hankey, B.F., Myers, M.H. and Young, J.L. Risk of leukemia associated with the first course of cancer treatment: an analysis of the surveillance, epidemiology, and end results program experience. *Journal of the National Cancer Institute*, **72**, 531–544 (1984)

149. Pedersen-Bjegaard, J. and Larsen, S.O. Incidence of acute, non-lymphocytic leukemia, preleukemia and acute myeloproliferative syndrome up to 10 years after treatment of Hodgkin's disease. *New England Journal of Medicine*, **307**, 965–971 (1982)

150. Morstyn, G., Campbell, L., Souza, L.M. *et al.* Effect of granulocyte colony stimulating factor on neutropenia induced by cytotoxic chemotherapy. *Lancet*, **i**, 667–672 (1988)

151. Butturini, A., De Souza, P.C., Gale, R.P. *et al.* Use of recombinant granulocyte-macrophage stimulating factor in the Brazil radiation accident. *Lancet*, **ii**, 471–475 (1988)

# 26

# Endocrine morbidity of cancer treatment

A. Grossman

As the treatments available for cancer have become more effective, so the actual morbidity associated with such therapies has assumed increasing importance. This is particularly true for endocrine changes, which are rarely life-threatening but may considerably affect the quality of the salvaged life. While little recognized for many years, the endocrine sequelae of radiotherapy and chemotherapy have assumed particular significance in terms of survival from childhood malignancy, especially leukaemias, lymphomas and intracranial neoplasia. Part of the delay in recognizing these problems has been the dominant concern to ensure and maintain survival at all costs, and the understandable concentration on diagnosing and treating tumour recurrence. In addition, there may be a considerable delay in the onset of certain, especially neuroendocrine, sequelae such that their presence may not necessarily be related to therapy far distant in time. Finally, in the case of a neuroendocrine diagnosis, only in the last decade or so have the requisite diagnostic and screening tests become generally available, such that subtle changes in growth and development may be quantified and treated. It should also be noted that many endocrine organs remain relatively impervious to cancer therapies, and abnormalities of the pancreatic islet cells, adrenals and parathyroids following such therapy have rarely been reported. Clearly, bilateral adrenalectomy for breast cancer will have endocrine implications for long-term replacement therapy, but this is dealt with in any standard endocrine text. Furthermore, there are numerous categories of endocrine neoplasia which will also have specific problems and consequences. However, what is currently under discussion is the endocrine effect of radiotherapy and chemotherapy for non-endocrine tumours, which may be, and

often is, distant in time from the associated endocrine defect induced by treatment. As such, there are two principal sites of possible endocrine failure, the gonads (following both radiotherapy and chemotherapy) and the hypothalamopituitary axis (mainly following radiotherapy). In addition, some modalities of therapy may cause changes in thyroid function and these will also be alluded to briefly.

## Gonadal function

### Radiotherapy

#### Testis

There is little doubt that radiotherapy causes marked changes in testicular function, although a large number of variables have to be taken into account. Thus, in addition to the total received dose, the fractionation regimen may be crucially important and there may well be significant effects of elapsed time, as there clearly is with respect to the neuroendocrine axis (see below). Furthermore, the pubertal status of the irradiated patient may also be of importance in determining the ultimate long-term effects of external beam radiotherapy, although this may only reflect a temporary masking of a gonadal defect.

In animal studies the germ cells themselves, particularly the type B spermatogonia, are most sensitive to the damaging effects of radiation. Similarly, in man, external irradiation to the testis results in a dose-dependent reversible (at low doses) fall in sperm count which may recover over periods up to 5 years [1]. Indeed, recovery has been seen at single doses as high as 600 cGy. In fractionated irradiation, total doses of up to 40 cGy over 7 weeks produced mild reversible germinal damage; complete, albeit temporary, azoospermia was seen at doses up to 150 cGy, while above this dose there might still be complete recovery although this could be long delayed in time [2]. Clinically, doses of this size will lead to temporary sterility in adults, but eventual recovery (at least to some extent) is probable. Thus, Smithers, Wallace and Austin [3] noted that approximately 50% of a group of men subject to 'dog-leg' radiotherapy to para-aortic and ipsilateral ilioinguinal nodes for testicular tumours eventually went on to father children despite a scatter dose to the testes of several hundred cGy. Certainly, 2400 cGy conventionally fractionated causes permanent sterility. It is therefore of considerable importance that the testes be protected from coincidental irradiation during treatment of para-testicular tumours in childhood such as Wilms' tumour and rhabdomyosarcoma. Such protection may include adequate and effective shielding regimens, or transposition operations during the therapy. Clearly, where future fertility is not a factor these considerations are not relevant, but damage to the endocrine tissues may then need to be taken into account (see below).

Endocrine dysfunction may also occur following external beam irradiation to the testis, but the threshold for damage to occur is set rather higher. Thus, Shalet [4] studied ten adult patients who received 270–1000 cGy to the testes via a fractionated regimen in childhood, and noted no long-term change in serum testosterone or luteinizing hormone (LH). At 2400 cGy, however, there was clear Leydig cell damage with low and unresponsive serum testosterone levels. He suggested that for practical purposes fractional doses below 1000 cGy may be considered as relatively safe with regard to Leydig cell function.

Pragmatically, any male patient who has had his gonads irradiated at any point in the past should have his serum testosterone and LH checked at intervals, reasonably every 1–5 years. A normal testosterone level in association with an elevated serum LH suggests compensated hypogonadism, and will only require treatment if there are clinical indications of sexual dysfunction; a frankly subnormal testosterone will almost always require treatment, except in the elderly, as long-term hypogonadism increases the risk of osteoporosis in later life. Treatment is with either injectable esters of testosterone (Primoteston, Sustanon), usually 500 mg intramuscularly every 3 weeks, or testosterone undecanoate (Restandol) by mouth. The latter is extensively converted to dihydrotestosterone, such that circulating levels of testosterone may not accurately reflect its biological effect. Sublingual testosterone is no longer available.

## Ovary

As for the testis, the germ cells of the ovary are highly susceptible to radiation-induced damage. However, whereas the testis is an organ capable of the continuous production of huge numbers of germ cells throughout adult life, in the female there is a reducing number of oocytes throughout life. The effects of radiotherapy in the female are therefore more likely to be irreversible compared with the male. Thus, while an ovarian dose of up to 150 cGy is unlikely to cause any problems, doses around 500 cGy may be permanently sterilizing in some patients, while around 1000 cGy is likely to cause permanent sterility in the majority of patients [2]. Generally speaking, the diminishing number of oocytes seen during life determines the fact that, at any given radiation dose, the risk of permanent sterility for any particular dose increases with age. However, it would appear that at doses above 1000 cGy, residual fertility is rare. It is therefore particularly important that whenever possible the ovaries are transposed during abdominal irradiation to receive the minimal dose in women of reproductive age; published data are variable in the case of Hodgkin's disease, but do suggest that such sparing may be possible [5].

There are few studies which differentiate the endocrine from the germinal effects of ovarian irradiation in women, and in general infertility is associated with amenorrhoea and often hot flushes. As in men, hormonal replacement therapy is used to prevent the long-term risks of osteoporosis, as well as the oestrogen-mediated loss of secondary sexual characteristics such as breast size. In addition, ovarian ablation may lead to vulval atrophy, dyspareunia, and an increased incidence of ischaemic heart disease. Hormone replacement therapy may be undertaken most physiologically with cyclical ethinyl oestradiol (10–30 µg daily) and medroxyprogesterone acetate (5–10 mg daily for 7–14 days each month), but alternative regimens using the mixed oral contraceptive pill or conjugated equine oestrogens have been used. Whatever the medication, if the uterus is *in situ* regular shedding of its lining is necessary, and oestrogens should always be combined with a progestagen. In women in whom oestrogens are contraindicated, e.g. when treated for carcinoma of the breast, hot flushes may sometimes be eased with clonidine (25–150 µg daily, although it may be sedative). Vaginal dryness can be helped with local K–Y jelly, but topical oestrogens should be avoided as they may be systemically absorbed.

## Chemotherapy

### Testis

Some cytotoxic chemotherapy has a profound effect on testicular structure and function which is both drug and age-dependent. While experimental data are most valuable in defining mechanisms and parameters using single agents, it should be realized that the majority of clinical trials employ multiple drug regimens, and are thus less suited to dissecting out which drugs on which occasion caused any degree of testicular damage. Furthermore, synergistic drug effects and the time variable render any simple description of cytotoxic-induced damage highly specious. Nevertheless, sufficient information is now available to allow the clinician reasonably to predict the gonadal effects of any course of chemotherapy.

Alkylating agents such as cyclophosphamide and chlorambucil appear to be most clearly damaging, with low-dose prolonged treatment with either drug associated with severe germinal damage which is only partially reversible on stopping treatment [6,7]. This may be a general property of alkylating agents. Antimetabolites such as methotrexate and spindle poisons like vincristine cause much less severe oligospermia which is generally reversible [8], although cytarabine (cytosine arabinoside) may be more damaging. Combinations of such relatively mild (in endocrine terms) drugs, as in methotrexate/mercaptopurine/vincristine/prednisolone for acute lymphoblastic leukaemia, also appears to spare the germinal epithelium; only if drugs such as cyclophosphamide are added does spermatogenesis become impaired, sometimes irreversibly [9]. Similarly, if nitrogen mustard is added to vincristine/procarbazine/prednisolone as in the MOPP regimen for Hodgkin's disease, severe germ cell damage can be expected, although it has been pointed out that these testes may not be normal pre-therapy. In postpubertal patients this damage may lead to feedback elevation in follicle stimulating hormone (FSH), although this does not invariably occur; indeed, no rise in FSH level is seen in prepubertal children even with very severe disruption of the germinal epithelium [10]. However, this does not imply germ cell sparing, and the evidence suggests that there will eventually be a rise in serum FSH [4].

Most recently, Tsatsoulis *et al.* [11] have studied the effects of cyclical MOPP on long-term gonadal function, and investigated changes in the tubule-derived peptide inhibin. Rather surprisingly they found that even in patients with considerably elevated serum FSH levels there was no change in circulating inhibin, and in fact inhibin correlated positively with the FSH. This suggests that germ cell damage may be associated with preserved Sertoli cell function, but leaves unexplained the endocrine regulator of FSH release in these patients.

In a large series of 74 postpubertal males, the group from St Bartholomew's Hospital confirmed the finding that mustine-containing chemotherapy led to severe germinal destruction with elevated FSH levels, with a return of spermatogenesis in only

a small minority of patients [12]. However, as was found for radiation-induced damage, the Leydig cell appears to be more resilient in the face of chemotherapeutic assault. Compensated Leydig cell failure was noted in the patients studied by Chapman *et al.* [12] and Whitehead *et al.* [13], while cyclophosphamide in childhood is also only rarely associated with permanent testosterone deficiency. Similarly, Waxman *et al.* [14] noted that 36 out of 46 men in prolonged remission following mustine/procarbazine-containing therapy for Hodgkin's disease had persistent azoospermia or profound oligospermia, but normal levels of testosterone and sex hormone binding globulin. Furthermore, even when serum LH levels are elevated, the Leydig cell may still respond to exogenous gonadotrophin. Thus, while alkylating agents may cause germ cell damage at any age, usually producing irreversible sterility, testosterone deficiency is a relatively rare finding. Most importantly, this implies that sperm banking should be considered in all patients undergoing either alkylating agent chemotherapy or sterilizing radiotherapy, who may wish to achieve fertility at some later time. Such techniques of cryopreservation may not always be successful, especially as sperm count and quality may be compromised even before treatment [15] but this at least allows the patient's wife the option of artificial insemination by husband (AIH), with or without *in vitro* fertilization.

## *Ovary*

As was found for the testis, the germ cells of the ovary are also exquisitely sensitive to alkylating agents, used both for immunosuppression and as cytotoxic chemotherapy. Thus, continuous cyclophosphamide 100 mg daily will generally cause complete amenorrhoea with a destruction of ovarian follicles, and similar results have been obtained with melphalan and busulphan [16] (but not methotrexate [8]). However, in the case of the ovary the gonadal steroid-producing cells appear to be more vulnerable than testicular Leydig cells, such that the resulting infertility is compounded by oestrogen deficiency. These damaging effects are predominantly seen in older women, such that single-agent chemotherapy with alkylating drugs may not interfere with menstrual function in prepubertal children or young women. Thus, low-dose cyclophosphamide in prepubertal girls was found not to interrupt later menstrual function [4]. It should be emphasized that few reports clearly differentiate hormone secretion from fertility, and usually relate gonadal dysfunction to menstrual disturbance, which is primarily an endocrine event. Thus, women with apparently retained menses may nevertheless fail to ovulate, or may ovulate with inadequate luteal function – in either instance fertility may be compromised.

Combination (alkylating agent-containing) chemotherapy for Hodgkin's disease was found to produce amenorrhoea or marked oligomenorrhoea in the majority of the 41 women assessed by Chapman *et al.* [12], the disruption appearing earlier after therapy in older patients. The mustine in the MOPP regimen was probably the principal cause of this effect, and as noted above the women with retained menses may still have decreased fertility. Again, in childhood even combination therapy may be less toxic, and Siris, Leventhal and Vaitukaitis [17] noted ovarian failure in less than 10% of girls with acute lymphoblastic leukaemia treated with vin-cristine/prednisolone/6-mercaptopurine/ methotrexate. Indeed, even when ovarian failure does occur it may be temporary.

Thus, in the female as in the male cytotoxic chemotherapy with alkylating agents may disrupt gonadal function, but this appears to be more frequently temporary when administered prepubertally. In contrast to the male, sex steroid deficiency is a more common sequel, and hormone replacement therapy should not be withheld for longer than 1 year other than in exceptional circumstances. There is a suggestion in the literature that in general the ovary is less susceptible to the damaging effects of chemotherapy compared with the testis, but this may simply reflect the difficulty in obtaining information with regard to germ cell function. As for the male, consideration should be given to cryopreservation of ovarian gametes or fertilized embryos whenever chemotherapy is being initiated in young women. It is probably unnecessary in prepubertal girls, or when no alkylating agent is being administered.

The apparent protective effects of the inactivity of the prepubertal gonad has suggested to several groups that enforced quiescence of the gonad in adult life may partially protect it from chemotherapy-induced damage. However, gonadal steroids do not influence the degree of damage to germinal tissue following radiotherapy or chemotherapy, and analogues of gonadotrophin releasing hormone (which 'down-regulate' the gonadotrophins) have shown no clinical utility [18].

## Radiotherapy and the thyroid

Generally speaking, at low doses radiation is oncogenic to thyroid tissue, whereas with higher doses there occurs thyroid failure with less risk of carcinogenesis (Figure 26.1). It has been suggested that the critical features in the development of thyroid malignancy post-radiotherapy are both the presence of radiation-induced DNA damage as well as continued and long-lasting stimulation by thyroid

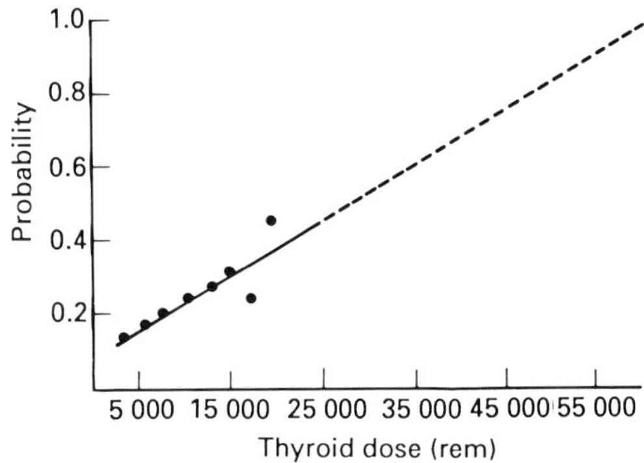


**Figure 26.1**  The probability of a patient becoming hypothyroid 5 years after a given dose of thyroid radiation (in rem). This is based on the total thyroid dose following $^{131}$I given as treatment for Grave's disease, and extrapolating to high doses. Note that at 60 000 rem all subjects will be rendered hypothyroid. Data taken from ref. [19] with permission

stimulating hormone (TSH) of the gland to produce a state of compensated euthyroidism.

Apart from animal studies carried out with radioactive iodine, the most important information has come from studies on children irradiated for enlarged tonsils, adenoids or thymus, the so-called 'status thymolymphaticus'. Maxon *et al.* [19] collated the available data on the incidence of thyroid malignancy following such exposure, demonstrating a 0.7% incidence of new cases of malignancy at a thyroid dose of 1600 rem (radiation dose equivalents); at the conventional thyroid dose of approximately 500 cGy the incidence was 2% (new cases per year). More recent studies have increased the incidence rate to 5% following similar radiotherapy, but with latent periods extending up to 25 years and beyond. At external radiation doses below 2000 rem it is estimated that there is a linear no-threshold risk of 4.2 cases/million persons/rem/year, but with a three times higher risk of total thyroid nodules (Figure 26.2). The malignant tumours, however, are usually well-differentiated papillary carcinomas and, although relatively large and often multifocal, are for the most part readily accessible to therapy [20]. At higher doses of radiation it has generally been reported that the sterilization of the thyroid leads to cell necrosis and atrophy, and thus above 2000 cGy the risk of tumour formation is extremely low. In such patients there may be multinodularity of the thyroid associated with low serum thyroxine and elevated TSH, but occasionally some thyroid tissue may survive producing compensated euthyroidism. However, any residual tissue is clearly at risk of tumour formation. Doniach *et al.* [21] described the

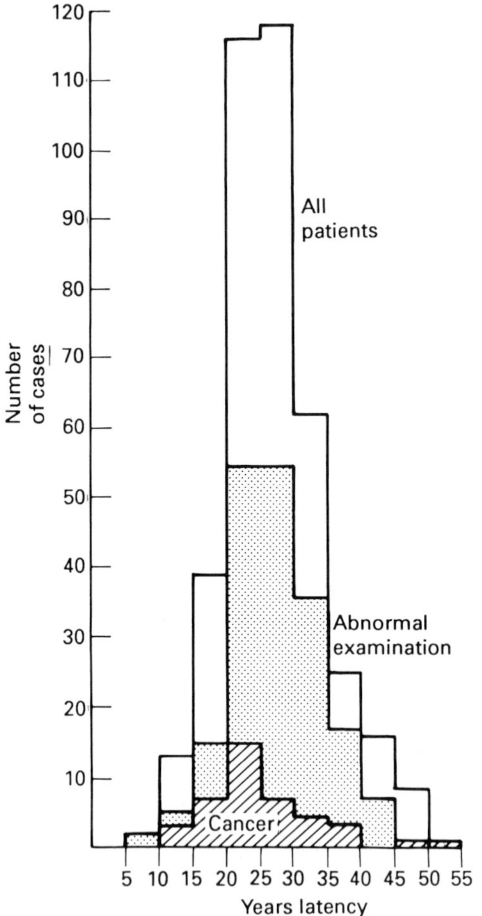



**Figure 26.2** Histogram of the presence of thyroid nodules or thyroid cancer in 416 patients with a history of radiation exposure to the thyroid for treatment of non-thyroid conditions. The data illustrate the high percentage of patients having an abnormal examination following external beam irradiation, and also the peak in cancer incidence at 20–25 years later. Data taken from ref. [20] with permission

case of an infant irradiated for a laryngeal rhabdomyosarcoma who received 5200 cGy to the thyroid; 12 years later he developed a papillary carcinoma in the remnant. Interestingly enough, the parathyroids in this surgical specimen were thought to demonstrate some degree of structural damage with functional compensation. Thus, even very high doses of irradiation to the thyroid, as is used for the treatment of Hodgkin's disease, may increase the risk of malignancy. We would suggest that any patient who has had irradiation in the region of the thyroid should have at least yearly TSH estimations,

with prompt institution of thyroid hormone replacement therapy at the first sign of an increased level; this will not only treat any incipient hypothyroidism but may also decrease the risk of malignant transformation. Late treatment with thyroxine is less valuable. Constine *et al.* [22] described transient hypothyroidism in 20 of 75 children given mantle irradiation for Hodgkin's disease, suggesting that spontaneous recovery may be relatively common. Nevertheless, we believe the risk of malignancy is sufficiently great that persistently elevated TSH levels should not be left untreated.

In adults the risk of radiation-induced thyroid malignancy is much less but is still present, necessitating monitoring of TSH levels. It has been estimated that the risk would be approximately 4 cases/million patients/rem/year respectively [19]. The role of chemotherapy in potentiating or aggravating radiation-induced thyroid dysfunction remains uncertain.

# Hypothalamopituitary axis

## Radiotherapy

The effects of radiotherapy on neuroendocrine function have only relatively recently been identified and, to some extent, quantified. Part of the delay in the realization of the potent effects of radiotherapy on the hypothalamus and pituitary can be ascribed to the relatively poor prognosis of many of the primary lesions, especially in childhood tumours. In addition, the neuroendocrine changes in growth and development take many years to become clinically manifest. Furthermore, many of the neuroendocrine screening procedures are of recent provenance, as radioimmunoassays have gradually spread into widespread use and our understanding has advanced of the mechanisms of action of dynamic testing. As the most sensitive function of the hypothalamopituitary axis to radiotherapy is growth, and as growth hormone (GH) plays no clear role in adult physiology, it is apparent that irradiated *childhood* tumours are most likely to demonstrate neuroendocrine sequelae. Changes in sexual function and fertility, especially if delayed in onset, may also be missed unless the clinician is sensitized to ask the right questions and order the most appropriate investigations.

In animal models high-dose irradiation can certainly cause pituitary cell necrosis, with the somatotrophs appearing to be most sensitive [23]. However, one must consider the effects of dose fractionation and time since exposure, as the total received radiation dose alone is inadequate to account for the observed changes [5]. These considerations also apply to radiation-induced damage to the central nervous system, which may be due to primary neuronal disturbance, interference with the supporting and surrounding glial tissue, or disturbance of the vitally important microvasculature. This latter phenomenon appears particularly important in the case of the hypothalamohypophyseal portal system, which may be especially vulnerable to damage. As will become apparent, many of the effects of radiotherapy, at least at relatively low doses, on neuroendocrine function appear to result from disturbances at the hypothalamus and its portal tributaries rather than from a direct onslaught on the pituitary; the pituitary *per se* will then suffer secondary changes from loss of its tropic hormones, although higher doses of irradiation may cause direct damage.

Shalet *et al.* [24] were among the first to observe that children with brain tumours (gliomas, ependymomas, medulloblastomas) tended to grow poorly after treatment. In an initial study of nine children aged 7–14 years, all of whom had been irradiated but only three of whom had received chemotherapy, they noted height retardation and a bone age delayed by 2 years or more (compared with the chronological age) in five of the nine. Six of the nine showed subnormal GH responses to dynamic stimulation with insulin. There was evidence that GH responsiveness was normal pre-treatment, and there was a tendency for the GH loss to increase with the dose of radiotherapy and duration of survival. This loss of GH reserve appeared to be relatively specific, since dynamic cortisol reserve, thyroid function, serum prolactin and gonadal function were essentially normal in a group of 20 adult patients treated with radiotherapy (2000–5000 cGy) in childhood [25]. This second study confirmed the progressive loss of GH with time and further suggested that it did not occur below a threshold of 2950 cGy. This finding was directly reinvestigated in 39 patients, all studied more than 2 years after completion of central nervous system radiotherapy. It was found that GH loss was correlated with the dose of radiotherapy; only a single patient treated with less than 2900 cGy showed a decrement in GH responsiveness [26] (Figure 26.3). These studies are particularly important as the achieved doses received by the hypothalamus and pituitary were carefully recalculated for each patient. Nevertheless, we now know that there may be progressive loss of GH reserve with time, such that a so-called threshold dose may not exist.

The suspicion that GH loss is a time-dependent phenomenon gains further support from the use of 'prophylactic' cranial irradiation given for childhood acute lymphocytic leukaemia. Relatively low doses of irradiation such as 2400 cGy (in 20 fractions) or 2500 cGy (in 10 fractions) led to a subnormal GH response to two dynamic stimulation tests in four of 15 children aged 7–11 years, often occurring only a few months after therapy [27]; the higher dose

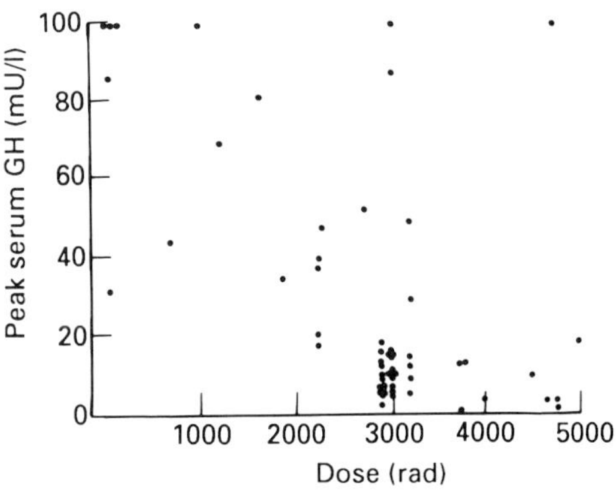



**Figure 26.3** Peak serum GH responses to hypoglycaemia in relation to the dose of irradiation received by the hypothalamopituitary region. Note that a significant fall in peak serum GH only occurs above 3000 cGy. Data taken from ref. [26] with permission

appeared to be more effective in lowering GH but this was confounded by differences in elapsed time. However, the clinical importance of these often small changes remains uncertain. In a group of 26 children, 14 out of 17 receiving 2500 cGy as leukaemia prophylaxis demonstrated subnormal GH responses to insulin-induced hypoglycaemia (only one of nine was subnormal in the 2400 cGy group), but no clear abnormalities in somatomedin-C levels or growth were apparent [28]. Thus, it was argued that minor changes in GH reserve may not be clinically important. Similarly, of 21 children in remission from acute lymphoblastic leukaemia for 3–5 years, random assignment to 2400 cGy cranial prophylaxis showed that while final height was significantly less compared with non-irradiated children, there was no significant difference compared with the control group [29]. Radiotherapy had caused a slight diminution in growth velocity during treatment, but this was transient with no obvious long-term sequelae.

Starceski *et al.* [30] found that in well-matched irradiated and non-irradiated children, both 2400 cGy (in 12 fractions) and 1800 cGy (in 10 fractions) caused significant growth retardation at 3 year follow-up but the effect was relatively minor – a fall in height percentile during therapy of 12 points which were not later 'caught up'. A recent large Italian study [31] also concluded that 2400 cGy was associated with a failure to catch up the growth failure during radiotherapy, although again the loss was relatively modest (Figure 26.4); this was associated with abnormal GH responses to L-dopa stimulation in 44% of these children (22% with absent responses). Unlike the earlier studies, these authors could find no endocrine or growth sequelae at a dose of 1800 cGy. Probably the main conclusion to draw

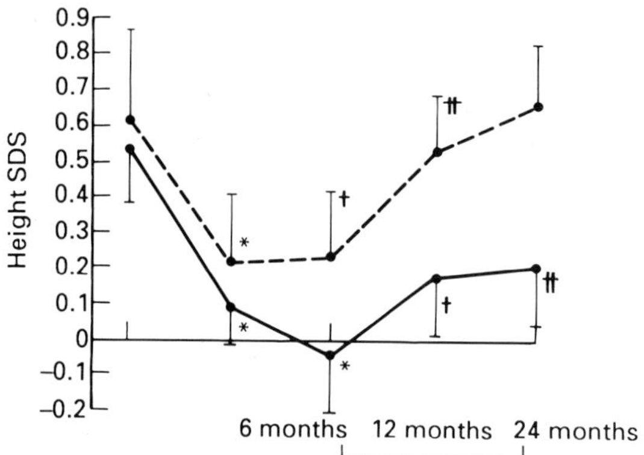

**Figure 26.4** Height standard deviation scores (SDS) in two groups of children given either 1800 cGy (-----) or 2400 cGy (———) at various times after treatment. *$P < 0.005$, †$P < 0.001$, ††$P < 0.025$, as compared with value at diagnosis. Note that following 1800 cGy there was a small decrease in height SDS which was effectively made up, but that the decrement in height remained in children treated with 2400 cGy. Data taken from ref. [31] with permission

from these studies is that failure to fulfil expected growth potential may occur at both 1800 cGy and, more frequently, at 2400 cGy, and seems to involve a failure to recover height lost during the treatment. The more marked and often progressive loss of GH reserve may well be a separate and less important phenomenon. This is even more surprising as 2400 cGy cranial prophylaxis leads to a massive fall in physiological pulsatile GH release even when pharmacological testing reveals a normal reserve [32,33], and biosynthetic GH may restore growth in such patients.

In a large Australian series, Kirk *et al.* [34] reported that at 6 years from diagnosis 71% of children treated with 2400 cGy showed a decrease in

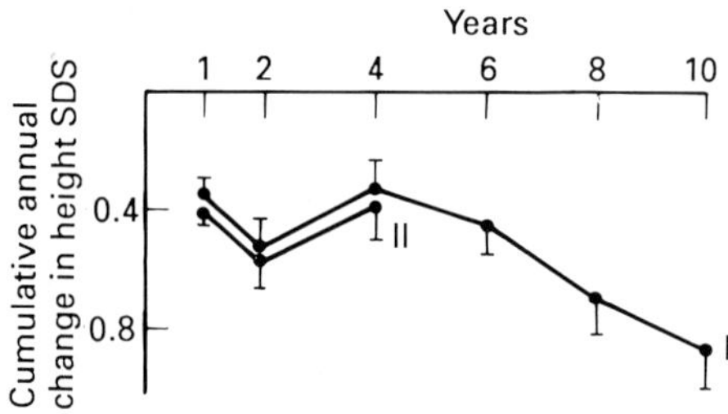

**Figure 26.5** Cumulative annual change in height SDS in 34 children receiving 2400 cGy prophylactic irradiation (Group I) or 1800 cGy (Group II). Note the small loss of height at 4 years, although this appears to increase in the small number of patients followed up for 10 years. Data taken from ref. [35] with permission

standing height of more than one standard deviation below the population mean; this was attributed to GH deficiency. Similarly, Costin [33] found that 1800–2500 cGy (in 19 fractions) led to a diminution in the pulsatile release of GH, and a fall in mean height by 1.5 standard deviation scores in 16 child survivors. In a review of 243 children treated with either 1800 cGy or 2100–2500 cGy, workers from Manchester were unable to replicate these findings [35]. They found a minimal loss of standing height even at 6 years in the higher dose groups, and ascribed the poor responses of the Australian patients to chemotherapy. However, the loss of height did appear to be progressive (Figure 26.5).

While the mechanism of growth retardation following low-dose irradiation remains unclear, and its importance controversial, there is general agreement that the growth hormone deficiency following higher doses is secondary to a defect in the synthesis, release or transport of growth hormone-releasing hormone (GHRH). Children treated for non-pituitary intracranial tumours show a retained GH response to GHRH even when their responses to insulin are grossly subnormal [36,37] (Figure 26.6). GHRH acts directly on the pituitary, while insulin is presumed to work via the hypothalamus. Eventually the pituitary, deprived of endogenous hypothalamic GHRH, loses its stores of GH and becomes refractory to the acute administration of GHRH. However, the precise site of the damage is unknown, as it may reflect either direct hypothalamic neuronal loss or a fibrosing vasculitis of the portal vessels.

The treatment of radiation-induced GH deficiency is by means of biosynthetic GH. Previously, the limited supplies of cadaveric GH meant that not all children who may have benefited from such treatment were eligible to receive it, but now that there are virtually unlimited supplies clinical requirements should be paramount, although it should be noted that the treatment is extremely expensive. Romshe *et al.* [38] assessed nine children with poor growth more than 2 years post-irradiation (2400–5000 cGy) and followed their response to conventional GH therapy; all grew in a similar manner to children with conventional idiopathic GH deficiency. Thus, there is little reason to doubt that children treated at a young age with radiotherapy, especially high doses, will show a progressive fall in GH reserve concomitant with a decline in growth velocity, and such children should respond well to GH treatment [39]. What is currently unclear is whether all such children will require treatment, what tests should be performed, at what stage therapy should be started, and whether a return to the 'expected' pre-morbid height is probable.

As mentioned previously, tests of GH reserve include insulin-induced hypoglycaemia (which probably acts by stimulating hypothalamic GHRH and

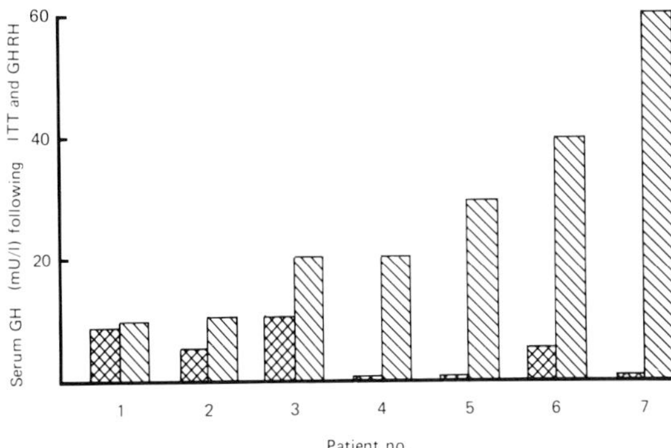



**Figure 26.6** Growth hormone responses to growth hormone releasing hormone (GHRH, right panel) and insulin-induced hypoglycaemia (ITT, left panel) in seven children given cranial irradiation. The abnormal responses to GHRH were only seen in children who were tested many years following radiotherapy. A. Grossman, A. Blacklay and P.N. Plowman (unpublished observations)

inhibiting somatostatin), clonidine, L-dopa, exercise and arginine; the mechanisms of these tests remain uncertain. Similarly, GHRH is not useful in the clinical, as opposed to the research, setting. Indeed, it has been suggested that all these pharmacological tests are inferior to 24 h GH profiles in terms of relevant physiological release, although this has been challenged. Shalet and his colleagues have suggested that even where mild GH deficiency is identified it may not necessarily require treatment, and changes in growth immediately after radiother-apy may not reflect GH deficiency [40]. They also argue that the prophylactic anti-leukemia prescrip-tions only cause an irreversible but relatively insigni-ficant non-progressive growth retardation during treatment, particularly at the preferred dose of 1800 cGy [35]. From the clinical standpoint, it would seem reasonable to assess the height and height velocity of all children treated with cranial irradia-tion at 6-monthly intervals, using properly designed auxological instruments and, preferably, trained personnel, with regular bone age estimations. Any child who then shows an unexpected decline in height percentile, especially if more than 1–2 years after treatment and involving a hypothalamic dose greater than 2500 cGy, will then require further evaluation. It may be that a 6-month therapeutic trial of biosynthetic GH will need to be given to assess responsiveness. The current optimal regimen is 2 units/kg GH subcutaneously daily, although this may require modification in the light of new information. It is also possible that synthetic GHRH, administered either by daily injection or, hopefully, by regular depot injection, may provide an effective alternative therapy. However, it should

be noted that spinal irradiation in childhood may lead to premature epiphyseal closure and produce an irreversible non-GH-dependent decrease in height velocity; this may be manifest by a relative decrease in sitting height compared with standing height. Whatever the threshold for intervention may be, all paediatric oncologists should be aware of the need for regular auxological assessment of cranially irradiated children.

Other radiation-induced neuroendocrine defects appear to be highly contingent upon the precise radiation prescription. Harrop *et al.* [41] looked at the effects of 2300–5200 cGy and, apart from GH deficiency seen in 11 of 15 patients (age range 6–60 years), several patients treated during childhood were also found to be hypogonadal, while others were noted to be unresponsive to clomiphene; this test is used to identify hypothalamic defects in the regulation of gonadotrophin release. Three out of 14 patients were said to show subnormal cortisol responses to hypoglycaemia, but no basal cortisol levels were given and this may not necessarily imply the need for corticosteroid replacement therapy. Thyroid function and serum prolactin levels were well maintained, and there was no evidence of diabetes insipidus in any patient. In a group of 20 patients studied by Shalet *et al.* [25] evaluated at a mean age of 24 years at 14 years post-irradiation, no neuroendocrine defect could be identified other than GH deficiency. The Hong Kong experience of the treatment of nasopharyngeal tumours by exter-nal beam radiotherapy is very extensive, and Karen Lam and her colleagues [42] have carefully moni-tored the hypothalamopituitary consequences of such treatment. In a study of 31 adult patients with irradiated nasopharyngeal tumours (two fields: hypothalamopituitary dose approximately 4000 cGy), serum prolactin, thyroxine, cortisol, testosterone and oestradiol levels were unchanged at 1 year. However, by 2 years four patients had developed hypopituitarism, but a much larger por-tion developed subtle changes in the neuroendo-crine axis such as a delayed hypothalamic TSH response to TRH, discordant gonadotrophin responses to LHRH and mild hyperprolactinaemia. An elevated serum prolactin is presumed to be a consequence of damage to the inhibitory dopamin-ergic pathway in the hypothalamus. At 5 years post-irradiation, eight of 34 patients showed endocrine disturbance, including subnormal thyroxine levels and impaired cortisol responses to hypoglycaemia. The particular nature of these changes suggested a hypothalamic defect in the synthesis or delivery of trophic hormone to the pituitary. Similarly, Samaan *et al.* [43] noted that 91 out of 110 patients, mean age 37 years, who received cranial irradiation for head or neck tumours had one or more endocrine defects; 43 had hyperprolactinaemia, 30 were TSH-deficient and 30 were ACTH-deficient. A high proportion of gonadal dysfunction (LH/FSH deficiency and/or high prolactin) was also noted by Huang, who investigated 12 women at 1–13 years post-radiotherapy [44]. In childhood, irradiation can also produce panhypopituitarism, but especially delayed or absent puberty; pubertal progression was abnormal in 14 out of 45 cases studied by Rappaport *et al.* at 5 years post-irradiation [45]. However, it should be noted that many of these patients received relatively high doses of hypothalamic irradiation, such as 5000, 5200 or even 6000+ cGy. At lower dosage regimens, growth hormone loss is followed by gonadotrophin deficiency in a variable number of patients, then cortisol and thyroid hormone deficiency in a few. Above 5000 cGy, direct pituitary damage may occur.

In a study of 36 women who had received 4500 cGy via three portals in 180 cGy fractions for small pituitary tumours, we noted that only one patient became hypothyroid and no patient became ACTH-deficient at a mean of 4 years post-radiotherapy [46]. More recently, at a mean 10 year follow-up we have noted an 11% incidence of hypothyroidism and 4% ACTH deficiency; gonadal function was marginally impaired in 48%, but only resulted in severe gonadotrophin deficiency in 16% [47]. Since these patients had pituitary lesions *ab initio*, it is surprising that the neuroendocrine defects are so much less than those reported in other series. It seems likely that it is not only the total dose which is important, but the fractionation of radiotherapy must be considered equally critical: thus, Lam *et al.* [42] used 200 cGy fractions delivered through parallel opposed fields.

In summary, most patients who receive cranial irradiation which includes the hypothalamopituitary axis may suffer at least some neuroendocrine sequelae. In childhood, regular assessment of height, growth and pubertal development is necessary in order rapidly to initiate treatment, as GH deficiency is common and occurs early. Otherwise, serum thyroxine, prolactin and testosterone/oestradiol should be checked yearly and appropriate replacement or treatment organized when required. Insufficiency of ACTH is relatively uncommon and more difficult to diagnose, but a 9 a.m. serum cortisol (with dynamic stimulation if levels are not unequivocally normal) should be performed 1–2-yearly, especially when the hypothalamus has received relatively high doses. Diabetes insipidus seems not to occur. As the neuroendocrine loss is progressive, follow-up should be for life.

### Chemotherapy

There are few data on the neuroendocrine impact of cancer chemotherapy, but the studies which have been carried out suggest that it is, at most, marginal.

Chemotherapy has been implicated in the transient disturbance of growth in children with acute lymphoblastic leukaemia, possibly by causing changes in somatomedin-C [35]. No growth disturbance was found following chemotherapy for childhood leukaemia at 3 years follow-up by Starceski *et al.* [30] (although these children were thought to be rather heavier than expected). Normal linear growth and weight gain following prednisolone, vincristine, 6-mercaptopurine, methotrexate or cyclophosphamide was noted in 21 children in another report [48]. Clayton *et al.* [35] considered that the poor growth observed in the Australian childhood leukaemia series was secondary to intensive chemotherapy, but there is no clear evidence for this suggestion. Costin observed no change in gonadal or thyroid function which he could attribute to chemotherapy [33]. Similarly, in adults there are few data indicating chemotherapeutic disruption of the thyroid or adrenal axes. As has been discussed, there are potent effects of such agents at the gonadal level, but the hypothalamopituitary axis appears to be relatively insensitive. Chapman *et al.* [12] reported a high prevalence of hyperprolactinaemia in women following chemotherapy for Hodgkin's disease, but this has not been confirmed.

In terms of individual agents, there are scattered reports of idiosyncratic pharmacological effects, such as the inappropriate secretion of vasopressin seen with vincristine. The long-term effects of prednisolone and related corticosteroids on growth and pituitary–adrenal suppression should also be remembered.

## Conclusions

The unwanted endocrine effects of radiotherapy and chemotherapy are principally exerted on the gonads and hypothalamopituitary axis. Radiotherapy at low doses can cause reversible damage to both testis and ovary, but at doses above approximately 1000 cGy permanent sterility may result in both men and women. In men the Leydig cells are a little more resistant, but at a sufficient dose even they will show eventual damage. Similarly, chemotherapy with alkylating agents will cause profound damage to the germ cells of both testis and ovary and, in females at least, may also affect the gonadal endocrine tissue. Profound damage to the Leydig cells in the male following chemotherapy appears to be less common. There is some doubt as to whether the effects of both forms of treatment are expressed in the prepubertal patient, but it seems wise to assume that the risk is present at all ages. However, due to the special case of the female in whom there is a diminishing pool of oocytes throughout life, the effects of chemotherapy are more intense in the older woman.

Radiotherapy, but probably not chemotherapy, also causes profound changes in pituitary function, particularly an early onset defect in the production of GH. There is no doubt that above 3000 cGy GH may be profoundly affected within a few years of treatment, while changes in the other pituitary hormones become more common with both an increase in radiation dosage and with increasing time. With regard to the prophylactic use of cranial radiotherapy for childhood leukaemias, the current dose of 1800 cGy appears to cause only a minor disturbance of growth which may not be hormone-dependent. Nevertheless, any patient receiving cranial irradiation will require monitoring of hormone status for life.

There is a clear relation between radiotherapy treatment including the thyroid and the late, sometimes very late, onset of thyroid malignancy. This may even occur at high doses of irradiation previously thought to be sterilizing. Thus, awareness of the possible endocrine complications of cancer therapy has increasingly become a vital part of the oncologist's clinical practice.

# Acknowledgements

I am most grateful to Miss Elzbieta Stawowska for secretarial assistance.

# References


1. Rowley, M., Leach, D.R., Warner, G.A. and Heller, C.G. Effect of graded doses of ionising radiation on the human testis. *Radiation Research*, **59**, 665–678 (1974)
2. Ash, P. The influence of radiation on fertility in man. *British Journal of Radiology*, **53**, 271–278 (1980)
3. Smithers, D.W., Wallace, D.M. and Austin, D.E. Fertility after unilateral orchidectomy and radiotherapy for patients with malignant tumours of the testis. *British Medical Journal*, **iv**, 77–79 (1973)
4. Shalet, S.M. Abnormalities of growth and gonadal function in children with malignant disease. *Journal of the Royal Society of Medicine*, **75**, 641–647 (1982)
5. Plowman, P.N. Endocrine effects of therapy. In *Endocrine Problems in Cancer* (eds R.T. Jung and K. Sikora), Heinemann Medical Books Ltd, London, pp. 255–272 (1984)
6. Fairley, K.F., Barrie, J.U. and Johnson, W. Sterility and testicular atrophy related to cyclophosphamide therapy. *Lancet*, **i**, 568–569 (1972)
7. Richter, P., Calamera, J.C., Morganfield, M.C. *et al.* Effect of chlorambucil on spermatogenesis in the human with malignant lymphoma. *Cancer*, **25**, 1026–1030 (1970)
8. Shamberger, R.C., Rosenburg, S.A., Seipp, C.A. and Sherins, R.J. Effects of high dose methotrexate and vincristine on ovarian and testicular functions in patients undergoing postoperative adjuvant treatment of osteosarcoma. *Cancer Treatment Reports*, **65**, 739–746 (1981)
9. Sherins, R.J., Olweny, C.L.M. and Ziegler, J.L. Gynecomastia and gonadal dysfunction in adolescent boys treated with combination chemotherapy for Hodgkin's disease. *New England Journal of Medicine*, **299**, 12–16 (1978)
10. Shalet, S.M., Hann, I.M., Lendon, M. *et al.* Testicular function after combination chemotherapy in childhood for acute lymphoblastic leukaemia. *Archives of Disease in Childhood*, **56**, 275–278 (1981)
11. Tsatsoulis, A., Shalet, S.M., Robertson, W.R. *et al.* Plasma inhibin levels in men with chemotherapy-induced severe damage to seminiferous epithelium. *Clinical Endocrinology*, **29**, 659–665 (1988)
12. Chapman, R.M., Sutcliffe, S.B., Rees, L.H. *et al.* Cyclical combination chemotherapy and gonadal function. *Lancet*, **i**, 568–569 (1979)
13. Whitehead, E., Shalet, S.M., Blackedge, G. *et al.* The effect of Hodgkin's disease and combination chemotherapy on gonadal function in the adult male. *Cancer*, **49**, 418–422 (1982)
14. Waxman, J.H.X., Terry, Y.A., Wrigley, P.F.M. *et al.* Gonadal function in Hodgkin's disease: long term follow-up of chemotherapy. *British Medical Journal*, **285**, 1612–1613 (1982)
15. Redman, J.R., Bajorunas, D.R., Goldstein, M.C. *et al.* Semen cryopreservation and artificial insemination for Hodgkin's disease. *Journal of Clinical Oncology*, **5**, 233–238 (1987)
16. Fisher, B., Sherman, B., Rockette, H. *et al.* L-Phenylalanine mustard in the management of premenopausal patients with primary breast cancer. *Cancer*, **44**, 847–857 (1979)
17. Siris, E., Leventhal, B.G. and Vaitukaitis, J.L. Effects of childhood leukaemia and chemotherapy on puberty and reproductive function in girls. *New England Journal of Medicine*, **294**, 1143–1146 (1976)
18. Morris, I.D. and Shalet, S.M. Endocrine-mediated protection from cytotoxic-induced testicular damage. *Journal of Endocrinology*, **120**, 7–9 (1989)
19. Maxon, H.R., Thomas, S.R., Saenger, E.L. *et al.* Ionizing irradiation and the induction of clinically significant disease in the human thyroid gland. *American Journal of Medicine*, **63**, 967–978 (1977)
20. DeGroot, L.J., Reilly, M., Pinnameneni, K. and Refetoff, S. Retrospective and prospective study of radiation-induced thyroid disease. *American Journal of Medicine*, **74**, 852–862 (1983)
21. Doniach, I., Kingston, J.E., Plowman, P.N. and Malpas, J.S. The association of post-radiation nodular disease with compensated hypothyroidism. *British Journal of Radiology*, **60**, 1223–1226 (1987)
22. Constine, L.S., Donaldson, S.S., McDougall, I.R. *et al.* Thyroid dysfunction after radiotherapy in children with Hodgkin's disease. *Cancer*, **5**, 878–883 (1984)
23. Lawrence, J.H., Nelson, W.O. and Wilson, H. Roent-

gen irradiation of the hypophysis. *Radiology*, **29**, 446–450 (1937)

24. Shalet, S.M., Beardwell, C.G., Morris-Jones, P. *et al.* Growth hormone deficiency in children with brain tumours. *Cancer*, **37**, 1144–1148 (1976)

25. Shalet, S.M., Beardwell, C.G., MacFarlane, I.A. *et al.* Endocrine morbidity in adults treated with cerebral irradiation for brain tumours during childhood. *Acta Endocrinologica*, **84**, 673–680 (1977)

26. Shalet, S.M., Beardwell, C.G., Pearson, D. and Morris-Jones, P.H. The effect of varying doses of cerebral irradiation on growth hormone production in childhood. *Clinical Endocrinology*, **5**, 287–290 (1976)

27. Shalet, S.M., Beardwell, C.G., Morris-Jones, P.H. and Pearson, D. Growth hormone deficiency after treatment of acute leukaemia in children. *Archives of Disease in Childhood*, **51**, 489–493 (1976)

28. Shalet, S.M., Price, D.A., Beardwell, C.G. *et al.* Normal growth despite abnormalities of growth hormone secretion in children treated for acute leukemia. *Journal of Pediatrics*, **94**, 719–722 (1979)

29. Wells, R.J., Foster, M.B., D'Ercole, A.J. and McMillan, C.W. The impact of cranial irradiation on the growth of children with acute lymphocytic leukaemia. *American Journal of Diseases of Children*, **137**, 37–39 (1987)

30. Starceski, P.J., Lee, P.A., Blatt, J. *et al.* Comparable effects of 100 and 2400 rad (18 and 24 Gy) cranial irradiation on height and weight in children treated for lymphocytic leukaemia. *American Journal of Diseases of Children*, **141**, 550–552 (1987)

31. Cicognani, A., Cacciari, C., Vecchi, V. *et al.* Differential effects of 18 and 24 Gy cranial irradiation on growth rate and growth hormone release in children with prolonged survival after acute lymphocytic leukemia. *American Journal of Diseases of Children*, **142**, 1199–1202 (1988)

32. Blatt, J., Berac, B.B., Gillin, J.C. *et al.* Reduced pulsatile growth hormone secretion in children after therapy for acute lymphoblastic leukaemia. *Journal of Pediatrics*, **104**, 182–186 (1984)

33. Costin, G. Effects of low-dose cranial radiation on growth hormone secretory dynamics and hypothalamic–pituitary function. *American Journal of Diseases of Children*, **142**, 847–852 (1988)

34. Kirk, J.A., Raphupathy, P., Stevens, M.M. *et al.* Growth failure and growth-hormone deficiency after treatment for acute lymphoblastic leukaemia. *Lancet*, **i**, 190–193 (1987)

35. Clayton, P.E., Shalet, S.M., Morris-Jones, P.H. and Price, D.A. Growth in children treated for acute lymphoblastic leukaemia. *Lancet*, **i**, 460–462 (1988)

36. Ahmed, S.R. and Shalet, S.M. Hypothalamic growth hormone releasing factor deficiency following cranial irradiation. *Clinical Endocrinology*, **21**, 483–488 (1984)

37. Blacklay, A., Grossman, A., Savage, M.O. *et al.* Cranial irradiation for cerebral and nasopharyngeal tumours in children – evidence for the production of a hypothalamic defect in growth hormone release. *Journal of Endocrinology*, **108**, 25–29 (1986)

38. Romshe, C.A., Zipf, W.B., Miser, A. *et al.* Evaluation of growth hormone release and human growth treatment in children with cranial irradiation-associated short stature. *Journal of Pediatrics*, **104**, 177–181 (1984)

39. Shalet, S.M., Whitehead, E., Chapman, A.J. and Beardwell, C.G. The effects of growth hormone therapy in children with radiation-induced growth hormone deficiency. *Acta Paediatrica Scandinavica*, **70**, 81–86 (1981)

40. Shalet, S.M., Beardwell, C.G., Aarons, B.M. *et al.* Growth impairment in children treated for brain tumours. *Archives of Disease in Childhood*, **53**, 491–494 (1978)

41. Harrop, J.S., Davies, T.J., Capra, L.G. and Marks, V. Hypothalamic pituitary function following successful treatment of intracranial tumours. *Clinical Endocrinology*, **5**, 313–321 (1976)

42. Lam, K.S.L., Tse, V.K.C., Wang, C. *et al.* Early effects of cranial irradiation on hypothalamic–pituitary function. *Journal of Clinical Endocrinology and Metabolism*, **64**, 418–424 (1987)

43. Samaan, N.A., Vieto, R., Schultz, P.N. *et al.* Hypothalamic, pituitary and thyroid dysfunction after radiotherapy to the head and neck. *International Journal of Radiation Oncology, Biology, Physics*, **8**, 1857–1867 (1982)

44. Huang, K. Assessment of hypothalamic–pituitary function in women after external head irradiation. *Journal of Clinical Endocrinology and Metabolism*, **49**, 623–627 (1979)

45. Rappaport, R., Brauner, P., Czernichow, P. *et al.* Effect of hypothalamic and pituitary irradiation on pubertal development in children with cranial tumours. *Journal of Clinical Endocrinology and Metabolism*, **54**, 1164–1168 (1982)

46. Grossman, A., Cohen, B.L., Charlesworth, M. *et al.* Treatment of prolactinomas with megavoltage radiotherapy. *British Medical Journal*, **288**, 1105–1109 (1984)

47. Grossman, A., Cohen, B.L., Harnett, A.N. *et al.* The effect of megavoltage radiotherapy on prolactinomas. *British Journal of Radiology* (Supplement 22), 27 (1988)

48. Sunderman, C.R. and Pearson, H.A. Growth effects of long-term anti-leukemia therapy. *Journal of Pediatrics*, **75**, 1058–1062 (1969)

# 27

# Psychiatric complications of cancer

E.J. Shakin, E. Heiligenstein and J.C. Holland

Patients show remarkable resilience in their ability to adapt to cancer and its treatment. When the stress related to the diagnosis and treatment of cancer is severe or persistent or when the patient's emotional resources are insufficient, psychological distress may result. When distress interferes with the patient's ability to participate in his treatment or to function adaptively, psychiatric complications may result and evaluation by a mental health professional is warranted.

Most patients with cancer are psychologically healthy. The prevalence of psychiatric disorders in 215 randomly assessed patients from three cancer centers was determined by the Psychosocial Collaborative Oncology Group using the Diagnostic and Statistical Manual-III (DSM-III) classification (see Table 27.1). Almost half of these patients (47%) had clinically significant symptoms that led to a specific psychiatric diagnosis. The remaining 53% were found to be adjusting normally and did not meet the criteria for a specific psychiatric diagnosis; 68% of those with a psychiatric diagnosis had adjustment disorders, i.e. some degree of anxiety and/or depression related to the cancer and its treatment. In fact nearly 90% of the psychiatric disorders (adjustment disorders, organic mental disorders and major depressions) were related to the diagnosis and treatment of cancer. Only 11% represented prior psychiatric problems, primarily personality disorders and anxiety disorders [1].

In a study of 546 patients seen for psychiatric consultation at Memorial Sloan-Kettering Cancer Center (MSKCC), 96% received a DSM-III Axis I diagnosis. The majority of these patients had adjustment disorders (54%); organic mental disorders (20%) and depression (9%) were less common. Axis II personality disorders were present in 17.5% of all patients [2].

**Table 27.1 Rates of DSM-III psychiatric disorders and prevalence of pain observed in 215 cancer patients from three cancer centers**

| Diagnostic category | Number in diagnostic class | Percentage of psychiatric diagnoses | Number with significant pain[a] |
|---|---|---|---|
| Adjustment disorders | 69 (32%) | 68% | |
| Major affective disorders | 13 (6%) | 13% | |
| Organic mental disorders | 8 (4%) | 8% | |
| Personality disorders | 7 (3%) | 7% | |
| Anxiety disorders | 4 (2%) | 4% | |
| Total with psychiatric diagnosis | 101 (47%) | | 39 (39%) |
| Total with no psychiatric diagnosis | 114 (53%) | | 21 (19%) |
| Total patient population | 215 (100%) | | 60 (28%) |

[a]Score greater than 50 mm on a 100 mm VAS for pain severity

In this chapter we describe the common psychiatric syndromes and their treatment in both the adult and child cancer patient. In the adult population these psychiatric complications are described in order of decreasing prevalence. Adjustment disorders with anxiety and/or depression, organic mental disorders, and depressive disorders occur in direct response to illness and are discussed first. The personality disorders, primary anxiety disorders and major mental illnesses are pre-existing conditions that are often exacerbated by illness (see Table 27.2)

**Table 27.2 Common psychiatric disorders in cancer patients**

Disorders directly related to illness:
1. Adjustment disorders:
   Anxiety
   Depression
   Mixed features
2. Major depression
3. Organic mental disorder (delirium)
4. Post-traumatic stress disorder

Pre-existing disorders exacerbated by illness:
1. Anxiety disorders:
   Phobias of needles, hospitals, enclosed spaces
   Panic disorders
   Agoraphobia
   Generalized anxiety
2. Personality disorders
   Paranoid, obsessive, dependent
   Borderline, histrionic
3. Schizophrenia
4. Bipolar disorder

and are, therefore, important in a discussion of the psychiatric complications of cancer.

Interventions for the psychiatric complications of cancer may involve the use of multiple disciplines and may include a variety of techniques, depending on the patient's needs. Psychiatrists, psychologists, psychiatric nurse clinicians, social workers, pastoral counselors and 'veteran' cancer patients may each make important contributions to the patient's psychosocial functioning. Specific interventions are discussed below.

# Psychiatric complications in adults

## Adjustment disorders

The diagnosis of cancer evokes many feelings related to sociocultural, patient-related and medically-related factors (see Table 27.3). Medical factors include tumor site, stage, associated pain,

**Table 27.3 Factors which influence patients' psychological adaptation to cancer**

Medical:
   Tumor site, stage at diagnosis
   Predicted outcome
   Symptoms, functional loss(es)
   Treatment(s) required
   Rehabilitation available
   Clinical course of illness
   Associated medical conditions

Patient-related:
   Level of cognitive and psychological development
   Ability to cope with life crises
   Emotional maturity
   Ability to accept altered or unachieved life goals
   Prior experience with cancer
   Concurrent life crises
   Support of family and others

Societal:
   Attitudes towards cancer and treatment
   Stigma associated with diagnosis
   Health care policy

required treatment(s), rehabilitation, clinical course of illness and associated medical conditions. Sociocultural factors include not only societal attitudes toward cancer and its treatment, but also how the patient perceives himself in light of the stigma associated with the diagnosis. Patient-related factors include the patient's level of cognitive development, ability to cope with stressful events, emotional maturity, disruptions in anticipated life goals, concurrent life stresses, and support from family, friends and others [3]. The psychiatric consultant must evaluate the relative contributions of these factors.

When the patient's emotional resources are inadequate to deal with the stress of the diagnosis and treatment of cancer, a variable degree of anxiety and/or depression may result. This is the most common reason for psychiatric referral. While adjustment disorders are seen in all types of cancer patients, an illustration of the complexity of these reactions is seen in the woman who discovers a lump in her breast. She must deal not only with the potential life-threatening nature of the cancer, but also with the consequences that a mastectomy or lumpectomy may pose in terms of her own self-image, body image, sexual functioning and social relations. She must make important treatment decisions at a time when anxiety is highest [4]. While societal supports have greatly increased in recent years, concurrent life stresses and/or a bad past experience with cancer may increase her stress.

In most cases the patient with an adjustment disorder will return to his normal level of social and occupational functioning soon after the stressor remits. If the stressor persists, the patient will attain a new level of adaptation. In the cancer patient the long duration of various treatments and the recurrent nature of the disease itself may prolong the duration of the maladaptive reaction. In cases where anxiety or depression is severe or persistent, a generalized anxiety disorder or a major depression must be ruled out (see also Depressive disorders and Anxiety disorders below).

### Treatment of adjustment disorders

When either the patient or a staff member perceives that the patient might benefit from psychosocial support to help relieve his/her emotional distress, psychiatric intervention may be sought. Although cancer patients are presumed to be emotionally healthy individuals, the anxiety and depression they experience in relation to their illness may pose several problems for themselves and their physicians. It may contribute to increased delays in seeking treatment and may impair a patient's ability to assimilate useful information from his physicians. This may lead to the breakdown of an adaptive patient–physician relationship and/or actual non-compliance. Interventions may help the patient, family members and staff deal with psychological issues related to or exacerbated by the cancer [5].

Interventions are directed at helping the patient and his family to adapt to ongoing stresses and to resume successful coping. By providing support, information and skills, the mental health professional can help the patient negotiate his way through a complex health care system. The therapist can clarify the medical situation, discuss the meaning of illness and help the patient re-establish appropriate and attainable life goals and expectations. 'Veteran' patients who have survived the cancer experience can reassure the patient that 'it is possible to get through all this'. Group therapy and self-help groups can provide additional information, reinforce positive coping strategies, and create a powerful milieu for sharing experiences. Religious counseling may provide additional support and spiritual guidance during times of emotional crisis. Relaxation, imagery and hypnosis may help reduce anxiety and thereby increase the patient's sense of control. Many of these interventions can also be used in patients with other psychiatric complications of cancer.

If the patient's symptoms warrant further intervention, a trial of benzodiazepines may be useful in controlling symptoms and facilitating other therapeutic interventions. Short-acting benzodiazepines such as lorazepam and alprazolam are commonly used. The fear of causing addiction to these drugs is unwarranted in terminal patients; medications can often be tapered as the stresses subside [6].

## Organic mental syndromes

Organic mental disorder is the second most frequent psychiatric complication of cancer (20% of psychiatric diagnoses in patients seen for psychiatric consultation) [2]. It is also the second most commonly cited reason for psychiatric consultation (18% of requests). The prevalence of delirium in cancer patients is quite variable and has been reported to be from 5 to 85%, depending on severity of illness [7].

The main disturbance in delirium is alteration in attention and disordered thinking [8]. Early symptoms of delirium include changes in the sleep-wake cycle, episodic disorientation, new onset memory loss, mild confusion, irritability, impulsivity and suspiciousness. Consultation requests are often solicited to evaluate 'depression', 'anxiety', or behavior problems. Symptoms progress to frank agitation, sleeplessness, assaultive behavior, delusions and hallucinations, and finally, if left untreated, death. The patient's response is labile, intense, often paranoid, and he may refuse reasonable requests.

Predisposing factors in the development of delirium include pre-existing brain disease, chronic organ dysfunction or failure, current or historic alcohol or drug addiction, environmental factors (sensory deprivation), and certain psychological predispositions. The hospitalized, older, terminal patient is most at risk [9].

In cancer patients indirect (i.e. non-structural) causes of brain dysfunction are the most common reason for delirium. Posner [10] estimates that 15–20% of patients on medical oncology units have cognitive impairments that are not recognized and are due to non-structural causes. Delirium is often related to multiple causes [7]: metabolic encephalopathy from vital organ failure or electrolyte imbalances; infection; vascular abnormalities; nutritional deficiencies; paraneoplastic syndromes; and treatment-related causes (chemotherapeutic agents, anticholinergic agents and radiation; see Table 27.4).

Of all medications, the ones most commonly associated with delirium in the cancer patient are analgesics and steroids. The analgesics most commonly used in the treatment of cancer pain include levorphanol, morphine and meperidine. Confusional states and delirium have often been reported with these agents, especially in the elderly and terminally ill. In addition to causing delirium, corticosteroids can cause minor mood lability, organic anxiety syndrome, organic mood syndrome (mania or depression), organic personality syndrome and dementia (usually reversible). Patients at higher risk for the development of severe symptoms with steroid administration include those on high-dose steroid treatment (>60 mg per day in adults) or those on rapidly tapering schedules. One should

Patients taking multiple medications with anticholinergic side effects may be at increased risk for anticholinergic delirium and a less anticholinergic antidepressant should be considered. Amitriptyline is available in a rectal suppository if the patient is unable to take oral medications. Amitriptyline, imipramine and doxepin can be given intramuscularly.

### Second generation antidepressants and heterocyclic antidepressants

If a patient does not respond to a TCA, or cannot tolerate its side effects, a second generation (trazodone, fluoxetine, buproprion) or heterocyclic (maprotiline, amoxapine) antidepressant can be used. The heterocyclic compounds have side effect profiles that are similar to the TCAs. Maprotiline should be avoided in patients with seizure disorders. The second generation antidepressants are generally considered to be less cardiotoxic than the TCAs [25]. Buproprion may be somewhat activating in medically ill patients, and trazodone is strongly sedating. Trazodone has been associated with priapism and should, therefore, be used with caution in male patients.

### Monoamine oxidase inhibitors (MAOIs)

A history of response to a MAOI may make these agents a logical choice in treating depression in the cancer patient. The actual use of MAOIs, however, is generally less well received as they impose further dietary restrictions on the patient who may already have nutritional deficiencies and dietary restrictions related to cancer. They are absolutely contraindicated in patients receiving meperidine and should be used cautiously in patients receiving other narcotics because of hypertensive reactions. Sympatheticomimetic agents and the chemotherapeutic agent procarbazine (also an MAOI) can cause hypertensive crises when used in combination with an MAOI.

### Psychostimulants

Dextroamphetamine and methylphenidate promote a sense of well-being, decrease fatigue, and stimulate appetite at low doses in cancer patients. Treatment is usually initiated at a dose of 2.5–5.0 mg at 8 a.m. and noon. The advantage is a rapid onset of action as compared with the TCAs. Some patients have been maintained on methylphenidate for up to a year without evidence of tolerance or abuse [26]. They potentiate the analgesic effects of the narcotic analgesics, while at the same time counteract unwanted daytime sedation. Occasionally they can produce nightmares, insomnia and even psychosis.

### Lithium

Lithium should be continued in patients who were maintained on it prior to the diagnosis of cancer. Medically ill patients may require lower therapeutic doses, and levels must be carefully monitored in patients undergoing rapid changes in fluid balance. It should be used cautiously in patients receiving other nephrotoxic agents (e.g. cisplatin). Lithium has been used to stimulate granulocyte production in neutropenic patients [27]. The leukocytosis is transient, however, and the functional capacity of these granulocytes has not been determined. No effect of lithium on mood has been reported in these patients.

### Benzodiazepines

The triazolobenzodiazepine alprazolam is effective in treating both anxiety and depression in cancer patients. Treatment is initiated with doses of 0.25 mg three times a day and titrated up to effective antidepressant doses, usually from 4 to 6 mg per day. The initial elan among physicians prescribing this drug has abated somewhat as patients find it difficult to taper off alprazolam. Abrupt discontinuation of alprazolam can lead to seizures.

### Electroconvulsive treatment (ECT)

ECT is useful when depression is life-threatening or accompanied by psychotic features, or if the patient's medical condition prohibits the use of antidepressant medication. Its effectiveness in treatment of depression in the medically ill has been well documented. Its use is contraindicated in patients with central nervous system tumors.

## Personality disorders

Patients with personality disorders have longstanding impairments in occupational or social functioning or experience ongoing subjective distress. Their maladaptive coping styles interfere with the ability to deal with the stress of cancer and its treatments. They tend to be inflexible in the face of the changing demands of their illness and its treatments. Staff often describe these patients as frustrating and difficult. The borderline patient will be unable to conform to hospital rules and will manipulate and polarize staff. The narcissistic patient may demand excessive attention that staff are unable to gratify. The dependent patient may require reassurance and support for even minor symptoms. The paranoid patient may make insinuations about a staff member's motives and threaten litigation. These behavior patterns cannot be significantly changed with psychiatric interventions during the crisis of medical illness. The mental health professional can, however, help the staff to understand the emotional distress underlying behavior and provide useful strategies for minimizing disruption of the medical ward.

## Treatment of personality disorders

The first goal of the psychiatric consultant is to identify the patient's habitual means of dealing with stress and to assess how it is interfering with his/her treatment. Legitimate complaints can be addressed via appropriate channels. Other complaints may reflect the patient's underlying emotional distress and character style. One staff member, preferably the patient's primary physician, should communicate all treatment decisions to the patient. Meetings should be held with all disciplines present to discuss the underlying motives for patients' behaviors and to plan logical approaches to managing disruptive behavior. The patient's medical problems and treatment plan should be outlined for all staff who are involved with the patient on a day-to-day basis. Priorities should be set to avoid power struggles between staff and patients. For example, a dependent patient may be allowed extended visiting time to decrease his anxiety and preserve staff resources. If the patient is self-destructive or assaultive, a 24 h companion can be ordered. This is often reassuring to both the patient and the staff. Finally, the psychiatric consultant may wish to reduce the patient's emotional distress with the use of psychotropic medication.

## Anxiety

Although 'anxiety' was the third most commonly cited reason (16%) for psychiatric consultation in the series reported by MSKCC, anxiety disorders were present in only 4% of the patients seen. This discrepancy is in part accounted for by other psychiatric disorders that include anxiety as a symptom. In fact, an additional 28% of patients had adjustment disorder, either with anxious mood or with mixed emotions [2].

In the cancer patient there are three basic sources of anxiety. Anxiety may be related to the diagnosis of cancer and the treatment it requires. It may have a physical cause such as an endocrine disturbance or a medication. Alternatively, it may be part of a long-standing problem that predates the cancer diagnosis, but is exacerbated during the course of treatment (panic disorder, generalized anxiety disorder, phobias).

Anxiety is commonly associated with various stages of illness and with specific treatments. For example, women completing radiation therapy for breast cancer often report increased anxiety at the end of treatment. This is frequently related to increased fears of recurrence without active treatment and to withdrawal of daily monitoring and reassurance by medical staff [28]. Similar issues exist for other types of cancer. The psychiatric consultant must determine if the anxiety is interfering with the patient's functioning and ability to cooperate with treatment. Psychotherapeutic interventions and/or anxiolytics are often helpful in patients who are not reassured by their primary physicians (see also Adjustment disorders).

Organic anxiety syndromes in adults with cancer are commonly related to pain, respiratory distress and a variety of medications. Patients in acute pain are often quite anxious and respond best to adequate pain control. The patient with respiratory distress responds well to oxygen and mild sedation.

The use of corticosteroids is often accompanied by anxiety and insomnia which can be treated with benzodiazepines. Patients in early stages of delirium and dementia may also appear anxious (see Organic mental syndromes). Withdrawal from alcohol and other drugs is often overlooked as a cause of anxiety, and the physician must be alerted to this during the first days of admission or if the patient is unable to take oral medications. Akathisia from antiemetics is commonly mistaken for anxiety or agitation and responds well to oral or parenteral lorazepam. Other medical conditions that should be considered in the differential diagnosis of anxiety include carcinoid, pheochromocytoma, hyperthyroidism, mitral valve prolapse, and primary and metastatic brain tumors.

Panic disorders, generalized anxiety disorders and phobias are distinguished from the other anxiety disorders as being long-lasting, often antedating the cancer diagnosis. They are characterized by the extreme fear of losing control and of being overwhelmed by various circumstances. Panic disorder occurs with or without agoraphobia and consists of unexpected, sudden anxiety attacks that are accompanied by shortness of breath, paresthesias, chest pain, palpitations, nausea and fear of dying. The patient with agoraphobia may require a family member to accompany him to procedures, to surgery, or even to come to the hospital. Patients with generalized anxiety disorder have excessive, pervasive and unrealistic anxiety that is manifested by motor tension, autonomic hyperactivity and an increased state of alertness. In the medical setting they tend to anticipate complications of treatment and fear that staff will not pay sufficient attention to their symptoms. Patients with specific phobias may avoid medical consultations and procedures because of severe anxiety. Patients with claustrophobia, for example, often report severe anxiety while in scanning devices. Relaxation and distraction techniques are often helpful in decreasing anxiety prior to procedures [29].

Post-traumatic stress disorder (PTSD) may ante-date the diagnosis of cancer or may be a result of particularly painful or frightening procedures. Symptoms often develop at the time of diagnosis and can elicit feelings about earlier traumas. PTSD results from a traumatic experience which is persistently re-experienced by a hypervigilant patient in a distressing and intrusive manner (nightmares, intrusive thoughts). Patients either avoid stimuli that they associate with the trauma or experience a sense of emotional detachment. PTSD has been described in adult cancer patients who are holocaust survivors.

## Treatment of anxiety disorders

Treatment of the anxiety disorders includes long-term behavioral interventions (e.g. relaxation techniques for needle phobias) and short-term psychopharmacological interventions. The mainstay of psychopharmacological intervention is the benzodiazepines. Other medications that can also be considered include antipsychotics, antihistamines, beta blockers and antidepressants.

### Benzodiazepines

The choice of benzodiazepine is dependent on desired half-life, route of administration, route of metabolism and presence or absence of active metabolites (see Table 27.6). In the medically ill patient drugs with shorter half-lives that have multiple routes of administration and no active metabolites are preferable. In patients with impaired liver function or patients taking other medications that are metabolized via the liver's oxidation system, the conjugated benzodiazepines are preferred (lorazepam, oxazepam and temazepam). Lorazepam is commonly chosen because it is short-acting, can be given orally or parenterally, and has no active metabolites; also, its metabolism is not altered by advanced age. The starting dose is determined by the degree of anxiety, the patient's hepatic and respiratory impairment, and the concurrent use of other central nervous system (CNS) depressants. Benzodiazepines can be prescribed if needed prior to procedures. For more long-standing anxiety, an around-the-clock schedule should be established. Unwanted sedation may diminish over time while anxiety remains under control on a constant dose. Persistent side effects of drowsiness, motor incoordination and confusion necessitate dose reduction or discontinuation. Behavioral disinhibition is rarely noted. These drugs should be tapered to avoid withdrawal phenomena.

### Other anxiolytics

In patients who do not respond to the benzodiazepines or who have cognitive impairments that make them more vulnerable to benzodiazepine-related confusion, a neuroleptic may be more useful in decreasing anxiety. Antihistamines are less effective anxiolytics but can be used in patients with respiratory compromise. Panic disorders have been treated with alprazolam, TCAs and MAOIs. Propranolol is useful in blocking the autonomic manifestations of panic. TCAs are also used in the treatment of PTSDs [5,6].

## Major mental illness

Schizophrenia and bipolar disorders make up 5% of the psychiatric diagnoses of patients seen for psychiatric consultation [2]. Although these conditions usually predate the onset of cancer, it is important to consider them in a discussion of the psychiatric complications of cancer because they are

**Table 27.6 Commonly prescribed benzodiazepines in cancer patients**

| Drug | Approximate dose equivalent | Initial oral dosage (mg) | Elimination half-life drug metabolites (h) | Active metabolite |
|---|---|---|---|---|
| Short-acting: | | | | |
| Alprazolam | 0.5 | 0.25–0.5 t.i.d. | 10–15 | Yes |
| Oxazepam | 10.0 | 10–15 t.i.d. | 5–15 | No |
| Lorazepam | 1.0 | 0.5–2.0 t.i.d. | 10–20 | No |
| Intermediate-acting: | | | | |
| Chlordiazepoxide | 10.0 | 10–25 t.i.d. | 10–40 | Yes |
| Long-acting: | | | | |
| Diazepam | 5.0 | 5–10 b.i.d. | 20–100 | Yes |
| Clorazepate | 7.5 | 7.5–15 b.i.d. | 30–200 | Yes |

often exacerbated by either the diagnosis of cancer or its treatments.

### Schizophrenia and its treatment

It is unusual for the first episode of schizophrenia to occur in a cancer patient. New onset psychosis in the young cancer patient is most commonly due to CNS complications of the disease and its treatment (e.g. steroid psychosis) or to drug or alcohol withdrawal or intoxication.

When the schizophrenic patient develops cancer, he may experience problems in several areas. First, patients with schizophrenia may respond inappropriately to warning symptoms of cancer and may delay coming for medical attention until their cancer is already quite advanced. Second, delusional beliefs may compromise understanding of illness and proposed treatment. Bizarre symptoms may not be recognized as cancer in the context of acute psychosis. Physicians must give special attention to issues of informed consent and competence. Third, paranoid distrust may interfere with expression of appropriate complaints of pain and discomfort. Fourth, they may have limited ability to participate in their care, especially at home where compliance is difficult to monitor.

Compliance can be optimized by the formation of a coordinated effort on the part of the family, physician, social worker, nurse and other medical staff. Early intervention by a psychiatric consultant can serve to assess the patient's understanding of his illness and proposed treatments, to educate staff about anticipated difficulties with treatment, and to monitor psychotropic medications. Medications may need to be raised under periods of acute stress or to be given by alternative routes if the patient cannot take oral medications.

### Bipolar illness and its treatment

Patients who have pre-existing bipolar disorder are at risk for relapse of their psychiatric symptoms under the stress of physical illness. Continuation of prophylactic lithium treatment is necessary during treatment for cancer (see p. 428). Episodes of acute mania often require the addition of an antipsychotic agent. Regular psychiatric care with appropriate psychopharmacological intervention can effectively reduce the morbidity and disruption caused by manic episodes.

# Psychiatric complications in children

The transition of pediatric cancer during the 1950s and 1960s from a neglected and hopeless illness to one of potential cure has generated interest in all aspects of the disease. In particular, there has been increased awareness of childhood cancer patients' emotional issues. Contributing to this were characteristics of general pediatrics such as concerns with comprehensive health care, acknowledgement of psychosocial influences on childhood development and the importance of the human aspects of medicine.

The child psychiatrist involved in pediatric consultation is frequently asked to diagnose and treat the psychiatric complications of pediatric cancer. These problems are not unique to tertiary care centers as more children with cancer are treated in the community and often spend the terminal phase of their illness at local hospitals.

## Adjustment disorders in children

Mild depression and anxiety in children with cancer are frequent responses to identifiable stressors and are not signs of underlying psychopathology. Adjustment symptoms are often evident when treatment is perceived to be worse than the disease. Common stressors include physical changes, such as alopecia and scarification, which serve as constant reminders of illness. Frequent clinic visits and hospitalizations disrupt a child's social life and most experience a decline in school performance or develop school phobia [30,31]. Hospital classes and home tutoring are offered by many school districts but the limited time available and discontinuity with teachers and peers diminishes the incentive for many children.

The acute and chronic uncertainty of childhood cancer poses significant stressors for the family. Initial reactions of anger, grief, hostility, guilt and disbelief remain prominent [32–34]. The diagnosis of cancer in a child is connected with death despite recent changes in prognosis of some neoplasms. Intellectual understanding does little to decrease parents' distress and fears. Parents must accept the rigors of treatment with no guarantee of success.

The chronicity of illness alters all aspects of family life. The parents' goals, wishes and expectations for their child and themselves are forever changed. The diagnosis of cancer in a child will most likely aggravate already existing family problems. However, the likelihood of divorce is not increased and couples are not usually brought closer together [35].

Adjustment disorders in children rarely require long-term individual or family therapy interventions. The preferred treatment goal is crisis intervention during the period of acute stress rather than achievement of long-term psychological changes. Adjustment issues that appear to be appropriate for individual child therapy include separation anxieties, self-esteem issues related to treatment (amputation, peer relations, sexual identity), and depression and anxiety resulting from diagnosis, relapse or prolonged hospitalization. Therapeutic interventions with parents are indicated to mediate family–staff conflicts, to reduce parental conflict that interferes with treatment objectives or quality of life, or to facilitate parental decision-making.

Technical problems related to individual psychotherapy in children with cancer are related to the realities of the treatment setting. The difficulties in performing psychotherapy on a hospital ward are self-evident. Lack of privacy, competition for time, and the degree of medical illness require the therapist to exhibit a great deal of flexibility and creativity. Playrooms make toys and activities commonplace. The therapist needs to determine what tools will best suit the therapeutic goals. Simplicity is usually the best approach and allows treatment to occur in a compromised setting. Often sessions cannot be planned and the therapist must use spontaneous meetings or impromptu interactions for therapeutic purposes.

## Organic mental syndromes in children

Organic mental syndromes are the most common psychiatric complications in children with cancer. Case reports frequently describe mental status changes from corticosteroids. Other chemotherapy agents are rarely cited. However, relatively little research has been performed to document these changes. The affective and neuropsychiatric effects of corticosteroids in children with other medical illnesses, particularly asthma, have resulted in increased symptoms of depression, anxiety and impaired verbal memory [36]. Children on doses greater than 40 mg/day appear to be at risk. Dramatic steroid-mediated psychiatric disturbances appear to be rare.

There are numerous recognized causes of delirium in children (Table 27.4). The syndrome generally presents with mood changes, emotional lability, social withdrawal and apathy. Medical staff concerns are consequently focused on depression or behavior problems but formal mental status examination reveals changes in attention, memory and concentration characteristic of delirium. For children of 6–12 years of age, we have developed a screening instrument, the Children's Cognitive Capacity Screening Examination (Figure 27.1), to quantify these deficits (Heiligenstein, Hamburg and Bowen, unpublished data).

Although delirium in children requires specific medical interventions, interim symptomatic treatment may be necessary. Children with 'quiet' delirium usually do not require psychopharmacological management. General care should include sensory stimulation to avoid sensory deprivation effects, provision of familiar stimuli such as family and use of companions to ensure patient safety, and proper nursing care. For patients who are agitated, overtly confused or hallucinating, or who represent a danger to themselves, high-potency neuroleptics such as haloperidol are effective. The safety record of haloperidol is excellent, as it has little effect on heart rate, blood pressure, respiration or cardiac output. Intravenous doses of 0.5 mg for children and 1.0 mg for adolescents may be repeated every 30 min. Dystonic reactions are uncommon but can be treated with anticholinergic agents such as diphenhydramine or benzotropine. If psychotic symptoms are reduced but agitation remains problematic, low-dose benzodiazepines (lorazepam 0.5–1.0 mg intravenously) can be added.

## Depressive disorders in children

Children with cancer are frequently referred for evaluation of sadness and depression. Mood disturbances resulting from a medical etiology (organic mood syndromes) are frequently misdiagnosed as 'depressive reactions' to cancer. However, the rarity of prepubertal major depressive disorder (depression without a medical etiology) mandates a thorough evaluation of potential medical etiologies that could lead to depressive symptoms. Prepubertal depressive disorder should be considered in children with a previous episode of depression prior to the diagnosis of cancer or with a history of affective disorders in a first- or second-degree relative.

The clinical features of depression in children with cancer include depressed mood, irritability, crying, anhedonia, social withdrawal, and morbid or suicidal ideation. The neurovegetative symptoms of depression (including sleep and appetite disturbances, fatigue, psychomotor retardation and physical complaints) have been found to overlap with symptoms of physical illness, thus limiting their diagnostic usefulness [37].

The distinctive feature of an organic mood syndrome is the presence of a specific medical etiology felt to be responsible for the depressive symptoms. In children with cancer these can include acute or chronic pain, chronic nausea, physical disability, and a wide variety of medications. Multiple agents are frequently responsible and a causal relationship between a specific factor and the onset of depression may be difficult to determine.

In addition to etiology, organic mood syndromes differ from prepubertal depressive disorders in natural history. Whereas prepubertal depressive disorders are unlikely to resolve either spontaneously or quickly, organic mood syndromes do remit quickly once the specific factor is removed. This is best seen in children with depression due to poorly treated acute pain. Proper analgesia with

Name:                                                    Chart #:

Age:                                                     Date of test:

Check items answered correctly.

*Instructions:*  "I would like to ask you a few questions. Some you will find very easy and others may be
                  hard. Just do your best."

"Let's see how many different animals you can think of before I say stop. You know, like cat and dog.
Ready, go." (Time for 20 seconds and record *all different* responses. ***Scoring:*** Child names 7 animals: check
#s 1, 2 and 3)

|     |                                                                              |            |
|-----|------------------------------------------------------------------------------|------------|
| 1)  | 5 animals                                                                    | __________ |
| 2)  | 6 animals                                                                    | __________ |
| 3)  | 7 animals                                                                    | __________ |
| 4)  | 8 animals                                                                    | __________ |
| 5)  | 9 animals                                                                    | __________ |
| 6)  | Repeat the numbers: 8, 7, 2.                                                  | __________ |
| 7)  | Say them backwards                                                           | __________ |
| 8)  | Repeat these numbers: 9, 6, 3, 1                                              | __________ |
| 9)  | An apple and an orange are both fruits. Red and blue are both ___________     | __________ |
| 10) | A penny and a dime are both ___________                                      | __________ |
| 11) | A table is made of wood; a window is made of ___________                     | __________ |

Three item recall. "Remember these three things: car, pencil, sixteen. I will ask for them later."

|     |                                                                              |            |
|-----|------------------------------------------------------------------------------|------------|
| 12) | What number is left out: 1-2-3-4-5-7-8-9                                      | __________ |
| 13) | When I say 5, 10, 20 . . . what comes next?                                   | __________ |
| 14) | How many 5-cent candy bars can you buy for a dime?                           | __________ |
| 15) | Carol was invited to a 3 o'clock party. She got there are 3:30. Was she early or late?__________ |

What were the things that I asked you to remember?

|     |                                                                              |            |
|-----|------------------------------------------------------------------------------|------------|
| 16) | Object #1                                                                     | __________ |
| 17) | Object #2                                                                     | __________ |
| 18) | Object #3                                                                     | __________ |
| 19) | If you have 9 pennies and lose 2 of them, how many will you have left?        | __________ |
| 20) | If I went to the store and bought a dozen apples, how many would that be?     | __________ |

Total Correct (maximum score = 20): ________

IF SCORE <13, SUSPECT DIMINISHED COGNITIVE CAPACITY

**Figure 27.1** Children's Cognitive Capacity Screening Exam

subsequent pain control can lead to resolution of depressive symptoms in days.

Previous reports of rapid improvement in childhood depressive disorders with low-dose tricyclic antidepressants may be more a reflection of the natural history of an organic mood syndrome than drug effect [38]. As a consequence, the pharmacological treatment of this group of depressive syndromes should only be considered if other interventions have failed. Due to less promising results in the treatment of depression in healthy children with tricyclic antidepressants, the psychostimulants may be a potential alternative.

## Anxiety disorders in children

Between 25% and 65% of children become sensitized to cancer chemotherapy and develop aversive symptoms [39]. Cognitive symptoms of aversion are described by children as feelings of hopelessness, insomnia, anxiety and dysphoria. Parents report behavioral changes such as social withdrawal, sad faces, anticipatory nausea and vomiting, and intense fear or panic. The symptoms become noticeable 1–2 days prior to clinic visits and diminish over the next few days. It is not unusual for parents to use physical force to maintain appointments.

Chemotherapy-related nausea and vomiting are frequently exacerbated. Non-compliance is a problem associated with aversive symptoms and can be a vehicle for maladaptive coping for both the patient and family. This can involve use of unorthodox therapies and unilateral decisions to stop treatment.

Post-traumatic stress disorder (PTSD) is a specific type of anxiety due to the effects of trauma. Such stressors include life-threatening illness. Recall of prior painful or frightening treatment is a common cause of PTSD in children with cancer. Illness can also exacerbate feelings about earlier traumas. This has been noted in childhood cancer patients who have been subjected to physical abuse. In the child with cancer, symptoms can develop at various stages of illness but are frequent at the time of diagnosis or following intensive care unit admissions. Variables that appear important in the development of the disorder are biological vulnerability to stressful events and severity of the stressor. Most important may be the developing emotional state of children which prevents them from using various adaptive strategies in dealing with trauma.

The typical presenting symptoms include frequent unwanted recollections of the stressful event (nightmares, intrusive thoughts) along with affective blunting. Children rarely experience a numbing response to the environment, often responding with anxiety, restlessness, hyperalertness, repetitive play and difficulty in concentrating. Use of denial is prominent and minimizes the painful event. The non-specific emotional symptoms can make the diagnosis difficult to distinguish from a generalized anxiety disorder, depression or panic disorder. Questions about intrusive phenomena assist in determining the specific diagnosis and many children are relieved to understand their symptoms are an expected response to severe stress. As a consequence, the psychiatric consultation can often have a major therapeutic impact.

Reduction of anxiety symptoms in children is crucial and can facilitate a sense of trust and optimism in the patient and family which can minimize maladjustment. Beneficial interventions for aversive symptoms include relaxation techniques, hypnosis, or cognitive distraction [39]. If symptom reduction is partially obtained, these techniques can be combined with anti-anxiety medications. Lorazepam at 0.5–1.0 mg orally q.i.d. can be started on the day symptoms are noted, with additional doses before the trip to the hospital or in the waiting area. The medication is continued for 1–2 days following the clinic visit and then stopped. The reduction in symptoms and decrease in chemotherapy-related side effects can be marked [40]. Treatment of PTSD can involve use of cognitive distraction techniques, supportive psychotherapy and judicious trials of benzodiazepines.

# Conclusions

Observations of the psychiatric complications of cancer in adults and children outlined above indicate the new interest in both the identification and management of these psychological consequences of cancer treatment. Research which further defines and tests effective therapies is needed in this new field of psycho-oncology.

# References


1. Derogatis, L.R., Morrow, G.R., Fetting, J. *et al.* The prevalence of psychiatric disorders among cancer patients. *Journal of the American Medical Association*, **249**, 751–757 (1983)
2. Massie, M.J. and Holland, J.C. Consultation and liaison issues in cancer care. *Psychiatric Medicine*, **5**, 343–359 (1987)
3. Rowland, J. Intrapersonal resources: coping. In *Psychological Care of the Patient with Cancer: A Handbook of Psycho-Oncology* (eds J.C. Holland and J. Rowland), Oxford University Press, New York, pp. 44–57 (1989)
4. Scott, D.W. Anxiety, critical thinking and information processing during and after breast biopsy. *Nursing Research*, **32**, 24 (1983)
5. Massie, M.J., Heiligenstein, E.L., Lederberg, M. and Holland, J.C. Psychiatric care of the cancer patient. In *Textbook of Clinical Oncology*, American Cancer Society, New York (1990) (in press)
6. Breitbart, W. and Holland, J.C. Psychiatric complications of cancer. *Current Therapy in Hematology-Oncology*, **3**, 268–274 (1988)
7. Massie, M.J., Holland, J. and Glass, E. Delirium in terminally ill cancer patients. *American Journal of Psychiatry*, **140**, 1048–1050 (1983)
8. Fleischman, C. and Lesko, L.M. Delirium and dementia. In *Psychological Care of the Patient with Cancer: A Handbook of Psycho-Oncology* (eds J.C. Holland and J.H. Rowland), Oxford University Press, New York, pp. 342–355 (1989)
9. Slaby, A.E. and Cullen, L.O. Dementia and delirium. In *Principles of Medical Psychiatry* (eds A. Stoudemire and B.S. Fogel), Grune and Stratton, New York, pp. 135–176 (1987)
10. Posner, J.B. Neurologic complications of systemic cancer. *Disease-a-Month*, **25**, 1–60 (1978)
11. Menza, M.A., Murray, G.B., Holmes, V.F. and Rafulo, W.A. Decreased extrapyramidal symptoms with intravenous haloperidol. *Journal of Clinical Psychiatry*, **48**, 278–280 (1987)
12. Stoudemire, A. and Fogel, B.S. (eds). *Principles of Medical Psychiatry*, Grune and Stratton, New York (1987)
13. Bukberg, J.B., Penman, D.T. and Holland, J.C. Depression in hospitalized cancer patients. *Psychosomatic Medicine*, **46**, 199–212 (1984)

14. Plumb, M. and Holland, J.C. Comparative studies of psychological function in patients with advanced cancer: I. Self-reported depressive symptoms. *Psychosomatic Medicine*, **39**, 264–276 (1977)

15. Holland, J.C., Hughes-Korzun, A., Tross, S. *et al.* Comparative psychological disturbance in pancreatic and gastric cancer. *American Journal of Psychiatry*, **143**, 982–986 (1986)

16. Shakin, E.J. and Holland, J.C. Depression and pancreatic cancer. *Journal of Pain Symptom Management*, **3**, 194–198 (1988)

17. Breitbart, W. Suicide in cancer patients. *Oncology*, **1**, 49–53 (1987)

18. Breitbart, W. Suicide in cancer patients. In *Psychological Care of the Patient with Cancer: A Handbook of Psycho-Oncology* (eds J.C. Holland and J.H. Rowland), Oxford University Press, New York, pp. 291–299 (1989)

19. Holland, J., Farsanello, S. and Ohnuma, T. Psychiatric symptoms associated with L-asparaginase administration. *Journal of Psychiatric Research*, **10**, 165 (1974)

20. Editorial. Drugs that cause psychiatric symptoms, *Medical Letter*, **28**, 81–86 (1986)

21. Editorial. Cancer chemotherapy. *Medical Letter*, **29**, 29–36 (1987)

22. Massie, M.J. and Holland, J.C. The cancer patient with pain: psychiatric complications and their management. *Medical Clinics of North America*, **71**, 243–258 (1987)

23. Lipsey, J.R., Robinson, R.G., Pearlson, G.D. *et al.* Nortriptyline treatment of post-stroke depression: a double-blind study. *Lancet*, **i**, 297–300 (1984)

24. Rifkin, A., Reardon, G., Siris, S. *et al.* Trimipramine in physical illness with depression. *Journal of Clinical Psychiatry*, **46**, 4–8 (1985)

25. Glassman, A.H. The newer antidepressant drugs and their cardiovascular effects. *Psychopharmacology Bulletin*, **20**, 272–279 (1984)

26. Fernandez, F., Adams, F., Holmes, V.F. *et al.* Methylphenidate for depressive disorders in cancer patients. *Psychosomatics*, **28**, 455–461 (1987)

27. Lyman, G.H., Williams, C. and Preston, D. The use of lithium carbonate to reduce infection and leukopenia during systemic chemotherapy. *New England Journal of Medicine*, **302**, 257–260 (1988)

28. Holland, J.C., Rowland, J., Lebovits, A. and Rusalem, R. Reactions to cancer treatment: assessment of emotional response to adjuvant radiotherapy as a guide to planned interventions. *Psychiatry Clinics of North America*, **2**, 347 (1979)

29. Massie, M.J. Anxiety, panic and phobias. In *A Handbook of Psycho-Oncology: Psychological Care of the Patient with Cancer* (eds J.C. Holland and J.H. Rowland), Oxford University Press, New York, pp. 300–309 (1989)

30. Lansky, S.B., Lowman, J.T., Vats, T. and Gyulay, J.E. School phobia in children with malignant neoplasms. *American Journal of Diseases of Children*, **129**, 42–46 (1975)

31. Deasy-Spinetta, P. The school and the child with cancer. In *Living with Childhood Cancer* (eds J.J. Spinetta and P. Deasy-Spinetta), C.V. Mosby, St. Louis, pp. 158–168 (1981)

32. Lascari, A.D. and Stehberns, J.A. The reactions of families to childhood leukemia. *Clinical Pediatrics*, **12**, 210–214 (1973)

33. Chodoff, P., Friedman, S.B. and Hamburg, D.A. Stress, defenses and coping behavior: observations in parents of children with malignant diseases. *American Journal of Psychiatry*, **120**, 743–749 (1964)

34. Powazek, M., Schijving, J., Goff, J.R. *et al.* Psychosocial ramifications of childhood leukemia: One year post-diagnosis. In *The Child with Cancer* (eds J.L. Schulman and M.J. Kupat), Charles C. Thomas, Springfield, Illinois, pp. 143–155 (1980)

35. Lansky, S.B., Cairns, N.U., Hassannein, R. *et al.* Childhood cancer: parent discord and divorce. *Pediatrics*, **62**, 184–188 (1978)

36. Bender, B.G., Lerner, J.A. and Kollasch, E. Mood and memory changes in asthmatic children receiving corticosteroids. *Journal of the American Academy of Child and Adolescent Psychiatry*, **27**, 720–725 (1988)

37. Heiligenstein, E. and Jacobsen, P.B. Differentiating depression in medically ill children and adolescents. *Journal of the American Academy of Child and Adolescent Psychiatry*, **27**, 716–719 (1988)

38. Pfefferbaum, B. Common psychiatric disorders in childhood cancer and their management. In *Psychological Care of the Patient with Cancer: A Handbook of Psycho-Oncology* (eds J.C. Holland and J.H. Rowland), Oxford University Press, New York, pp. 544–561 (1989)

39. Redd, W.H. Anticipatory nausea and vomiting and their management. In *Psychological Care of the Patient with Cancer: A Handbook of Psycho-Oncology* (eds J.C. Holland and J.H. Rowland), Oxford University Press, New York, pp. 423–433 (1989)

40. Greenberg, D.B., Suzman, O.S., Clarke, J. and Baer, L. Alprazolam for phobic nausea and vomiting related to cancer chemotherapy. *Cancer Chemotherapy Reports*, **71**, 549–550 (1987)

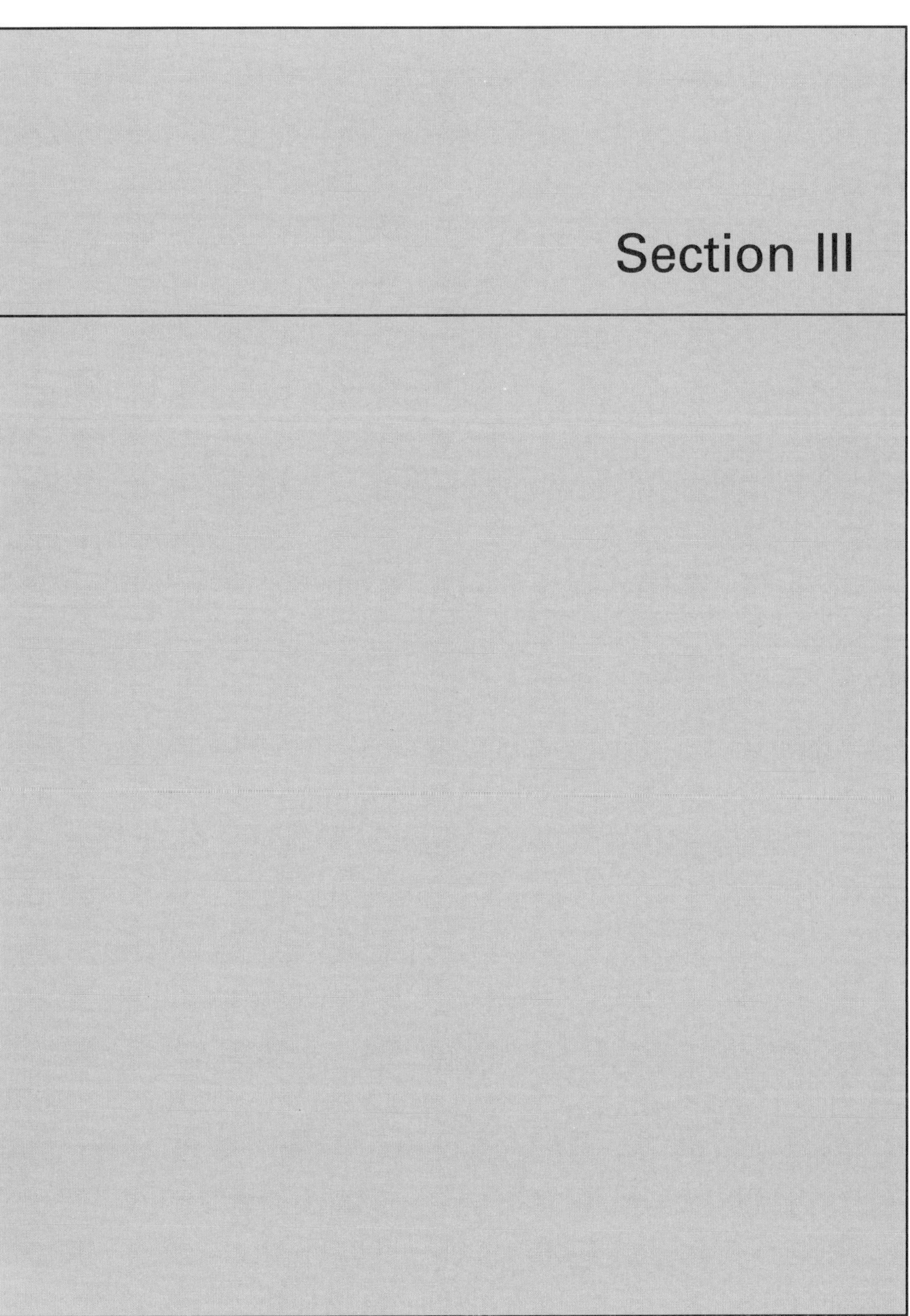
Section III

# 28

# Adaptation after radical gastrointestinal surgery

S. Raimes and H.B. Devlin

To cure rarely, to relieve sometimes, to comfort always.
'Hippocratic' maxim

Surgery remains the treatment of choice for most gastrointestinal cancers; it is at present the only treatment that has the potential to cure the patient. Gastrointestinal malignancies have often spread beyond the primary organ by the time the patient presents, however, if spread is confined to adjacent organs or to local, and even regional, lymph nodes then complete excision is possible. Curative surgery, therefore, has usually to be radical and by definition includes excision of the cancer together with as wide a margin of normal tissue as possible and as much of the lymphatic drainage as is feasible. Radical surgery along these lines remains controversial, but the weight of evidence shows that it is a decisive factor in the attainment of cure for some gastrointestinal malignancies.

Many patients cannot be cured by radical surgery, though this may not be apparent at the time of surgery. When there are metastases to other organs, in particular the liver, surgery cannot bring about a cure. For these patients the most we can do is to provide the best palliation possible. Realizing this fact we have to decide whether the benefit to the patient from a major surgical procedure is worthwhile in terms of survival and, more importantly, to their quality of life. Unfortunately quality of life is a difficult concept to define and it is apparent that there remains a conflict between a scientific approach to cancer surgery and a humanistic one [1].

The gastrointestinal tract has a fundamental role in the ingestion, digestion and absorption of food. The upper tract is particularly important in the assimilating of nutrients and operations on this part of the gastrointestinal system have effects on nutrition. Radical surgery of the upper gastrointestinal tract may lead to weight loss and deficiencies of vital vitamins and minerals due to either malabsorption of food or to the physiological effects caused by the anatomical derangement that results from the surgery. These derangements are different for each operation and it is important to be aware of the pathophysiology associated with these procedures in order to understand and treat the resulting side effects.

In contrast the lower gastrointestinal tract is largely involved in the elimination of wastes and unused foodstuffs. This requires a complex and coordinated physiological process that is ultimately under conscious control. The act of defaecation is a uniquely private one and is a 'taboo' subject for most people. The rectum and anal canal are the most important parts for control of defaecation and the side effects of their removal with the need for a colostomy are, understandably, predominantly psychological in contrast to the side effects of surgery to the upper tract which are predominantly physiological. The loss of the ability to control defaecation and the change in the patient's body image caused by the stoma may have profound effects on their psyche.

Radical surgery for cancer causes side effects that are specific to each procedure and also effects that are common to any major surgical procedure. The patient may sense a loss of personal dignity after major surgery; the need for a stoma exacerbates this further. The knowledge that the operation was for malignancy itself produces anxiety, fear and even depression. When the prognosis is guarded, as it often is for gastrointestinal cancers, this inevitably heightens the anxiety. Even when the patient is given a good prognosis the diagnosis of cancer induces a degree of uncertainty. It is common for patients to underplay their postoperative side effects because their dominant fear is disease progression and any unusual symptoms invoke a fear of recurrent disease. The psychological and physiological consequences of these radical operations are interrelated and may interact; for instance, the patient who is depressed will tend to eat less and thus further compromise their nutrition. Many patients develop a sense of dependence on their surgeon and this is accompanied by a fear of displeasing him. The patient may, therefore, appear passive, uncomplaining and overly cooperative at follow-up visits while they actually have problems that are markedly diminishing their quality of life. The surgeon may be tempted to feel self-gratified that he has got the patient through such a major procedure without problems, but it is important to ask direct questions and to search for significant postoperative side effects.

It is important that the patients should not lose confidence in the early postoperative phase when they are at their lowest ebb. The operations are disfiguring to the patients and their wounds are painful. Patients are often scared to look at their wounds; they may also feel insecure about them and have an unrealistic fear of the wound bursting. These patients have large wounds and they may suffer discomfort for several months, so it is important to reassure them and allay their fears. Operations through the chest commonly cause persistent pain from damage to intercostal nerves; this post-thoracotomy neuralgia can usually be abolished by intercostal nerve blocks.

Weight loss is inevitable in the early postoperative period after radical cancer surgery. The patient is in a catabolic phase in which fat stores and both skeletal and visceral muscle are mobilized to provide energy. Provided that there are no operative problems this period is short, but if complications occur then it may be prolonged and can lead to serious malnutrition and delayed recovery. The syndrome of postoperative fatigue is becoming increasingly recognized [2]. Even minor uncomplicated operations may lead to a state of functional impairment that lasts several weeks so it can be appreciated that after major radical procedures this period of fatigue may continue for many months. This should be explained to the patient so that they do not interpret this as being due to cancer. The postoperative fatigue syndrome is peculiar to man and is not seen in animals. More research is required to fully explain it but it does appear to be due to a combination of physical and psychological processes [3].

The aims of the surgeon are to cure the patient if possible and to obtain the optimum quality of life for all patients whether they have been cured or not. This requires adequate preoperative preparation, good surgery and thorough postoperative follow-up. In the following sections we describe the rationale and results of radical surgery for cancer of the thoracic oesophagus, stomach, exocrine pancreas and rectum. The abnormal physiological state that results from each procedure is reviewed and the diagnosis and treatment of the most common side effects outlined.

## Cancer of the thoracic oesophagus

Oesophageal cancer is a feared disease because of the high operative mortality of oesophagectomy and the dismal overall prognosis.

The majority of oesophageal cancers arise from squamous epithelium. Most so-called adenocarcinomas of the oesophagus have spread upwards from the proximal stomach; true adenocarcinomas of the oesophagus are uncommon. Squamous carcinomas show a marked tendency to spread longitudinally and there may even be skip lesions at a distance from the main tumour. Curative surgery has, therefore, to be extensive and an operative margin of 12 cm on either side of the visible tumour has been recommended. In addition, the lymphatic spread does not follow a segmental pattern and node metastases may be found anywhere between the external jugular vein and the coeliac axis even when the nodes adjacent to the tumour are clear [4]. If surgery is to have any chance of being curative then it has to be radical and should include removal of most of the oesophagus together with an en bloc resection of as much of the lymphatic drainage as is technically feasible.

Reconstruction after oesophagectomy requires mobilization of the stomach, or a segment of the colon, or a length of small intestine up into the chest or neck to restore continuity (Figure 28.1). The most commonly performed procedure is oesophago-gastrostomy, either as a two- or three-stage operation. The colon is usually second choice, being used when there is insufficient stomach to replace the oesophagus [5].

Oesophagectomy has the highest mortality of any routinely performed operation – in the UK an average of 30% when performed for squamous cancers [6]. Unfortunately less than one in six of the operative survivors can be expected to survive for 5 years. The mortality of resection for adenocarcinoma involving the lower oesophagus is considerably lower but the long-term prognosis is even worse. It should be emphasized that the high operative mortality of oesophagectomy is largely because many surgeons perform this operation

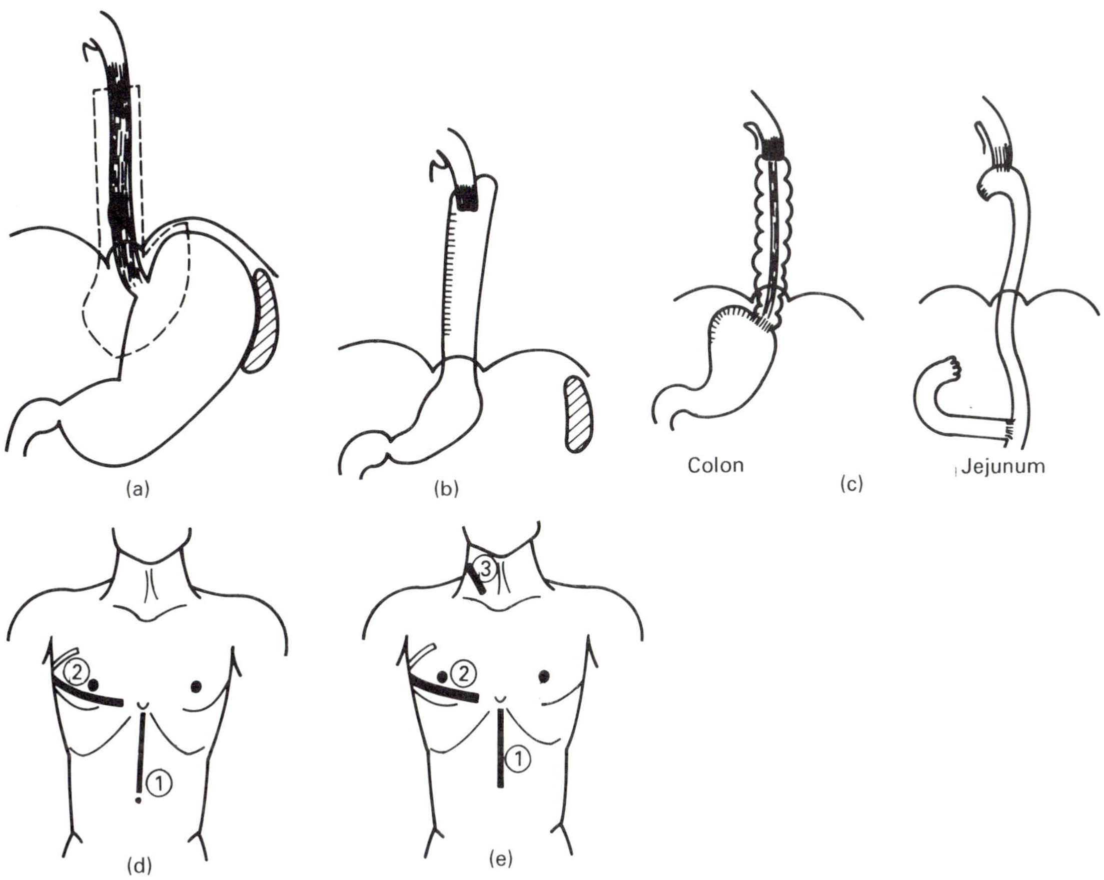



**Figure 28.1** Oesophagectomy: **a** radical oesophagectomy involves removal of the oesophagus and adjacent lymphatics and nodes. Excision should extend to 12 cm on either side of the visible tumour if cure is to be achieved; **b** reconstruction using stomach drawn up into chest and anastomosed to proximal stump; **c** an isolated segment of colon can be used to reconstruct the oesophagus; **d** reconstruction of oesophagus using a jejunal stump and Roux-en-Y anastomosis; **e** for lower oesophagus lesions a laparotomy and right thoracotomy incision affords good access; **f** for more proximal oesophageal lesions a three-stage procedure with cervical anastomosis is used

infrequently; the mortality rates of those surgeons who specialize in this field is much better with an average mortality of less than 10% [7]. Operative mortality does increase with the age of the patient but, if patients are carefully selected, oesophagectomy may still be indicated in the elderly [8].

The obvious question is whether the considerable risks of oesophagectomy are worthwhile in terms of survival and quality of life. At present surgery remains the only treatment that provides a chance of cure, albeit in only a small group of patients. However, for the less fortunate there is evidence that it does provide good palliation, in particular from dysphagia [9]. Other treatments carry less immediate risk to the patient but are never curative and, in general, provide poorer palliation. In the elderly and unfit radiotherapy is useful but does

produce significant short and long-term morbidity [10]. Intubation of the oesophagus to relieve dysphagia is a lesser procedure but has a significant mortality and an appreciable incidence of late complications. In addition, it generally produces poor palliation [11]. The use of lasers to re-cannulate the blocked oesophagus may prove to be the most effective alternative to surgery for the relief of dysphagia in those who are unfit or who have incurable disease [12].

Radical oesophagectomy remains the treatment of choice for cancer of the oesophagus provided that the surgeon is proficient and the patients are carefully selected. It is important to be aware of the common side effects of this procedure because they may considerably diminish the patient's quality of life.

## Pathophysiology

The oesophagus is a conduit for passage of food from the oropharynx to the stomach; this is not merely a passive action, but involves coordinated motor function in the muscle layers of the oesophagus. Physiological sphincter zones at either end of the oesophagus protect the pharynx and respiratory tract from regurgitation of damaging digestive juices. The lower oesophageal sphincter protects the oesophageal mucosa from reflux of gastric, and in some patients duodenal, contents both of which are damaging and can cause severe inflammation, ulceration and subsequently fibrosis.

An inevitable consequence of radical oesophagectomy is that the thoracic vagi are divided and the stomach and bowel are denervated. There is also a partial abdominal sympathectomy if coeliac axis nodes are excised en bloc with the oesophagus.

When the stomach is used to replace the thoracic oesophagus it shows no evidence of peristalsis when either liquids or solids are ingested whereas the colon, and to a lesser extent the small intestine, may contribute to active transit [13]. The resting pressure in colon and jejunal replacements is always subatmospheric, but that in the stomach is always greater than atmospheric despite lying within the thoracic cavity. This may explain why reflux problems are more common when the stomach is used in the reconstruction [14]. Although the stomach is vagally denervated it does show receptive relaxation to a meal but this is poorer than normal and may contribute to postprandial fullness.

Gastric emptying is faster than normal if a pyloroplasty or pyloromyotomy has been performed to counteract the effect of vagotomy. It is slower than normal, especially for solids, if there is no drainage procedure but this delay is rarely of clinical significance.

Both basal and maximal acid output are markedly reduced after oesophagogastrectomy, some patients becoming virtually achlorhydric [15]. Most patients develop an atrophic gastritis which occasionally progresses to gastric ulceration, this being more common when the patient has also received radiotherapy [16]. Gastritis appears to be less common if there is no drainage procedure [17].

## Postoperative problems

### Dysphagia

Inability to swallow food is not only distressing, it also has a deleterious effect on nutrition. Most patients with oesophageal cancer have presented with this as their main symptom and it is very demoralising if dysphagia recurs after surgery. Oesophagogastrectomy is successful in producing normal, or at least satisfactory, swallowing in up to 90% of patients; nearly all can eat their meals at a normal rate, although only about half can eat whatever they want [18]. Symptoms include pain on swallowing, the feeling of food sticking and regurgitation of undigested food.

Recurrence of dysphagia after surgery may be due to fibrosis at the anastomosis, recurrent cancer at the anastomosis or external compression by mediastinal recurrence. While the first is relatively easy to manage the latter two causes are ominous and usually signal a rapid deterioration in the patient's condition.

Anastomotic strictures usually present clinically in the first few weeks after surgery and occur in about 20% of patients [19]. Fortunately these fibrotic strictures dilate fairly easily either endoscopically or with radiologically placed pneumatic balloons. In most cases only one or two dilatations are required. Although the circular stapling devices have proved extremely useful in oesophageal surgery they do appear to cause a higher incidence of anastomotic strictures unless the largest sizes are used [20]. Strictures associated with stapled anastomoses may be more resistant to dilatation and require repeated regular interventions. It must be stressed that simple measures, such as ensuring the patient eats solid foods and chews properly, are important in maintaining the anastomotic lumen; replacement of ill-fitting dentures and treatment of oral or pharyngeal candidiasis can be of immense benefit.

Later development of dysphagia may be due to stricturing caused by reflux or due to recurrent cancer. It should be investigated urgently by barium swallow, endoscopy with biopsy, cytology brushing of the anastomotic area and computed tomography or nuclear magnetic resonance imaging. Very rarely, when there is local recurrence without evidence of spread, a second resection may be contemplated in the younger patient. Strictures caused by reflux respond to repeated dilatation but cancer recurrence responds poorly and the emphasis must then fall on effective palliation; the patient may benefit from radiotherapy, endoscopic intubation or laser therapy.

### Reflux

When gastric juice, or more importantly bile or duodenal contents, reflux above the anastomosis the patient may develop distressing symptoms that lead to food avoidance and a low morale. In severe cases there may be spillover into the respiratory tract, especially during the night, with a risk of aspiration pneumonia. Persistent reflux may lead to stricturing at or above the anastomosis.

Reflux is relatively common after intrathoracic oesophagogastrostomy; the lower the anastomosis in the chest the higher the incidence. When the anastomosis is made in the neck reflux appears to be less common provided that the upper oesophageal sphincter functions normally [21]. When the jejunum is used to replace the oesophagus reflux is rarely a problem but the results after colon replacement may be marred by reflux and regurgitation [22].

Reflux problems are much more common when there is a drainage procedure because this allows duodenal juices and bile to reflux into the stomach and subsequently into the oesophagus. Many oesophageal surgeons believe that for this reason alone it is best to avoid a pyloroplasty or pyloromyotomy, recognizing that a small number of patients may experience problems from slow gastric emptying [5].

Reflux should initially be treated by simple measures. Minor dietary adjustments may be sufficient and the patient should be instructed to avoid eating or drinking for at least 2 h before bed. The patient should be advised on posture and, if nocturnal reflux is a problem, to use extra pillows, wedge their mattress or place blocks under the head of their bed. Medical treatment should be reserved for resistant cases. The histamine receptor antagonists are of no value because these patients produce little acid. Useful preparations are those that bind bile acids or coat the oesophageal mucosa; these include aluminium-containing antacids and alginate or dimethicone and antacid combinations. In patients who have not had a drainage procedure reflux may be due to regurgitation precipitated by poor gastric emptying. In such cases regular metoclopramide or domperidone may be helpful.

### Postprandial symptoms

The most common symptom after oesophagectomy is early fullness. This is due partly to removal of part of the proximal stomach and partly to the poorer receptive relaxation as a result of vagotomy. Fullness may be more troublesome if a drainage procedure has not been performed but only rarely do patients experience serious problems from delayed emptying [20]. It is most important that this symptom is tackled relentlessly as it may lead to progressive malnutrition due to inadequate calorie intake. Expert dietary advice is important to maintain nutrition; in general smaller meals taken more frequently will suffice. Patients who do not have a drainage procedure may benefit from metoclopramide or domperidone; very rarely is it necessary to re-operate in order to drain the stomach.

Most other postprandial symptoms are due to the drainage procedure and are discussed in the section on gastrectomy.

### Nutrition

Most patients with cancer of the oesophagus have lost weight preoperatively and all lose some weight immediately after surgery. This weight loss may continue for some months but is gradually reversed provided that good nutritional advice is given. At best only half the survivors will have reached their preoperative weight a year after surgery; far fewer will have regained their pre-illness weight. Some patients continue to lose weight due to early recurrence of cancer.

Investigation of malnutrition after oesophagectomy has shown that carbohydrate, protein and vitamin $B_{12}$ absorption are near normal [23]. However, nearly all patients show an increase in faecal fat levels which is thought to be due to vagotomy [24]. This loss is not clinically important as long as the losses are replaced by increasing the calorie intake. In fact, post-oesophagectomy malabsorption is relatively mild and it is probably true to say that it is of greater physiological interest than of practical importance [25].

Dysphagia severely limits calorie intake; reflux symptoms may lead to food avoidance and postprandial fullness may make it difficult to take sufficient calories. These problems can usually be dealt with provided that they are identified, adequate time is spent with the patient and their diet is adjusted accordingly.

## Cancer of the stomach

Although gastric cancer shows a decreasing incidence in most parts of Europe and the United States, it remains one of the most prevalent malignancies. Cancer of the stomach responds poorly to either radiotherapy or chemotherapy and, therefore, radical surgery holds the only chance of cure at present. In common with most other gastrointestinal malignancies gastric cancer rarely presents at an early stage. Spread outside the stomach has often occurred – to adjacent organs, the peritoneal cavity or via the lymphatics or bloodstream – by the time the patient presents clinically. When spread is confined to lymph nodes or adjacent organs the cancer is still curable. Current knowledge suggests that lymphatic spread is in a progressive pattern away from the stomach. The Japanese have described four 'tiers' of lymph nodes at increasing distances from the stomach. The first 'tier' of nodes to be involved are the perigastric nodes and spread then appears to follow a centrifugal pattern into the subsequent 'tiers' of nodes. For a gastrectomy to be regarded as being curative at least one 'tier' of nodes must be removed beyond the 'tier' involved [26]. A radical gastrectomy includes, by definition, removal

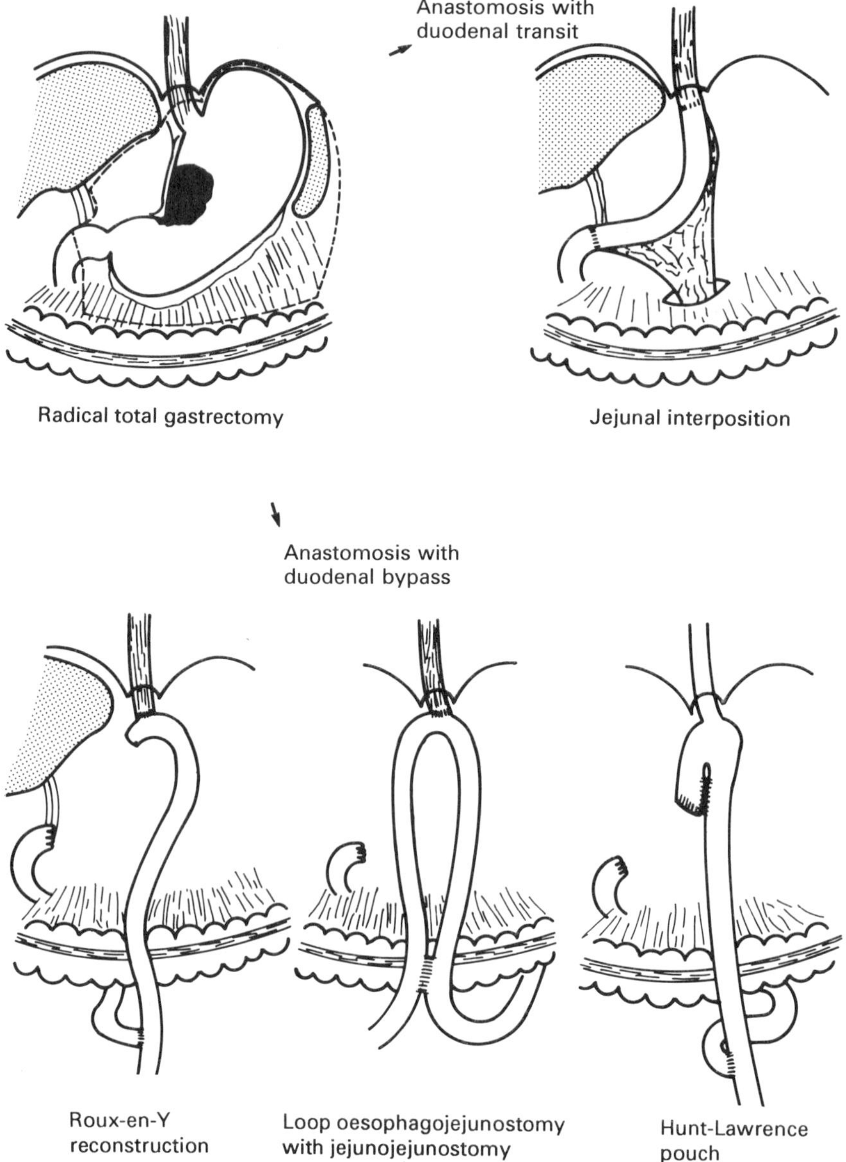


**Figure 28.2** Reconstructions following gastric resection

of the second 'tier' of nodes ($R_2$ resection) and preferably the third 'tier' ($R_3$ resection) [27].

The ultimate procedure for gastric cancer is total gastrectomy with anastomosis of the distal oesophagus to the jejunum. Lesser resections may lead to local recurrence in the remaining stomach; however, the mortality of total gastrectomy is 5–10% and is about double that of a subtotal resection. In poorer risk patients with distal gastric cancers a subtotal gastrectomy is acceptable provided that there is a clearance of at least 6 cm proximal to the tumour.

There are a large number of reconstructions described following gastric resection (Figure 28.2). It is not within this chapter to discuss the relative merits of each reconstruction; basically they can be divided into those that bypass the duodenum and those that restore continuity between the oesophagus and duodenum by interposing a length of jejunum. The reconstructions may utilize the small bowel pouch with the aim of creating a neo-stomach although the value of this is debatable.

In the UK less than 20% of patients with gastric

cancer undergo a potentially curative procedure and the overall survival of gastric cancer patients is only 5% at 5 years [28]. Of those who undergo a total or subtotal gastrectomy about half will die within a year of surgery and only 20–30% survive for 5 years; it must be emphasized that these are the average results in the West and the Japanese are able to produce figures that are about 20% better – gastric cancer is the commonest malignancy in Japan and their experience is consequently superior to our own. Their better survival figures can only be partly attributed to earlier diagnosis and in the absence of any evidence that gastric cancer is a 'different' disease in the East it has to be concluded that their surgical policy is an important factor [29]. Radical lymphadenectomy is advised for all gastric cancers as a small number of patients with early cancers may have involved nodes [30]. Aggressive resection of involved adjacent organs is advocated and impressive survival figures have been shown, even in advanced tumours [31]. Western surgeons seem reluctant to adopt these methods although most would accept that a higher percentage of curative procedures would probably be performed. At present we seem unable to reproduce the Japanese results and the onus is on us to determine why this should be [32].

Although surgical cure of gastric cancer remains elusive, patients should not be denied the possible benefits of gastrectomy provided that the operative mortality is acceptable. Gastrectomy often provides good palliation and prevents the distressing symptoms of pain, vomiting, dysphagia and acute or chronic blood loss [33]. A recent study has confirmed that most patients who have undergone a total gastrectomy experience a good quality of life [34]. However, gastrectomy produces a profound physiological alteration in the upper gastrointestinal tract and may lead to troublesome long-term side effects; these must be recognized and treated if the patient is to obtain the optimum quality of life.

## Pathophysiology

The stomach is a complex organ that functions as a reservoir for ingested food and is involved in absorption and digestion. When a meal is ingested the stomach is able to dilate to accommodate it without a marked rise in intraluminal pressure. This is known as receptive relaxation. The stomach alters the foodstuffs to some extent by mechanical mixing and grinding and also initiates the digestive process by releasing acid and enzymes. The most important function of the stomach is to release food to the intestine at a controlled rate that allows adequate mixing with bile and pancreatic secretions and thus the most efficient absorption of nutrients by the

small bowel. The rate of delivery to the duodenum is controlled by a complex humoral and neural feedback from the small gut.

The reservoir function of the stomach is lost after gastrectomy and this limits the size of the meal that can be eaten. Although the proximal jejunum shows dilatation following gastrectomy it can never completely replace the gastric reservoir and all patients experience fullness and have to limit their meal size. The ingested food also passes immediately into the small intestine in an unprepared state and out of synchronization with the biliary and pancreatic secretions. The rapid filling of the small intestine with large amounts of hypertonic food triggers a neurohumoral response that in some patients may present clinically as a mixture of unpleasant gastrointestinal and cardiovascular symptoms commonly known as the 'early dumping syndrome'. Why it is that only some patients experience these symptoms when all are exposed to the same abnormal stimuli remains a perplexing mystery. The presence of hypertonic material in the upper small intestine causes a rapid movement of fluid into the gut from the extracellular compartment contributing to the postprandial symptoms. Gastric cancer operations inevitably cause vagal denervation of the small intestine and this appears to further alter the already abnormal physiology and leads to a very rapid movement of hypertonic foodstuffs through the small bowel and may precipitate violent diarrhoea attacks ('post-vagotomy diarrhoea').

Excision of the pyloric sphincter mechanism allows reflux of bile and duodenal contents into the residual stomach after subtotal gastrectomy. This is very damaging to the gastric mucosa and causes severe gastritis. After total gastrectomy the lower oesophageal sphincter mechanism is also removed and unless the duodenal contents are prevented from refluxing into the oesophagus by a diversion or interposition procedure, the patient may develop severe inflammation and subsequent stricturing of the lower oesophagus.

Gastric acid is important in protecting the gastrointestinal tract from ingested harmful bacteria. This is lost after gastrectomy and additionally the reconstruction procedure may lead to blind loops of small intestine and stasis of the contents, this being more common when a pouch is constructed. This leads to bacterial overgrowth of both aerobic and anaerobic organisms that are normally present only in the large bowel. These faecal bacteria may produce toxins that damage the brush border enzymes vital for digestion; they may also utilize important nutrients such as the B vitamins. Some anaerobes deconjugate and dehydroxylate bile acids that are essential for normal fat absorption by the small intestine. Significant bacterial overgrowth may, therefore, result in profound malabsorption, diarrhoea and steatorrhoea.

Provided there is no bacterial overgrowth the absorption of nutrients is remarkably little affected by gastrectomy [35]. Carbohydrate absorption is near normal although the pattern of absorption is abnormal with hyperglycaemia and hyperinsulinaemia in the early postprandial period and then a hypoglycaemic phase about 2 h after eating. After a carbohydrate-rich meal the hypoglycaemic phase may be quite profound and the patient becomes clinically hypoglycaemic; this has been badly labelled the 'late dumping syndrome'.

Protein absorption is also decreased and this is reflected by an increase in faecal nitrogen; this is rarely clinically important [36]. Fat malabsorption may be more of a problem. On average post-gastrectomy patients absorb only 80% of ingested fat. This produces mild steatorrhoea but does not usually lead to malnutrition; indeed the degree of fat malabsorption correlates poorly with weight change after gastrectomy. More marked steatorrhoea and subsequent weight loss should raise the possibility of small intestinal bacterial overgrowth. There is also some malabsorption of the fat-soluble vitamins. Vitamin A deficiency is detectable [37] but remains a subclinical problem even many years after surgery [38]. Vitamin D malabsorption leads to decreased calcium absorption and long-term survivors should, therefore, be monitored as some will develop clinical osteomalacia though this may take many years [39]. There is no evidence of either vitamin E or vitamin K deficiency.

Gastric acid is necessary to release vitamin $B_{12}$ from foodstuffs and, more importantly, the gastric parietal cells secrete intrinsic factor which is essential for $B_{12}$ absorption in the terminal ileum. After total gastrectomy patients absorb virtually no vitamin $B_{12}$ and body stores are gradually depleted though it may take several years before they develop the clinical signs of deficiency with megaloblastic abnormalities. Iron absorption after total gastrectomy is not as abnormal as may be expected. Even when the duodenum is bypassed it appears that the jejunum can adapt to absorb iron provided that there are sufficient naturally occurring chelating agents in the food [40]. Iron absorption shows a gradual improvement after gastrectomy and provided intake is adequate is near normal 1 year after surgery [41].


## Postoperative problems

### *Early dumping syndrome*

This is a common postprandial problem following gastrectomy. It occurs during eating or within about 15 min of completing a meal. The patient experiences a number of symptoms, predominantly cardiovascular, at the beginning of the attack with

**Table 28.1 Symptoms of the early dumping syndrome**

| *Cardiovascular and vasomotor* | *Gastrointestinal* |
| --- | --- |
| Sensation of warmth | Nausea |
| Flushing | Vomiting |
| Sweating | Eructations |
| Palpitations | Epigastric fullness |
| Breathlessness | Borborygmi |
| Weakness | Diarrhoea |
| Feeling of faintness | |
| Loss of consciousness | |

Most patients with the syndrome experience more than one of these symptoms.

gastrointestinal symptoms occurring later (Table 28.1). Most patients have some of these symptoms in the first few weeks after operation, but in most they are relatively mild and improve considerably with simple dietary adjustments which the patients usually discover for themselves.

The diagnosis of early dumping can usually be made by taking a careful history. In less clear cases it is helpful to ask the patient to fill in a diary card recording foods eaten and symptoms experienced. When there is real doubt or the symptoms seem atypical then a 'dumping provocation test' is useful as it will reproduce the patient's symptoms and also give objective evidence of early dumping [42]. The patient is given a drink of hypertonic glucose which may produce a severe attack. For this reason it is advisable to perform the test in a hospital ward with medical attendance throughout.

The majority of patients can be treated quite simply. A thorough dietary assessment is mandatory and should be carried out by a dietician. It is important to identify foods that tend to precipitate attacks such as those with a high carbohydrate content and hypertonic liquids, particularly soups, gravies and sweet drinks. These substances should obviously be avoided and, in addition, the patient advised to take liquids separately from their meals. Hot, sweet beverages are notorious for precipitating attacks and patients should be advised to avoid sugar or to replace sugar by a proprietary sweetener. Small frequent meals are better than large ones. When patients experience severe cardiovascular symptoms they should be advised to lie down immediately after eating if this is socially acceptable.

In severe cases other measures may be necessary although the patient should be reassured that this syndrome shows a marked tendency to improve. Guar gum or pectin taken before a meal may be helpful but tend to exacerbate fullness and may also precipitate diarrhoea attacks in some patients. The only drug which appears to have a useful effect is a somatostatin analogue and this has yet to be fully evaluated [43,44]. Obviously further surgery should be avoided although in rare cases a jejunal interposition procedure may be warranted.

## Postprandial fullness ('small stomach syndrome')

The feeling of early satiety, epigastric discomfort, bloating or even pain is extremely common after gastrectomy. In some patients it leads to regurgitation or vomiting of undigested food and in most patients it limits meal size. There are several possible causes for postprandial fullness. In the majority of cases it is probably due to distension of the proximal jejunum, but in some it is a manifestation of early dumping. A less common cause in patients who have a Roux-en-Y reconstruction is when there appears to be a defect in normal peristalsis in the long limb and this produces a functional hold-up in propulsion of the meal resulting in pain and vomiting soon after eating [45].

It is important to take a careful history from the patient. In the absence of other dumping symptoms the patient should be advised to take smaller meals more frequently. In more difficult cases a dumping provocation test may be helpful but can give false positive results. When there is a suspicion of a functional problem then meal transit can be studied using a radiolabelled semi-solid meal.

The use of jejunal pouches in the reconstruction undoubtedly decreases the incidence of early satiety; however, good dietary advice is usually all that is required to alleviate this problem and ensure adequate calorie intake.

## Reflux

Reflux of bile and alkaline juices may cause epigastric discomfort, heartburn and bile vomiting. In the worst cases these symptoms are unremitting and the patient avoids eating in order not to exacerbate the problem further. Persistent reflux may result in oesophageal stricturing leading to dysphagia.

The diagnosis is usually made on clinical grounds. If objective evidence is required the best test is a 99m-technetium-HIDA scan [46]. We advise endoscopy in patients with reflux to assess the degree of mucosal damage. Treatment is often unsatisfactory and along the same lines as that described for reflux after oesophagectomy. Patients with severe unresponsive symptoms may well warrant further surgery to divert their bile.

Reflux is most common after loop oesophagojejunostomy and is largely avoided by making the reconstruction with a long Roux-en-Y limb.

## Diarrhoea

Diarrhoea attacks may occur as part of early dumping attacks but more commonly are typical of the type seen after truncal vagotomy. Post-vagotomy diarrhoea is usually episodic, the patient complains of discrete attacks of explosive, watery diarrhoea associated with extreme urgency. They may occur every day, usually in the morning, but many patients only suffer attacks at intervals of a few days or even weeks. Patients may become socially restricted because of the fear of having an attack in a public place [47]. Unlike early dumping attacks that occur after a large hypertonic stimulus, post-vagotomy diarrhoea is usually precipitated by a relatively small osmotic load such as a cup of sweet tea. Avoidance of such stimuli, especially refined carbohydrates, is the first step in the treatment of this problem. Resistant cases should be treated with small doses of loperamide given on a regular basis, not once attacks have started as this is too late. We advise starting 2 mg taken first thing in the morning and increasing in 2 mg steps; rarely does a patient need more than 4 mg to prevent attacks.

Diarrhoea that persists for several days at a time is more likely to be due to bacterial overgrowth in the proximal small intestine. In such cases faecal fat levels are markedly elevated and the patient may have steatorrhoea. The diagnosis may be made by intubating the jejunum and aspirating small intestinal juice for culture. Alternative non-invasive tests are the $^{14}$C-glycocholate breath test and the end-expired hydrogen breath test. We have found that the latter test has to be interpreted with care after gastric surgery because carbohydrate malabsorption due to rapid small bowel transit may give a false positive result.

Bacterial overgrowth appears to be more common when an intestinal pouch is created [48]. Overgrowth should be treated with courses of antibiotics such as neomycin or metronidazole. In resistant cases which show evidence of nutritional insufficiency further surgery should be contemplated.

## Malnutrition

Malabsorption is rarely the cause of malnutrition after total gastrectomy unless there is bacterial overgrowth [49]. With few exceptions patients who lose weight or fail to regain their preoperative weight do so because they fail to ingest sufficient calories. The commonest cause for an inadequate intake is the occurrence of postprandial symptoms, in particular early satiety and the early dumping syndrome. Correction of these problems is usually sufficient to correct malnutrition [35]. It is a fallacy that post-gastrectomy patients inevitably lose weight; on the other hand most fail to ever regain their pre-illness weight [50].

We advise that patients should be kept under regular dietary surveillance for a minimum of 12 months after surgery. They have to be re-educated about eating habits and should continue to see an experienced dietician as outpatients. While patients will take sufficient calories when in hospital, their intake usually decreases on going home [49]. Nutrition appears to improve over the first 6 months after surgery by which time more than half of the patients are taking their recommended calorie intake [51].

Of the different types of reconstruction after gastrectomy none has yet proved to be superior [52]. Despite the theoretical advantages of intestinal pouches they do not produce significantly better nutritional results [38].

All gastrectomy patients should receive regular vitamin $B_{12}$ in the form of hydroxycobalamin 1 mg intramuscularly every 3 months [53]. The only other supplement we recommend is oral iron which we give for 12 months or longer if intake is poor.

# Cancer of the pancreas

Cancer of the exocrine pancreas has a dreadful prognosis and should be differentiated from peri-ampullary cancers and endocrine islet cell tumours which tend to have a better prognosis. Cancer of the pancreas spreads at an early stage and has nearly always done so before it presents clinically. At least 70% of patients have clinical or radiological evidence of spread at the time of presentation. Of the remainder less than a third, or even less in some countries including the UK, will undergo a potentially curative procedure. Overall, 90% of those with pancreatic cancer will die within 1 year of diagnosis.

The results of treatment with radiotherapy and chemotherapy are dismal and at present the only chance of cure remains radical surgery [54]. The results, even from specialized centres, are hardly impressive; at best the operative mortality is around 10% with only 8% of those with cancer in the head of the pancreas surviving for 5 years and none with cancer in the body or tail of the gland surviving that long [55].

Peri-ampullary tumours (being defined as any tumour within 1 cm of the ampulla of Vater) are less common than adenocarcinomas. They can arise from the papilla, adjacent duodenal mucosa, distal common bile duct or proximal pancreatic duct [56]. As many as 95% of these lesions are resectable and the 5-year survival for those who undergo radical surgery is 30–50%.

The radical operations for cancer of the pancreas are shown in Figure 28.3. Pancreaticoduodenectomy is the most commonly performed and is often called

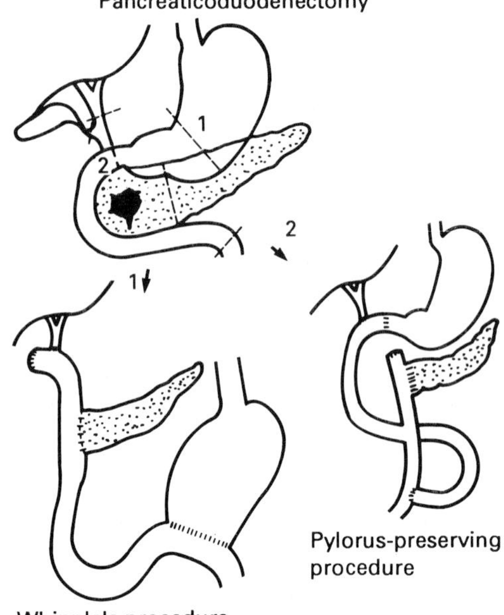


**Figure 28.3** Pancreatectomy for malignant disease of the pancreas head or body, or of the distal biliary tree or ampulla, involves resection of the duodenum as well. It may be possible to preserve the pylorus allowing a Roux-en-Y reconstruction, however usually the classic Whipple's operation with anastomosis of the bile duct, pancreatic duct and stomach to proximal jejunum is performed

Whipple's operation after the surgeon who was one of those foremost in the development of radical pancreatic excision. A partial gastrectomy, usually with truncal vagotomy, is also performed as an acid lowering procedure to decrease the problem of stomal ulceration. Over the last 10 years there has been a swing towards preservation of the pylorus so decreasing the incidence of side effects associated with rapid gastric emptying [57]. Although the operative mortality of pancreaticoduodenectomy decreases with increasing experience it still averages 15%. In addition there is a high complication rate, particularly from biliary and pancreatic leaks, leading to prolonged hospitalization.

Total pancreatectomy has been advocated because it allows a wider lymphadenectomy than Whipple's procedure; it also removes multicentric disease which is present in one-third of cases and avoids pancreatic leaks. Despite this, operative mortality is higher and survival has not been shown to be improved. In addition, all patients become insulin-dependent diabetics and have pancreatic exocrine insufficiency [58].

The most radical procedure is that of regional pancreatectomy which involves an en bloc lymphadenectomy including resection and reconstruction of the adjacent major vessels [59]. This procedure is not widely accepted as it has an unacceptably high mortality and morbidity.

The results of surgery for pancreatic cancer show little improvement and the appalling results encourage nihilism. Pancreatic excision remains the only chance of cure at present. More importantly, it is the treatment of choice for peri-ampullary tumours and for some cases of carcinoma of the head of the pancreas. This operation causes a considerable disturbance in upper gastrointestinal physiology and thus has significant side effects.

## Pathophysiology

The physiological disturbances that occur after pancreaticoduodenectomy are due to excision of part or all of the pancreas gland and also to the gastrectomy and vagotomy if these have been performed as part of the procedure. Abnormalities in bile secretion are not seen unless there is a technical problem at the choledochojejunal anastomosis.

Endocrine insufficiency is inevitable after total pancreatectomy but diabetes is rare after partial pancreatectomy unless the patient had underlying chronic pancreatitis. However, while blood glucose levels are normal both the insulin and glucagon response to glucose infusion are delayed. This subclinical abnormality does not appear to improve or deteriorate with time [60].

Exocrine insufficiency is clinically evident in 20–30% of patients after pancreaticoduodenectomy. Most patients show an improvement in exocrine function because the blockage of the pancreatic duct is relieved. The commonest cause for postoperative insufficiency appears to be stenosis at the pancreaticojejunal anastomosis [61]. In the absence of stenosis there is no evidence of deterioration of exocrine function [62].

Fat absorption is impaired in all patients but few have problems with steatorrhoea or malnutrition [63]. Excessive loss of faecal nitrogen is seen in virtually all patients but nitrogen balance is nevertheless usually positive. Iron absorption is not decreased despite removal of the duodenum. Although faecal calcium levels are increased serum levels remain normal and there are no long-term reports of bone problems [64].

Gastric acid secretion is increased after Whipple's procedure and this, together with a decrease in pancreatic production of bicarbonate, is responsible for the problem of stomal ulceration.

Many of the side effects of this operation are, in fact, due to the gastrectomy or vagotomy described previously. Pylorus-preserving pancreaticoduodenectomy avoids the vagotomy and drainage procedure and the gastric emptying of both solids and liquids is not significantly different from normal [65]. There were fears that preserving the pylorus would lead to problems with gastric stasis but these have not occurred. In the immediate postoperative period there is a delay in emptying [66] but this is only transient and soon returns to normal [67].

Jejunogastric reflux is very common after Whipple's procedure and may cause symptoms. Although reflux can be demonstrated after the pylorus-preserving operation it is not as marked and is rarely a problem clinically [68].

## Postoperative problems
### Nutrition

Most patients begin to put on weight soon after the operation. Failure to gain weight is usually due to exocrine insufficiency but may be related to post-gastrectomy side effects or residual cancer.

The most common clinical signs of pancreatic exocrine insufficiency are weight loss and steatorrhoea [35]. In some cases it may not occur for some time after surgery and careful follow-up is important if it is to be identified. When insufficiency is suspected additional tests may be useful in planning treatment; faecal fat estimations are markedly increased and response to treatment may be monitored by measuring fat levels although this is not a very precise method. We avoid the use of intubation studies for measuring pancreatic function and prefer an indirect PABA (*N*-benzyl-tyrosyl-*p*-aminobenzoic acid) test. This can also be used to make the diagnosis and monitor treatment.

Treatment of insufficiency is with pancreatic exocrine extract (pancreatin) taken with meals. This can be given as granules, tablets or in enteric-coated capsules; the latter are indicated for patients who experience abdominal discomfort and nausea with this treatment. There is also some evidence of increased efficacy when pancreatin is given in capsule form. There are several commercial preparations of pancreatin with little to choose between them. Treatment should be started at two tablets or capsules three times a day with meals and increased depending on the clinical response, faecal fat levels and PABA testing. It has been suggested that histamine type 2 receptor antagonists should be given with pancreatin as they increase gastric pH and should decrease destruction of the pancreatic enzymes. The evidence is, however, contradictory and we suggest that these drugs are only given if there is a poor response to the pancreatin alone. They are more likely to be useful after the pylorus-preserving procedure when gastric acid secretion is not reduced, unlike the standard pancreaticoduodenectomy. Commercially available pancreatic extracts do not contain sufficient lipase activity to completely correct fat malabsorption but do allow increased consumption of fat to counteract the calorie loss.

### Diarrhoea

This is a fairly common problem after pancreatectomy. It may be due to steatorrhoea, post-vagotomy diarrhoea if a truncal vagotomy has been performed, or less commonly due to bacterial overgrowth in the jejunal limb used for the reconstruction.

Patients with steatorrhoea pass fat-laden stools which are foul smelling and bulky. They may complain of colicky abdominal discomfort with frequency and sometimes urgency of defaecation. In the absence of any evidence of pancreatic insufficiency the simplest treatment is to reduce the amount of fat in the diet. However fat is an important source of calories and if the patient shows evidence of malnutrition they will require pancreatin. An alternative is to give dietary supplements of medium chain triglycerides (MCTs) which do not require lipase activity for digestion and absorption.

Post-vagotomy diarrhoea has already been discussed. It is important to think of this if the history is suggestive or if the diarrhoea is out of proportion to the degree of fat malabsorption. Some unfortunate patients have both steatorrhoea and post-vagotomy diarrhoea.

If diarrhoea does not respond to simple measures and if faecal fat levels are high and do not respond to pancreatic extracts, then the possibility of bacterial overgrowth should be investigated as described in the previous section.

### Postprandial symptoms

Any patient who has had a partial gastrectomy, with or without truncal vagotomy, as part of their pancreaticoduodenectomy may develop unpleasant postprandial symptoms. The commonest are fullness, early dumping and post-vagotomy diarrhoea. These symptoms may affect the patient's quality of life and also their nutrition by leading to food avoidance. The treatment is similar to that already described; however great care is needed with dietary manipulation if the patient has pancreatic exocrine insufficiency or diabetes. In such cases we would strongly recommend inpatient investigation and treatment.

These side effects are much less common after the pylorus-preserving procedure and this has to be strongly recommended provided it does not compromise the cancer excision.

### Diabetes mellitus

Iatrogenic insulin-dependent diabetes is rarely a problem except after total pancreatectomy. Most patients can be controlled on conventional insulin regimens. About one in five patients develop a brittle form of diabetes that is difficult to control and may require repeated admissions to hospital and may even prove fatal. It is extremely important that the patient is carefully counselled and assessed before embarking on total pancreatectomy; this operation is contraindicated if the patient would be incapable of managing the diabetes.

### Stomal ulceration

Ulceration at the gastrojejunal anastomosis occurs in 5–10% of patients after Whipple's operation. Ulceration would be expected to be more common after the pylorus-preserving operation as there is no acid lowering procedure; however most series have not confirmed this fear [69]. Ulceration is more common after total pancreatectomy due to reduced levels of bicarbonate in the jejunum and possibly the loss of pancreatic hormones.

Stomal ulceration is dangerous and it seems an unnecessary tragedy for a patient to die from a bleeding or perforated ulcer having survived such a radical procedure [70]. Epigastric pain or dyspeptic symptoms should be investigated urgently by endoscopy. Fortunately most patients respond well to histamine type 2 receptor antagonists.

## Cancer of the rectum

Cancer of the rectum is common in western countries and has shown little change in incidence over the last 30 years. Although rectal cancer often shows some response to radiotherapy, surgery remains the treatment of choice. Unlike cancers of the upper gastrointestinal tract the patient can be offered a reasonably good prognosis after excision of the tumour provided that distant spread has not occurred.

Rectal cancer spreads around the bowel wall and proximally up the rectum. Fortunately it rarely spreads downwards for more than 1 or 2 cm and this often allows the tumour to be removed with an adequate margin of normal tissue to leave sufficient rectum for anastomosis with the proximal colon. The operation of choice for rectal cancer is an anterior resection (Figure 28.4); this allows the patient to avoid a colostomy and remain continent. Tumours in the upper and middle thirds of the rectum are treated by this operation with excellent functional results. The introduction of circular stapling devices in the 1970s has allowed resection and anastomosis of tumours low in the rectum with conservation of the sphincter mechanism [71].

The functional results of low anterior resections have yet to be fully assessed and there also remains some concern that local recurrence of the tumour

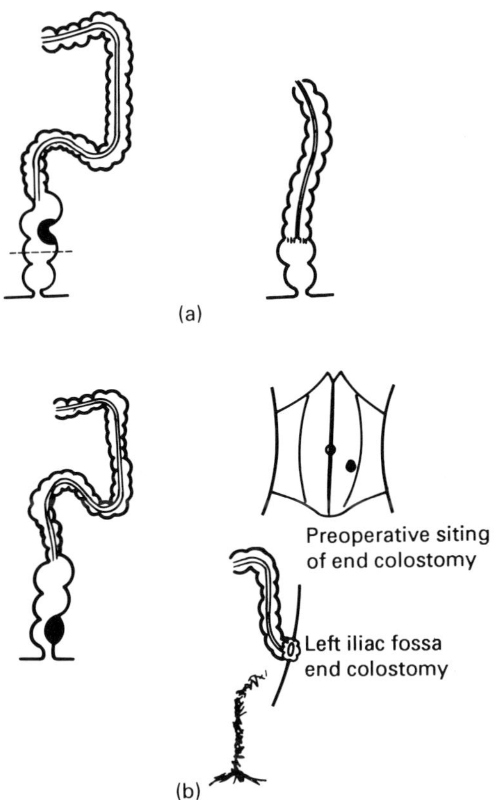



**Figure 28.4** Resection of the rectum: **a** anterior resection; **b** abdominoperineal resection

may be more common as resection margins become narrower [72]. However this is contentious; occasional reports of high local recurrence rates contrast with other series which show low rates [73–75]. When the tumour lies very low in the rectum or in the anal canal a sufficient margin cannot be obtained and the entire anorectum has to be excised as an abdominoperineal resection. After this procedure the patient has a permanent end colostomy. Fortunately the number of patients requiring this operation has decreased since the acceptance of the low stapled anatomosis [76]. Hartmann's procedure is basically an anterior resection of the rectum but without the anastomosis; it is usually performed in emergency situations which make joining the bowel ends dangerous. Continuity is re-established at a subsequent elective operation and the patient, therefore, has a temporary end colostomy.

Radical surgery of rectal cancer has to include the perirectal tissues into which these tumours tend to spread and which contain the lymphatics that drain the rectum. Lymphatic spread of rectal cancer is predominantly along the inferior mesenteric artery

to the pre-aortic nodes. Tumours in the lower rectum may also spread into the internal iliac group of nodes. A radical procedure should include an en bloc resection of as much of the lymphatic drainage as is feasible. Classically, the inferior mesenteric artery is ligated at its origin but at present there is little evidence that this is significantly better than ligating it lower down. The studies are only retrospective, but it seems that once the cancer has spread to the more proximal nodes it has virtually always spread beyond [77]. Extended lymphadenectomy has been advocated for cancer in the lower rectum and includes stripping of the lymphatic tissue and nodes from the pelvic side walls and internal iliac arteries. This inevitably leads to a greater chance of damage to adjacent organs and results in a high incidence of urinary and sexual problems because of damage to the pelvic autonomic nerves [78]. This procedure has not been widely adopted in the west, but the Japanese have reported long-term survival in patients with involved iliac nodes who have had an extended lymphadenectomy so it is of possible benefit in some patients.

The mortality of rectal excision does not vary as widely as that for upper gastrointestinal cancer; in most series it is below 5% and this includes a considerable proportion of elderly patients. There is evidence that anterior resection now has a higher mortality than abdominoperineal excision due largely to the risk of a serious anastomotic breakdown.

The prognosis of rectal cancer has changed little over the years, tending to suggest that more radical procedures are not necessarily producing better results. When the cancer is confined within the rectum the prognosis is excellent with up to 95% of patients surviving for 10 years without recurrence. When the tumour has spread into the perirectal tissue, but the lymph nodes are not involved, 75% of patients will survive for 5 years only, falling to 70% at 10 years. When the lymph nodes contain cancer deposits the prognosis is much worse and only 30% survive for 5 years. If distant metastases are present then virtually no patients survive for 5 years [79].

The side effects of excision of the rectum are most commonly related to the colostomy. All operations in which part or all of the rectum is resected may cause damage to the pelvic autonomic nerves resulting in problems with the urinary bladder and sexual organs.

## Pathophysiology

The primary function of the rectum is to store faeces until a convenient time for defaecation. As faeces enter the rectum from the colon there is an accommodation response with receptive relaxation of the rectum to allow storage without a rise in the intrarectal pressure. The afferent endings for this reflex are in the wall of the ampulla of the rectum which lies immediately above the anal canal, and also in the levator ani muscle. The accommodation response occurs at a subconscious level but once the rectum is full the intrarectal pressure rises and there is a conscious desire to defaecate. When this occurs there is a reflex sampling of the rectal contents in which the upper anal canal relaxes to allow the faeces or flatus to come into contact with the somatic sensory epithelium of the canal. Unlike the large bowel mucosa which is only sensitive to distension the anal canal is sensitive to other stimuli. If the rectum contains flatus this may be released if the situation permits. If the rectum contains faeces then defaecation may be initiated or, if this is not socially acceptable, the urge may be suppressed at a conscious level in which case the internal and external anal sphincter tone is maintained and the pressure within the anal canal remains higher than that in the rectum [80].

Resection of the upper part of the rectum does not significantly alter accommodation and defaecation so the patient does not usually notice a change in bowel function; however, if the resection is low in the rectum then the rectal reservoir is small and accommodation is subsequently diminished resulting in more frequent defaecation. Although the colon does not show receptive relaxation the levator ani receptors are still stretched and a feeling of rectal fullness is experienced and the defaecation reflex is intact; while continence is normal in many patients, older patients may have problems.

Patients with a colostomy are incontinent of both faeces and flatus because they have lost their anal sphincter mechanism. They also have no sensory component in the colon and are thus unaware of when their stoma will function. The activity of the colostomy is dependent on the natural activity of the colon; this usually takes several months to become established and varies with such factors as the eating pattern, diet and level of physical activity. Some colostomates have only one or two actions each day, often after a meal or hot drink in the morning, while others have an almost continuous flow of faeces.

## Postoperative problems

### *Living with a colostomy*

In the UK most colostomates use the natural method of colostomy control. This entails careful dietary manipulation and sometimes the use of drugs to induce the colostomy to act once or twice a day. Only about one-third of the patients achieve this ideal and most have to wear a stoma appliance all the time because the colostomy action is unpre-

dictable [81,82]. In contrast, control of the colostomy by intermittent irrigation of the colon is popular in the USA where only a minority rely on natural evacuation. Irrigation can be performed once each day in most cases and involves about an hour of time [83]. Between 0.5 and 1.5 litres of warm water are run gradually into the colon via a spout inserted into the colostomy. This stimulates the colon into mass peristalsis and the contents are then evacuated via a large bore tube or a drainage sleeve into the lavatory. Controlled studies have confirmed that irrigation is superior to natural evacuation in that it produces better regulation of the colostomy (some patients wear only a lightweight stoma cap), less odour, fewer skin problems and a reduction in psychosocial problems [84,85]. We would urge that all colostomates who are mentally alert, have good eyesight, manual dexterity and time, facilities and motivation should be taught this method. It should be avoided if there are surgical colostomy problems, in particular parastomal herniation.

Most colostomates have to restrict their diet to some degree, either to maintain a regular colostomy output or to avoid excessive flatus [86]. Odour is mainly caused by fermentation of undigested carbohydrate in the colon and foods such as beans and onions may have to be restricted. Fizzy drinks and beer also cause excessive flatus and eggs may cause an unpleasant odour. We encourage the patient to experiment with foodstuffs and only exclude the troublesome ones. A strictly controlled diet may be socially restricting and a sensible balance must be struck. Odour is a particular cause of anxiety to ostomates and every effort should be made to control this so that the patient does not become socially isolated. Many modern stoma appliances incorporate activated carbon filters to deodorize flatus and prevent the stoma bag inflating. Oral preparations, such as chlorophyll tablets, are sometimes prescribed but their true value is doubtful. There are various commercial additives that can be placed in the bags that will mask odours.

We do not recommend the routine use of drugs to control colostomy function; simple dietary manipulation is usually all that is required. If the patient has an excessive output from the stoma then either codeine phosphate or loperamide is usually effective. Bulking drugs such as methylcellulose and ispaghula husk are useful in the management of constipation; in general purgatives should be avoided. It should be remembered that other drugs may have an effect on colostomy function. Drugs with anticholinergic actions, including the tricyclic antidepressants and cardiac drugs such as disopyramide and quinidine bisulphate, may cause constipation. Oral antibiotics may alter the bowel flora and can cause unpleasant diarrhoea. Colostomates should be advised to avoid them if possible.

## Skin problems

Modern stoma appliances have greatly reduced the incidence of skin problems. Dermatitis around the stoma may be due to effluent leaking onto the skin or due to a contact allergy. Effluent dermatitis is uncommon with left-sided end colostomies although it may be a problem if the patient has diarrhoea. Contact dermatitis is caused by an allergy to part of the appliance and has a clearly demarcated geometric outline. The patient often has a history of skin problems or hypersensitivity. The correct diagnosis of the cause of skin damage is important if treatment is to be effective.

Both types of dermatitis lead to hyperaemia and sogginess of the skin and this often leads to secondary infection. The inflamed skin should be swabbed for culture of bacteria and fungi and then cleaned with a bland soap and carefully dried. It should be protected from further damage with a waterproof adhesive material such as karaya gel or carboxymethylcellulose and, if leakage has caused the problem, the area of leakage built up to allow full contact by the appliance. Problems with leakage can be avoided by correct siting of the colostomy in a position away from scars and skin creases on a flat area of the abdominal wall. In severe cases the stoma may need to be refashioned or even resited. For contact dermatitis the appliance should be changed and patch testing performed. Maceration of the skin by sweat trapped beneath the appliance can be prevented by a cotton appliance cover. A short course of a mild local corticosteroid cream such as 0.1% betamethasone may be helpful but prolonged use should be avoided. If there is a superadded fungal infection an antifungal agent can be used either alone or with the steroid cream. Topical antibiotics are notorious for causing hypersensitivity reactions and should be avoided if possible.

## Surgical problems

Most surgical problems are due either to faulty construction technique or poor siting of the stoma: the importance of correct siting cannot be overemphasized.

Paracolostomy herniation is the most common complication occurring in up to 20% of patients [87,88]. The incidence is considerably reduced if the colostomy is brought out through the rectus muscle [89]. The incidence is also lower when the colostomy follows an extraperitoneal route. Many of these hernias are of little significance, but serious complications can occur. The hernia may interfere with fitting an appliance and lead to leakage with skin and odour problems, irrigation may become impossible and there is also a risk of perforation by the irrigation spout. As with all hernias there is always the risk that bowel may strangulate within them. In most cases surgical repair of the hernia is indicated; in some it may be necessary to resite the colostomy.

Prolapse of the colostomy may occur, being most likely when the opening in the abdominal wall is too large. The stoma can be reconstructed at a local operation by mobilizing it down to the peritoneal cavity, excising the excess and fixing the colon mesentery to the peritoneum before refashioning the stoma. Colostomy stenosis may be due to the abdominal wall opening being too narrow or due to ischaemia. In severe cases of ischaemia the stoma may retract; this also happens if the stoma is under tension. Stenosis can be dealt with by a local operation with refashioning of the colostomy, but this may not be enough for cases of retraction which may require a further laparotomy and mobilization of the left colon.

Carcinomas may develop on a colostomy; this may be due to an insufficient margin being left proximal to the original cancer and the colostomy is involved by spread in the mural lymphatics, or because of metachronous cancer. In intraperitoneal carcinomatosis metastatic cancer may grow out through the colostomy incision to involve the stoma. Bleeding from a colostomy is often due to local minor trauma, but the stoma should be carefully examined and the bleeding investigated further if the appearances are suspicious.

## Psychosocial problems

However careful the preoperative counselling, patients are universally shocked to see their stoma; their immediate response is virtually always one of denial. Some patients with denial also experience a 'phantom rectum' (a sense of rectal fullness associated with a desire to defaecate). The patient's own body image is distorted and they commonly regard themselves as mutilated, fragile and weak. Some patients develop profound feelings of horror, shame, degradation and a fear of rejection by others.

In general, the ostomate develops a new order of living with some change in personality characterized by a conscious control of the range and type of their social participation. There may be a tendency towards regression in thought and behaviour resulting in a restriction in their interests and a withdrawal from emotional involvement. Others may become obsessively involved in trying to live a 'normal life'. The elderly, in particular, may become socially isolated. Depression is the commonest psychological problem and a proportion of patients will require psychiatric treatment.

Even with the most careful care and support it is disappointing to find that many colostomates do not resume the same quality of life that they previously experienced [90]. Stoma care after discharge from

40. Fischermann, K., Harly, S., Worning, H. and Zacho, A. Pancreatic function and the absorption of fat, iron, vitamin $B_{12}$ and calcium after total gastrectomy for gastric cancer. *Gut*, **8**, 260–266 (1967)

41. Bradley, E.L. and Isaacs, J. Post-resectional anaemia. *Archives of Surgery*, **111**, 844–848 (1976)

42. Ralphs, D.N.L., Thomson, J.P.S., Haynes, S. *et al.* The relationship between the rate of gastric emptying and the dumping syndrome. *British Journal of Surgery*, **65**, 637–641 (1978)

43. Hopman, W.P.M., Wolberink, R.G.J., Lamers, C.B.H.W. and van Tongeren, J.H.M. Treatment of the dumping syndrome with the somatostatin analogue SMS 201–995. *Annals of Surgery*, **207**, 155–159 (1988)

44. Primrose, J.N. and Johnston, D. Somatostatin analogue SMS 201–995 (Octreotide) as a possible solution to the dumping syndrome after gastrectomy or vagotomy. *British Journal of Surgery*, **76**, 140–144 (1989)

45. Mathias, J.R., Fernandez, A., Sninsky, C.A. *et al.* Nausea, vomiting and abdominal pain after Roux-en-Y anastomosis: motility of the jejunal limb. *Gastroenterology*, **88**, 101–107 (1985)

46. Donovan, I.A., Fielding, J.W.L., Bradby, H. *et al.* Bile diversion after total gastrectomy. *British Journal of Surgery*, **69**, 389–390 (1982)

47. Raimes, S.A., Smirniotis, V., Wheldon, E.J. *et al.* Post-vagotomy diarrhoea put into perspective. *Lancet*, **ii**, 851–853 (1982)

48. Troidl, H., Kusche, J., Vertweber, K.-H. *et al.* Pouch versus oesophagojejunostomy after total gastrectomy: a randomized clinical trial. *World Journal of Surgery*, **11**, 699–712 (1987)

49. Bradley, E.L., Isaacs, J., Hersh, T. *et al.* Nutritional consequences of total gastrectomy. *Annals of Surgery*, **182**, 415–429 (1975)

50. Cristallo, M., Braga, M., Agape, D. *et al.* Nutritional status, function of the small intestine and jejunal morphology after total gastrectomy for carcinoma of the stomach. *Surgery, Gynecology and Obstetrics*, **163**, 225–230 (1986)

51. Braga, M., Zuliani, W., Foppa, L. *et al.* Food intake and nutritional status after total gastrectomy: results of a nutritional follow-up. *British Journal of Surgery*, **75**, 477–480 (1988)

52. Hugier, M., Lancret, J.M., Bernard, P.F. *et al.* Functional results of different reconstructive procedures after total gastrectomy. *British Journal of Surgery*, **63**, 704–708 (1976)

53. Chipping, P.M. Vitamin $B_{12}$ deficiency. *Prescribers' Journal*, 117–124 (1988)

54. Trede, M. Treatment of pancreatic carcinoma: the surgeon's dilemma. *British Journal of Surgery*, **74**, 79–80 (1987)

55. Matsumo, S. and Sato, T. Surgical treatment for carcinoma of the pancreas. *American Journal of Surgery*, **152**, 499–503 (1986)

56. Robertson, J.F.R., Imrie, C.W., Hole, D.J. *et al.* Management of peri-ampullary carcinoma. *British Journal of Surgery*, **74**, 816–819 (1987)

57. Traverso, L.W. and Longmire, W.P. Preservation of the pylorus in pancreatoduodenectomy. *Surgery, Gynecology and Obstetrics*, **146**, 959–962 (1978)

58. van Heerden, J.A. Pancreatic resection for carcinoma of the pancreas: Whipple versus total pancreatectomy – an institutional perspective. *World Journal of Surgery*, **8**, 880–888 (1984)

59. Fortner, J.G. Regional pancreatectomy for cancer of the pancreas, ampulla and other related sites. *Annals of Surgery*, **199**, 418–425 (1984)

60. Miyata, M., Yamamoto, T., Hamagi, M. *et al.* Pancreatic endocrine function in long term survivors after pancreatoduodenectomy: special reference to reversibility of insulin and glucagon secretion. *World Journal of Surgery*, **12**, 651–657 (1988)

61. Fish, J.C., Smith, L.B. and Williams, R.D. Digestive function after radical pancreaticoduodenectomy. *American Journal of Surgery*, **117**, 40–47 (1969)

62. Tanaka, T., Ichiba, Y., Fujii, Y. *et al.* Clinical and experimental study of pancreatic exocrine function after pancreaticoduodenectomy for peri-ampullary carcinoma. *Surgery, Gynecology and Obstetrics*, **166**, 200–205 (1988)

63. Lerut, J.P., Gianello, P.R., Otte, J.B. and Kestens, P.J. Pancreaticoduodenal resection. *Annals of Surgery*, **199**, 432–437 (1984)

64. Griffen, W.O. Metabolic consequences of pancreatectomy. In *Metabolic Surgery* (eds H. Buchwald and R.L. Varco), Grune and Stratton, New York, pp. 111–124 (1978)

65. Fink, A.S., De Souza, L.R., Mayer, E.A. *et al.* Long term evaluation of pylorus preservation during pancreaticoduodenectomy. *World Journal of Surgery*, **12**, 663–670 (1988)

66. Warshaw, A.L. and Torchiana, D.L. Delayed gastric emptying after pylorus preserving pancreaticoduodenectomy. *Surgery, Gynecology and Obstetrics*, **160**, 1–4 (1985)

67. Patti, M.G., Pellegrini, C.A. and Way, L.W. Gastric emptying and small bowel transit of solid food after pylorus preserving pancreaticoduodenectomy. *Archives of Surgery*, **122**, 528–531 (1987)

68. Itani, K.M.F., Coleman, R.E., Akwari, O.E. and Myers, W.C. Pylorus preserving pancreaticoduodenectomy. *Annals of Surgery*, **204**, 655–664 (1986)

69. Grace, P.A., Pitt, H.A. and Longmire, W.P. Pancreaticoduodenectomy with pylorus preservation for adenocarcinoma of the head of the pancreas. *British Journal of Surgery*, **73**, 647–650 (1986)

70. Grant, C.S. and van Heerden, J.A. Anastomotic ulceration following sub-total and total pancreatectomy. *Annals of Surgery*, **190**, 1–5 (1979)

71. Heald, R.J. Towards fewer colostomies – the impact of circular stapling devices on the surgery of rectal cancer in a district hospital. *British Journal of Surgery*, **67**, 198–200 (1980)

72. Jeekel, J. Can radical surgery improve survival in colorectal cancer? *World Journal of Surgery*, **11**, 412–417 (1987)

73. Hurst, P.A., Prout, W.G., Kelly, J.M. *et al.* Local recurrence after low anterior resection using the staple gun. *British Journal of Surgery*, **69**, 275–276 (1982)

74. Heald, R.J., Husband, E.M. and Ryall, R.D.H. The meso-rectum in rectal cancer surgery – the clue to pelvic recurrence. *British Journal of Surgery*, **69**, 613–616 (1982)

75. Williams, N.S., Durdey, P. and Johnston, D. The outcome following sphincter saving resection and abdominoperineal resection for low rectal cancer. *British Journal of Surgery*, **72**, 595–598 (1985)

76. Foster, M.E., Leaper, D.J. and Williamson, R.C.N. Changing patterns in colostomy closure: the Bristol experience. *British Journal of Surgery*, **72**, 142–145 (1985)

77. Pezim, M.E. and Nicholls, R.J. Survival after high or low ligation of the inferior mesenteric artery during curative surgery for rectal cancer. *Annals of Surgery*, **200**, 729–733 (1984)

78. Glass, R.E., Ritchie, J.K., Thompson, H.R. and Mann, C.V. The results of surgical treatment of cancer of the rectum by radical resection and extended abdomino-ilial lymphadenectomy. *British Journal of Surgery*, **72**, 599–601 (1985)

79. Goligher, J.C. *Surgery of the Anus, Rectum and Colon*, Bailliere Tindall, London (1984)

80. Duthie, H.L. Dynamics of the rectum and anus. *Clinics in Gastroenterology*, **4**, 467–478 (1975)

81. Devlin, H.B., Plant, J.A. and Griffin, M. Aftermath of surgery for anorectal cancer. *British Medical Journal*, **iii**, 413–418 (1971)

82. Williams, N.S. and Johnston, D. The quality of life after rectal excision for low rectal cancer. *British Journal of Surgery*, **70**, 460–462 (1983)

83. Laucks, S.S., Mazier, W.P., Milsom, J.W. *et al.* An assessment of colostomy irrigation. *Diseases of the Colon and Rectum*, **31**, 279–282 (1988)

84. Williams, N.S. and Johnston, D. Prospective controlled trial comparing colostomy irrigation with 'spontaneous action' method. *British Medical Journal*, **281**, 107–109 (1980)

85. Doran, J. and Hardcastle, J.D. A controlled trial of colostomy management by natural evacuation, irrigation and foam enema. *British Journal of Surgery*, **68**, 731–733 (1981)

86. Gazzard, B.G., Saunders, B. and Dawson, A.M. Diets and stoma function. *British Journal of Surgery*, **65**, 642–644 (1978)

87. Burgess, P., Mathew, V.V. and Devlin, H.B. A review of terminal colostomy complications following abdomino-perineal resection for carcinoma. *British Journal of Surgery*, **71**, 1004 (1984)

88. Leslie, D. The parastomal hernia. *Surgical Clinics of North America*, **64**, 407–415 (1984)

89. Turnbull, R.B. and Weakley, F.L. *Atlas of Intestinal Stomas*, C.V. Mosby, St. Louis (1967)

90. MacDonald, L.D., Anderson, H.R. and Bennett, A.E. *Cancer Patients in the Community: Outcomes of Care and Quality of Survival in Rectal Cancer*, DHSS, HMSO, London (1982)

91. Rubin, G.P. Aspects of stoma care in general practice. *Journal of the Royal College of General Practitioners*, 369–372 (1986)

92. Kinn, A.-L. and Ohman, U. Bladder and sexual function after surgery for rectal cancer. *Diseases of the Colon and Rectum*, **29**, 43–48 (1986)

93. Janu, N.C., Bokey, E.L., Chapius, P.H. *et al.* Bladder dysfunction following anterior resection for carcinoma of the rectum. *Diseases of the Colon and Rectum*, **29**, 182–183 (1986)

94. Balsev, I. and Harling, H. Sexual dysfunction following operation for carcinoma of the rectum. *Diseases of the Colon and Rectum*, **26**, 785–788 (1983)

95. Hjorstrup, A., Kirkegaard, P., Friis, J. *et al.* Sexual dysfunction after low anterior resection for mid-rectal cancer. *Acta Chirurgica Scandinavica*, **150**, 687–688 (1984)

96. Devlin, H.B. and Plant, J.A. Sexual function, an aspect of stoma care. *British Journal of Sexual Medicine*, **6**, 33–37 (1979)

97. Danzi, M., Ferulano, G.P., Abate, S. and Galifano, G. Male sexual function after abdomino-perineal resection for rectal cancer. *Diseases of the Colon and Rectum*, **26**, 665–668 (1983)

# 29

# Minimizing morbidity in cancer surgery

G. Westbury and M.W. Kissin

## Introduction and general overview

The principal function of the surgeon in the treatment of cancer as of the radiotherapist is locoregional control. Failure to achieve control precludes cure and even when metastases supervene persistent disease at the primary and/or lymph node sites often shortens life and causes major misery. In spite of increasing surgical radicality, cure rates for most solid tumours have been unaltered for many decades except where influenced by adjuvant therapy. In accepting that the surgical contribution to cure has generally reached a plateau, surgeons have turned increasingly towards improving the cost/benefit ratio of their treatment by attempting to reduce its morbidity.

All categories of surgical patients have benefited from improvement in perioperative management including nutritional support, intensive care, the control of wound pain and the rational use of antibiotics. Current emphasis is upon reduction of operative blood loss and consequent transfusion requirement, not only to avoid the risk of transmitting the hepatitis B virus and HIV, but because of as yet unsubstantiated suspicion that metastatic spread might be enhanced [1].

More specifically and in relation to technical aspects of cancer surgery, two contrasting themes can be identified. The first is conservation surgery in which radical clearance of tumour is achieved sparing uninvolved tissues which are functionally or aesthetically important, e.g. sphincter-conserving resection of the rectum; limb-sparing surgery for sarcoma; conservation of the mandible in surgery for tongue cancer. Such procedures depend on accurate knowledge of the surgical pathology of specific cancers together with scrupulous case selection in which clinical and histological evidence is supported by appropriate imaging investigations. The second major line of development is in the area of reconstructive surgery where tissue deficits attending unavoidable sacrifice of important structures are restored. Considerable advances have been made throughout this field which involves many specialities. Noteworthy are the development of pedicled, axial pattern flaps and microvascular free tissue transfer for immediate, one-stage repair of soft tissue, bone or visceral defects, and the design of procedures which impart continence following loss of anal or urinary sphincters. For the future, organ and limb transplantation may well take their place in the reconstructive armamentarium if the problems of rejection can be overcome without the need for generalized immunosuppression with its tumour-enhancing effects.

Increasing understanding of the biology and surgical pathology of solid tumours has allowed a more rational and precise prescription of the extent of operation required. Case selection for sphincter conservation surgery in rectal cancer and reduction in the width of excision margins for melanoma are good examples, as are the selective avoidance of elective lymph node dissection based on the characteristics of the primary lesion in cutaneous melanoma and squamous carcinoma of the oral cavity.

The extent of surgical resection and its ensuing disability may also be reduced by adjuvant irradiation or chemotherapy. Radiotherapy reduces the local failure rate following localized excision for breast cancer and limb-sparing surgery for soft tissue sarcomas; it provides an effective alternative to elective neck dissection for N0 squamous carcinoma of the head and neck. Chemotherapy not only reduces mortality from metastatic disease in osteosarcoma of the limbs but influences the primary tumour to enable limb-conserving resection with bone replacement in suitable cases. Chemotherapy, sometimes in association with local irradiation, has likewise markedly curtailed the need for mutilating surgery in embryonal sarcomas of the head and neck and of the urogenital tract in infancy and childhood.

Finally technological advances of a wide variety have contributed to the minimization (and sometimes avoidance) of surgery and its consequent morbidity. Fine needle aspiration cytology or needle biopsy of the Tru-Cut® type have substantially reduced the need for open surgery to establish tumour tissue diagnosis; ultrasound or computed tomographic (CT) guidance places deeply seated visceral lesions within the range of these techniques, e.g. lung and pancreas. Fibreoptic instrumentation has made possible the endoscopic control of colonic polyps and papilliferous tumours within the renal pelvis, and the per duodenal placement of stents within the biliary outflow system to relieve obstructive jaundice from cancer of the pancreas or major bile ducts.

The laser provides an alternative to the scalpel for certain tumours of the eye and skin while the ultrasonic beam minimizes blood loss in hepatic resection and reduces normal tissue damage in the removal of tumours of the brain and spinal cord.

These themes will be further elaborated for cancer surgery at selected anatomical sites.

**Table 29.1 Minimizing morbidity in breast cancer surgery**

| Complication | Methods to minimize morbidity |
|---|---|
| Seroma | Use suction drains; anchor skin flaps |
| Neurovascular damage | Preserve pectoral and intercostobrachial nerves; preserve nerve and blood supply to latissimus dorsi and serratus anterior |
| Lymphoedema | Avoid radiotherapy to axilla after axillary clearance |
| Shoulder stiffness | Avoid radiotherapy to axilla after axillary clearance |
| Cosmetic deformity | Where possible hide scars below bra line; involve patient in treatment decisions; select breast conservation according to size and position of tumour, and shape of breast; offer reconstruction after mastectomy |
| Psychological problems | Involve patients in treatment decisions; use nurse counsellors |

# Breast cancer

As for most cancer procedures, surgical morbidity can be considered in terms of general and specific complications. General complications such as chest infection and venous thromboembolism are seldom the source for concern when treating superficial tumours like breast cancer. Instead there are a number of specific early and late complications consequent on surgical technique and subsequent use of radiotherapy. Some of these are detailed in Table 29.1 and are discussed below.

## Axillary morbidity

The optimum management of the axilla remains controversial. Since the pathological status of the axillary lymph nodes remains a key prognostic factor, the surgeon must remove nodes for examination. However, there is considerable morbidity attendant on over-enthusiastic lymphadenectomy. Clearly, the surgeon has to refine operative technique so that maximum information is gained at minimum expense. Moreover, to minimize long-term side effects, a close liaison with the radiotherapist is required in order to avoid unnecessary irradiation. Like many other areas in cancer therapy, the axilla demands teamwork and selective use of treatments.

## Seroma

Seroma formation is a troublesome complication that may require repeated outpatient aspiration. It occurs in 40% of patients after extended mastectomy and 30% after wide local excision plus axillary dissection. It appears to be related to the use of adjuvant tamoxifen therapy, age of the patient, surgical technique and early mobilization of the shoulder [2]. Seroma formation can be significantly discouraged by using suction drains and by anchoring the skin flaps to the chest wall [3; M.W. Kissin and A.J. Webb, 1988, personal communication].

## Lymphoedema and shoulder mobility

Of all the complications of treating breast cancer, lymphoedema of the upper limb is one of the most distressing and unpleasant for the patient and is particularly frustrating for the surgeon (Figure 29.1). Moreover, it may lead to lymphangiosarcoma. The incidence of lymphoedema is similar after axillary sampling plus radiotherapy, radiotherapy alone and axillary clearance alone (7–9%).

However, radiotherapy should be avoided after axillary clearance, as the incidence of lymphoedema rises significantly to 38% [4]. Irradiating the node-negative axilla is unnecessary, and the same is true for the node-positive axilla after axillary clearance, since it does not prolong survival and the incidence of axillary recurrence is extremely low after total clearance alone. Furthermore, it must be borne in mind that radiotherapy used to complement surgery carries its own hazards. These include radiation-induced sarcoma formation [5], brachial plexus neuropathy [6] and, on the left side, an increase in late deaths from myocardial damage. With the adoption of a more rational combined approach to the breast and the axilla it might be imagined that the risk of shoulder immobility, like that of lymphoedema, has decreased. However, Aitken *et al.* [7] have recently shown that shoulder mobility is significantly reduced following combined treatment of the axilla by node sampling and radiotherapy when compared with axillary clearance alone.

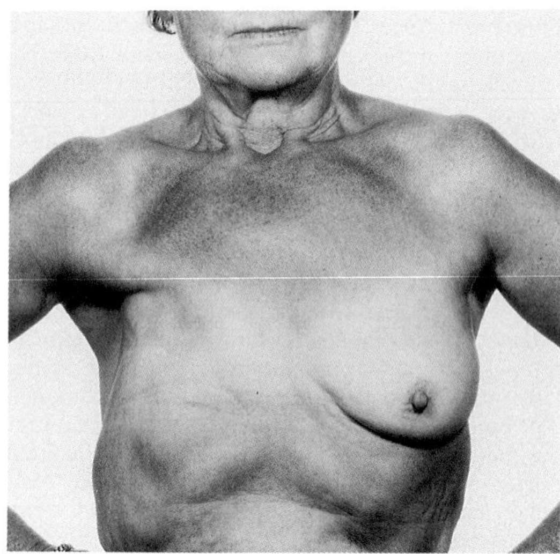

**Figure 29.2** Atrophy of the lower portion of the right pectoralis major muscle 2 years after modified radical mastectomy for a T1,N0 breast cancer

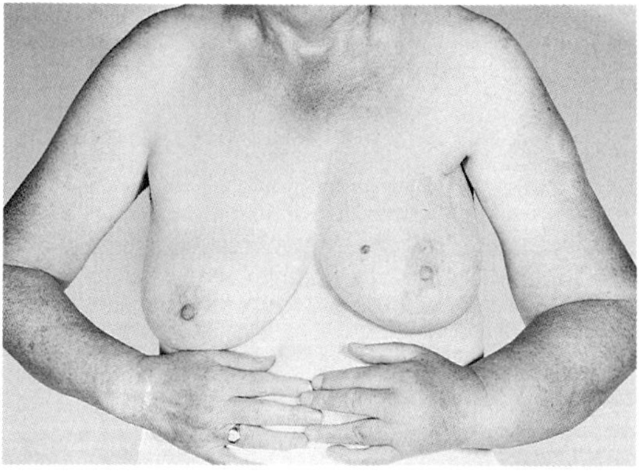

**Figure 29.1** Lymphoedema of the left upper limb 3 years after wide local excision, axillary sampling and external beam irradiation for a T2,N1 breast cancer

## Operative neurovascular damage

The technique of axillary dissection demands identification and preservation of the nerves supplying the serratus anterior, pectoralis major and minor and latissimus dorsi muscles. Damage to the first of these causes winging of the scapula (a minor deformity). Damage to the pectoral nerves causes atrophy of the anterior axillary fold (Figure 29.2), and this may make submuscular post-mastectomy breast reconstruction more difficult [8]. Inadvertent damage to the blood supply of the latissimus means that this muscle cannot be used in flap reconstruction. During the course of axillary dissection the

intercostobrachial nerve is usually sacrificed, and this can result in unpleasant sensory changes on the inner aspect of the upper arm. This problem can be avoided by preserving the nerve [9].

## Breast morbidity

The extent of surgery to the breast itself is amongst the most controversial topics in cancer therapy. The surgeon and patient have to reach a mutual understanding based on information derived from known prognostic factors. The psychological morbidity associated with breast loss has to be balanced against the possibility of local recurrence. Importantly, local recurrence following conservative excision and irradiation may be impossible to diagnose in its early, salvageable stage, either by clinical examination, cytology or mammography. Optimum results, in terms of control of disease and cosmesis, call for close teamwork between surgeon and oncologist.

## Psychological sequelae

Women who develop breast cancer and undergo operation experience a prolonged and mounting burden of psychological stress. In a group of 75 women studied 1 year after mastectomy, 25% needed treatment for anxiety or depression and 3%

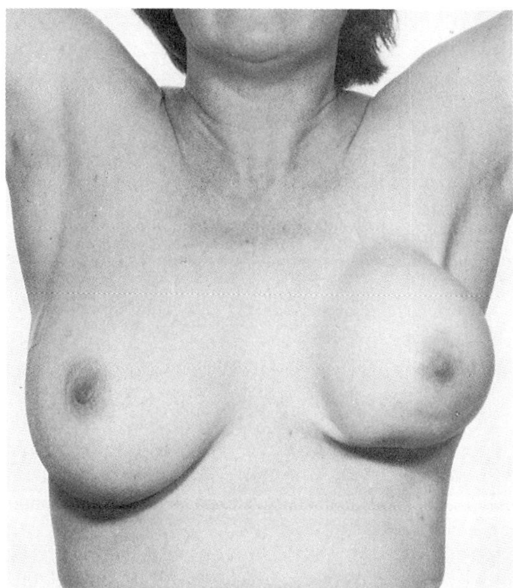

**Figure 29.3** Marked capsule formation around a subcutaneous silicone implant inserted 2 years after a subcutaneous mastectomy for lobular carcinoma *in situ*

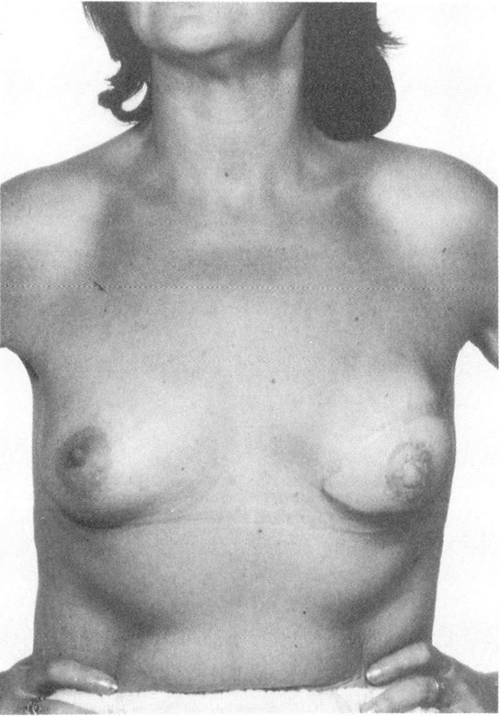

**Figure 29.4** Reconstruction of the left breast 2 years after mastectomy and axillary dissection for T2,N0 breast cancer. The breast mound has been restored by insertion of a silicone prosthesis. Extra skin and soft tissue is provided by transposition of a latissimus dorsi myocutaneous flap. The nipple complex has been refashioned using labial skin

had sexual difficulties [10]. It is widely assumed that breast conservation is associated with a decrease in these problems, but controlled studies suggest that this may not always be the case [11]. Although breast conservation reduces body image problems, it seems to increase anxiety concerning local recurrence. While the development of post-mastectomy counselling services has failed to prevent psychological morbidity, it does permit its early diagnosis and has a favourable impact on social recovery [12]. In addition, the benefits in terms of population survival produced by breast screening must be balanced by unnecessary heightening of anxiety in large groups of well women.

## Cosmetic appearance

### Breast reconstruction

Many women who choose to have mastectomy can now benefit from immediate or delayed breast reconstruction. Since considerable technical experience is required to obtain a satisfactory result, such procedures should be carried out in specialist centres. Some women simply desire the restoration of a breast mound and cleavage, but others require recreation of the nipple and contralateral reduction mammoplasty for symmetry. The ideal prosthesis should be inert, easy to insert and resemble the normal breast in appearance and texture. These objectives remain largely unfulfilled, but the 'low bleed' thick walled silicone implant is currently the prosthesis of choice. The widespread introduction of breast reconstruction has itself led to several new surgical complications. The prosthesis inevitably induces capsule formation which can be painful and distort the new breast and may eventually require surgical revision (Figure 29.3). The inflatable variety of prosthesis is prone to sudden deflation, and when this occurs replacement is necessary. When skin and soft tissue cover is adequate subcutaneous or submuscular insertion may suffice, but often more complex procedures are required [13]. These include the use of myocutaneous flaps (Figure 29.4) to add bulk and cover [14], and enlargement of the submuscular cavity using tissue expanders [15].

Subcutaneous mastectomy plus reconstruction is perhaps the optimum method of avoiding cosmetic deformity and reducing psychological morbidity [16]. However, this technique is only suitable for patients with small, peripheral, good prognosis tumours. It is possible that the widespread use of radiotherapy in young women with natural good survival prospects may in time produce a crop of radiation-induced sarcomas of the breast [17]. In addition, the ability of implanted foreign material to induce sarcoma formation, both in animals and in man, raises the possibility that insertion of a prosthetic silicone implant may also carry some measure of risk [18].

### *Breast conservation*

Breast conservation surgery, usually combined with radiotherapy, has become established as a definite therapeutic option in certain cases of breast cancer, and this is supported by the results of several randomized trials which have shown comparable rates of local control to mastectomy. The term 'local excision' is applied to a large variety of breast conservation procedures ranging from 'tumourectomy' to removal of the entire quadrant of origin. This leads to considerable variation in aesthetic results and makes reports from different centres difficult to compare [19]. The techniques involved may not be as simple as they sound, and do not guarantee a satisfactory appearance (Figure 29.5). Adequate reflection of the skin is required to enable the surgeon to dissect safely through non-malignant tissue, resection down to and including the pectoral

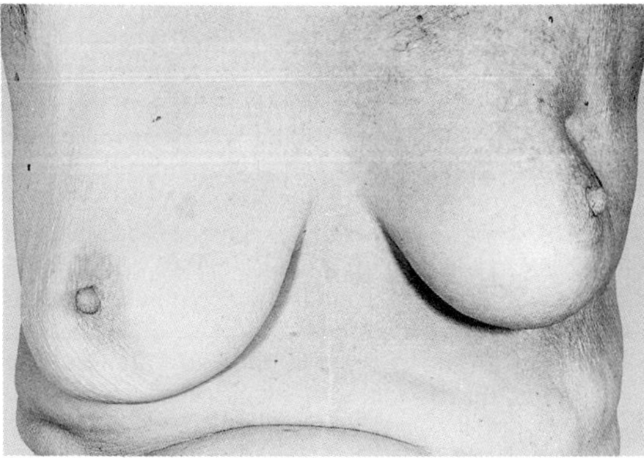

**Figure 29.5** Unsatisfactory cosmetic result 1 year after breast conservation therapy for a T1 breast cancer. This patient had wide local excision, external beam irradiation plus an iridium wire implant boost to the tumour bed

fascia is advisable, skin excision may be necessary, and macroscopic contamination of the wound should be avoided. Indeed, even when these points are adhered to, it is still possible to retrieve viable tumour cells from the resulting cavity [20]. Technical details such as the skin incision (radial or circumferential), reconstruction of the breast parenchyma and the use of drainage, have yet to be standardized [19]. These are problems for the future.

## Sarcomas of the limbs

Surgical ablation of limb sarcoma, whether arising in bone or in soft tissues, was traditionally achieved by amputation proximal to the involved bone or musculofascial compartment. Most osteosarcomas arise around the knee joint and the majority of soft tissue sarcomas in the thigh so the resulting mutilation and disability were considerable and, certainly for bone sarcoma, balanced by slender prospects of cure. Cade [21] showed that adjuvant radiotherapy extended the ability of surgeons to obtain local control of soft tissue sarcoma by limb-sparing soft part resection and, when given preoperatively, could convert large, fixed tumours to a state of operability. The demonstration of the effect of chemotherapy in osteosarcoma, not only for metastases but also on the primary bone lesion, opened up the possibility of limb-conserving bone resection and replacement in some of these patients.

### Soft tissue sarcoma

The pathological basis for limb-sparing surgery in soft tissue sarcoma is the tendency for these often grossly well demarcated tumours to spread microscopically within the confines of anatomical compartments but not readily to penetrate their fascial boundaries. Compartmental resection is therefore the logical radical surgical management. Not all soft tissue sarcomas arise within defined compartments (the axilla, groin, antecubital and popliteal fossae do not have complete fascial boundaries) and some of those which do originate within a compartment ultimately transgress those confines. For high grade sarcomas treated by surgery alone, radical limb-sparing compartmentectomy succeeds locally in only approximately 75% of patients. With diminishing margins of clearance the incidence of local recurrence progressively rises so that enucleation of the tumour in the temptingly deceptive plane of the pseudo-capsule virtually guarantees local failure [22].

Strict criteria of selection to achieve a reasonable control rate by surgery alone therefore necessarily condemns many patients to amputation. The capacity of radiotherapy to reduce local failure even after enucleation has been clearly demonstrated, so much so that some groups advocate a deliberate policy of surgical clearance with limited margins in order to preserve maximum limb function [23]. Local failure after limb conservation can usually be salvaged by further local resection or by amputation and this delay does not appear to prejudice survival [24]. In an attempt further to reduce the local failure rate, intra-arterial infusion of doxorubicin has been added to radiotherapy and surgery [25]. Initial reports of this trimodality approach quoted an extremely low rate of local failure but the incidence of limb morbidity was unacceptably high. Brennan *et al.* [26] claim excellent tumour control by local resection with interstitial radiotherapy with iridium wire after-loading. This technique obviates the need for prolonged outpatient irradiation but wound complications are increased. There is little to choose between these various combined treatment methods in terms of limb salvage and it requires long-term studies of late functional results coupled with cost and hospitalization time to determine which is the best approach. When further local resection is required for recurrence following radiotherapy, flap repair may be essential to ensure sound healing and good function [27].

While amputation achieves a lower local failure rate than combined modality management, survival is not improved [24] and few patients would elect to lose a limb where conservation can be offered. The finding in two studies that amputees scored better in terms of psychological morbidity than those managed by multi-modality limb-sparing treatment is puzzling and requires further elucidation [28,29]. There are obvious analogies with the current trends and controversies in the management of breast cancer.

## Osteosarcoma

This occurs most commonly at the lower end of the femur or upper end of the tibia of children and young adults. Amputation needs to be at mid-thigh level or, where there is extensive involvement of the femoral shaft, through the hip joint. Advances in chemotherapy together with developments in the field of bio-engineering permit limb conservation in selected cases by resection of an appropriate length

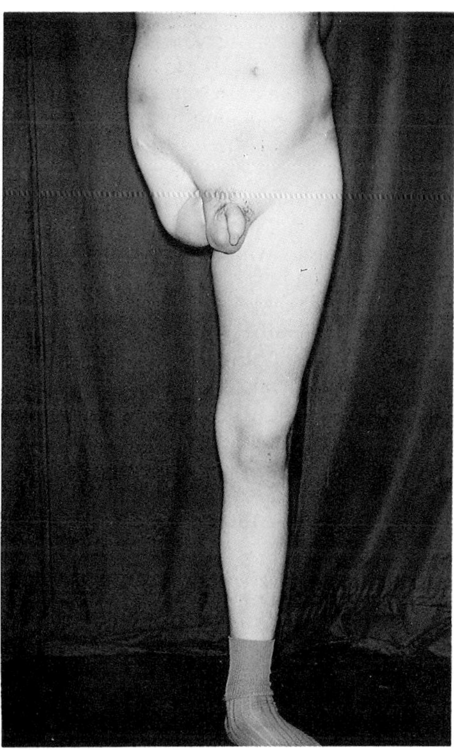

**Figure 29.6** Osteosarcoma of right femur treated by disarticulation through the hip joint

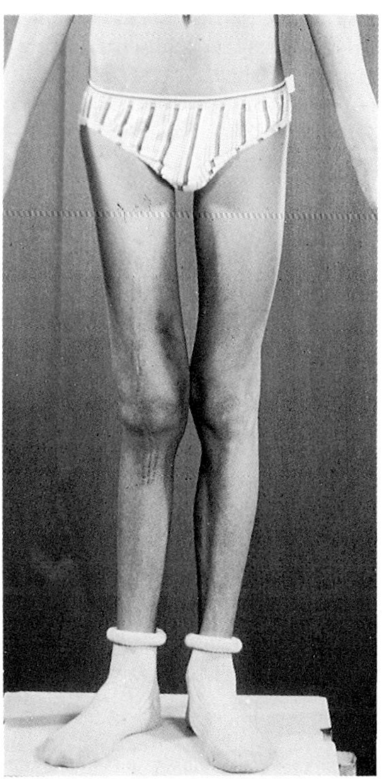

**Figure 29.7** Osteosarcoma of right femur. Local resection and replacement of lower two-thirds of femur and knee joint

of femur together with the knee joint and their replacement with a custom-built metallic endoprosthesis [30]. For children the femoral component is adjustable so as to allow lengthening at intervals to keep pace with normal limb growth. Limb-sparing surgery is contraindicated in the presence of extensive extraperiosteal spread into the soft tissues and there is then little alternative to major amputation (Figures 29.6 and 29.7).

## Sarcomas of the limb girdles

The most major and mutilating limb ablations in the surgical repertoire are the forequarter and the hindquarter amputation. Satisfactory limb-sparing resections of shoulder or pelvic girdle can sometimes be achieved provided the major nerves and vessels at the limb root are not involved by tumour. Such surgery is most readily undertaken in the upper limb where the shoulder girdle is non-weight-bearing and mobile. Scapulectomy, with or without resection of the upper end of the humerus and clavicle, are as effective cancer operations as amputation in appropriate cases and while resulting in a stiff or flail shoulder they leave the important functions of the arm, forearm and wrist unimpaired [31].

Osseous and cartilaginous tumours of the iliac blade or pubic bone may be locally resectable and this type of surgery produces relatively little disability. Where disease is more aggressive and involves the acetabulum, total excision of the hemi-pelvis

with limb conservation may still be possible provided the major nerves and vessels can be spared [32]. The subsequent gait resembles that of an untreated congenital dislocation of the hip but function is infinitely superior to that of an artificial limb fitted after hindquarter amputation. Function is further improved by use of a specially constructed 'saddle' endoprosthesis [33].

In the classical hindquarter amputation the ilium is sectioned close to the sacroiliac joint. Where the extent of disease permits, bone section can be performed at a more distal level, above the acetabulum (Figure 29.8). This not only conserves the contour of the iliac crest but leaves a stump of bone to provide valuable counter pressure for the prosthesis and thus considerably enhances function.

## Melanoma

Traditional management of the primary lesion was by wide excision including the underlying deep fascia, a policy based on an early post-mortem study of a patient dying of advanced disease [34]. Such clearance, which certainly in the limbs requires closure by split skin grafting, is greatly in excess of requirement for most melanomas which present for surgery. Breslow, whose staging system is based on the thickness of the primary tumour, found that for lesions less than 0.85 mm thick local recurrence and metastases were not seen even when excision margins were 1 mm or less [35]. Subsequent studies have established the safety of narrower than traditional margins of clearance graded according to Breslow microstaging [36]. Even for thick lesions many surgeons limit the normal tissue margin to 3 cm and conserve the deep fascia whose sacrifice confers no local or survival benefit [37]. Rationalization of surgery according to the biology of the individual melanoma has greatly reduced the need for mutilating excision and skin grafting with resulting diminution of deformity and hospital stay.

Controversy still surrounds the place of elective node dissection for N0 patients. This is especially the case in the lower limb because of the substantial morbidity following groin dissection both in terms of wound healing and subsequent lymphoedema. Veronesi *et al.* [38] found no survival benefit from elective node dissection while others have claimed reduced mortality though only for primary tumours of intermediate thickness [39]. These arguments will be resolved by prospective trials which are currently in progress but at present even the protagonists of elective dissection are selective in their choice of patients and exclude those with thin and very thick tumours from an unprofitable intervention. On the other hand, when the inguinal or axillary nodes are clinically involved and operable, radical dissection is

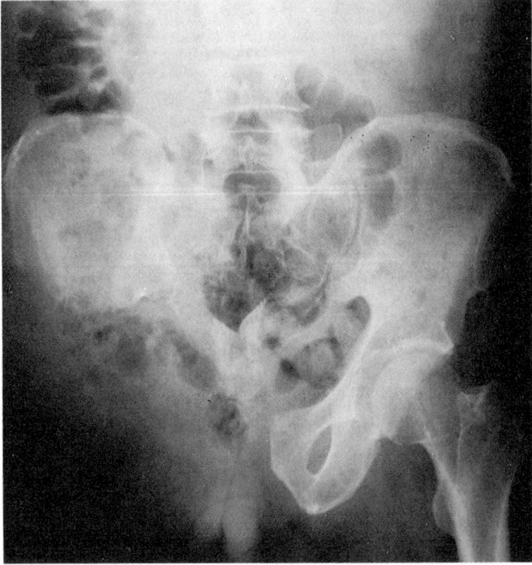

**Figure 29.8** Modified hindquarter amputation. Bone resected transversely above acetabulum

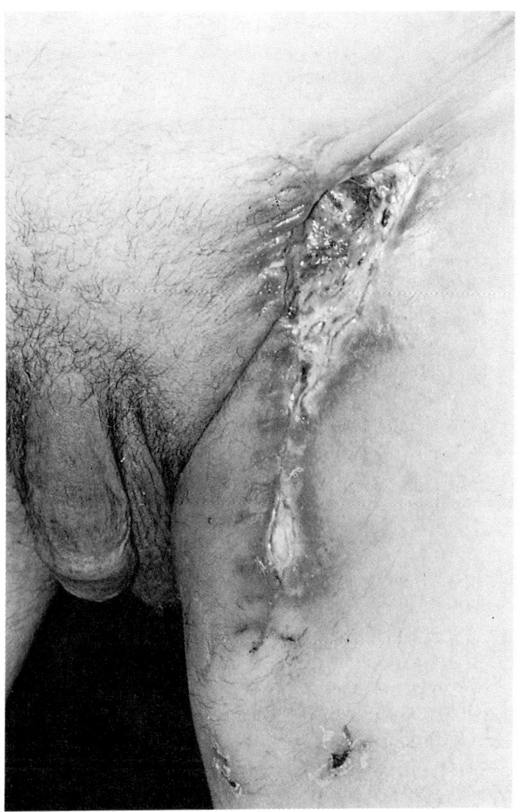

**Figure 29.9** Groin dissection showing extensive skin sloughing. The skin edges were not excised

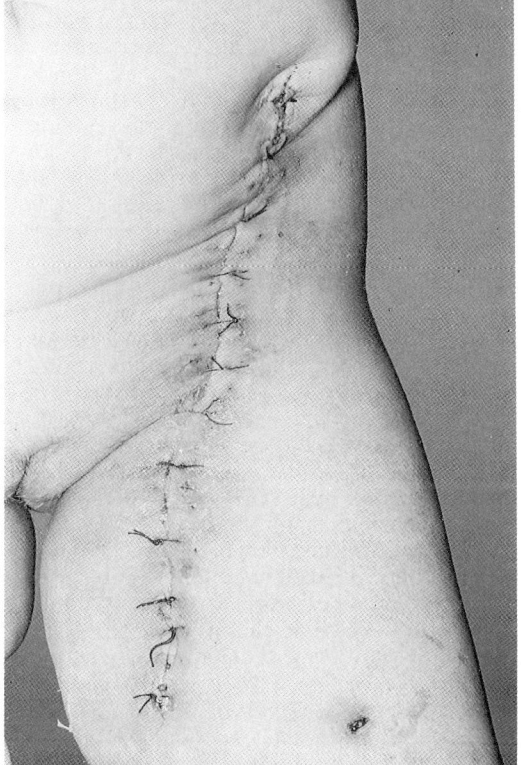

**Figure 29.10** Groin dissection showing per primam healing. The skin edges were excised prior to wound closure

mandatory to avoid the tragedy of uncontrolled nodal disease. For the lower limb ilio-inguinal dissection is superior to inguinal dissection in terms of local tumour control and carries no extra risk of lymphoedema [40]. The incidence of wound complications can be minimized by attention to important technical details, notably sacrifice of potentially ischaemic skin edges bordering a vertical incision [41] (Figures 29.9 and 29.10).

Major amputation in melanoma is now seldom undertaken, since such major mutilation cannot improve survival in the early case or achieve it when the disease is locoregionally advanced. Isolated limb perfusion plays a valuable role in the palliation of the latter group of patients [42].

# Gastrointestinal cancer

Surgical resection for gastrointestinal malignancy is commonly associated with a protracted recovery phase. During this time the general complications of intestinal surgery such as wound infection, chest infection and anastomotic leakage may cause considerable morbidity. Although cure rates have remained static over the last 50 years, advances in technology and technique have doubled the resection rate and halved the morbidity. The improved results from specialized centres throughout the world in all aspects of gastrointestinal cancer, as with most technically demanding surgery, depend on high standards of excellence and are achieved by treating large numbers of patients. In these centres the limits of surgery have almost been reached [43]. However, there is a disturbingly wide variation in results, both for cure and for surgical complication rates, outside these centres and a strong case can be made for specialization even within the overall confines of gastrointestinal tract surgery [44].

## Upper gastrointestinal cancer

### *Oesophageal cancer*

Surgical advances for oesophageal cancer emphasize the points made above. Because the 5-year survival rates are generally poor, the principal aim is to restore the ability to swallow food. The best functional results are obtained by resection and anastomosis rather than with irradiation. When the tumour is too advanced for curative therapy, palliative bypass or direct laser coagulation produce a better quality of life than simple intubation [45]. The traditional surgical approach for middle third tumours has been a staged trans-thoracic procedure, but recently, trans-hiatal oesophagectomy has become fashionable [46]. The main advantages of this approach rest on the avoidance of thoracotomy in elderly patients with reduced pulmonary reserve. However, the trans-hiatal procedure involves 'blind' dissection and this may cause rupture of the oesophagus or surrounding vessels when the tumour is fixed. For these reasons it should be restricted to selected cases where the tumour lies at either end of the gullet, when the patient is unfit for thoracotomy and when CT scanning shows no para-oesophageal invasion. Sugimachi *et al.* [47] stress that the prognosis of patients with oesophageal cancer is related to the resectability of lesion and the extent of postoperative complications. Though 53% of 123 patients developed postoperative complications, the vast majority of these were related to pulmonary infection and failure (32%) whereas only 7% developed anastomotic leakage. Meticulous refinements in technique and perioperative care have allowed other Japanese authors to report 38% 5-year survival rates with a mortality rate of less than 2% [48]. Such results were accomplished by working free from stress imposed by theatre time restrictions, use of a diathermy knife, avoidance of blood loss and transfusion, and extensive use of stapling devices. Results of this order place an obligation on the occasional resectionist to refer patients to a specialized centre.

## Gastric cancer

New technology and technique are also important in gastric cancer, but in addition demographic factors play a role. The prognosis is much better in Japan than in Europe, and is explained by the higher incidence of early gastric cancer. This has, paradoxically, been accompanied by the development of more radical types of gastrectomy which include extensive dissections away from the perigastric lymph nodes [49]. In the UK, gastric cancer has a gloomier outlook since the majority of patients present with advanced disease, and the 5-year survival rate is only 20%. Less extensive gastrectomy is recommended because there are few cases that satisfy the Japanese criteria for radical cure [50]. Moreover, radical resection is associated with increased operating time, blood loss and postoperative stay without any proven survival benefit [51].

Thus, outside Japan, standard partial or total gastrectomy is the preferred means of improving quality of life without causing excessive morbidity.

## Pancreatic cancer

The incidence of pancreatic cancer is rising. It is a disease which carries a very poor prognosis and palliative treatment is all that can be offered for most patients. Pancreatectomy, when possible, is attended by considerable morbidity and mortality even in experienced hands [52]. When resection seems feasible the choice of procedure rests between total pancreatectomy (which renders the patient devoid of exocrine and endocrine function), Whipple's operation (which includes resection of the pylorus, duodenum and antrum but maintains distal pancreatic function), and pylorus-preserving pancreatectomy [53]. Conservation of the pylorus has been claimed to improve functional results. In patients presenting with obstructive jaundice the overall 5-year survival rate is in the order of 5%. The morbidity and mortality for major surgery in the presence of chronic biliary obstruction is considerable and appears to be especially related to the effects of hepato-renal failure. It was hoped that a period of biliary decompression by external drainage prior to surgery would reduce the risk of this complication, but the study of McPherson *et al.* [54] showed that this potential benefit was not realized. However, the advent of the biliary endoprosthesis does offer an alternative to surgical decompression of the common bile duct. Stents can be introduced either by the endoscopic [55] or transhepatic routes [56]. Although survival remains unaffected, patients so treated have shorter hospital stays. Internal stenting also shows promise as a means to improve biliary drainage prior to Whipple's operation for ampullary tumours [57].

## Colorectal cancer

Although surgical resection might seem to be a standardized procedure, the extent of local and lymph node dissection and the effectiveness of measures preventing local or systemic spread during the operation are not well defined [58]. Furthermore, surgical management differs for elective cases and those patients presenting with large bowel obstruction. For right-sided obstructing cancers, resection and primary anastomosis is the universally accepted practice. However, for left-sided obstructing cancers, the introduction of on-table lavage to achieve safe restorative resection without covering colostomy has yet to convince many surgeons to abandon the time-honoured two-stage approach with preliminary relieving colostomy [59,60].

### Avoiding colostomy and local recurrence

In the last decade there has been a technical revolution in the surgical management of rectal cancer. The introduction of stapling instruments has allowed conservation of the anal sphincter in many more patients than previously. The resulting quality of life is far superior to that associated with a permanent colostomy, although frequency of bowel action may still be an inconvenience for some patients with very low anastomoses [61]. However, even this relative imperfection may now be circumvented by the construction of a colonic pouch [62,63]. The construction of small bowel pouches has little place in the management of invasive colorectal cancer, but may be of use in avoiding a permanent ileostomy in patients requiring total colectomy for premalignant conditions such as ulcerative colitis, Crohn's disease and polyposis coli. It is, however, disturbing that despite these advances, local recurrence after rectal excision varies from less than 5% to more than 20%, depending on the expertise of the surgeon [64]. Some of these differences may depend on case selection, but they are more likely to be due to variations in the extent of local tissue removal. The mesorectum and pararectal tissues often contain microscopic tumour deposits, and failure to remove these tissues favours local recurrence.

### Avoidance of anastomotic recurrence

At the time of presentation, 60% of patients with large bowel cancer are suitable for a 'curative' resection [65]. Unfortunately, anastomotic recurrence develops in 5–18%, and is associated with substantial morbidity and mortality. Residual tumour cells in the mesorectum which spread back towards the anastomosis may be responsible in some cases. It seems unlikely that anastomotic recurrence results from incomplete mucosal resection because distal intramural spread is uncommon and only affects a few millimetres of rectum [66]. Alternative mechanisms include implantation of exfoliated cancer cells liberated at the time of operation [67] and metachronous carcinogenesis at a site of proliferative instability [68]. Steps used to reduce implantation include cleansing the bowel ends with chlorhexidine-cetrimide or povidone-iodine solutions prior to suturing and irrigating the distal bowel prior to mobilizing the tumour and on completion of the anastomosis [69]. Metachronous carcinogenesis may explain why anastomotic recurrence is more likely to develop at colocolic or colorectal anastomoses (10%) than at ileocolic anastomoses (<1%), as the small bowel appears to be relatively resistant to the effects of carcinogens. Increased adoption of subtotal colectomy would decrease the incidence of metachronous tumours, reduce the risk of anastomotic leak due to tenuous blood supply, and simplify follow-up, since only sigmoidoscopy would be required [70]. Such an approach would necessitate leaving sufficient distal bowel to avoid the problems of frequent bowel action.

### Prevention and treatment of hepatic metastases

Clumps of tumour cells may be shed into the portal circulation during manipulation of the tumour and produce hepatic metastases. Implantation may be enhanced by blood loss, transfusion and anaesthesia. Turnbull, in 1970, reported that the incidence of liver metastases was reduced by preliminary division of the lymphovascular pedicle coupled with minimal handing of the bowel (so-called 'no-touch' technique) prior to tumour mobilization [71]. Although Turnbull's hypothesis has been disputed, Wiggers *et al.* [72] recently reported a similar improvement using an identical technique.

Longitudinal studies of CT scanning of the liver have demonstrated that occult hepatic metastases are present in 15–35% of patients at the time of laparotomy [73]. Median survival time in untreated patients is between 4.5 months and 15 months. In all, 16% of untreated patients with solitary liver secondaries will survive for 5 years, while up to 40% selected with less than four metastases will survive after resection. In order to justify the high risks of hepatic resection, considerable expertise is required and this type of surgery should only be performed in specialized centres where morbidity is at an acceptable level and mortality is less than 5% [74]. New technology, such as the use of perioperative ultrasonography, provides supplementary information to the surgeon to help select those who might benefit from this procedure [75]. Unfortunately, less than 7% of all patients with liver metastases are suitable for such surgery [76].

## Urological cancer

Patients with cancer of the urinary tract have benefited from improvements in instrumentation and in surgical technique. The renal pelvis and calyces can be inspected with a telescope inserted under radiological control through a small incision in the loin and superficial epithelial tumours destroyed under vision by diathermy or laser. This 'minimally invasive surgery', developed originally as an alternative to open surgery for calculous disease of the kidney, is of particular value in patients with a solitary kidney and those who are poor operative risks. Major surgery is especially hazardous in the presence of renal impairment due to chronic urinary obstruction. In the case of resectable cancers drainage of the kidneys can be established quite simply by minimal surgery of the above type and this has replaced the major procedure of formal bilateral nephrostomy. Where there is ureteric obstruction from inoperable extrinsic compression due to malignant retroperitoneal masses, the kidneys can be decompressed by the cystoscopic insertion of ureteric stents. The resultant improvement in renal function may permit treatment of the obstructing pathology, e.g. testicular tumour metastatic to the para-aortic lymph nodes, so that the stents can subsequently be removed.

## Continent urinary diversion

The operation of total cystectomy, whether undertaken alone for primary bladder cancer or as a component of partial or total exenteration, must be completed by some form of urinary diversion. This is most commonly achieved by implanting the ureters into a conduit of ileum which drains at the skin surface into a bag. The use of a drainage bag is an embarrassment to some patients so that there is considerable interest in methods of achieving continent urinary reservoirs. These are of two main types. In the first the ureters are implanted into a Kock pouch of ileum where the bowel is intussuscepted to form a valvular stoma (as originally used to fashion a continent ileostomy following total colectomy). In the second the Mitrofanoff principle is applied in which the appendix or an isolated segment of ureter or fallopian tube is used as a conduit from the urinary reservoir to the skin, continence being achieved by tunnelling the conduit sub-mucosally into the segment of small or large bowel in valvular fashion. In either method the patient catheterizes the stoma intermittently. These are time-consuming procedures to follow a major resection and carry their own complications, though less for the Mitrofanoff than for the Kock operation [77]. Their use should be restricted to patients who are fit and have a reasonable life expectancy in terms of their age and malignant disease.

## Cancer of the prostate

Although British urologists have in the past been reluctant to consider radical prostatectomy for early stage cancer, this approach is beginning to attract attention in some centres in the UK. While the role of this type of surgery is still controversial, its application is clearly restricted to disease confined within the prostatic capsule. Case selection is therefore of crucial importance and clinical assessment is considerably sharpened by the use of trans-rectal ultrasound imaging. Among the objections to classical radical prostatectomy is the morbidity of impo-

tence and incontinence. A modified dissection of the gland which spares the neurovascular bundle to the corpus cavernosum [78], coupled with conservation or careful repair of the bladder neck, avoids these two distressing sequelae in the majority of cases.

## Lung cancer

Measures to reduce morbidity for surgery in lung cancer can be considered in terms of preoperative evaluation, intraoperative measures and postoperative management.

## Preoperative evaluation

General clinical assessment of cardiopulmonary function is supplemented by split lung function studies and exercise testing with electrocardiographic monitoring to uncover asymptomatic ischaemic heart disease. These measures are important because of the association of smoking with chronic bronchitis and coronary artery disease, and the fact that lung cancer generally affects the older age groups.

More specifically, careful staging of intrathoracic disease is essential to exclude inoperable cases from futile thoracotomy [79]. Computed tomography of the chest and mediastinoscopy are important measures in the patient with a normal chest radiograph. Mediastinoscopy is especially valuable when computed tomography shows an abnormality in the mediastinum since not all abnormalities are due to malignancy. This procedure carries a very small morbidity and virtually no mortality. The adoption of these investigations has considerably reduced the incidence of failed thoracotomy with its attendant morbidity and mortality, and pulmonary resection rates greater than 90% are regularly achieved.

## Intraoperative measures

The essential surgical procedure is resection of the primary tumour and of the regional lymph nodes. Sacrifice of normal lung tissue should be avoided as far as is technically possible. The results of lobectomy in terms of cancer control match those of pneumonectomy and carry a much lower morbidity and mortality; sleeve resection of the bronchus extends the scope of lung conservation in suitable cases [80]. For selected patients with T1,N0 tumours, segmental resection is as effective as lobectomy. The complication of bronchopleural fistula has been largely eliminated as the result of careful surgical handling of the tissues and the use of polypropylene sutures or staples for bronchial closure. Application of the cryoprobe to the intercostal nerves on either side of the thoracotomy incision prior to chest closure reduces postoperative pain and greatly assists deep breathing and clearing of sputum in the postoperative period.

### Postoperative management [81]

The importance of pain control has been mentioned and intercostal nerve cryoablation should be supplemented by the use of effective analgesics. The problem of sputum retention in the early postoperative period has been greatly diminished by the mini-tracheostomy tube which can be readily inserted through the cricothyroid membrane under local anaesthesia. In certain cases, e.g. following tracheal resection or in elderly patients with impaired pulmonary function, mini-tracheostomy is often established at the time of operation.

Infection is not commonly a major complication of pulmonary surgery but antibiotics are especially important in pneumonectomy where there is a large dead space, or in patients whose ability to resist sepsis has been impaired by cytotoxic therapy. Supraventricular tachyarrhythmias may complicate pulmonary resection especially in the elderly, following right pneumonectomy, intrapericardial manipulation or hypoxia. Prophylactic digoxin is indicated in the presence of these risk factors.

# Head and neck cancer

This anatomical area is small in volume but crowded with organs of specialized function in relation to the special senses, speech and swallowing. Cancer, and the surgery required for its control, may inflict devastating disabilities. Conservation and reconstruction are both employed in their mitigation.

### Conservation surgery

In the classical radical neck dissection the specimen includes the sternomastoid muscle, the internal jugular vein and the accessory nerve. Loss of the accessory nerve is disabling in many patients causing drooping and weakness of the shoulder, sometimes associated with considerable pain. With appropriate case selection modifications of the classical operation which spare the nerve have shown no detriment to control of disease in the neck [82]. Where bilateral simultaneous neck dissection is required conservation of one internal jugular vein prevents the gross facial congestion and oedema and occasional cerebral symptoms which follow bilateral ligation.

Carcinoma of the tongue seldom invades the mandible yet mandibular resection has, in the past, been a component of the composite (commando) operation for those tumours unsuitable for peroral

removal. Loss of a segment of mandible is deforming and disabling, especially in the region of the chin. Perfect access for composite resection without loss of the mandible can be attained in most cases either by median mandibulotomy with mandibular swing or by the pull-through procedure [83]. Where carcinoma of the tongue or of the floor of the mouth is adherent to but not frankly invading the inner table, adequate surgical clearance can be obtained with maintenance of the arch by splitting the mandible sagittally with the power saw and removing the detached portion of inner table in continuity with the soft tissue specimen.

### Reconstruction

The subject of reconstruction following major surgery in this region has undergone a major revolution in the past 20 years [84]. In particular the development of regional, axial patterned, cutaneous and myocutaneous flaps, and more recently the ability to transfer free flaps with microvascular anastomosis, has enabled surgeons to undertake complete restoration of major defects at the same session as the resection. Patients, who in the past spent months in hospital undergoing multistage tube pedicle transfer, are now able to leave hospital with their repair completed within a few weeks of operation. The introduction of well vascularized tissue into the repair is of particular value after radiotherapy. Wound breakdown with salivary fistula and its potentially lethal risk of secondary carotid arterial haemorrhage is now rarely seen.

# Central nervous system cancer

Improvements in general care including anaesthesia, the establishment of intensive therapy units and the use of steroids have all contributed to the reduction in morbidity associated with the surgery of the central nervous system. Modern imaging techniques have replaced invasive radiology which had its own hazards, and have also helped in case selection and the correct allocation of treatment. The ultrasonic aspirator and the laser permit surgical ablation of tumours with less damage to normal brain tissue than the use of conventional instruments.

### Brain tumours

Prior to the availability of computed tomography and magnetic resonance imaging, biopsy carried a 15% mortality with a successful diagnosis in only 85% of cases. Now with stereotactic guided biopsy of the Tru-Cut needle type, mortality is less than 1%, morbidity which is mainly reversible in the order of 5% and the positive diagnosis rate over 90%.

Surgical resection for operable tumours can be undertaken either by image-directed stereotactic techniques [85] or freehand using the operating microscope. The surgeon is thereby able to operate close to the tumour and avoid unnecessary damage to the normal brain.

## Childhood brain tumours

The majority of these are located in the posterior fossa and children usually present with hydrocephalus, vomiting and dehydration. Formerly treatment involved a limited resection and the insertion of a shunt to reduce intracranial pressure, followed by radiotherapy. The preferred approach now is to remove sufficient tumour to restore the drainage of cerebrospinal fluid. This avoids the complications of a shunt and at the same time leaves less residual tumour for the radiotherapist and medical oncologist to deal with.

## Spinal tumours

The commonest cause of extradural compression of the cord is metastatic tumour. Surgery is indicated in the presence of progressive paraparesis in patients with a reasonable life expectancy from their cancer. In general, complete paraplegia of more than 12 h duration is accompanied by a decreasing chance of recovery and after 24 h the prospects are extremely poor. The purposes of surgery are relief of pain, preservation of neurological function and, where appropriate, stabilization of the associated fracture. Operation carries a not insignificant mortality and morbidity in the patient with carcinomatosis [86]. Modern imaging has enabled more rational and accurate planning of operation than hitherto. When the tumour is situated predominantly posterior to the cord, classical laminectomy is indicated. When, however, most of the tumour lies anteriorly as is more commonly the case, a lateral or anterior approach has gained favour, with removal of part of the involved vertebra where necessary and mechanical stabilization.

## References


1. Francis, D.M.A. and Judson, R.T. Blood transfusion and the recurrence of cancer of the colon and rectum. *British Journal of Surgery*, **74**, 26–30 (1987)
2. Bryant, M. and Baum, M. Postmastectomy seroma following mastectomy and axillary dissection. *British Journal of Surgery*, **74**, 1187 (1987)
3. Cameron, A.E.P., Ebbs, S.R., Wylie, F. and Baum, M. Suction drainage of the axilla: a prospective randomized trial. *British Journal of Surgery*, **75**, 1211 (1988)
4. Kissin, M.W., Querci della Rovere, G., Easton, D. and Westbury, G. Risk of lymphoedema following the treatment of breast cancer. *British Journal of Surgery*, **73**, 580–584 (1986)
5. Davidson, T., Westbury, G. and Harmer, C.L. Radiation-induced soft-tissue sarcoma. *British Journal of Surgery*, **73**, 308–309 (1986)
6. Barr, L.C. and Kissin, M.W. Radiation-induced brachial plexus neuropathy following breast conservation and radical radiotherapy. *British Journal of Surgery*, **74**, 855–856 (1987)
7. Aitken, R.J., Gaze, M.N., Rodger, A. *et al.* Arm morbidity within a trial of mastectomy and either nodal sample with selective adjuvant radiotherapy or axillary clearance. *British Journal of Surgery*, **76**, 568–571 (1989)
8. Hoffman, G.W. and Elliott, L.F. The anatomy of the pectoral nerves and its significance to the general and plastic surgeon. *Annals of Surgery*, **205**, 504–506 (1987)
9. Teicher, I., Poulard, B. and Wise, L. Preservation of the intercostobrachial nerve during axillary dissection for carcinoma of the breast. *Surgery, Gynecology and Obstetrics*, **155**, 891–892 (1982)
10. Maguire, G.P., Lee, E.G., Bevington, D.J. *et al.* Psychiatric problems in the first year after mastectomy. *British Medical Journal*, **i**, 963–965 (1978)
11. Fallowfield, L.J., Baum, M. and Maguire, G.P. The effects of breast conservation on psychological morbidity associated with diagnosis and treatment of early breast cancer. *British Medical Journal*, **293**, 1331–1334 (1986)
12. Maguire, P., Brooke, M., Tait, A. *et al.* The effect of counselling on physical disability and social recovery after mastectomy. *Clinical Oncology*, **9**, 319–324 (1983)
13. Ward, D.J. Breast reconstruction. *Hospital Update*, **13**, 725–734 (1987)
14. Mansel, R.E., Horgan, K., Webster, D.J.T. *et al.* Cosmetic results of immediate breast reconstruction post-mastectomy: a follow-up study. *British Journal of Surgery*, **73**, 813–816 (1986)
15. Dickson, M.G., Sharpe, D.T., Dickson, W.A. *et al.* Breast reconstruction by tissue expansion. *Annals of the Royal College of Surgeons of England*, **68**, 18–21 (1986)
16. Hinton, C.P., Doyle, P.J., Blamey, R.W. *et al.* Subcutaneous mastectomy for primary operable breast cancer. *British Journal of Surgery*, **71**, 469–472 (1984)
17. Laskin, W.B., Silverman, T.A. and Enzinger, F.M. Postradiation soft tissue sarcomas: an analysis of 53 cases. *Cancer*, **62**, 2330–2340 (1988)
18. Jennings, T.A., Peterson, L., Axiotis, C.A. *et al.* Angiosarcoma associated with foreign body material: a report of three cases. *Cancer*, **62**, 2436–2444 (1988)
19. Aspegren, K., Holmberg, L. and Adami, H-O. Standardization of the surgical technique in breast-conserving treatment of mammary cancer. *British Journal of Surgery*, **75**, 807–810 (1988)

20. Lucarotti, M., White, H. and Leaper, D.J. The role of intraoperative breast cytology to assess the extent of conservative surgery. *European Journal of Surgical Oncology*, **14**, 710 (1988)

21. Cade, S. Soft tissue tumours: their natural history and treatment. *Proceedings of the Royal Society of Medicine*, **44**, 19–36 (1951)

22. Cantin, J., McNeer, G.P., Chu, F.C. and Booher, R.J. The problem of local recurrence after treatment of soft tissue sarcoma. *Annals of Surgery*, **168**, 47–53 (1986)

23. Suit, H.D., Mankin, H.J., Schiller, A.L. *et al.* Results of treatment of sarcoma of soft tissue by radiation and surgery at Massachusetts General Hospital. *Cancer Treatment Symposia*, **3**, 43–47 (1985)

24. Potter, D.A., Kinsella, T., Glatstein, E. *et al.* High-grade soft tissue sarcomas of the extremities. *Cancer*, **58**, 190–205 (1986)

25. Eilber, F.R., Morton, D.L., Eckardt, J. *et al.* Limb salvage for skeletal and soft tissue sarcomas. Multidisciplinary preoperative therapy. *Cancer*, **53**, 2579–2584 (1984)

26. Brennan, M.F., Hilaris, B., Shiu, M.H. *et al.* Local recurrence in adult soft-tissue sarcoma. A randomised trial of brachytherapy. *Archives of Surgery*, **122**, 1289–1293 (1987)

27. Stotter, A., McLean, N.R., Fallowfield, M.E. *et al.* Reconstruction after excision of soft tissue sarcomas of the limbs and trunk. *British Journal of Surgery*, **75**, 774–778 (1988)

28. Sugarbaker, P.H., Barofsky, I., Rosenberg, S.A. and Gianola, F.J. Quality of life assessment of patients in extremity sarcoma clinical trials. *Surgery*, **91**, 17–23 (1982)

29. Weddington, W.W. Jr., Segraves, B.K. and Simon, M.A. Psychological outcome of extremity sarcoma survivors undergoing amputation or limb salvage. *Journal of Clinical Oncology*, **3**, 1393–1399 (1985)

30. Kemp, H. Limb conservation for osteosarcoma and other primary bone tumours. *Baillière's Clinical Oncology*, **1**, 111–136 (1987)

31. Malawer, M.M., Sugarbaker, P.H., Lampert, M. *et al.* The Tikhoff-Linberg procedure: report of ten patients and presentation of a modified technique for tumors of the proximal humerus. *Surgery*, **97**, 518–528 (1985)

32. Sweetnam, R. Limb preservation in the treatment of bone tumours. *Annals of the Royal College of Surgeons of England*, **65**, 3–7 (1983)

33. Steinbrink, K. and Neider, E. Total femoral replacement and the saddle prosthesis. In *Bone Tumour Management* (eds R. Coombs and G. Friedlaender), Butterworths, London, pp. 159–165 (1987)

34. Handley, W.S. The pathology of melanotic growths in relation to their operative treatment. *Lancet*, **i**, 927–933, 996–1003 (1907)

35. Breslow, A. and Macht, S.D. Optimal size of resection margin for thin cutaneous melanoma. *Surgery, Gynecology and Obstetrics*, **145**, 691–692 (1977)

36. Taylor, B.A. and Hughes, L.A. A policy of selective excision for cutaneous malignant melanoma. *European Journal of Surgical Oncology*, **11**, 7–13 (1985)

37. Kenady, D.E., Brown, B.W. and McBride, C.M. Excision of underlying fascia with a primary malignant melanoma: effect on recurrence and survival rates. *Surgery*, **92**, 615–618 (1982)

38. Veronesi, U., Adamus, J., Bandiera, D.C. *et al.* Inefficacy of immediate node dissection in stage 1 melanoma of the limbs. *New England Journal of Medicine*, **297**, 627–630 (1977)

39. Balch, C.M., Soong, S.-J., Milton, G.W. *et al.* A comparison of prognostic factors and surgical results in 1,786 patients with localised (Stage I) melanoma treated in Alabama, USA and New South Wales, Australia. *Annals of Surgery*, **196**, 677–684 (1982)

40. Kissin, M.W., Simpson, D.A., Easton, D. *et al.* Prognostic factors related to survival and groin recurrence following therapeutic lymph node dissection for malignant melanoma. *British Journal of Surgery*, **74**, 1023–1026 (1987)

41. Westbury, G. Axillary and inguinal node clearance. In *Rob and Smith's Operative Surgery: Plastic Surgery* (eds J. Watson and R.M. McCormack), Butterworths, London, pp. 433–438 (1980)

42. Rosin, R.D. and Westbury, G. Isolated limb perfusion for malignant melanoma. *Practitioner*, **224**, 1031–1036 (1980)

43. Williams, N.S. Changing patterns in the treatment of rectal cancer. *British Journal of Surgery*, **76**, 5–6 (1989)

44. Anonymous. Rectal cancer should be treated by experts. *Lancet*, **i**, 1476 (1986)

45. Steger, A.C. and Hira, N. The palliative endoscopic treatment of inoperable oesophagogastric and rectal cancers: a low power contact laser technique. *Annals of the Royal College of Surgeons of England*, **69**, 166–168 (1987)

46. Wong, J. Transhiatal oesophagectomy for carcinoma of the thoracic oesophagus. *British Journal of Surgery*, **73**, 89–90 (1986)

47. Sugimachi, K., Matsuoka, H., Ohno, S. *et al.* Multivariate approach for assessing the prognosis of clinical oesophageal carcinoma. *British Journal of Surgery*, **75**, 1115–1118 (1988)

48. Khoury, G. Oesophageal surgery under Akiyama. *Lancet*, **i**, 91 (1989)

49. Kodama, Y., Sugimachi, K., Soejima *et al.* Evaluation of extensive lymph node dissection for carcinoma of the stomach. *World Journal of Surgery*, **5**, 241–248 (1981)

50. Irvin, T.T. and Bridger, J.E. Gastric cancer: an audit of 122 consecutive cases and the results of $R_1$ gastrectomy. *British Journal of Surgery*, **75**, 106–109 (1988)

51. Dent, D.M., Madden, M.V. and Price, S.K. Randomized comparison of $R_1$ and $R_2$ gastrectomy for gastric cancer. *British Journal of Surgery*, **75**, 110–112 (1988)

52. Trede, M. Treatment of pancreatic carcinoma: the

surgeon's dilemma. *British Journal of Surgery*, **74**, 79–80 (1987)

53. McMahon, M.J. Operative techniques – pylorus-preserving pancreaticoduodenectomy. *Surgery*, **58**, 1393–1394 (1988)

54. McPherson, G.A.D., Benjamin, A.S., Hodgson, H.J.F. *et al*. Pre-operative percutaneous transhepatic biliary drainage: the results of a controlled trial. *British Journal of Surgery*, **71**, 371–375 (1984)

55. Shepherd, H.A., Royle, G., Ross, A.P.R. *et al*. Endoscopic biliary endoprosthesis in the palliation of malignant obstruction of the distal common bile duct: a randomized trial. *British Journal of Surgery*, **75**, 1166–1168 (1988)

56. Speer, A., Russell, R.C.G., Hatfield, A. *et al*. Randomized trial of endoscopic vs percutaneous stent insertion for malignant obstructive jaundice. *Lancet*, **i**, 57–61 (1987)

57. Neoptolemus, J.P., Talbot, I.C., Carr-Locke, D.L. *et al*. Treatment and outcome in 52 consecutive cases of ampullary carcinoma. *British Journal of Surgery*, **74**, 957–962 (1987)

58. Sugarbaker, P.H. and Corlew, S. Influence of surgical techniques on survival in patients with colorectal cancer. *Diseases of the Colon and Rectum*, **25**, 545–547 (1982)

59. Thompson, W.H.F. and Carter, S.St.C. On-table lavage to achieve safe restorative rectal and emergency left colonic resection without covering colostomy. *British Journal of Surgery*, **73**, 61–63 (1986)

60. Huddy, S.P.J., Shorthouse, A.J. and Marks, C.G. The surgical treatment of intestinal obstruction due to left sided carcinoma of the colon. *Annals of the Royal College of Surgeons of England*, **70**, 40–43 (1988)

61. Williams, N.S. The rationale for preservation of the anal sphincter in patients with low rectal cancer. *British Journal of Surgery*, **71**, 575–581 (1984)

62. Lazorthes, F., Fales, P., Chiotasso, P. *et al*. Resection of the rectum with construction of a colonic reservoir and coloanal anastomosis for carcinoma of the rectum. *British Journal of Surgery*, **73**, 139–141 (1986)

63. Parc, R., Tiret, E., Frileux, P. *et al*. Resection and coloanal anastomosis with colonic reservoir for rectal carcinoma. *British Journal of Surgery*, **73**, 139–141 (1986)

64. Phillips, R.K.S., Hittinger, R., Blesovsky, L. *et al*. Local recurrence following curative surgery for large bowel cancer: the overall picture. *British Journal of Surgery*, **71**, 12–16 (1984)

65. Umpleby, H.C. and Williamson, R.C.N. Anastomotic recurrence in large bowel cancer. *British Journal of Surgery*, **74**, 873–878 (1987)

66. Kirwan, W.O., Drumm, J., Hogan, J.M. and Keohane, C. Determining safe margin of resection in low anterior resection for rectal cancer. *British Journal of Surgery*, **75**, 720 (1988)

67. Umpleby, H.C., Fermor, B., Symes, M.O. and Williamson, R.C.N. Viability of exfoliated colorectal cancer cells. *British Journal of Surgery*, **71**, 659–653 (1984)

68. Williamson, R.C.N., Davies, P.W., Bristol, J.B. and Wells, M. Intestinal adaptation and experimental carcinogenesis after partial colectomy: increased tumour yields are confined to the anastomosis. *Gut*, **23**, 316–325 (1982)

69. Skipper, D., Cooper, A.J., Marston, J.E. and Taylor, I. Exfoliated cells and *in vitro* growth in colorectal cancer. *British Journal of Surgery*, **74**, 1049–1052 (1987)

70. Marston, A. Treatment of cancer of the colon: a non-specialist's point of view. *British Journal of Surgery*, **76**, 71 (1989)

71. Turnbull, R.B. Jr. Cancer of the colon. The five- and ten-year survival rates following resection utilizing the isolation technique. *Annals of the Royal College of Surgeons of England*, **46**, 243–250 (1970)

72. Wiggers, T., Jeekel, J., Arends, J.W. *et al*. No-touch isolation technique in colon cancer: a controlled prospective trial. *British Journal of Surgery*, **75**, 409–415 (1988)

73. Finlay, I.G. and McArdle, C.S. Occult hepatic metastases in colon cancer. *British Journal of Surgery*, **73**, 732–735 (1986)

74. Greenway, B. Hepatic metastases from colorectal cancer: resection or not. *British Journal of Surgery*, **75**, 513–519 (1988)

75. Traynor, O., Castaing, D. and Bismuth, H. Peroperative ultrasonography in the surgery of hepatic tumours. *British Journal of Surgery*, **75**, 197–202 (1988)

76. Taylor, I. Colorectal liver metastases – to treat or not to treat. *British Journal of Surgery*, **72**, 511–516 (1985)

77. Cumming, J., Worth, P.H.L. and Woodhouse, C.R.J. The choice of suprapubic continent catheterisable urinary stoma. *British Journal of Urology*, **60**, 227–230 (1987)

78. Walsh, P.C. and Mostwin, J.L. Radical prostatectomy and cystoprostatectomy with preservation of potency. Results using a new nerve-sparing technique. *British Journal of Urology*, **56**, 694–697 (1984)

79. Spiro, S.G. and Goldstraw, P. Editorial. The staging of lung cancer. *Thorax*, **39**, 401–407 (1984)

80. Deslauriers, J., Gaulin, P., Beaulieu, M. *et al*. Long-term clinical and functional results of sleeve lobectomy for primary lung cancer. *Journal of Thoracic and Cardiovascular Surgery*, **92**, 871–879 (1986)

81. Goldstraw, P. Postoperative management of the surgical patient. *Baillière's Clinical Anaesthesiology*, **1**, 207–231 (1987)

82. Byers, R.M., Wolf, P.F. and Ballantyne, A.J. Rationale for elective modified neck dissection. *Head and Neck Surgery*, **10**, 160–167 (1988)

83. Westbury, G. Carcinoma of the tongue. In *Rob and Smith's Operative Surgery: Plastic Surgery*, 4th edn (eds T.L. Barclay and D.A. Kernahan), Butterworths, London, pp. 483–494 (1986)

84. McGregor, I.A. and McGregor, F.M. In *Cancer of the Face and Mouth: Pathology and Management for Surgeons*, Churchill Livingstone, Edinburgh, pp. 5–54 (1986)

85. Kelly, P.J., Alker, G.J. Jr. and Goerss, S. Computer-assisted stereotactic laser microsurgery for the treatment of intracranial neoplasms. *Neurosurgery*, **10**, 324–331 (1982)

86. Findlay, G.F.G. Adverse effects of the management of malignant spinal and compression. *Journal of Neurology, Neurosurgery and Psychiatry*, **47**, 767–788 (1984)

# 30

# Minimizing the morbidity from radiotherapy

**P.N. Plowman**

Radiotherapy currently holds a cardinal place in the local/regional control of many cancers, but the increasing awareness of radiation morbidity, the causation of which is nowadays so much better understood, has made critical auditing of the practice of radiation therapy an important subject. Take, for example, the patient whose retinoblastoma was cured in early childhood by a single fraction of radiotherapy from a lateral orthovoltage portal (Figure 30.1). The punched out, poorly developed temporal region and the atrophic, telangiectatic skin bear witness to an unfractionated radical dose in childhood. In this review we must study the use of fraction size in reducing morbidity. Take as another example the child whose flank radiation planning following nephrectomy for Wilms' tumour was carried out to a very low technical standard (Figure 30.2). Figure 30.2a demonstrates that the patient was simulated but the radiation therapist was ignorant of or failed to observe the recommendation to encompass both vertebral growth centres in the portal. The consequence of the therapist's oversight is shown in Figure 30.2b where the plain X-ray 10 years following the radiotherapy demonstrates the scoliosis that has resulted. From this example it is obvious that radiation technique must be reviewed; the radiation technique will involve the discussion of the target volume, the modality of radiotherapy employed and the arrangement of external beam portals with particular regard to the specific organ tolerance of viscera within the target volume or abutting it. The best modality of radiotherapy must be chosen: Figure 30.3 shows the late result of high-dose orthovoltage neuraxis radiation for medulloblastoma with its disproportionate photoelectric bone dose absorption. The narrow sacrum and low,

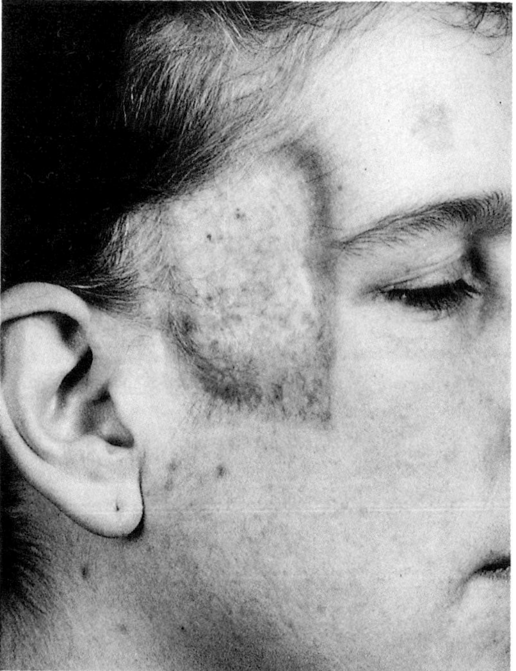

**Figure 30.1** Lateral orthovoltage radiotherapy portal used for treatment of retinoblastoma in infancy. A single radiation treatment was delivered. The punched out skin portal, the atrophic and telangiectatic skin and growth stunting are obvious

maldeveloped lumbar vertebrae are obvious late sequelae.

The current views of radiation tolerance of different human structures is a most important area to

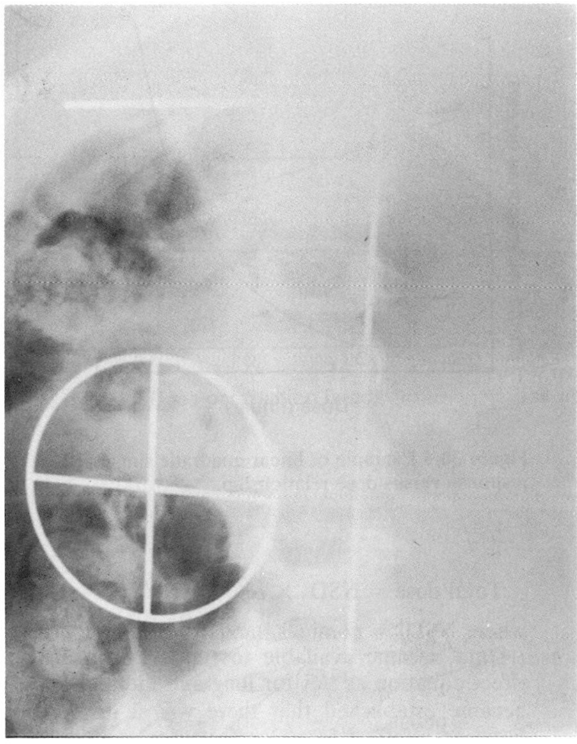

(a)

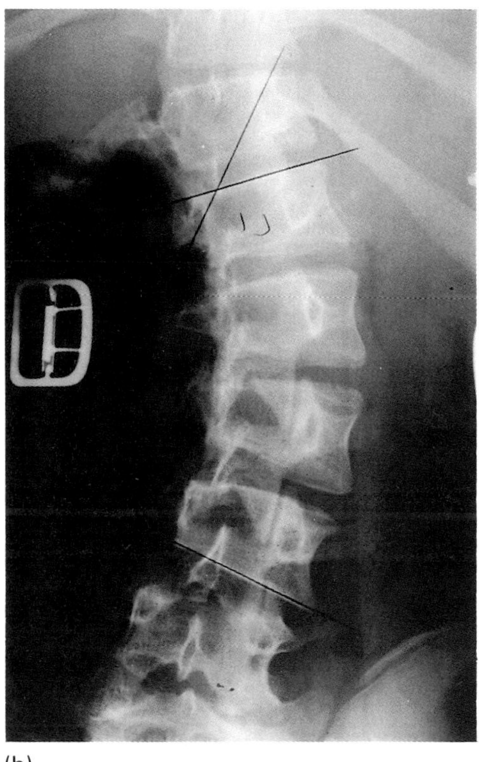

(b)

**Figure 30.2 a** The simulation film for the radiation portal to the flank of this young child following right nephrectomy for Wilms' tumour. The sloping medial border, which fails to encompass most of the vertebral growth epiphyses on the left side, is obvious. **b** Ten years later the growth stunting of the right side of the lumbar vertebrae and the normal growth of the (unirradiated) left lumbar vertebral epiphyses has led to scoliosis

review with regard to reducing morbidity; the possibility of synergized toxicity by chemoradiotherapy is also potentially important. Lastly, the introduction of special radiation techniques to supplant conventional external beam therapy may also reduce radiation morbidity.

# Fractionation

The 'manipulation' of fractionation (and time) in radiotherapy prescriptions may allow a reduction in the severity of early and late morbidity following radiation to normal tissues per given total dose delivered.

With regard to the acute tolerance of normal pig skin, Fowler *et al.* [1] observed that a given level of acute skin reaction could be effected by applied superficial X-ray dose prescriptions of 3500 cGy in five fractions over 5 days or by 5500 cGy in 21

fractions over 28 days. The critical experiment with regard to the relative importances of fraction size and overall time was to give five fractions distributed evenly over 28 days. For the previously observed level of skin reaction, would the required total dose be nearer 3500 cGy or 5500 cGy? They found that 4200 cGy was required. They concluded that whilst overall time and fraction size both contributed, fraction size was more important.

Ellis [2] derived, from experiments such as the above and clinical radiotherapy of skin cancer data, an isoeffect equation suitable for equating different dose prescriptions (total dose, number of fractions, overall time) with respect to acute skin tolerance as the end point:

$$\text{Total dose (rad or cGy)} = \text{NSD} \times N^{0.24} \times T^{0.11}$$

Where NSD = nominal standard dose (rets), $N$ = number of fractions and $T$ = overall time (days).

The 'NSD equation' has been widely used in clinical practice to alter the total dose prescribed when, for example, changing a radical radiotherapy

**Table 30.1** Estimates of $\alpha/\beta$ values and flexure doses ($D_f$) for normal tissues. $D_f$ values calculated as 10% of $\alpha/\beta$. Data adapted from ref. [5]

|  | $\alpha/\beta$ (Gy) | $D_f$ (Gy) |
|---|---|---|
| Early reactions: | | |
| Skin desquamation | 12 | 1.2 |
| Hair follicles (depilation) | 7 | 0.7 |
| Lip mucosal desquamation | 8 | 0.8 |
| Jejunal epithelium[a] | 13 | 1.3 |
| Colon epithelium[a] | 8 | 0.8 |
| Seminiferous epithelium[a] | 14 | 1.4 |
| Bone marrow | 9 | 0.9 |
| | | |
| Late reactions: | | |
| Transverse myelitis: | | |
|    cervical | 3 | 0.3 |
|    lumbar | 4 | 0.4 |
| Brain ($LD_{50}$/10 months) | 2 | 0.2 |
| Cataracts | 2 | 0.2 |
| Radiation nephritis | 1.5–4 | 0.2–0.4 |
| Pneumonitis | 3 | 0.3 |
| Bowel stricture/perforation | 4 | 0.4 |
| Liver | 1 | 0.1 |
| Heart | 1 | 0.1 |

[a] Clonal assays in which repopulation may affect result obtained

The major clinical question is whether we can manipulate this to our advantage in reducing the incidence of late morbidity. If we reduce the dose per fraction by several large decrements, will we continue to see equal reductions in the damage to late responding tissues? Due to the linear quadratic (or similar) nature of the response curve, the answer is of course, no, and thus in order to approach the critical clinical question posed above, we need to know the size of fraction for each tissue below which no further increase in tissue repair or dose sparing occurs with greater subdivision of the total dose into yet more fractions [6–8]. This led to the definition of the 'flexure' dose ($D_f$): the dose per fraction at which a significant departure from an initially straight to a curved dose-response curve can be detected as the dose (per fraction) is increased. As Fowler, Joiner and Williams [8] state, this flexure dose occurs gradually rather than at a precise dose; nevertheless, the range of $D_f$ for any tissue would be relevant to clinical practice. Without attempting here to mathematically derive the answer [5,8], suffice it to say that the range of $D_f$ appears to be $0.05\alpha/\beta$–$0.15\alpha/\beta$ and may be most simply stated as $0.1\alpha/\beta$ or 10% $\alpha/\beta$. This is tabulated for normal tissues in Table 30.1. Thus, again, the flexure dose is smallest for late responding tissues (0.13–0.5 Gy) and largest for early reactions (0.5–2 Gy).

All the foregoing strengthens our 'handle' on the relative importance of fraction size on morbidity in different human tissues. It does, however, assume the linear quadratic model and must expect that tumour response does not demand more than a critically low fraction size. Not many data on human tumours and their response to radiation have yet been analysed in this manner. However, those that have conform to the conclusions reached by Williams, Denekamp and Fowler [9] who reviewed the data on experimental tumours; there did appear a tendency for $\alpha/\beta$ values to exceed those for late responding tissues and in some cases also those of early reacting tissues. The data of Fowler [10] extend and confirm these observations.

Fowler, Joiner and Williams [8] concluded that the consequences of low $D_f$ values for late responding tissues lead to the following recommendations for radiotherapy where *late* damage to normal tissues is a potential problem:

1. The theoretical advantage of sparing late injury by using more fractions of smaller size might persist until doses per fraction down to 1–50 cGy are used, depending upon which normal tissue is at risk and whether tumour $D_f$ values are really significantly higher.
2. It would be better to use a partial transmission block over late reacting normal tissues with every fraction, rather than to use standard doses per fraction and then to block/shield out the critical tissue part way through the treatment course. This topic has recently been reviewed [11].
3. Every radiation portal should be treated every day.

The important complicating caveat to all the foregoing is that the linear quadratic mathematics may not be entirely correct and the time factor between intervals may be more important than envisaged when the inter-fraction repair kinetics of tissue damage was thought to obey first order kinetics (rather than a several component repair as is now thought likely). The model also takes no account of the 'time factor' or the 'volume factor' in clinical radiotherapy, e.g. the volume factor in CNS radiation tolerance [12,13].

## The target volume

The target volume for a radiotherapy plan will vary not only according to the palpable, imageable or operative description of a tumour's extent, but also by one's knowledge of the local and locoregional patterns of spread of that particular tumour type. Thereafter the delicate practice of screening vital organs (see below) abutting or within the target volume must be practised such that the radiotherapy is executed safely but effectively.

The benign pituitary adenoma provides a good opening example and the practice at St. Bartholomew's Hospital is described. Following operative resection of a macroadenoma (which is almost always via the trans-sphenoidal route), the target volume is planned from the preoperative CT scans (the reconstruction sagittal and coronal views being most important in this regard). A three-field plan (two laterals and one superior or anterosuperior) is then devised. This assessment of target volume is made despite the frequent operative description of 'all macroscopic tumour removed and diaphragma seen to descend into the fossa', and despite the known radiosensitivity of the optic chiasm and hypothalamus lying just rostral to the pituitary fossa. We have examples of 'standard' $4 \times 4$ cm postoperative portals centred on the pituitary fossa at other centres where an unirradiated (and unresected) rostral part of the tumour was omitted and has regrown to cause late relapse. The observance of the optic chiasmal and hypothalamic tolerance is made here by the dose prescription (45 Gy in 25 fractions) and not by screening. However, where a large prolactinoma has been medically shrunk by dopamine agonist therapy our target volume is based on the CT scan appearances following dopamine agonist, the rationale here being that medical therapy causes shrinkage of the whole tumour.

We believe that such a belief in medical therapy is not justified in many malignant tumours and despite good shrinkage of a paediatric rhabdomyosarcoma with initial chemotherapy, we believe some dose must still be delivered to the initial imageable extent of the tumour; this philosophy must remain under review as drug regimes improve.

For early carcinoma of the uterine cervix, external beam therapy to the pelvis precedes intracavitary boost. The regional nodes are at risk and the whole pelvis is irradiated – even for Figo $I_b$ disease. This whole pelvis target volume may seem large, particularly for the early stage disease, but is justified by the preponderance of lymphatic regional spread over blood spread and the necessity for first-time cure in this disease.

Early stage paediatric and perhaps adult Hodgkin's disease differs in that first-time cure may not be all-important due to the efficacy of chemotherapy for relapse. This has caused radiotherapists to think long and hard concerning the target volume for Stage I–II$_A$ patients. Should we treat such children with mantle radiotherapy in the knowledge that the disease spreads by contiguity to adjacent node regions and that the highest 'first-time' cure rates are so achieved, or can we safely use involved fields knowing that by curing the majority by this method (and reducing the late morbidity to the whole population) the minority who relapse can be salvage cured by chemotherapy? The target volume for early stage Hodgkin's disease in children has now

been reduced to involved fields, and the introduction of effective non-alkylating containing chemotherapy makes us even happier with this decision (as even salvage therapy will not involve alkylating agent chemotherapy).

In head and neck cancer, the clinical question arises as to when one can decide to give just brachytherapy to a very limited volume versus all external beam or external beam and a brachytherapy boost, and when the target volume should include the nodes, for here too is a condition that spreads preferentially to the regional nodes. The answers here must lie in the past experiences of others and thereby a knowledge of the natural history of the particular cancers. For example, an early carcinoma of tongue may be safely treated by brachytherapy alone and, with careful follow-up, salvage cure (by block dissection) of nodal relapse or hemiglossectomy for local relapse remain curative. A larger carcinoma of the floor of mouth should preferably be given 50 Gy through opposed lateral portals to the whole floor of the mouth prior to a brachytherapy boost to a shrunken primary. With regard to the nodes, the incidence of nodal metastases from carcinoma of the lip, true cords or small cancer of the tongue is so low not to warrant inclusion of these in the target volume, but for carcinoma of the tonsil or pharynx it is so high that it must be done.

Far more difficult comes the problem of a large right-sided Wilms' tumour infiltrating the liver, a chordoma abutting the brainstem or cervical cord, a retroperitoneal sarcoma infiltrating the small bowel mesentery, etc. We will approach these particular target volume difficulties (all of which relate to adjacent normal tissue tolerance) in the subsequent sections on the arrangement of portals, special techniques and, of course, the dose prescription.

## Arrangement of portals and avoidance of organs at risk

In external beam radiotherapy, the arrangement of radiation portals may be used to great advantage to allow a target volume to be treated to radical dose without danger to an adjacent and critically radiosensitive normal tissue. Many examples could be given but two have been selected: the first is the unusual optic nerve meningioma.

The optic nerve meningioma classically causes major deterioration in vision when it begins to expand the nerve within the fixed confines of the optic canal. The alternative to radical surgery is radical radiotherapy and yet the dose that is delivered is at least 50 Gy in 6 weeks which is a dose that approaches optic chiasmal tolerance. However,

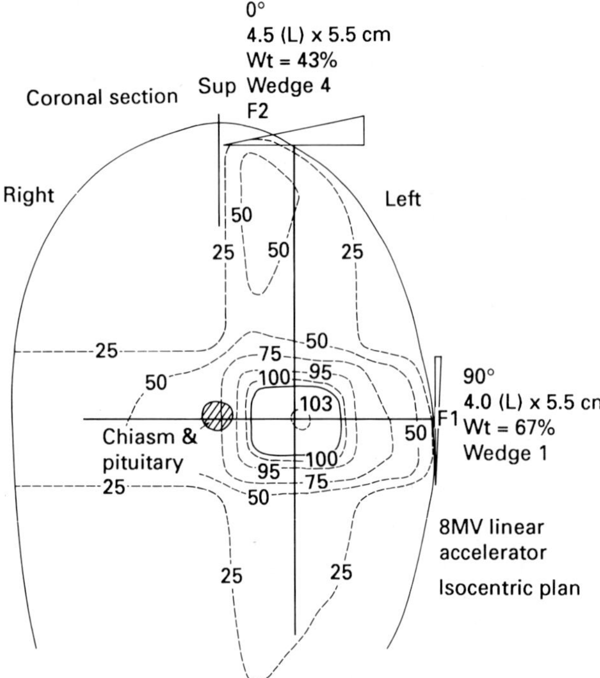


**Figure 30.7** Radiotherapy isodosimetric plan for treatment of optic nerve meningioma. The target volume, which must include the entire length of the nerve within the optic canal, abuts the optic chiasm (whose tolerance to radiotherapy is considered below that desired for the target volume). A highly precise lateral and superior wedge pair of fields are used to fully irradiate the optic canal but not the chiasm

the optic chiasm's radiation tolerance must be respected because damage here would harm vision in the only healthy eye and, yet, the radiation target volume must include the optic canal and thus abut the optic chiasm. Figure 30.7 demonstrates the radiation plan used with success in these patients. A wedged pair of direct superior and lateral (actually, lateral with a 7° posterior angulation) MV X-ray portals have been employed, displayed in the coronal plane for the figure illustrated. The midline optic chiasm is obviously outside the high-dose volume. Such a careful set-up as this, of course, requires an excellent close fitting mask and exact reproducibility of patient positioning together with modern radiation simulator and linear accelerator facilities.

The second example illustrates the usefulness of CT scanning to define the tumour or the critical normal tissue and, by so doing, CT planning of the radiation portals allows the therapist to directly view how the critical tissues will be dosed. Figure 30.8 shows a planned oesophageal cancer target volume abutting but sparing the spinal cord, mediastinum and lungs from full dose.

A conceptually simpler method of avoiding irradiation of critical tissues would be to displace them during radiotherapy. Thus an intraoral stent is used to displace the mandible downwards during radiotherapy to the floor of the mouth or tongue and the palate and upper dentition are thus out of the fields. Conversely for malignancy of the palate, such a stent displaces the tongue and floor of the mouth outside the portals – thereby considerably improving the acute radiation tolerance of the mouth. In young children, the dentition (particularly the permanent dentition) may be protected by such manoeuvres. In the radical radiation of localized prostate cancer, patients are asked to attend each day with a full bladder; thus the majority of the bladder is displaced outside the radiation portals and radiation cystitis does not occur – again demonstrating simple organ displacement.

More sophisticated attempts at organ displacement have been attempted. Small bowel radiation tolerance is below the dose prescription desired by therapists for many pelvic malignancies and displacement of most of the pelvic small bowel by omentum or water-filled balloons has been attempted to obviate radiation enteritis. In children, particularly with pelvic Ewing's sarcoma, a method of bowel displacement is used which has been found safe and effective [14]. Polyglactin (Vicryl) material is an absorbable compound used for surgical suturing. A mesh of polyglactin became available and has been used to displace pelvic small bowel outside the pelvis by operative suture of the mesh around the peritoneum to form a diaphragm at the pelvic brim below which the small bowel is unable to prolapse

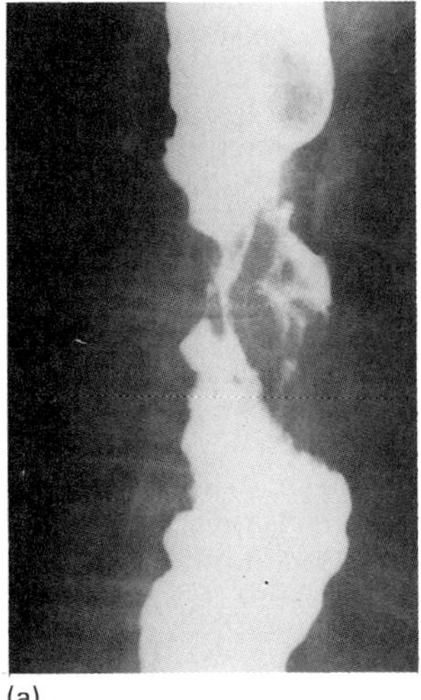

(a)

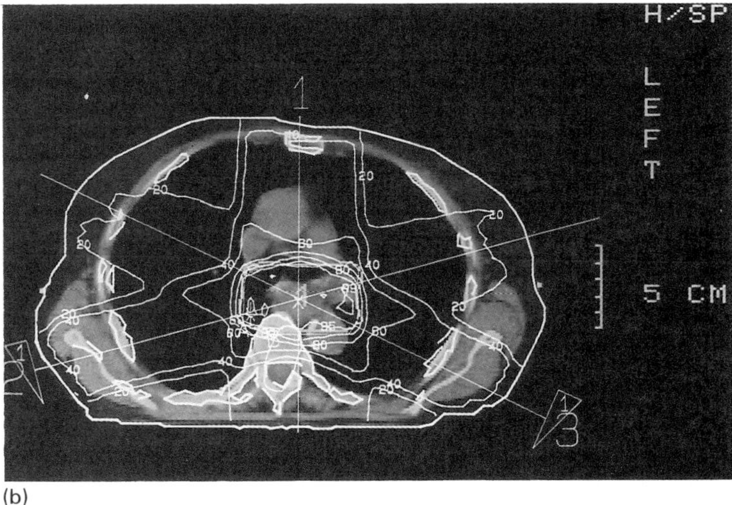



(b)

**Figure 30.8** Computed tomographic (CT) plan scan for localized oesophageal cancer. **a** The barium swallow shows the localized lesion and the plan scan (**b**) shows the isodosimetric 6 MV X-ray therapy plan superimposed on the CT scan image

(a)

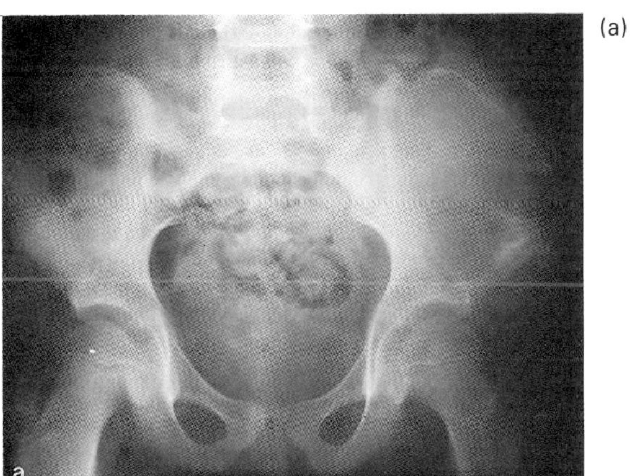

(b)

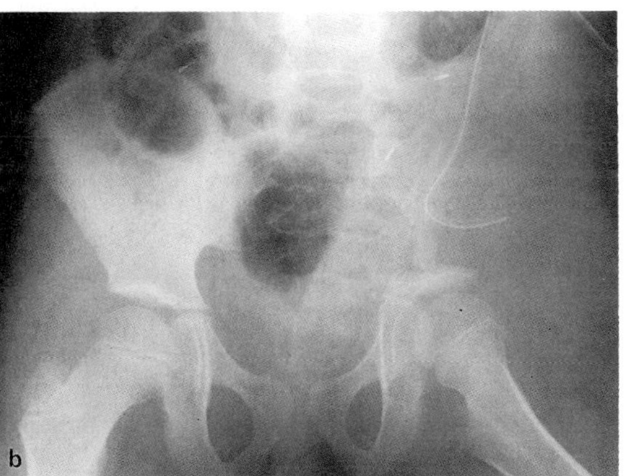

**Figure 30.9** Bowel displacement by polyglactin mesh prior to radiation. **a** Plain X-ray showing huge iliac crest Ewing's sarcoma involving sacrum. Following chemotherapeutic mass shrinkage, operative resection of the iliac bone was performed. Polyglactin mesh was used to hold bowel away from radiation target volume in A-P plane. Tumour was to resection margins. **b** The level of the polyglactin mesh is shown by the radio-opaque clips. All bowel is superior to this plane. The region of the tumour bed (below the mesh) was irradiated to 50 Gy. Radiation enteropathy was avoided [14]

(Figure 30.9). After approximately 6 weeks *in vivo*, the mesh decays and absorbs such that a second operation is unnecessary and the bowel descends back into the pelvis in the post-radiation period.

Another example of operative displacement of organs is ovarian displacement prior to pelvic radiotherapy. Children with vaginal or uterine rhabdomyosarcoma have an excellent prognosis with chemotherapy (often nowadays excluding an alkylating agent) and radiotherapy. Although the uterine radiation dose will probably prevent pregnancy, operative displacement of the ovaries to the level of the kidneys (a relatively easy procedure as their vascular supply is derived from the aorta at that level) saves ovarian function (see Figure 30.13 on p. 484) [15].

If the organ at risk cannot be moved, can it be specifically screened? Standard radiation portals for nasopharyngeal carcinoma 'generously' encompass the skull base and the hypothalamus and mastoids are often in the radiation volume. We have documented hypothalamus neuroendocrine morbidity following such radiation [16]. Recently, during our neoadjuvant cisplatin-containing chemotherapy for childhood nasopharyngeal carcinoma, enhanced sensorineuronal deafness caused by cisplatin plus radiation to the cochlea has been observed. With modern immobilization and set-up sophistication, the day-to-day set-up reproducibility is now excellent, so we have considered it safe to encompass the skull base less generously in our radiation portals for T1–2 disease (Figure 30.10) [17]. As cisplatin chemotherapy may be part of the treatment programme for both pineal germinoma and infantile medulloblastoma, and as the radiation target volume in both these malignancies abuts the mastoid, particular attention to screening the cochlea is again important as we have shown elsewhere [17].

More common examples of specific organ screening are the lung blocks in total body irradiation work and the renal screens when giving whole abdominal radiotherapy.

The 'shrinking field' technique of several phases of radiotherapy – the first taking a wide area around the tumour to a modest dose and the next taking the tumour with less generous margins to a high dose followed perhaps by a third phase boost to a small volume to a very high dose – is a well recognized technique to reach high doses to tumours whilst respecting the radiation tolerance of adjacent organs. Variations on this theme include the introduction of blocks into treatment fields at various stages of treatment; for example, in the famous Stanford mantle radiation portals for Hodgkin's disease, a spinal cord block from the posterior field is introduced at 20 Gy and a subcarinal block to screen the heart at 30–35 Gy. The 'thin lung block' also introduced by Kaplan allowed low fraction doses to treat the lungs during mantle radiotherapy. This is a superior technique to leaving 'high risk

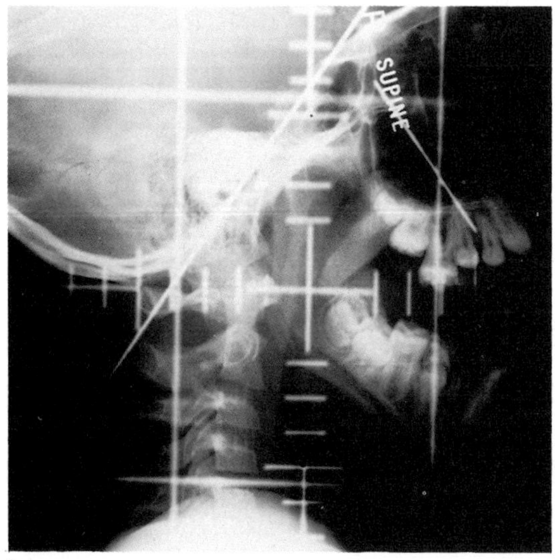


(a)

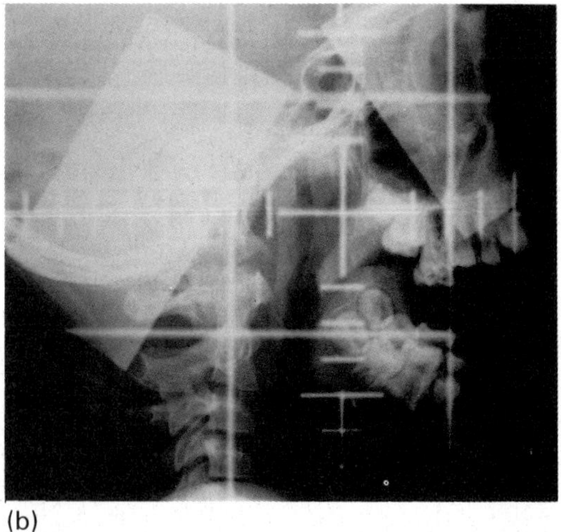

(b)

**Figure 30.10 a** Phase I and **b** phase II lateral radiation portals for T1 nasopharyngeal carcinoma. This child had presented with T1,N3 disease and therapy had commenced with cisplatin-containing chemotherapy. The shielding of the inner ear and hypothalamus are noted, and represented by the diagonal lines across the supero-posterior field corners [17]

lungs' unblocked until a critical dose and then screening them 'completely', because of the greater sparing effect of low fraction sizes on late lung morbidity.

A comparable example from recent experience is as follows. A 10-year-old child had a large right-sided Wilms' tumour invading the liver, and on MRI CT scans the liver appeared abnormal up to its diaphragmatic surface. The child commenced AVA chemotherapy (actinomycin D, vincristine and doxorubicin (Adriamycin)) and, after partial response, came to delayed nephrectomy. The histology still showed active tumour at resection margins and invading the liver. Postoperative radiotherapy commenced (1 month since last AVA) with parallel opposed (anterior and posterior) 6 MV X-ray portals. A thin liver block was used to deliver a dose of 3000 cGy in 20 fractions to the majority of the right flank whilst the area of liver at risk received 2000 cGy in 20 fractions over the same time period (Figure 30.11). The actinomycin and doxorubicin were not reintroduced for a further 3 weeks, to avoid the recall phenomenon.

Thus, strategically placed 'thin blocks' allowing partial transmission and the lower daily fractions may allow critical tissues to be relatively spared from radiation morbidity. This partial transmission block is replacing classic 'shrinking field technique' in paediatric radiotherapy in this centre [11].

Avoidance of 'uncontrollable' drug/radiation interactions is important.

## Special radiation methods

Under this heading radiation techniques will be discussed that involve great precision and enable the

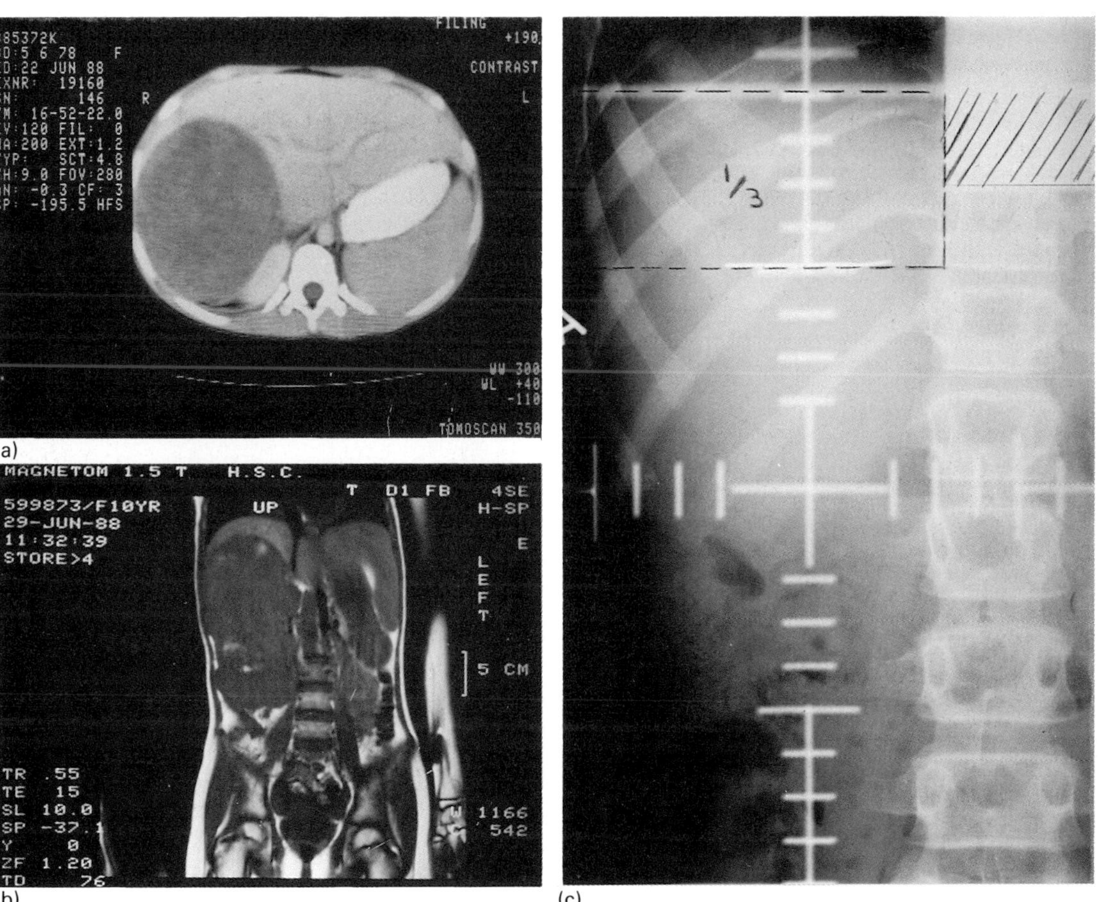

**Figure 30.11** Partial transmission block technique. **a** Transaxial CT and **b** coronal MR appearances of a huge Wilms' tumour invading the liver. Following induction chemotherapy (including actinomycin D), operative removal left microscopic tumour at the superior border. **c** The radiotherapy portal shows the partial screening of part of the portal containing liver throughout treatment

therapist to deliver a radical dose to a tumour whilst respecting the radiation tolerance of normal tissues abutting the target volume.

Schipper pioneered a sophisticated megavoltage photon technique that treats the retina up to the ora serrata where an abrupt field margin drops the dose immediately such that the lens and anterior ocular structures are spared radiation. This method avoids the cataracts and anterior ocular complications seen after whole eye radiotherapy and has proved an important advance in retinoblastoma therapy [18]. Put simply, a beam splitting technique and collimation out to almost target distance together produce a very sharp beam edge anteriorly with little penumbra and no divergence. By use of a contact lens to locate the cornea and a rod connected to the contact lens (and indirectly to the linear accelerator via a scaled groove rigidly mounted from the machine head) the sharp anterior beam edge is brought in, with 0.5 mm accuracy, to a known distance behind the cornea (Figure 30.12). This technique is an excellent example of a modern radiotherapy method of reducing morbidity.

Brachytherapy is a time-honoured radiotherapy method for localizing the radiation dose and its role has already been discussed in carcinoma of the tongue. Another example which fits in with the ovarian transposition exemplified earlier is in the treatment of the favourable risk paediatric botryoid sarcoma of the vagina that is most commonly seen in young children [18]. With non-alkylating agent chemotherapy (vincristine, actinomycin D), and

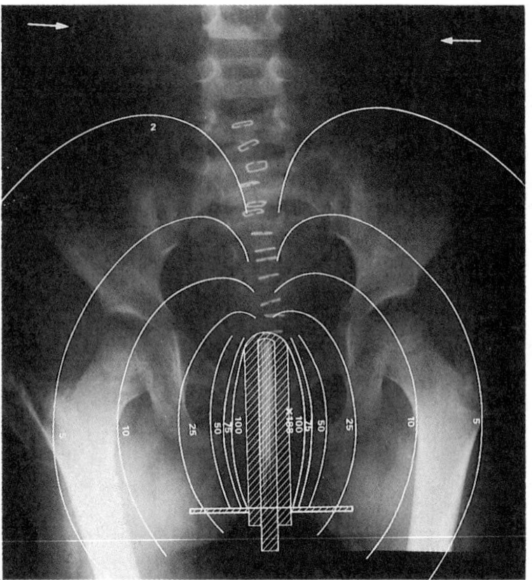

**Figure 30.13** Plain radiograph of the abdomen of a child with vaginal rhabdomyosarcoma. The repositioned ovaries (marked by arrows) are away from the vaginal brachytherapy radiotherapy – isodosimetry superimposed – and received less than 2% of the surface vaginal dose [15]

following ovarian transposition, vaginal brachytherapy delivers a radical dose to the vaginal wall with rapid fall-off of the dose towards the pelvic contents (Figure 30.13).

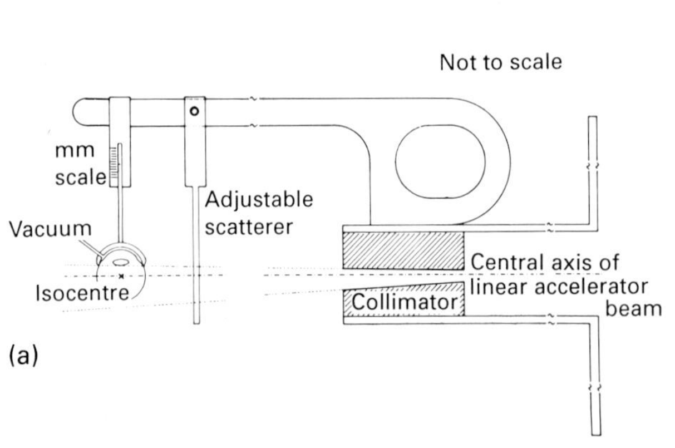


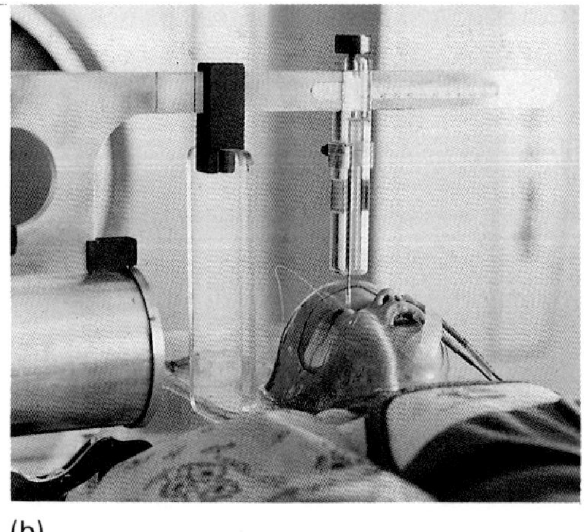


**Figure 30.12** Lateral radiotherapy, lens-sparing technique for retinoblastoma. A penumbra trimmed and non-divergent beam, whose anterior edge represents almost the central axis beam from a linear accelerator, is positioned with 0.5 mm accuracy at a selected distance behind the cornea using a contact lens and system connecting this ocular reference point to the beam. The retina up to the ora serrata is thus irradiated and the lens and anterior ocular structures are spared (St Bartholomew's method). **a** Diagrammatic representation of the set-up and **b** child on set-up [18]

Focal brain radiotherapy has only recently been available with a degree of sophistication and appears suitable for discrete recurrences of low-grade gliomas or even boosts after conventional external beam radiotherapy. The modern stereotactic frame coupled to modern CT and computing facilities allows a highly precise and preplanned brain brachytherapy programme to be established (Figure 30.14b). A stereotactic external beam rotational therapy facility is a second method of focal brain radiotherapy (Figure 30.14) that has already established itself as highly effective and safe for small deep-seated cerebral arteriovenous malformations. At St Bartholomew's Hospital we are currently comparing these two techniques in the treatment of brain tumours [19,20]. Both techniques have the advantage of delivering very high doses to the tumour but a fast falling dose gradient at the tumour perimeter (Figure 30.14).

The electron beam has other characteristics that may be used to advantage to reduce late morbidity. For example, a sarcoma arising in the sacrum or buttock may be treated with a posterior electron beam portal. This capitalizes on the dose distribution of megavoltage electrons. A full dose is achieved to the desired depth; then, a very sharp cut off in beam penetration allows all peritoneal structures to be spared.

Lastly, the Boston group have demonstrated clearly that the proton beam's Bragg peak may be used to deliver radical curative doses to tumours whilst sparing adjacent structures. They have demonstrated this most clearly for ocular melanoma [21] and chordoma [22]. Focal brain radiotherapy has enormous promise for the future [23].

Whether the high KERMA for fat makes neutrons a selective treatment for liposarcoma (and indeed whether the neutron beam has any useful role in radiotherapy), whether pi-mesons or other exotica have advantageous roles or whether hyperthermia and radiation together improve the therapeutic ratio, remain controversial issues beyond this review.

## References


1. Fowler, J.F., Morgan, M.A., Silvester, J.A. *et al.* Experiments with fractionated X-ray treatment of the skin of pigs. I. Fractionation up to 28 days. *British Journal of Radiology*, **36**, 188–196 (1963)
2. Ellis, F. Fractionation in radiotherapy. In *Modern Trends in Radiotherapy*, Volume 1 (eds T. Deeley and C. Wood), Butterworths, London, pp. 34–51 (1967)
3. Sheline, G. Irradiation injury of the human brain: a review of clinical experience. In *Radiation Damage to the Nervous System* (eds H.A. Gilbert and A.R.


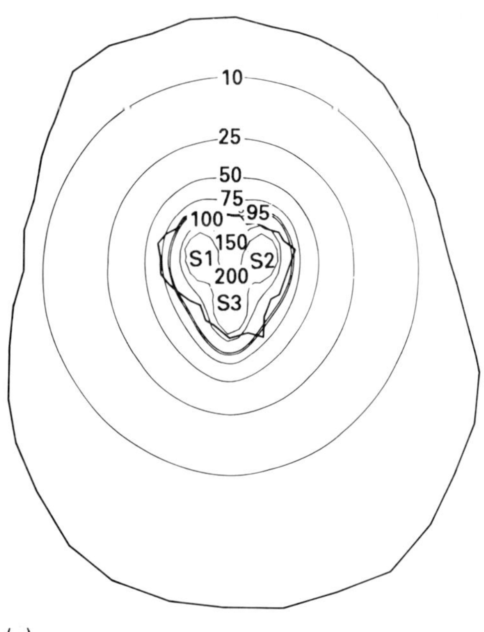


(a)

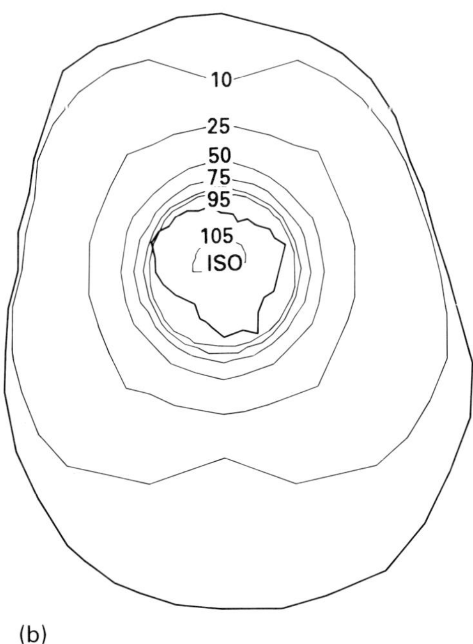


(b)

**Figure 30.14** Comparison of two methods of focal brain radiotherapy. For a paediatric low grade glioma, locally recurrent after conventional external beam radiotherapy, two isodosimetric plots for stereotactic implant brachytherapy (**a**) and stereotactic rotational external beam radiotherapy (**b**). Courtesy of Mr E. Thomson, St Bartholomew's Hospital

talk about one's feelings about mastectomy – I think there should be – and when I got home I had to adjust as best I could . . . . Some help, someone to talk to before and in the months following the operation would have helped, I'm sure. In the months which followed I went through a phase of extreme hypochondria – to me everything even slightly odd possibly represented a return of the cancer. I knew with about 80% of my mind that I was being a fool, but I worried, how I worried. If only I'd had a doctor who'd said "Come whenever you are worried – I shan't think you're a fool and it only takes a minute to put your mind at rest". But I knew my doctor would be of no help, so I worried through alone' [6].

Another patient, a physician suffering from lymphoma, wrote:

'Today's oncologists need to be encouraged to derive feelings of self-esteem and career satisfaction from improving the quality as well as the quantity of their patient's existence. By addressing the emotional problems associated with chemotherapy they can diminish their patient's feelings of abandonment and rage and prevent the despair which patients suffer . . . . The central point regarding chemotherapy from the standpoint of the patient is that these powerful drugs interfered with body functions which most people take for granted, making me feel as though I had surrendered bodily control to a group of external agents. That helpless feeling, rather than any individual side-effect, was what occasioned the need for the greatest adjustment' [7].

A psychologist suffering from embryonal testicular carcinoma with pulmonary metastases described similar feelings of helplessness:

'I also realized that my lack of control over, and information about, when chemotherapy would end and whether or not it would be followed by radiation had kept me feeling helpless . . . . patients with cancer do not feel effective or even have control over their own bodies. Their very cells seem to be rebelling and going crazy. It is essential, therefore, for them at least to exercise some form of control over their treatment and their hospital environment. If they are not given appropriate ways for participation, they may see no alternative except resistance to therapy as a method of exercising control. When patients are given a sense of choice and responsibility, rather than a sense of having to do it for someone else, they can accept and decide that they want even a painful treatment'.

Fiore concluded:

'Fighting cancer must come to mean more than excising a tumor and focusing the latest weapons on the metastases. It must include a recognition, by both the medical professionals and the patient, that the patient's mind and body are powerful factors in this fight. Failure to use these potential allies can mean losing them to the 'enemy' through patient resistance to treatment, depression and loss of will to live. Effective cancer therapy must treat the healthy portion of the patient's body and psyche as well as combat the diseased cells' [8].

# Major psychological problems related to cancer

Despite advances in treatment, many cancers still entail various distressing consequences which patients fear such as the debilitating effects of chemotherapy, extensive and somtimes mutilating surgery, recurrence of the disease, progressive weakness, pain and, finally, death. It is hardly surprising, therefore, that the experience of cancer leads to considerable psychological ill-health [9]. But it is not merely the physical consequences of cancer which determine the occurrence and degree of psychological morbidity. The personal meaning of the disease and the individual's coping style are critical aetiological factors. This point is fundamental to an understanding of cancer-related psychological morbidity and to the development of psychotherapeutic methods designed to improve the quality of life of patients. The way in which patients appraise the threat of cancer will, of course, vary according to the individual. Nonetheless, there are certain major psychological problems which commonly beset cancer patients.

## Loss of control

According to a survey of the literature [10], the single most important psychological problem reported by patients is loss of personal control. This refers to feelings of powerlessness, of being unable to influence the disease or to take an active part in its treatment. Loss of control is engendered by uncertainty about disease outcome, by feelings that one's body cells are out of control [8] and by high technology treatments which seemingly leave no room for initiatives by the patient. Feelings of loss of control, if severe and persistent, will lead to feelings of helplessness, hopelessness and depression. Hence, it is important for patients to be able to counter this sense of loss of control. A recent study has shown how changes in clinical practice which gave patients personal control over choice of treatment resulted in significant psychological benefit. Women with early breast cancer were offered or not offered a choice of mastectomy versus wide local excision plus radiotherapy. Morris and Ingham [11] reported that whether or not patients were given a choice was of greater relevance to psychosocial outcomes than the type of operation performed. Providing a choice led to improved adjustments with respect to work ability, attitudes towards the future, beliefs about coping and in physical and psychological functioning.

## Threat to survival

Despite some advances in treatment, the diagnosis of cancer still represents, for many people, a catastrophic threat amounting to a death sentence. At the very least, the occurrence of cancer forces each of us to face the possibility of death. Furthermore, it is not merely the possibility of death but the process of dying from cancer which is a frightening prospect.

## Threat to the self-image

The morbidity associated with cancer and its treatments can result in major disruption of the patient's life. Included under this heading are the painful and debilitating symptoms of many cancers, disfigurement (e.g. mastectomy, maxillofacial surgery, limb amputation), loss of body function (e.g. ostomies, radical gynaecological surgery) and the side effects of chemotherapy (e.g. alopecia, nausea, vomiting, lassitude, depression, intercurrent infections, the 'moon face' associated with steroids). These and other adverse consequences of cancer may threaten the patient's self-image in various areas such as work ability, earning capacity, social activities, role in the family, sexuality and emotional relationships.

As emphasized earlier, the extent to which the patient's quality of life is impaired will depend partly on how these threats are perceived by the individual. For example, a longitudinal study of patients with breast cancer and lymphoma who were receiving chemotherapy [12] showed that the same side effect of chemotherapy could be perceived as either harmful (e.g. 'the pain means the cancer is growing and destroying my bones') or helpful (e.g. 'the pain means the drug is killing cancer cells'). The authors found that some patients gauged the effectiveness of their treatment by the occurrence of side effects: the absence of side effects was taken to mean that chemotherapy was ineffective. By contrast, other patients were distressed by failure to control the drugs' side effects which raised doubts about the overall effectiveness of treatment.

# Adjustment to cancer

Clinical observations indicate that patients' initial reactions upon discovering that they have cancer are often numbed shock and disbelief, anger with or without guilt ('why me?'), anxiety and depression [13–16]. This sequence of reactions is commonly seen following various severe life crises and is said to constitute a coping process which eventually leads to readjustment [17]. But, clearly, this does not always happen. In the case of cancer, between 22% [18] and 44% [9] go on to develop psychiatric disorders which may persist for years even in the absence of disease [19]. These disorders are discussed in Chapter 27. Here we shall consider the kind of adjustment cancer patients make following the initial stress reactions.

## Coping

Coping is defined as contending successfully or dealing competently with a person, situation, task or problem [20]. Coping is used synonymously here with *mental adjustment* which refers to the cognitive and behavioural responses made by an individual to the diagnosis of cancer. Mental adjustment comprises:

1. Appraisal: how the patient perceives the implications of cancer; and
2. The ensuing reactions: what the patient thinks and does to reduce the threat posed by cancer.

In a seminal paper on coping, Pearlin and Schooler [21] identified three coping functions:

1. Eliminating or modifying conditions giving rise to problems.
2. Perceptually controlling the meaning of the experience in a manner that neutralizes its problematic character.
3. Keeping the emotional consequences of problems within manageable bounds.

How do these functions apply to cancer patients? Taking the first, clearly patients cannot eliminate cancer. Nevertheless they can, to a limited extent, modify conditions giving rise to problems by participating in decisions regarding treatment. For example, women with breast cancer may ask for mastectomy, thereby reducing their fear that less extensive surgery will not remove the cancer completely; alternatively, they may choose lumpectomy and avoid feelings of loss of femininity associated with breast amputation. The second and third coping functions mentioned by Pearlin and Schooler are of direct relevance for cancer patients. The ways in which patients attempt to control the meaning of their disease and its emotional consequences are described below.

Coping is a complex process. In studying how

patients cope with cancer, two different but complementary approaches have been used:

1. The macroscopic in which we have attempted to delineate global categories of adjustment or 'coping styles' [18,22].
2. The microscopic in which the various separate cognitive and behavioural responses made by patients were identified and rated [23].

In a study of women with early, non-metastatic breast cancer, we delineated several broad categories of adjustment to cancer.

## Fighting spirit

The patient accepts the diagnosis, adopts a hopeful attitude, is determined to fight the disease, and tries to obtain as much information as possible.

### *Examples*

1. 'I won't let the cancer beat me, I'm trying everything to get better. I go to classes to learn to relax and to think positively'.
2. 'At first I was devastated, but now I realize that I've got too much to live for . . . . I believe with the help of the doctors I can get well'.

## Avoidance (denial)

Patient refuses to accept the diagnosis and avoids using the word 'cancer', or admits the diagnosis but minimizes its seriousness and any associated anxiety. Such patients are usually very guarded when asked about their disease and restrict discussion of the subject.

### *Examples*

1. 'The doctors just took my breast off as a precaution'.
2. 'There could have been a few cancer cells, but it wasn't serious, there's nothing to worry about'.

## Fatalism (stoic acceptance)

Patient accepts the diagnosis, does not seek further information and adopts a resigned attitude.

### *Examples*

1. 'I know what it is, I know it's cancer, but I've just got to carry on as normal. There's nothing I can do'.
2. 'It's cancer, I don't dwell on what's going to happen; I leave it all to the doctors'.

## Anxious preoccupation

Patient reacts to the diagnosis with marked, persistent anxiety with or without depression; seeks information about the disease but interprets it pessimistically; often monitors bodily symptoms and worries that aches and pains indicate spread or recurrence of cancer.

### *Examples*

1. 'I keep worrying about it coming back – I get this pain in the shoulder here, what do you think it is, doctor?'
2. 'I know it's cancer. I can't stop thinking about it; I've gone to a man who does acupuncture and someone has told me about meditation; do you think it helps?'

## Helplessness/hopelessness

Patient is engulfed by knowledge of the diagnosis, adopts a wholly pessimistic attitude; daily life is disrupted by fears about cancer and dying.

### *Examples*

1. 'There's nothing they can do, I'm finished'.
2. 'I feel hopeless a lot of the time, I keep worrying about it and cry a lot . . . can't seem to get it out of my mind, I don't know what to do'.

It should be emphasized that these are broad categories of adjustment. They do not include every possible kind of adjustment, nor are they always mutually exclusive. For example, patients may show anxious preoccupation as well as helplessness/ hopelessness. Nevertheless, when patients are rated according to their predominant coping style, more than 90% can be grouped in one of the above categories with a high level of agreement (85%) between independent raters [24].

What are the components of these global categories of adjustment? In a study of newly diagnosed patients with breast cancer, Hodgkin's disease and lymphoma, Morris, Blake and Buckley [23] rated cognitive and behavioural responses elicited from a semi-structured interview. A total of 68 separate responses were obtained. These comprised:

1. Appraisal responses, e.g. believes cancer will not have adverse consequences, passively accepts cancer, attributes cancer to a specific factor, sees cancer as a challenge, sees cancer as a severe threat, claims more pressing concern(s) than that of the cancer.

2. Palliating responses, i.e. strategies for reducing the impact of cancer such as using prayer, using humour, trying to expunge from the mind thoughts and feelings associated with cancer, directing anger towards doctors and others, counterbalancing the stress of cancer with positive aspects of life.
3. Confronting responses, e.g. planning positive events and activities, adopting a positive approach by self-exhortation.
4. Behavioural responses, e.g. uses distraction, keeps busy, puts on a brave front, behaves in a self-indulgent way, musters the support of others, avoids others' sympathetic responses, seeks or avoids information about cancer.

A principal components analysis comprising all 68 cognitive and behavioural responses and psychological data clearly identified four factors (accounting for 65.5% of the variance) corresponding to our global categories of fighting spirit, fatalism, helplessness/hopelessness (including anxious preoccupation) and avoidance. These results lend support to the validity of our global categories of adjustment.


# Measurement of adjustment to cancer

The assessments of adjustment to cancer described so far were based on clinical interviews. There can be no doubt that a skilful, searching clinical interview is the best method of assessing the individual patient's adjustment. But this method is costly and laborious; hence its use is impractical in studies involving large numbers of patients attending busy oncology clinics. For large systematic studies a self-rating questionnaire is required. We have developed such a questionnaire – the MAC (Mental Adjustment to Cancer) scale [25,26]. This scale has now been given to more than 600 patients with a wide variety of early and advanced cancers. It is acceptable to almost all patients and easy to administer. The MAC scale provides a quantitative measure of fighting spirit, fatalism, anxious preoccupation and helplessness/hopelessness. However, we have not succeeded in measuring avoidance/denial. Our original clinical studies began in the early 1970s when the topic of cancer was still relatively unmentionable. It may be that changes in public health education and medical practice which now encourage frank discussion of cancer have made it more difficult for patients to deny that they have cancer; alternatively, self-rating scales may be unsuitable for measuring denial. Further work on the measurement of denial is required.

# Clinical implications
## Quality of life

Though difficult – if not impossible – to define comprehensively, from a clinical standpoint quality of life refers to the physical and emotional (psychosocial) well-being of patients. Both aspects should be taken into account in clinical trials of cancer treatments [27]. One important determinant of emotional well-being is the mental adjustment of patients to cancer.

In a study of women with newly diagnosed breast cancer [28], denial – assessed clinically – was found to be negatively correlated with anxiety and general mood disturbance – as measured by the State-Trait Anxiety Inventory [29] and the Profile of Mood States [30]. In other words, patients who denied the diagnosis of cancer or its serious implications experienced less psychological morbidity. Hence, denial may be a useful coping strategy providing, of course, that it does not lead to refusal of treatment. In the cited study, no patient refused treatment. In a subsequent study involving male and female patients with cancers of various types and stages, mental adjustment was measured by the MAC scale and anxiety and depression by the Hospital Anxiety and Depression Scale [31]. Fatalism and helplessness/hopelessness were found to be significantly associated with depression and anxious preoccupation with depression and anxiety [25]. These findings, if confirmed, suggest that certain coping responses, viz. fatalism, anxious preoccupation and helplessness/hopelessness are associated with psychiatric symptoms and hence impaired quality of life.


## Duration of survival

In 1979 we reported the results of a 5-year prospective study of women with non-metastatic breast cancer whose mental adjustment to cancer had been assessed clinically 3 months after mastectomy. Disease outcome was found to be significantly correlated with mental adjustment; recurrence-free survival was commonest among women who had responded with fighting spirit and least common among women with a helpless/hopeless response [22]. These results held good at 10-year follow-up [32]. We have just completed a 15-year follow-up of these patients: mental adjustment remains a significant predictor of disease outcome.

Could this result be an artefact due to initial differences in stage of disease between patients who showed different types of mental adjustment? There was no evidence to support this explanation, since patients in each of the mental adjustment categories were found to be similar in terms of clinical stage, histological grade, approximate tumour mass and mammographic appearance [33]. Oestrogen receptor status was not measured when we began our study in 1971, but the prognostic significance of oestrogen receptor status remains uncertain [34]. Of greater relevance is the absence of data on axillary lymph node status. The latter is recognized as an important prognostic indicator in patients with primary breast cancer, although this prognostic influence appears to be largely confined to the first 5 years [35]. Despite the length of follow-up, therefore, our results should be interpreted with caution. The relationship between axillary lymph node status and mental adjustment has been examined in a subsequent study which we reported recently [36]. In this latest study of patients with early (T0–2, N0–1, M0) breast cancer, mental adjustment assessed 3 and 12 months after diagnosis was shown to be unrelated to the number of lymph nodes found at operation, number of nodes pathologically involved, as well as clinical stage, histological grade, size of tumour and extension to chest wall and skin. These results confirm our previous findings that mental adjustment is independent of other known prognostic factors; in particular, there is no evidence of any association with local lymph node involvement.

The results of our studies provide support – though not conclusive proof – for the hypothesis that mental adjustment to cancer affects disease outcome in women with early, non-metastatic, breast cancer. Di Clemente and Temoshok [37] replicated our original prospective study in patients with malignant melanoma (86% clinical stage I) who were followed up for 18 to 29 months. Partial confirmation of our results was reported: fatalism (stoic acceptance) in women and helplessness/hopelessness in men were each significantly associated with poor outcome, i.e. disease progression. These psychological predictors of outcome were unrelated to the two biological prognostic factors, viz. tumour thickness and clinical stage. To date, no other replication study has been reported. However, several investigators, using different methods and psychological measures, have examined the effects of coping responses, emotional support, stress and psychiatric symptoms on disease outcome [38–49]. The duration of follow-up ranged from 12 months to a maximum of 5 years. The cited studies involved mainly patients with early and advanced cancers of the breast, cervix and malignant melanoma. A detailed review of the literature [50] has revealed differences in methodology – particularly divers measures of given psychological factors – which make it difficult to compare reported results. Consequently, any conclusions drawn can only be regarded as tentative:

1. There is no convincing evidence that coping responses or other psychological factors influence outcome in patients with advanced disease.
2. In patients with certain early, non-metastatic cancers, there is evidence that disease outcome is correlated with coping responses as well as other psychological factors, viz. fighting spirit and emotional support are significantly associated with good outcome and fatalism, helplessness/hopelessness and anxiety/depression with a poor outcome.

It must be stressed that these tentative conclusions are based entirely on correlational studies which, by their very nature, cannot provide conclusive proof. But the consistent trend reported in several independent studies indicates at least the strong possibility that coping responses are significant prognostic indicators in patients with early cancers.

## Psychotherapy

Since, as we have seen, the kinds of mental adjustment or coping responses which patients make affect their quality of life and, possibly, duration of survival, there is clearly a need for psychological therapy for patients whose poor coping responses are likely to have adverse effects. Such therapy should be designed specifically for patients with cancer, based on the premise that, generally speaking, these patients are not suffering from underlying psychopathology but are normal individuals subjected to severe stress. It follows that psychodynamic psychotherapy is inappropriate for, and probably unacceptable to, cancer patients. More relevant is a cognitive-behavioural approach which focuses on the specific problems faced by these patients and teaches them active coping skills.

Some progress is being made in this relatively new field. Several clinical trials of brief psychotherapy and so-called 'counselling' have been published [51–54]. Given the formidable methodological and practical problems involved in evaluation studies of psychotherapy [55], it is hardly surprising that conflicting results have been reported. Additional studies of counselling and general psychological support are unlikely to prove fruitful. Further advances require the development of *specific* psychotherapeutic procedures – based on a rational theoretical framework – and evaluation of these procedures in randomized, controlled trials. One such study is currently being undertaken by the author and his colleagues [50,56]. Although the study is still at an early stage, it is encouraging to note that significant alterations in coping responses have been obtained. However, these are preliminary observations; our study will not be completed until 1991. Other studies along similar lines are needed to provide a sound basis for psychological therapy designed to promote active coping responses in patients with cancer.

# Acknowledgements

My thanks are due to Professor T.J. McElwain for his support and encouragement, to Keith Pettingale, Tina Morris, Maggie Watson and Stirling Moorey for their invaluable contribution to the research underpinning this chapter, to Gill Chesney for her unstinting help in preparing the manuscript and to the many patients who have taught me much. Funding by the Cancer Research Campaign is gratefully acknowledged.

# References

1. Mitchell, G.W. and Glicksman, A.S. Cancer patients: knowledge and attitudes. *Cancer*, **40**, 61–66 (1977)

2. Dunkel-Schetter, C. Social support and cancer: findings based on patient interviews and their implications. *Journal of Social Issues*, **40**, 77–98 (1984)

3. Neuling, S.J. and Winefield, H.R. Social support and recovery after surgery from breast cancer: frequency and correlates of supportive behaviours by family, friends and surgeons. *Social Science and Medicine*, **27**, 385–392 (1988)

4. Mackillop, W.J., Stewart, W.E., Ginsburg, A.D. and Stewart, S.S. Cancer patients' perceptions of their disease and its treatment. *British Journal of Cancer*, **58**, 355–358 (1988)

5. Cooper, A. Disabilities and how to live with them: Hodgkin's disease. *Lancet*, **i**, 612–613 (1982)

6. George, B. Cited by Greer, S. Psychological consequences of cancer. *Practitioner*, **222**, 173–178 (1979)

7. Cohn, K.H. Chemotherapy from an insider's perspective. *Lancet*, **i**, 1006–1009 (1982)

8. Fiore, N. Fighting cancer – one patient's perspective. *New England Journal of Medicine*, **300**, 284–289 (1979)

9. Derogatis, L.R., Morrow, G.R., Fetting, J. *et al.* The prevalence of psychiatric disorders among cancer patients. *Journal of the American Medical Association*, **249**, 751–757 (1983)

10. Northouse, P.G. and Northouse, L.L. Communication and cancer: issues confronting patients, health professionals and family members. *Journal of Psychosocial Oncology*, **5**, 17–46 (1987)

11. Morris, J. and Ingham, S. Choice of surgery for early breast cancer: psychosocial considerations. *Social Science and Medicine*, **27**, 1257–1262 (1988)

12. Leventhal, H., Easterling, D.V., Coons, H.L. *et al.* Adaptions to chemotherapy treatments. In *Women with Cancer* (ed. B.L. Andersen), Springer, New York, pp. 172–203 (1986)

13. Aitken-Swan, J. and Easson, E.C. Reactions of cancer patients on being told their diagnosis. *British Medical Journal*, **i**, 779–783 (1959)

14. Senescu, R.A. The development of emotional complications in the patient with cancer. *Journal of Chronic Diseases*, **16**, 813–832 (1963)

15. Peck, A. Emotional reactions to having cancer. *American Journal of Roentgenology Radium Therapy and Nuclear Medicine*, **114**, 591–599 (1972)

16. Holland, J.C. Psychological aspects of cancer. In *Cancer Medicine* (eds J.F. Holland and E. Frei), Lea and Febiger, Philadelphia (1973)

17. Falek, A. and Britton, S. Phases in coping: the hypothesis and its implications. *Social Biology* (Chicago), **21**, 219–239 (1974)

18. Morris, T., Greer, H.S. and White, P. Psychological and social adjustment to mastectomy: a two year follow-up study. *Cancer*, **40**, 2381–2387 (1977)

19. Fobair, P., Hoppe, R.T., Bloom, J. *et al.* Psychosocial problems among survivors of Hodgkin's disease. *Journal of Clinical Oncology*, **4**, 805–814 (1986)

20. *Concise Oxford Dictionary*, Clarendon Press, Oxford (1976)

21. Pearlin, L.I. and Schooler, C. The structure of coping. *Journal of Health and Social Behaviour*, **19**, 2–21 (1978)

22. Greer, S., Morris, T. and Pettingale, K.W. Psychological responses to cancer: effect on outcome. *Lancet*, **ii**, 785–787 (1979)

23. Morris, T., Blake, S. and Buckley, M. Development of a method for rating cognitive responses to a diagnosis of cancer. *Social Science and Medicine*, **20**, 795–802 (1985)

24. Greer, S., Moorey, S. and Watson, M. Patients' adjustment to cancer: the Mental Adjustment to Cancer (MAC) scale versus clinical ratings. *Journal of Psychosomatic Research*, **33**, 373–377 (1989)

25. Greer, S. and Watson, M. Mental adjustment to cancer: its measurement and prognostic importance. *Cancer Surveys*, **6**, 439–453 (1987)

26. Watson, M., Greer, S., Young, J. *et al.* Development of a questionnaire measure of adjustment to cancer: the MAC scale. *Psychological Medicine*, **18**, 203–209 (1988)

27. Selby, P. and Robertson, B. Measurement of quality of life in patients with cancer. *Cancer Surveys*, **6**, 521–543 (1987)

28. Watson, M., Greer, S., Blake, S. and Shrapnell, K. Reaction to a diagnosis of breast cancer: relationship between denial, delay and rates of psychological morbidity. *Cancer*, **53**, 2008–2012 (1984)

29. Spielberger, C.D., Gorsuch, R.C. and Lushene, R.E. *The State-Trait Anxiety Inventory*, Consulting Psychologists Press, Palo Alto (1970)

30. McNair, D., Lorr, M. and Droppleman, L. *Manual for Profile of Mood States*, Educational and Industrial Testing Service, San Diego (1971)

31. Zigmond, A.D. and Snaith, R.P. The Hospital Anxiety and Depression scale. *Acta Psychiatrica Scandinavica*, **67**, 361–370 (1983)

32. Pettingale, K.W., Morris, T., Greer, S. and Haybittle, J.L. Mental attitudes to cancer: an additional prognostic factor. *Lancet*, **i**, 750 (1985)

33. Pettingale, K.W., Philalithis, A., Tee, D.E.H. and Greer, S. The biological correlates of psychological responses to breast cancer. *Journal of Psychosomatic Research*, **25**, 453–458 (1981)

34. Butler, J.A., Bretsky, S., Menendez-Botet, C. and Kinne, D.W. Estrogen receptor status protein of breast cancer as a predictor of recurrence. *Cancer*, **55**, 1178–1181 (1985)

35. Fentiman, I.S., Cuzick, J., Millis, R.R. and Hayward, J.L. Which patients are cured of breast cancer? *British Medical Journal*, **289**, 1008–1011 (1984)

36. Pettingale, K.W., Burgess, C. and Greer, S. Psychological response to cancer diagnosis. I. Correlations with prognostic variables. *Journal of Psychosomatic Research*, **32**, 255–261 (1988)

37. Di Clemente, R.J. and Temoshok, L. Psychological adjustment to having cutaneous malignant melanoma as a predictor of follow-up clinical status. *Psychosomatic Medicine*, **47**, 81 (1985)

38. Weisman, A.D. and Worden, J.W. *Coping and Vulnerability in Cancer Patients*, Massachusetts General Hospital, Boston (1977)

39. Derogatis, L.R., Abeloff, M.D. and Melisaratos, N. Psychological coping mechanisms and survival time in metastatic breast cancer. *Journal of the American Medical Association*, **242**, 1504–1508 (1979)

40. Rogentine, G.N., Van Kammen, D.P., Fox, B.H. *et al*. Psychological factors in the prognosis of malignant melanoma: a prospective study. *Psychosomatic Medicine*, **41**, 647–655 (1979)

41. Temoshok, L. and Fox, B.H. Coping styles and other psychosocial factors related to medical status and to prognosis in patients with cutaneous malignant melanoma. In *Impact of Psychoendocrine Systems on Cancer and Immunity* (eds B.H. Fox and B.H. Newberry), C.J. Hogrefe, Toronto, pp. 258–287 (1984)

42. Cassileth, B.R., Lusk, E.J., Miller, D.S. *et al*. Psychological correlates of survival in advanced malignant disease? *New England Journal of Medicine*, **312**, 1551–1555 (1985)

43. Goodkin, K., Antoni, M.H. and Blaney, P.H. Stress and hopelessness in the promotion of cervical intra-epithelial neoplasia to invasive squamous cell carcinoma of the cervix. *Journal of Psychosomatic Research*, **30**, 67–76 (1986)

44. Hislop, T.G., Waxler, N.E., Coldman, A.J. *et al*. The prognostic significance of psychosocial factors in women with breast cancer. *Journal of Chronic Diseases*, **40**, 729–735 (1987)

45. Jamison, R.N., Burish, T.G. and Wallston, K.A. Psychogenic factors in predicting survival of breast cancer patients. *Journal of Clinical Oncology*, **5**, 768–772 (1987)

46. Cella, D.F. and Holland, J.C. Methodological considerations in studying the stress-illness connection in women with breast cancer. In *Stress and Breast Cancer* (ed. C.L. Cooper), John Wiley, Chichester, pp. 197–214 (1988)

47. Levy, S.M., Lee, J., Bagley, C. and Lippmann, M. Survival hazards analysis in first recurrence breast cancer patients. *Psychosomatic Medicine*, **50**, 520–528 (1988)

48. Temoshok, L., Sweet, D.M., Blois, M.S. and Sagebiel, R.W. Psychosocial factors related to outcome in malignant melanoma: a matched samples design. *Oncology News Update*, May/June (1987)

49. Wirsching, M., Georg, W., Hoffmann, F. *et al*. Psychosocial factors influencing health development in breast cancer and mastopathia: a general systems study. In *Stress and Breast Cancer* (ed. C.L. Cooper), John Wiley, Chichester, pp. 97–107 (1988)

50. Moorey, S. and Greer, S. *Psychological Therapy for Patients with Cancer*, Heinemann, Oxford, pp. 41–52 (1989)

51. Gordon, W.A., Freidenbergs, I., Diller, L. *et al*. Efficacy of psychosocial intervention with cancer patients. *Journal of Consulting and Clinical Psychology*, **48**, 743–759 (1980)

52. Maguire, P., Tait, A., Brooke, M. *et al*. Effect of counselling on the psychiatric morbidity associated with mastectomy. *British Medical Journal*, **281**, 1454–1456 (1980)

53. Linn, M.T., Linn, B.S. and Harris, R. Effects of counseling for late stage cancer patients. *Cancer*, **49**, 1048–1055 (1982)

54. Cain, E.N., Kohorn, E.I., Quinlan, D.M. *et al*. Psychosocial benefits of a cancer support group. *Cancer*, **57**, 183–189 (1986)

55. Greer, S. Psychotherapy for the cancer patient. *Psychiatric Medicine*, **5**, 267–279 (1987)

56. Greer, S. and Moorey, S. Adjuvant psychological therapy for patients with cancer. *European Journal of Surgical Oncology*, **13**, 511–516 (1987)

# Index